Adaptive
Health Management Information Systems

Concepts, Cases, and Practical Applications

FOURTH EDITION

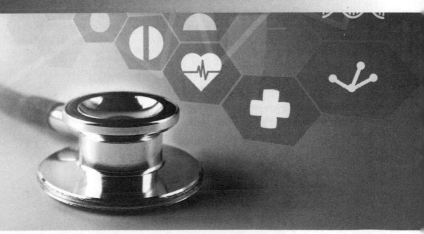

D1194248

Joseph Tan

Professor, McMaster University
DeGroote School of Business
Hamilton, ON, Canada

with

Phillip Olla
(& Joshia Tan)

JONES & BARTLETT
LEARNING

World Headquarters
Jones & Bartlett Learning
5 Wall Street
Burlington, MA 01803
978-443-5000
info@jblearning.com
www.jblearning.com

Jones & Bartlett Learning books and products are available through most bookstores and online booksellers. To contact Jones & Bartlett Learning directly, call 800-832-0034, fax 978-443-8000, or visit our website, www.jblearning.com.

Substantial discounts on bulk quantities of Jones & Bartlett Learning publications are available to corporations, professional associations, and other qualified organizations. For details and specific discount information, contact the special sales department at Jones & Bartlett Learning via the above contact information or send an email to specialsales@jblearning.com.

15401-6

Production Credits

VP, Product Management: Amanda Martin
Director of Product Management: Cathy Esperti
Product Manager: Danielle Bessette
Product Assistant: Tess Sackmann
Project Specialist: Kelly Sylvester
Digital Project Specialist: Rachel Reyes
Senior Marketing Manager: Susanne Walker
Manufacturing and Inventory Control Supervisor: Amy Bacus
Composition: codeMantra U.S. LLC

Project Management: codeMantra U.S. LLC
Cover Design: Kristin E. Parker
Senior Media Development Editor: Shannon Sheehan
Rights Specialist: Rebecca Damon
Cover Image (Title Page, Part Opener, Chapter Opener):
   © phasin/Getty Images and © gonin/Getty Images
Printing and Binding: Sheridan Books
Cover Printing: Sheridan Books

Library of Congress Cataloging-in-Publication Data
Library of Congress Cataloging-in-Publication Data unavailable at the time of printing.
LCCN: 2019946986

6048

Printed in the United States of America
23 22 21 20 19   10 9 8 7 6 5 4 3 2 1

Contents

PART I Emergent HMIS Perspectives 1

Chapter 1 Emerging Perspectives in Health Information Systems/Technologies (Health IS/IT) 3

Joseph Tan

Chapter 2 Precision Medicine: Decoding the Biology of Health and Disease 25

James M. Snyder with case scenario by Joseph Tan

Technology Review I

Review on Big Data Analytics in Health Care. . . 44

Abir Belaala, Labib Sadek Terrissa, Noureddine Zerhouni, Christine Devalland, and Joshia Tan

Chapter 3 Adoption and Commercialization of Digital Health 69

Greg Moon and Phillip Olla

Policy Review I

Online Health Information Seeking: Recasting Access and Digital Equity 81

Fay Cobb Payton and Lynette Yarger

Mini-Case (Part I)

Ginger.io: Mental Health Behavioral Analytics 93

Phillip Olla and Greg Moon

PART II HMIS Technology and Applications   95

Chapter 4 Data in Digital Health Systems. 97

Siti A. Arshad-Snyder

Technology Review II

Big Data, Geospatial Technology, IoT, and Cloud Computing for Health Systems. 112

Prabha Susy Mathew, Anitha S. Pillai, and Joseph Tan

Chapter 5 Digital Health Enterprise Software: SCM, CRM, and ERP. 125

Joshia Tan with Joseph Tan

PART III HMIS Planning and Management   189

Chapter 8 Digital Health Strategic Planning and Strategies for Health Systems 191

Joseph Tan and David Pellizzari

Policy Review II
Roles and Responsibilities of Health Systems Leaders and Managers 208

Joseph Tan with Phillip Olla and Joshia Tan

Chapter 9 Decision Aiding and Predictive Systems: A Framework for Data Mining and Machine Learning for Health Systems Management 217

Saumil Maheshwari, Anupam Shukla, and Joseph Tan

Chapter 10 The Role of Informatics in Public Health 241

April Moreno Arellano

Chapter 11 Health IS/IT Project Implementation, Innovation Procurement, and Services Management 255

Joseph Tan with Phillip Olla and Joshia Tan

Mini-Case (Part III)
Physician Intervention in Reducing Readmissions and Tele-Health Solution. 282

Jacqueline S. Jones, Sam Kazziha, and Mohan Tanniru

PART IV HMIS Standards, Policy, Governance & Future 289

Chapter 12 Clinician Confidentiality, Privacy, and Ethical Issues in the Digital Age 291

Charie Faught

Policy Review III
Health IT Standards Adoption in Health Systems 310

Sanjay Sood and Joseph Tan

Chapter 13 AI and Social Media Analytics for Health Systems: Understanding Consumers' Preferences in Healthcare Services 319

Adela S. M. Lau, Kristine Baker, Katherine Kempf, Katie Grzyb, Sijuade Oke, Eric Tsui, Liege Cheung, Marie-Claire Slama, and Min Su

Chapter 14 Health Care Globalization Through Health Information Technology Enabled Initiatives 343

Anantachai Panjamapirom and Philip F. Musa

Chapter 15 Exploring Healthcare Futures: Emerging Technology in Health Care 367

Phillip Olla, Rajib Biswas, and Joseph Tan

New to This Edition

Adaptive Health Management Information Systems, Fourth Edition, is for those instructors needing and wanting to keep pace with rapidly evolving perspectives in the field of healthcare management information systems (HMIS) and e-health digitalization. Not just a regular update of the previous edition, this new edition is vastly reorganized, revised, and reformatted with numerous contributed pieces from experts in all HMIS-related fields. To improve the previous edition, we have added much needed discussions in contemporary topics, such as precision medicine, digital health commercialization, pharmacy informatics, big data analytics, and AI (artificial intelligence). Therefore, this new edition, containing new motivating scenarios related to digital health technology applications, is also packed with creative developments and designs of real-world examples; stimulating chapter questions; glossary; illustrative graphics, tables, and exhibits; and additional readings. Significant updates and complete revisions have been incorporated throughout the text—so much so that readers familiar with the previous editions of this work would not have recognized this work as a derivative of the previous ones.

Specific updates:

- **Content.** Rich, extensive coverage of topics in HMIS and Health IT/IS domains across all dimensions, with contemporary perspectives, emerging technological applications, and implementations from developed and developing countries to serve as examples in enhancing the understanding of topics.

- **Scenarios.** Real-world, realistic scenarios set the stage for topic discussion and motivate student readers. A short reflection is also provided at the end of each scenario to develop students' imagination.

- **Technology Reviews.** Background readings on technological topics to enhance understanding of contemporary research and developments in Health IT/IS domains.

- **Policy Reviews.** Background readings on policy-related areas to enhance understanding of policy implications for trends in Health IT/IS domains.

- **Mini-Cases.** Reflective readings for students to draw lessons from various parts of the major sections of the text.

- **Chapter Questions.** Short and long questions to stimulate classroom discussion and promote learning of various topics discussed in the text.

- **New Major Cases.** A range of relevant new cases to enhance understanding of the materials and promote further interactions among students and between student groups and instructors.

Dedication

To the memory of all those loved ones, who have since passed away as I worked through various editions of this enduring text; to my students and colleagues, who have contributed to my near 30 years of teaching and learning; and those who have enjoyed my works in the fields of health services administration, health informatics, business and e-health information systems, e-Business informatics and strategies; and to my inner and expanding circle of friends and relatives, especially my own beloved family members who have all assisted me one way or another to hone my thinking and fuel my lengthy academic publishing and writing career.

—Joseph Tan

Acknowledgments

Above and beyond those to whom I am indebted while assembling previous editions of this text, I must acknowledge the generous help of those newly added academic and professional contributors, including those who were brought on board by my co-editor, Dr. Philip Olla. Dr. Olla has personally assisted in revising parts of the writing of various contributed pieces in this new edition. Sincere gratitude is also to Mr. Joshia Tan for his insights and copyediting efforts in making this revised edition not only a more appealing text, but one that would be more readable and valuable for both students and instructors.

There are several individuals whom I must especially thank: first, the publisher, who swiftly agreed to the need for an update of the text, and very patiently waited for the contributions to come in, who was flexible with the submission of the final overdue manuscript when loved ones passing away caused delays, when there were challenges connecting with some of the previous contributors, and when awaiting new contributors to complete their follow-up revisions after receiving feedback from the editorial team members (myself, Olla, and Josh). Finally, several of my students (Dr. Michael Dohan, Chloe Nyitray, Grace Simpson, Brandon Nixon, and Mr. David Pellizzari) also collaborated at different times for adding the new content of the book.

I am thankful to all who contributed for volunteering their time, efforts, and patience with my ongoing disruptive returns to them for more details and changes, and I am also particularly grateful to my wife, Leonie Tan, and son, Joshia Tan, who have ceaselessly encouraged me in every way possible to go on with my revising the text when all of us were going through very challenging times of overseeing the passing away of two beloved brothers—one, my own elderly brother, Paul and the other, my wife's younger brother, Peter—throughout the duration of this project.

To all of these individuals and to my family members, friends, students, and relatives, I offer my many thanks for the support and encouragement provided to me. Much of the value of this work is due to their contributions and assistance.

—*Joseph Tan*

Foreword

Dr. & Professor Norm Archer
McMaster University
Hamilton, ON, Canada

As you can see from the chapters in this volume, we are living in times where there are rapid advances in information and communication technologies (ICT). These may surpass our ability to quickly adapt them to meet practical needs. Health care often lags in terms of technology adaptation. This is due to a variety of barriers, but technology can provide some solutions:

- In the absence of widespread accepted standards, initial surges of HMIS development resulted in the growth of information silos that cannot intercommunicate. Efficient service provision requires information sharing. This problem is slowly being overcome by interoperability solutions. A less expensive solution is the DHIS 2 (District Health Information System) open source system. It is in use in 60 countries, including 40 countries in Africa, Asia, and Latin America. Many have adopted DHIS 2 as a nationwide standard, thus eliminating problems such as interoperability, retraining mobile staff, and healthcare system integration.
- The adoption of new technology supports rapid and efficient record keeping, data retrieval, communications, and applications in a variety of devices, resulting in massive floods of (Big) Data about patient health and management. A barrier is often a lack of trained and experienced staff to organize these data and to develop efficient methods that use health data analytics, including machine learning and/or decision support through deep learning.
- A barrier in many healthcare institutions is that they have been distracted by data breach and data hostage problems, requiring much time and money to be spent on improving data security. A resulting side benefit is better management of patient privacy.
- Precision medicine looks promising, and has been used effectively in some cases. A barrier is the high cost of specialized molecules to treat small groups of people, resulting in unaffordable treatments. There is no practical solution in sight as of yet.
- Personal computing has radically changed the dynamic of written communications. But physicians now work longer hours to do tasks formerly done by assistants. This barrier prevents spending sufficient time with patients; as a result, the strongest predictor of physician burnout is the amount of time spent doing computer documentation. Artificial intelligence (AI) solutions may eventually be able to reduce this documentation load.
- Computer system support affects physicians through work structuring, thereby reducing practice flexibility. This is not necessarily a barrier; well-designed systems may in fact help physicians to make better decisions from evidence-based medicine, improving care quality.

- Intelligent digital assistants, such as Alexa and Cortana can understand voice and be activated by voice commands to accomplish basic tasks. This improves user adaptability, and may take over some of the documentation needs of healthcare professionals.

Ultimately, virtual care (telemedicine) allows individuals to connect online anytime, anywhere with healthcare providers and other health professionals through secure text and video. A barrier to this approach is the shortage and the cost of highly trained professionals, which may have to be supplanted partially by a combination of AI and online health self-management, including prevention and treatment of chronic disease among older adults and the elderly.

Biography

Norm Archer, PhD (Physics), is *professor emeritus* of the DeGroote School of Business, McMaster University. He teaches courses in electronic health (eHealth) and information systems and has published widely on eGovernment, eBusiness, and eHealth; more specifically, Professor Archer and his students conduct research on eHealth applications and systems; eBusiness; identity theft; supply chain management; project management; change management in eGovernment; and mobile commerce. He has a major responsibility in the collaborative MSc eHealth program that is a joint undertaking by the DeGroote School of Business, Faculty of Health Sciences, and the Computing and Software Department in the Faculty of Engineering.

Preface

*A*daptive Health Management Information Systems: Concepts, Cases, and Practical Applications, Fourth Edition is finally here to aid students and instructors who want to take the next big leap in digital healthcare transformation. Indeed, just as with previous editions, this new edition is not simply an update, but a complete makeover—clearly a reorganized, expanded, and fully revised manuscript with new and logically ordered contributions, still divided into the five common major themes connecting a 15-chapter series, supplemented with Technology and Policy Reviews as well as Cases and Mini-Cases. Several short, medium, and long cases are therefore assembled to promote a wide range of class discussions from the readings and beyond. Put simply, significant updates and complete revisions to all parts of the previous edition have been generated throughout the text so that readers of previous editions would not have recognized this work as a derivative of the other. It is no longer just a new hybrid vehicle that the co-editors have decided to usher in this time; instead, what we got is a "self-driving" vehicle that does away with most, if not all, of the parts powering the old model design that is driver-dependent.

As we begin to witness the power of big health data analytics, geospatial data analytics, and social media analytics, we become more conscious of how the massive data around and about us are changing our behaviors—the way we think, the way we work, and the way we interact with each other. The jobs that we currently do in the ever-growing healthcare systems are gradually fading away, as new roles are defined with advances in technological interventions and ubiquitous computing. To this end, it is hoped that this newly minted HMIS text will continue to motivate its readers to seek new perspectives, bringing together state-of-the-art knowledge as well as best practices that incorporate the benefits of emerging and innovative technologies discussed throughout this text. As evidenced both in the Contents and the range of shorter and longer cases provided in this text, the ever-growing spectrum of topics to be covered in a health information systems/information technology (health IT/IS) or health informatics courses is expanding. In this new edition, we have attempted to aggregate the different theories, methodologies, and practices into a five-part cluster that readers would be familiar with from previous editions.

Part I, comprising Chapters 1–3 (supplemented with a *Mini-case*, a *Technology Review*, as well as a *Policy Review*), offers emergent perspectives on HMIS. Part II, covering Chapters 4–7 (accompanied by two *Technology Reviews*), concentrates on HMIS technology and applications, whereas Part III, covering Chapters 8–11 (supplemented by a *Policy Review* and a *Mini-case*), shifts focus to HMIS planning and management. Part IV, which encompasses Chapters 12–15, addresses HMIS standards, governance, policy, globalization, and future, and is also supplemented with a *Policy Review* and a *Mini-case*. Finally, a range of shorter and longer cases highlighting HMIS practices and implementation are presented in Part V. Each of these major themes progressively flows from one topic to another to unveil diverse and critical aspects of the hidden HMIS gem.

It is the hope of the editorial team members that this *Fourth Edition* will open eyes, stimulate conversations, and further extend the possibilities and opportunities of future theorists, methodologists, and practitioners in the HMIS, health IT/IS, and health informatics areas.

Joseph Tan with Philip Olla (& Joshia Tan)

About the Editors

Joseph Tan

Primary author and editor, Joseph Tan, PhD (MIS), MS (Industrial and Management Engineering), BA (Maths/Computer Science), Dip (Civil Engineering), formerly *Wayne C Fox Chair* of eBusiness Innovation, is Professor of eHealth Innovation, eBusiness Strategies, Entrepreneurship & Informatics, DeGroote School of Business, McMaster University. He is the founding and ongoing Editor-in-Chief (EIC), *International Journal of Healthcare Information Systems and Informatics* (*IJHISI*), as well as the co-EIC, *International Journal of Applied Research on Public Health Management* (*IJARPHM*), with a professional background that spans a broad spectrum of interdisciplinary, multidisciplinary, and trans-disciplinary research areas. He is also EIC, *SpringerBriefs for Healthcare Economics & Management*, and the Senior Associate Editor (eHealth Informatics) of *HLPT: Health Technology & Policy*.

Joseph Tan's 30-year academic and administrative experiences include employment in academia and private and non-profit sector organizations, as well as consulting and program development activities catering to executives and foreign delegation. His management philosophy is to motivate others to work collaboratively on available opportunities (and challenges) so as to effect transformative change; he regularly mentors junior faculty, staff, and adult students. He has been named among the Top 10 most influential professors of informatics with an overall career focus to reshape the landscape of IS/IT applications and promotion in eBusiness/eHealth informatics through cross-disciplinary thinking/project partnering with diverse practitioners, clinicians, researchers, and a variety of user communities. His leadership style is to influence and inspire others to become self-made leaders, continually achieving higher quality, effective, productive, and respectful contributions in terms of realizing the shared vision and negotiated goals.

Professor Tan has published over 150 papers, abstracts, books and book chapters, editorials, and reviews. His work has appeared in over 30 refereed journals, including *AJHP; Applied Ergonomics; CMI; Computer Graphics Forum; Comm. of the ICISA; CACM; CAIS; Decision Sciences; Encyclopedia of IS; HSMR; HCMF; HCMR; H&HSA; HLPT, Hospital Topics; ISR; Inf. Res.; IJHTM; IJEH; IJHCI; IJMC; IJMTP; IJT&LD; JAMIA; JCIS; Journal of Digital Imaging; JHAE; JHCQ; JMS; Methods of Information in Medicine; Nature, Neural Computing & Applications,* and *THIM,* as well as numerous local, national, and international conference proceedings. Just as with time spent on compiling this revised fourth edition, Professor Tan is currently compiling a new *case text* to bring together insights and lessons learned from various sources during his many years of teaching and learning in the *Connected Health* discipline, including *eBusiness strategies, entrepreneurship, and innovation* areas. Again, this work will be collaborated with other authors, co-editors, and contributors. Another key work being planned is the *Road to Heaven on Earth,* to be released in the coming future.

Dr. Tan has demonstrated skills and ability to serve in both academia and for-profit and non-profit industry. He has achieved recognized scholarship in teaching and learning with students' nominations for teaching excellence awards. Dr. Tan also appears as an invited keynote speaker for a number of local as well as major national and international conferences across North America, Asia, Africa, and elsewhere, and networks widely with key decision executives and policymakers apart from academic scholars and practitioners at local, provincial/state, national, and international levels, including private, public, and nongovernmental organizations and universities. As a well-established educator and negotiator, he has continued to play an active leadership role in curriculum and program accreditation, peer-reviewed journal publications, encyclopedia works and book reviews, online education and programming, planning and organization of symposiums and conferences, development of book series, special issue journals, federal grant proposals, and large-scale international interdisciplinary grant-funded programs.

Phillip Olla

Contributing author and co-editor, Dr. Phillip Olla is a Digital Health specialist with over 20 years of experience working at the leading edge of technology innovation. He is currently the CEO of Audacia Bioscience, a life science company incorporating biomarkers, AI, and smartphone technology to develop innovative diagnostic solutions. Prior to founding Audacia Bioscience, he was the Executive Director of Mobile Diagnostic Services, a social enterprise which created point-of-care diagnostic technology for low-resource global health settings. His professional experience and consulting services span an array of industries and disciplines such as Oracle, 02, Roche Diagnostics, and NASA. Dr. Olla has completed over 50 client consultancy engagements with Fortune 100 companies in 12 countries, successfully assisting with corporate education, technology deployments, business development, competitor analysis, portfolio analysis, and strategic technology roadmaps. Dr. Olla is an Adjunct Professor at the University of Windsor, and was previously the Director of Research and Professor of Health Informatics at Madonna University in Livonia, Michigan.

Dr. Olla is a public speaker who has presented extensively within the domains of industry and academia and even for nongovernmental organizations such as the World Health Organization and the United Nations. Dr. Olla has a PhD in Information Systems from Brunel University in the United Kingdom. His publications include numerous peer-reviewed journal articles, industry reports, seven book chapters, and three books; *Mobile Health Solutions for Biomedical Applications*. He is a Chartered Engineer registered with British Engineering Council and a Fellow of the Chartered Institute of Information Technology.

Joshia Tan

Editorial consultant, Joshia Tan hails from a banking and commercial background. Over the last decade or so, Joshia has held a number of leadership, strategy, sales, and commercialization roles across Brazil, Canada, China, Singapore, and the United States with HSBC—including coverage of some of the largest technology and healthcare/pharmaceutical corporates in the world. Currently, he serves as Senior Vice President of Business Development in Singapore, covering the evolving trade financing needs of Fortune 100 clients across 19 markets in the Asia Pacific region.

Joshia maintains a keen interest in the Digital Health landscape and has authored or co-authored a number of case studies and book chapters; he has also served on various advisory boards for non-profits and holds a Bachelor of Science in Business Administration from Washington University in St. Louis.

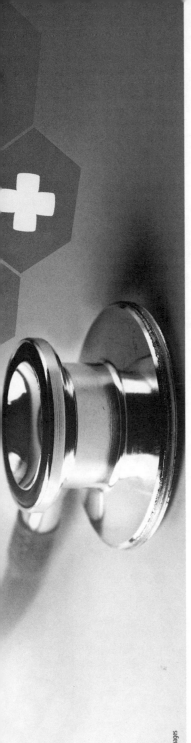

PART I

Emergent HMIS Perspectives

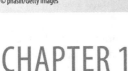

CHAPTER 1

Emerging Perspectives in Health Information Systems/ Technologies (Health IS/IT)

Joseph Tan

LEARNING OBJECTIVES

- Overview the field of health information systems/technologies (health IS/IT) to showcase emergent thinking and perspectives
- Highlight major health IS/IT components
- Outline key health IS/IT themes vis-à-vis the organization of this text
- Conceptualize health IS/IT cultures

CHAPTER OUTLINE

Scenario: Charting the Future of Philips HealthSuite Digital Platform: Toward a New Vision of Connected Health

 I. Introduction
 II. Scoping the HMIS Field: A Digital Health Ecosystem Perspective
- *Routine Business vs. Health (Clinical) Data, Information, and Knowledge*
- *The Need for and Challenge of a Digital Health Ecosystem*

- *An EHR: Defining the Basic Functions of a Typical Health IS/IT System*
III. Major Health IS/IT Components
IV. HMIS Cultures
 V. Conclusion

Notes
Chapter Questions

Scenario: Charting the Future of Philips HealthSuite Digital Platform Toward a New Vision of Connected Health[1]

Amsterdam-based Royal Philips has recently announced joining hands with Seoul-based Samsung Electronics Co. Ltd. to usher in a new era of connected health on a global scale. Notably, this collaboration involves linking both the Philips *HealthSuite digital platform* and the Samsung *ARTIK Smart IoT platform* seamlessly to advance the evolving healthy living ecosystem of connected Philips' health-assistive devices effectively and to allow previously stored health information contained in Philips HealthSuite to be securely accessed and shared via the Samsung's cloud platform.

Directing a new vision for connected health, these shared platforms will enrich each other in terms of value-added capabilities to deliver e-care services anywhere, anytime for subscribing patients in the following innovative ways:

- Critical and relevant health information can be continuously gathered, compiled, stored securely, and analyzed from a mix of different device types, apps, and sensors ranging from medical system such as image scanning and lab test reporting systems, personal health records (PHRs), and electronic medical records (EMRs), to wearables and device-linked mobile apps such as portable heart rhythm sensors, health-fitness trackers, smart watches, blood glucose monitors, and other Philips–Samsung connected health consumer products and gadgets;
- Not only will subscribing patients have easy and secure access to their own health and clinical information anytime, anywhere, but they will also be empowered to better monitor their status of health and well-being with the use of Philips–Samsung platforms jointly with their caregivers to achieve a seamless continuum of care;
- Care providers will now have real-time, holistic, and digital information when attending to their subscribing patients so as to support timely and effective clinical decision making. Moreover, care teams can be guided toward the most appropriate care vis-à-vis their patients' specific situation(s) through meaningful health analytics while abnormal test observations of individual patients can be flagged automatically and care providers alerted before the impending conditions become acute; and
- Third-party developers will also be empowered to swiftly generate interoperable connected health as well as Internet of Things (IoT) solutions by leveraging the use of integrated datasets stored within both these Philips–Samsung platforms, thereby allowing leaders of health systems to gain evidence-based insights in pursuing organizational and financial decisions to benefit their patient populations and society.

Altogether, as noted by James Stansberry, the Senior VP and GM of ARTIK IoT, Samsung Electronics:

This is an incredibly exciting time in health care, as the industry begins to harness the power of data to bring better care to consumers. Samsung ARTIK-enabled devices and cloud services integrated with Philips HealthSuite can address the growing need for connected health platforms that can safely access, share, and analyze information, helping health systems and providers achieve their goal of delivering better care to consumers, from prevention and detection to diagnosis and treatment (Ibid).

Visualize how this new Philips–Samsung collaboration will impact the future of virtual delivery of global healthcare services in light of rapidly increasing mobility of patients on the one hand, and for older adults and the elderly who may be less mobile on the other. Additionally, reflect upon why and how third-party developers, designers, and informaticians may now be empowered to generate better and more useful apps that will bridge the gap between professionally and personally relevant health datasets across the health continuum. Finally, what other innovative health services may also be potentially supported on the Philips–Samsung platforms and how will such collaborative efforts usher in a new era of connected health?

▶ I. Introduction

The historical evolution and cumulative knowledge development of health IS/IT over the last several decades have been meaningfully converging and have continued to transform traditional healthcare services delivery systems and health organizational informatics environments both in North America and globally.[2] Specific to the healthcare industry, administrators, clinicians, researchers, and other health practitioners, including health informaticians, are being increasingly pressured to adapt health IS/IT and applications of health informatics (HI) to growing public and private sector expectation. Major sources of concerns include the escalating costs of traditional care delivery systems; decreased funding from governments and third parties; better informed patients regarding treatment alternatives, including more patient-centric and ethical approaches to applying clinical informatics (CI) and information processing methods; as well as increased participation and expectation from new and emerging forms of health organizational governance and community-based digital health reporting structures.

Today, new perspectives in health management information systems (HMIS) have evolved because of rapid and exciting breakthroughs in health IS/IT and communication networks, including new media. Specifically, such thinking calls for more productive and effective health data sharing, big data analytics to guide and improve the coordination of healthcare services delivery, and the application of precision medicine to redefine health care and shared clinical decision making via more integrated and interoperable health IS/IT systems. Accordingly, a critical effort to bridge the concepts of corporate digitization of CI and systems, on the one hand, and the negotiated management of healthcare services delivery, on the other, has called for a major revision of this adaptive health IS/IT text. Indeed, those who understand health IS/IT and informatics concepts, trends and challenges, and the potential benefits of related applications will be better prepared to work collaboratively using agent-based groupware, artificial intelligence, and net appliances during the current era of knowledge explosion and shared data digitization to achieve greater group productivity, improve health organizational agility, and cultivate a more positive inter-organizational partnership in the context of the growing number of electronic health (e-health) services delivery networks that are beginning to inter-connect.[3]

In this chapter, the primary objective is to overview the major underlying themes of health IS/IT within the context of the need for and challenge of building a sustainable digital health ecosystem. Section II focuses on scoping the health IS/IT field by emphasizing the basic heath vs. business data concepts and showing how e-technology and HI application concepts are contributing to the push toward health organizational digitization and transformation. Section III then surveys major components of health IS/IT and highlights the key themes in the health IS/IT field to show how the various chapters in the latest edition of this text are linked and organized. Section IV highlights cornerstones of health vs. business IS/IT cultures for driving current healthcare organizational digitization and transformation, while Section V concludes the chapter with a focus on how the different themes may be combined to achieve effective health IS/IT best practices in the coming era.

▶ ## II. Scoping the HMIS Field: A Digital Health Ecosystem Perspective

Healthcare (and clinical) informatics, or more generally for readers of this text, HMIS, may be viewed as an eclectic field. In this context, a typical health IS/IT system may be conceived as an integrated health information processing engine that links interrelated human–computer components for the accurate and rapid collection of various patient-related data, information, and knowledge elements to generate aggregated, well-classified, and needed administrative and clinical information, knowledge, and insights so as to aid users in shared decision making, including detection, control, analysis, diagnosis, treatment planning and evaluation, and many other subsequent health-related physical and cognitive activities. Other terms referring to a related or similar conceptualization of health IS/IT systems that are commonly encountered in the extant HMIS literature include health or healthcare information systems (HIS or HCIS), CI, medical information systems (MIS), medical informatics (MI), HI and telematics, e-health, and more recently, digital health (D-health).

Aside from the Affordable Care Act's mandate to measure meaningful use of various health IS/IT enterprise systems (primarily, the use of EHRs throughout the daily operations across many U.S. hospitals and health services centers), the core health IS/IT field integrates multifaceted concepts to be intelligently deployed in various connected domains. These core domains include strategic health IS/IT planning and management, the design and development of health IS/IT corporate infrastructure, application portfolios, and end-user interfaces, as well as practical implementation and ongoing evaluation of the impact of health IS/IT resources management on clinical decisions, including policy oversights on standards adoption, data and systems security and sharing, health data stewardship, privacy, and confidentiality.

Pertinent health IS/IT resources management encompasses routine health database administrative chores, CI apps and telematics, specialized health operational analysis and computer modeling, health data analytics as well as mostly automated user-assisted health information management, laboratory testing and radiological imaging systems, and decision aid systems. As with previous editions, we intend here to extend the term *adaptive* HMIS (and health IS/IT) to emphasize the need for an agile approach to health information administration and management. Health IS/IT students must learn how to apply data science thinking, HI and CI methods, and health IS/IT planning strategies from an adaptive but integrated perspective.

Routine Business vs. Health (Clinical) Data, Information, and Knowledge

On the basis of this generalization of the health IS/IT field, health (clinical) data, information, and knowledge (insights) are therefore uniquely differentiated from business data, information, and knowledge (insights) in specific terms, that is, the emphasis toward the need for complex professional "expertise" and higher-level processing to have taken place in order to convert static health data being gathered to aid useful clinical interpretation and insightful decision making under increasingly complex and risky situations. While a lot of business data, information, and knowledge elements are also non-trivial and often require expert judgments at a strategic level, at the operational level, it is common for raw business data gathered at the source to be conveniently automated for routine processing. Yet, unlike routine business data applications that can often be easily automated, health data and informatics applications are largely textual in nature and cannot be easily automated as these data elements must involve some form of expert input, yielding a resulting decisional interpretation that will eventually impact best practices. Healthcare-related knowledge, as the term suggests, refers to the cumulative experiences of applying health information to clinical decisions, thereby producing "wisdom," "rules of thumb" (heuristics), and "associations" to be used for future health-related consults.

Health data elements, in and of themselves, are specific facts and parameters. A good piece of datum is characterized by its accuracy, reliability, completeness, accessibility, timeliness, and security. Accuracy is achieved when health data recorded are true, correct, and valid about the status of a patient's condition; for example, a temperature of 104°F recorded as 101°F is inaccurate, constituting a medical recording error. Reliability means that the recorded data are trustworthy and consistent; for example, if the allergy list of a patient exists in the food services system, the same list should appear in the pharmacy system. Completeness entails that all required health data should (and must) be recorded; for example, a unique identifier must exist in the patient master index (PMI) for each patient recorded in a database to differentiate one patient from the other. Accessibility refers to empowering appropriate personnel with valid access authorization and authentication to view the relevant data wherever and whenever required; for example, physicians should be able to view the electrocardiography (EKG or ECG) or electroencephalography (EEG) reports of their patients following their rounds in the wards. Timeliness ensures that the available

health data are current for the decision tasks at hand, while security and privacy stipulate that only designated persons with valid access rights and verifiable authenticated identities can view or make changes to any or all relevant aspects of the recorded data. This will ensure patients' data privacy, confidentiality, and safeguard against data misuse.

Clinical datasets are unique. Unlike financial and accounting data, clinical data are typically non-transactional. Indeed, data about a patient may be entered by different personnel, by different departments, and at different times to show the progression of health status of the patient; for example, a nurse may jot down the demographics of a patient when he or she first arrives, then the physician or other specialists may record their observations and diagnoses about the patient. These data are mainly textual in nature, although many of the patient's monitored health indicators, such as weight, temperature, blood pressure, and glucose level, can be measured quantitatively. The physician and specialists may also send the patient for laboratory tests and other scans which will give rise to other types of quantitative and qualitative (interpretative) data once results are being aggregated. Put together, clinical data can range from health-related data derived from statistical and complex simulation models and tabular and graphical presentation data to digitized images to subjective opinions and interpretations of the same underlying data. Similarly, when a patient is discharged, the process will create further clinical (e.g., changes to their health status information) and administrative–financial data (e.g., billing and accounting data).

In the context of present-day health organizational digitization and transformation, health IS/IT are therefore used primarily to gather and analyze patients' clinical and financial records, following which these various sources of data elements are aggregated and manipulated using necessary and relevant models (including built-in knowledge elements as needed) to support health providers (e.g., health administrators, clinicians, nurses, and other healthcare professionals) in making timely decisions to improve the efficiency, effectiveness, and efficacy of health services rendered or to be rendered to the patients. Health data collected must be meaningful and worthwhile. While health databases must be properly organized and be made available to their users in a timely fashion, it is critical to consider and understand the needs of their users prior to the data collection process. Otherwise, managing and maintaining inappropriate and unnecessary data, especially in large medical databases, may drain valuable health organizational resources. Users of medical and health-related data range from patients to care providers, government agencies, healthcare planners, judicial agents, educators, researchers, and third-party funders/payors. Different types of users may also require different scopes, formats, and presentations of data. To design and build an effective health IS/IT, it is critical to fully comprehend the need for and challenge of a digital health ecosystem in which health IS/IT systems basically function seamlessly to improve the quality of patient care services being delivered anywhere, anytime.

The Need for and Challenge of a Digital Health Ecosystem

A 2018 Federal Ministry for Economic Cooperation and Development (BMZ) report to encourage strategic partnership for a Digital Africa[4] notes that attempts to invest in digital healthcare infrastructure and build toward a future digital health ecosystem are critical. The BMZ report further argues that such efforts will lead to a seamless exchange of health information among care provider organizations and improve the coordination of care delivery services nationwide. Such investments can also ultimately benefit the health and well-being of the entire targeted population, aside from both enhanced national productivity and wealth. One part of this cited BMZ report notes: "Digital health ecosystems and applications will deliver an additional dimension to support national health services. It will enable individual providers to offer better quality health care and, as a long-term vision, ensure innovation, safety and value in addition to quality in health care."[5(p. 9)]

Conceivably, a digital health ecosystem may be best structured as a holistic linking of ecologically consistent embedded units of health IS/IT applications to support and improve well-coordinated, integrative care delivery across the relevant geographic biosphere. As shown in **FIGURE 1-1**, this digital health ecosystem[6] can function via complex physical–biological components interacting at various levels, including: (a) the clinical care and practice level, (b) the public health and policy level, and (c) the clinical research level.

The simple logic behind promoting a vision of a healthy, interoperable, and learning health IS/IT ecosystem is to achieve the right channeling of health information; in short, it is to create an environment where the right information will continually be made available to the right people at the right time "across products and organizations in a way that can be relied upon and meaningfully used by recipents."[7(p. 2)] At the clinical care and practice level, therefore, the key health data exchanges involve quality measures captured from patients to be provided to the care practitioners as the practitioners interact actively with health decision support systems (HDSS) to offer guidance for patients' diagnosis, therapies, and rehabilitative activities. Here, both individual patients and care providers will be able to access, share, and meaningfully capture, store, and use relevant health information for care delivery to maintain the desired patient health outcomes. Importantly, the emphasis on health IS/IT will be to focus on quality and safety in the care delivery process.

At the public health and policy level, the focus of health IS/IT will shift toward population-based health statistics with

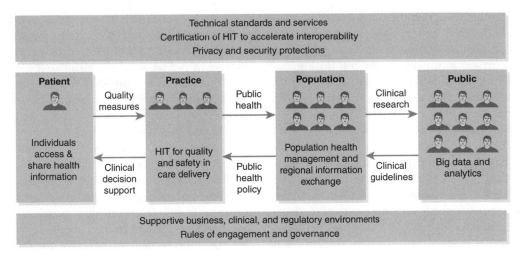

FIGURE 1-1 Health IS/IT Ecosystem.

Data from Connecting Health and Care for the Nation: A 10-Year Vision to Achieve an Interoperable Health IT Infrastructure. https://www.healthit.gov/sites/default/files/ONC10yearInteroperabilityConceptPaper.pdf

emphasis on regional information management and exchange. Here, data derived from population health analysis will dictate public health policies, which will in turn be used to guide ongoing and evolving professional services and best practices. Beyond this and at the clinical research level, big data and analytics will then be channeled to benefit both healthcare organizations and the public communities by enabling better insight into clinical practice guidelines about various care services such as pain management and alternative cancer treatments for various forms of cancer. While the use of a commonplace health IS/IT such as an EHR is clearly meaningful in recording medical histories for individual patients to aid clinical diagnosis and therapeutic treatments at the clinical care and practice level, the big data generated by EHRs has the potential to improve research analysis and provide analytical insights toward boosting overall public health at the clinical research level.

Even so, the key challenge in digital health ecosystem-based management is the need to achieve seamless connectivity and interoperability among different components within and among ecosystems. This entails the ability to steer key stakeholders toward an operational digital health strategy, the ability to translate a viable and sustainable e-health strategy into a strong digital health ecosystem, and the need to monitor and evaluate outcomes and results being achieved to guide future directions. Unlike other service sectors, such as banking, insurance, and retailing, which have successfully implemented powerful, connected e-business ecosystems globally, the challenges for building an e-healthcare ecosystem have to do with the difficulties faced in sharing and exchanging clinical data across often diverse systems. This is chiefly due to the uniqueness of individual health data, characterized by these recordings being largely textual, poorly structured, and kept separately in siloed systems which are not easily interoperable. Moreover, different care providers tend to abbreviate as well as interpret the same or almost similar medical terminology quite differently.

Aside from increased health data and health IS/IT complexity, many health processes, regulatory factors, and emergency health decisions, by their very nature, are also non-trivial, sometimes excessively complex, and multifaceted. For example, unlike well-structured routine business decisions, treatment pathways for older and elderly adult patients often differ substantially even for patients diagnosed with similar symptoms due to the tendency for these patients to become multi-morbid.

Nonetheless, just as with many other industries, a growing trend toward emphasizing big data analytics has already begun to revolutionize the healthcare industry in more ways than one could imagine. Today, owing to the extensive adoption of technologies such as EHR, computerized physician order entry (CPOE), and clinical decision support systems (CDSS) across hospitals and clinics in North America and elsewhere, care providers can better meet the changing needs of patients by coordinating care in a more efficient and effective manner via big data tracking and disease pattern analytics. Similarly, healthcare administrators and office managers can better account for expenses, eliminate waste, and compute income generated from different forms of services rendered due to the implementation of enterprise resource planning (ERP), supply chain management (SCM), and customer relation management (CRM) systems. The growing complexity of the health IS/IT landscape as well as increased complexity of the regulatory mechanisms, especially for health data confidentiality and privacy, storage, dissemination, and use, continue to impact the challenges faced in building a sustainable digital health ecosystem. Owing to the unpredictability of these various interacting components within the digital health ecosystem, it is further argued that the management of such an ecosystem simply has to be adaptive, including the need for broad representations and participation from major stakeholders, and its future sustainability being dependent on the quality of leadership that will be defined from evolving health IS/IT governance.[8–10]

An EHR: Defining the Basic Functions of a Typical Health IS/IT System

To understand the basic functions and capabilities expected of a typical health IS/IT system,

we focus here on the EHR—one of the premier and most used health IS/IT systems for clinical care services.[11] **TABLE 1-1** depicts the 2015 base EHR definition of the most basic capabilities for operating an EHR,[12] highlighting the changes that have evolved since the 2014 edition.

A basic function of the EHR is to identify and maintain a patient record, in particular, changing patient demographics and clinical health information such as historical records of events and episodes. In other words, appropriate and sufficient individual patient data must be gathered and tracked over time from various sources before any clinician (EHR user) can meaningfully interpret the data to satisfy the long-term administrative and clinical needs of patients and/or their respective care providers. The fundamental value of such a system lies in properly managing its data collection and verification processes as well as providing an overall picture of the progression of health and well-being of the patient over his or her lifetime. Therefore, EHR data collection is not just about collecting every piece of information, but rather, collecting only those pieces that are meaningfully connected and vital to assist patients, providers, and other secondary users (e.g., third-party funders and researchers).

Another key function is to manage the patient's problem, medication, and medication allergy lists based on interactions with a clinician, including physicians and/or specialists, along a longitudinal basis. In the 2015 edition, documentation of smoking status and implantable device list have been added as highlighted in Table 1-1. To improve data timeliness, validity, and integrity, the preferred strategy in data collection methods for problem diagnosis is to use automated and direct data input at the source, such as the use of a point-of-care barcode scanner, and to warehouse the data either centrally or via online distributed network technology. Such approaches would require that the acquired input data first be converted into standardized

TABLE 1-1 2015 Base EHR Definition

Capabilities	Criteria	Changes from Earlier Office of the National Coordinator (ONC) for Health IT Requirements
Includes patient demographic and clinical health information, e.g., medical history and problem lists	Demographics	Gender identification and sexual orientation fields added
	Problem list	Minor update (SNOMED CT VERSION)
	Medication list	No change as with previous ONC requirements
	Medication allergy list	No change as with previous ONC requirements
	Smoking status (new)	New smoking status documentation
	Implantable device list (new)	Unique device ids linked to a patient's implantable device
Capacity to offer CDS (Clinical Decision Support)	CDS	Standard Information button
Capacity to support computerized physician order entry (CPOE)	CPOE (Meds, Labs, Rads)	No change as with previous ONC requirements—use of CPOE
Capacity to capture/query information relevant to healthcare quality	Clinical quality measures (CQMs)	CQMs being meaningfully derived from captured data; ability to export CQM data
Capacity to exchange e-health information with, and integrate such information from, other sources	Transition of care	Transport requirements updated to allow easier navigation of an inbound CCDA received from another provider
	Data export	Export summaries for single patient, subset of patients, or for all patients
	Application access (new)	EHRs to have open interfaces so as to permit other systems to access certain patient data
	Direct project	Send/Receive with EHRs/Patient Portals (PPs) via EDGE Protocol

Data from 2015 Edition Base EHR Definition - Certification Criteria Required to Satisfy the Definition. https://www.healthit.gov/sites/default /files/2015edition_base_ehr_definition_ml_11-4-15.pdf codes. This strategy is preferred over traditional manual and mechanical input and conversion methods that rely chiefly on clerical transcription of patient data from various self-reports and handwritten documents via the keyboard or some other input devices that are also prone to human errors. Regardless of the way patient-related data are gathered, coded, and entered into an EHR, the input data elements should be cleaned and meticulously verified for accuracy and validity before these data can be helpful in aiding the EHR users in clinical diagnosis.

A third function is to manage the clinical documents and notes with the capacity to support physician order entry. Here, different types of clinical documents and notes may be captured in the EHR; these include, among others, patient-specific care plans, guidelines, and protocols; tracked patient-specific instructions and orders for diagnostic tests; tracked order sets based on provider inputs or system prompts; records of test results, consents, and authorizations; and external clinical documents such as reports or scanned images. CPOE is the primary technology of choice here to be extended from the EHR so as to support administration of medications, laboratory testing, and/or diagnostic imaging in coordinating the continuing care of the patients.

Another technology to enhance EHR functions is the capacity to provide clinical decision support. Here, three common forms of health data management technologies are often employed to aid clinical decisions. Database management enhances data collection and storage activities, improves data integrity, reduces data update anomalies, and promotes preservation and structuring of data for efficient data processing and effective data retrieval activities. Data analytics construct, establish, manage, and interrelate models that may be needed by the health IS/IT users to rationalize the data being linked, analyzed, or computed. In fact, not all data collected are directly useful in the healthcare delivery process. Some information is collected merely to assist in the organization and generation of comparative data and statistics, or simply for research. More intelligent HDSS can assist care providers and clinicians in making more complex decisions that may require expertise within a specialized domain. In this case, apart from the use of database management technology and analytics, knowledgebase management systems come into play. Knowledgebase management assembles, stores, accesses, updates, and disseminates knowledge elements that may enhance the processing of such specialized decisional processes.

Additionally, quality displays and most appropriate representations of health data are important because not only can inappropriate representations of data slow down the process of data interpretation, but the decisions made from poorly represented data could also be error-prone and could generate unwanted and/or inappropriate clinical interventions. Hence, the capacity to capture and query information relevant to healthcare quality is pertinent. Application of a poor image compression technique or the use of an inadequate digital image resolution, for example, may not only slow down the reading of a scanned image for a radiologist, but it can easily lead to risky misdiagnosis on a patient's health condition. Accordingly, computerized software and intelligent graphical interfaces can be built to compact large amounts of information conveniently and to support individual users in filtering out the irrelevant information that may not be needed for a particular or specialized task application.[13]

Finally, interoperability or the capacity to share e-health information with, and integrate such information from, other sources cannot be overemphasized. Such a capability would be important not only for proper data export and transitions of care but also for access to previously recorded data stored in other systems and for the purpose of integrating and aggregating data from diverse data systems.

▶ III. Major Health IS/IT Components

An understanding of the adaptive but integrated health IS/IT begins with differentiating among its five major components and their interrelationships:

1. Data/information/knowledge (Content and Data Component)
2. Hardware/software/firmware/server (Infrastructure Component)
3. Process/task/system (Data Analytics Component)
4. Systems Network Integration/ Media Interoperability (Network Compatibility and Communications Component)
5. User/administration/management facing (Platform/Interface Component)

The content (and data) component, which we have discussed, forms the central core of all health IS/IT. It encompasses the specification of, organization on, and interrelationship among data, information, and knowledge elements required of integrated HMIS. Raw data form the basic building blocks for generating useful information that is to be stored; processed data are transformed into information that serves as useful output to inform end users deliberating on various types of decisions (identification, diagnostic, therapeutic, and consultative or second opinions). Some pieces of data about children may be that of the medication that they are allergic to (e.g., penicillin). Another example would be their vaccination records, including immunization dates and types. Having these data readily available will help determine when and whether the child is due for a particular vaccine, and such knowledge should be passed on to new care providers who may be assigned for future care delivery.

The combination of effective data, information, and knowledge resource management involves designing the critical databases and instituting various intelligent data-mining algorithms, rule engines, and online analytical processing (OLAP) tools to manage the increasingly complex and information-intensive care decision situations physicians are faced with daily. In other words, organized information and captured experience will, in turn, yield the essential knowledge (and intelligence) for guiding future clinical services. **FIGURE 1-2** shows the conceptual flow of the data–information–knowledge paradigm within the HMIS organizational and changing healthcare provider decision-making contexts.

Ultimately, the health IS/IT used to support key decision-making functions of care providers and administrators within the organization must be reformed to achieve greater integration of data, information, and knowledge across organizational stakeholders. The Philips–Samsung's newly proposed integrated platforms, discussed in the chapter-opening scenario, are examples of how innovative health IS/IT applications can better integrate enterprise databases (such as EHR) and other uncoordinated data systems such as CPOE and HDSS/CDSS to support integrated healthcare delivery at a regional or even global level. In an integrated and well-designed health IS/IT, the goal is to distribute these information-related elements efficiently, effectively, and appropriately throughout the organization for enriching learning among organizational users and for enhancing the delivery of care services across different providers.

The "infrastructure" component is elaborated next. Here, the hardware/software/ network component features prominently as it entails the choice deployment of various information and computing-related technologies to support health IS/IT and CI applications and use. Briefly, this component involves configuring various hardware, software, user interface, and communication-enabling infrastructures,

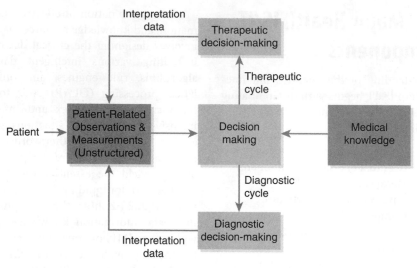

FIGURE 1-2 A Data/Information/Knowledge Decision System.

associated devices, and applications in such a way as to best achieve seamless information services integration throughout while connecting individuals, groups, and organizations.

The Philips–Samsung initiative, for example, is the joining of two major platforms created for integrating and securely storing as well as distributing data and information from both enterprise and related health IS/IT systems such as connected medical devices and wearables. It would be important to ensure that all such connected consumer-assistive devices can access the HMIS infrastructure seamlessly, better yet, these devises can access a "virtual" version of an application customized to a user-friendly interface. In this sense, for any patient and/or care provider, the infrastructure layer must and will be supportive of the end users, aiding the performance of tasks to be accomplished by these users and helping them to thrive when interacting within the ecosystem of the resulting technology-driven environment. Furthermore, new and emerging health IS/IT technologies and methods play an increasingly significant role in enhancing healthcare organizational delivery of patient care–related services. This brings us to the third basic HMIS component.

The data analytics component exemplifies the primary data processing and internalized data analytic engine for health IS/IT. Here, the focus shifts from just having information to informing (or descriptive analytics as to describe "what happened?"), from having a vague understanding to providing a highly probable diagnosis (or diagnostic analytics as to explain "why did it happen?") and from merely guessing to offering rational insights such as a prediction (or predictive analytics as to project "what will happen?"), and finally, from repeated analysis to an optimization of task analytics such as toward a prescription (or prescriptive analytics as to surmise "how can we make it happen?").

In practical terms, existing administrative-based health IS/IT, such as financial IS/IT, human resources IS/IT, facility utilization and scheduling systems, materials management systems, facilities management systems, and office automation systems, as well as clinical-based health IS/IT, such as EHR, CPOE, and HDSS/CDSS, must all be designed to collect relevant data and accumulate useful information for organizational data analytics processing that encompasses the entire spectrum of human–computer decision-making activities

The Analytics Spectrum

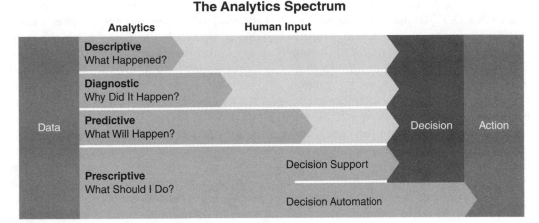

FIGURE 1-3 Stages of HMIS analytics.

Reproduced from Gartner Data & Analytics Summit Presentation, The Foundation of Data Science and Machine Learning: Achieving Advanced Insights and AI for Analytics, Peter Krensky, 29-30 May 2019.

as depicted in **FIGURE 1-3**. It is possible, too, that over time organizational, structural, and procedural changes and/or regulatory changes may require different analytics processes previously instituted to be altered or completely deleted—yielding to new processes, tasks, and applications. Therefore, a systems perspective is critical in order to achieve optimality among the different analytics processes and applications.

Surely, the integration/interoperability (network compatibility and communications) component that is discussed next serves as a key determinant of HMIS success from an enterprise view. Often, the key to positioning today's healthcare services organizations for future success is to ensure the interoperability of systems used in managing existing and ongoing healthcare information services vis-à-vis its competitive marketplace environment. The ONC has done a tremendous job in pushing U.S. hospitals and health centers to comply with the 2014–2015 "interoperability" mandates, creating a vision of stepping-stone compliance in the U.S. healthcare provider organizational environments to achieve efficient, effective, and excellent delivery of healthcare services. This creates a learning system for care providers on how the different organizational health IS/IT could be designed to fit well together to

achieve an integrated, enterprise-wide solution. On a global scale, this is exactly what the collaboration between Philips and Samsung platforms is doing so as to provide care services to subscribing consumers anywhere, anytime.

As early as 1980, Lincoln and Korpman recognized the difficulties with computer applications in healthcare services delivery.[14] In their classic paper, "Computers, Healthcare, and Medical Information Science," they argued that the goals for medical information science, although easy to state, are difficult to achieve for several reasons. First, adapting well-tested information processing procedures and methods from other fields into medicine is difficult because of the uncertainty and sophistication surrounding the medical context, the wide spectrum of medical data, and the vagueness, disparity, and variation of organizational healthcare objectives. Second, this challenge is further exacerbated by the apparent dissonance between the often-embedded ambiguity in medical data structure and the rigidity of computer logic structure. Specifically, in medicine, the materials cover the entire range of patient care data and the methods used span a wide range of disciplines, including the management, behavioral, and fundamental sciences, not just information processing and communications.

This brings us to the final but most critical health IS/IT component, the platform/interface component, which brings together and intelligently coordinates all of the other health IS/IT components. Based on a shared technological infrastructure, for example, various users are, in turn, empowered to perform designated tasks and activities that will support the overall business goals of the care provider organization—that is, to serve their clients (patients, clinicians, administrators, and more) both inside and outside the organization in the most efficient, productive, and effective manner. The function of this critical user component, when blended appropriately with all the other health IS/IT components, is to engender a holistic conceptualization that absorbs the many insights and interactions inherent in any organizational health IS/IT endeavor. It is the gateway for users to access all of the available health IS/IT features, functions, and capabilities.

Altogether, an adaptive, interoperable health IS/IT perspective encompasses a combined interaction of data-related elements, appropriate technologies and methods, designated task and analytics processes, and intended users' facing to inform and supply the needed information to support key organizational decision-making activities. The health IS/IT is an integral part of the organizational system, a mechanism that is central to integrating the enterprise and its various components. Every unit of that enterprise, which presumably is interrelated, must necessarily complete its purpose by working in unity. Like a jigsaw puzzle comprising a mass of irregularly shaped pieces that form a picture when fitted together, an adaptive, interoperable health IS/IT emerges when the different components of the enterprise fit together. The relationships among these major enterprise components are illustrated in **TABLE 1-2**, which may be further used to outline the different parts of this text.

TABLE 1-2 *Adaptive HMIS Text (4e):* Content and Organization

Part I Emergent HMIS Perspectives	
	Chapter 1. **Emerging Perspectives in health information systems/technologies (Health IS/IT)** *Joseph Tan*
	Chapter 2. **Precision Medicine: Decoding the Biology of Health and Disease** *James M. Snyder with case scenario by Joseph Tan*
	Technology Review I. **Review on Big Data Analytics in Healthcare** *Abir Belaala, L. S. Terrissa, N. Zerhouni, Christine Devalland, and Joshia Tan*
	Chapter 3. **Digital Health Commercialization** *Greg Moon and Phillip Olla*
	Policy Review I. **Online Health Information Seeking: Recasting Access and Digital Equity** *Fay Cobb Payton and Lynette Yarger*
	Mini-Case (Part I). ***Ginger.io: Mental Health Behavioral Analytics*** *Phillip Olla and Greg Moon*

(continues)

TABLE 1-2 *Adaptive HMIS Text (4e):* Content and Organization *(continued)*

Part IV **HMIS** **Standards,** **Policy,** **Governance,** **Ethics, and** **Future**	*Chapter 12.* **Clinical Confidentiality, Privacy, and Ethical Issues in the Digital Age** *Charie Faught* *Policy Review III.* **Health IS/IT Standards Adoption in Health Systems** *Sanjay Sood and Joseph Tan* *Chapter 13.* **Can AI Determine Consumers' Preferences on Healthcare Services? A Case Study of Zocdoc Using Social Media Analytics** *Adela Lau, Kristine Baker, Katherine Kempf, Katie Schwalm, Sijuade Oke, Eric Tsui, Liege Cheung, Marie-Claire Slama, and Min Su* *Chapter 14.* **Healthcare Globalization through Health Information Technology–Enabled Initiatives** *Anantachai Panjamapirom and Philip F. Musa* *Chapter 15.* **Healthcare Futures: Emerging Healthcare Technology** *Phillip Olla, Rajib Biswas, and Joseph Tan* *Mini-Case (Part IV).* **The Leadership of Future Health** *Joseph Tan with Joshia Tan*
Part V **HMIS** **Practices and** **Cases**	*Case 1.* **Digital Health Technology Commercialization Strategies** *Greg Moon and Phillip Olla* *Case 2.* **The Impact of Electronic Medical Records (EMRs) on Clinical Workflow and Practices: Perspectives of MS, a Physician Resident in Ottawa, Canada** *Brandon Lam with Joseph Tan* *Case 3.* **St. Joseph Mercy Oakland (SJMO): Digital Leadership in Health Care** *Mohan Tanniru, Jack Weiner, and Monica Garfield* *Case 4.* **Theranos: Innovating an Industry Primed for Innovation** *Chloe Nyitray, Brandon Nixon, Grace Simpson, and Joseph Tan* *Case 5.* **Patients Like Me (PLM): Social Media in Public Health** *Phillip Olla, Brianna Mozariwskyj, and Vickee Le*

Five major themes underlie this multi-disciplinary HMIS field—these themes help structure the scenarios, chapters, reviews, mini-cases, and major cases sequenced in this revised fourth edition of *Adaptive HMIS*: (1) emergent health IS/IT perspectives; (2) health IS/IT technologies and applications; (3) health IS/IT planning and health services management; (4) health IS/IT standards, policy, governance, ethics, and future; and (5) health IS/IT cases and practices.

Part I, comprising Chapters 1–3, emphasizes emergent HMIS perspectives. *Chapter 1* overviews the field of health IS/IT from currently developing perspectives of health IS/IT and clinical informatics, in particular how health organizational digitalization is transforming health services delivery locally, regionally, and globally. *Chapter 2* discusses the concepts of Precision Medicine as a new approach to decoding the biology of health and disease. This is followed by *Technology Review I* to unveil fundamental (but contemporary) thinking on the nature of big health data analytics, including key concepts on big health data and datasets, their sources and emerging analytic techniques, as well as the complex step-by-step process needed to extract meaningful insights from such massive data captured and accumulated in health warehouses, including streaming datasets. *Chapter 3* then delves into unveiling the intricacies and cognitive barriers challenging the digital health commercialization process. Following this, *Policy Review I* discusses the access and digital equity issues for seekers of online health information. Finally, we close Part I by incorporating a mini-case for class discussions that offers a challenging perspective on mental health behavioral analytics. Together, these chapters, shorter reviews, and the mini-case will set the stage for readers to reflect on how emerging trends and diverse perspectives in health IS/IT education, research, and development may be applied to transform the traditional healthcare services delivery.

Part II, comprising Chapters 4–7, surveys the technology and application layers of HMIS. *Chapter 4* focuses on the fundamental building blocks of digital health systems, that is, the digital data. This is supplemented by *Technology Review II*, an in-depth look into the broader area of geospatial data, geospatial technology, IoT, and cloud computing for health systems. *Chapter 5*, which introduces the readers to key digital health enterprise software, details three health organization management systems: SCM, CRM, and ERP. *Technology Review III* emphasizes the transformative power of SCM for health systems. *Chapter 6* familiarizes readers with four key patient-care coordination technologies, namely, EHR, CPOE, CDS, and PP. This is supplemented by *Chapter 7* focusing on the critical domain of pharmacy informatics with illustrative details on technologies for the medication use process and professional education. Finally, we close Part II by incorporating a mini-case for class discussions that offers illustrative examples of a mobile fitness device known as Lose IT! Altogether, these chapters, the appended review, and the mini-case are meant to broaden the readers' thoughts on how HMIS applications have significantly and will continue to impact our daily lives and well-being, both individually and socially.

Part III, which encompasses Chapters 8–11, informs readers about HMIS planning, design, and management issues. *Chapter 8* covers digital health strategic planning and strategies, accompanied by *Policy Review II* on the roles and responsibilities of health systems leaders and managers. *Chapter 9* presents decision aiding and predictive systems, re-affirming a framework for data mining and machine learning for health systems management, whereas *Chapter 10* offers professional and practical advice on the role of informatics in public health services. We then followed this with *Chapter 11* by reinforcing the concepts of health IS/IT implementation from the different perspectives, including those of project management, innovation procurement, and IT services management. Finally, we close Part III by incorporating a mini-case for class discussions that offers a challenging perspective on physician intervention in reducing readmission and tele-health. Together with these chapters, the policy review and the mini-case aim to challenge our thinking on how best to manage HMIS, the need to plan in advance, and the type of strategies available for us to begin generating new approaches toward implementing health IS/IT solutions for increasing health and well-being for ourselves, our communities, and our world.

Part IV of the text, which covers Chapters 12–15, acquaints the readers with HMIS standards, policy, governance, ethics, and the future. *Chapter 12* presents clinical confidentiality, privacy, and ethical issues in the digital era and is supplemented with *Policy Review III* focusing on the health IT standards adoption in health systems; *Chapter 13* opens up the scope of earlier discussions on data analytics by transitioning into artificial intelligence (AI) and social media analytics to studying consumers' preferences on healthcare services; *Chapter 14* surveys healthcare globalization through health information technology–enabled initiatives, while *Chapter 15* jumps forward with the futures of health services by projecting from current and emerging health technology innovation and diffusion. A mini-case on the challenging perspective of future health leadership at the societal and community level closes Part IV of the text.

Part V is devoted to assembling a series of selective cases intended to pull together parts and pieces of HMIS perspectives, methods, and applications as presented throughout the earlier parts of the text. In no particular order, these cases are intended primarily to stimulate class discussions and interactions among students and instructor(s). *Case 1, Digital Health Technology Commercialization Strategies,* focuses on digital health technology commercialization strategies, essentially illustrates and extends the thinking of *Chapter 3* on digital health commercialization

(in alignment with Part I on HMIS emergent perspectives). *Case 2, The Impact of Electronic Medical Records (EMRs) on Clinical Workflow and Practices: Perspectives of MS, a Physician Resident in Ottawa, Canada,* offers insights into the acceptance, use, benefits, and challenges of a patient-record oriented system to aid routine decision making for clinicians vis-à-vis their daily clinical workflow activities (in alignment with Part II on HMIS technology and applications). Interestingly, *Case 3, St. Joseph Mercy Oakland (SJMO): Digital Leadership in Health Care,* zooms in on HMIS planning and management (in alignment with Part III theme). *Case 4, Theranos: Innovating an Industry Primed for Innovation,* touches on key HMIS dimensions of standards, governance, politics, and ethics, aligning with topics covered largely in Part IV. *Case 5, Patients Like Me (PLM): Social Media in Public Health* attempts to integrate the emerging healthcare technologies alongside a more down-to-earth practice-based viewpoint, essentially integrating views toward future health from the current digital age with a focus on the patients and their social contacts, thereby combining thoughts from Part I *through* Part IV and bringing a closure to the entire text.

At this point, it appears timely to close the chapter discussions with a brief review on HMIS cultures.

▶ IV. HMIS Cultures

Why do HMIS cultures matter? A health information system exists as part of a larger system to support one or more of a combination of administrative, financial, clinical, research, or managerial activities occurring within a health organization. Yet, it is the culture of the health services organization that largely determines the appropriate product mix, roll out, and use of HMIS solutions within the organization. More likely than not, existing and traditional HMIS applications often tend to be disintegrated so that critical information embedded in the different parts of the organization is not going to be transparent among employees of the organization.

In terms of HMIS cultures, based on what we now know about successful and effective health IS/IT leadership, a healthcare services organization may intentionally or unintentionally adopt and nurture one of four cultural orientations: an information-functional culture, an information-sharing culture, an information-inquiring culture, and an information-discovery culture.[15] Understanding the different characteristics of each of these cultures is important to guide managers, administrators, and systems analysts in generating appropriate health IS/IT solutions for the organization.

An information-functional culture essentially takes the traditional view that information is power and that giving up information implies a power loss in terms of controlling others. It also follows that as most organizations are structured functionally, information-functional culture therefore limits the flow of information within a functional area such as human resources, accounting and finance, sales and marketing, and IT. For example, nurses in an emergency unit of a health system adopting an information-functional culture will attempt to safeguard their own use of patient-gathered information as well as limit the sharing of patient records as a way of exerting power over nurses in other units. Thus, whenever nurses from the acute care unit or other units need to schedule a care routine of a discharged patient from the emergency unit, they will have to involve the emergency nurses.

In contrast, an information-sharing culture promotes trust among employees of different units within the same system. While needing to be sensitive as to the privacy, confidentiality, and security of particular information under his or her safeguard, it is important that nurses, physicians, and others be able to share certain types of information with fellow employees for the benefit of the entire system.

For example, the chief medical officer (CMO) of a hospital who wants to see that his or her direct reports work collaboratively to benefit the efficient and effective running of the entire hospital must not only encourage sharing of information among individual physicians, but he or she should also focus on making information—especially on procedural problems and patient care process failures—transparent among the individual physicians in the hospital.

An information-inquiring culture essentially makes transparent the core values, beliefs, and purpose of the organization and ensures that critical information about the due processes, procedures, and functioning of the system is easily accessible for all employees throughout the system. Employees are also encouraged and trained to actively monitor such information and to align their daily actions and behaviors with the trends and new leadership directions of the system. For instance, all nurses and doctors of a health system could be asked to greet and politely interact with incoming and discharged patients to promote its reputation as a united system that is focused on patient care and customer satisfaction. All employees are also clear about how conflicts should and can be resolved quickly and the due procedures for attending to patient complaints.

Finally, an information-discovery culture entails that the system is able to share insights freely and encourages its employees to collaborate in offering new products and/or services that meet the needs of existing and new clients. Employees throughout the system are also provided with a comprehensive view of how the system functions and how it will support them in their attempt to deal with crises and radical changes and/or finding ways to achieve competitive advantages against its competitors. For health learning systems, it is necessary to start moving toward the adoption of an information-discovery cultural orientation, especially among the physicians, because of the need for a learning system to move away from strong traditional roots in which physicians are only accustomed to make their decisions independently about the patients under their care, when they are, in fact, having the need to coordinate that care among multiple caregivers within the system that they practice.

Understanding HMIS applications begins with having an appreciation of how health systems function and how IT should be deployed productively within these systems. The complexity of health learning systems and the intricacy of its myriad processes often are the root cause of IT failures in health systems. Many health executives thought that slapping a complex HMIS on top of the problems encountered in a health learning system would resolve its woes when, in many cases, it not only worsens them but also adds unnecessary expenses when the root causes of these problems are not well understood. It is far more important to map out the processes, simplify the complexity, consolidate the needs, and identify the core IT requirements. From here, management has to nurture, cultivate, and respect the working of the HMIS culture and implement appropriate health IS/IT solutions accordingly.

▶ V. Conclusion

This chapter starts out with a real-world scenario describing the emergent perspectives of HMIS and how these perspectives are impacting the futures of health services delivery. It briefly highlights the major components of a typical health IS/IT system and outlines key health IS/IT themes that aided in providing an organizing structure to group the wide-ranging

contributions submitted to this revised fourth edition of *Adaptive HMIS*. Importantly, students should appreciate the strategic, tactical, and operational functioning of a health learning system, including the HMIS cultures, before championing appropriate health IS/IT solutions that can be efficiently and effectively deployed in these systems to be used toward their intended capacity, thereby achieving the overarching goals and objectives of the health learning systems.

For the rest of Part I and beyond, it is hoped that the emergent HMIS perspectives on new medicine will open up the readers' minds in showcasing how the new technology of precision medicine (Chapter 2) and digital health commercialization (Chapter 3) are rapidly changing the landscape of medicine, bringing about more targeted healing to individuals impacted by different forms of diseases while monetizing digital health analytics. It is hoped that instructors will find these initial chapters in Part I helpful in encouraging students to become excited about the new world of HMIS. The scenario at the beginning of each chapter, the Technology Reviews, the Policy Reviews, and the mini-case(s) at the end of each part, together with the specific chapter questions and citations noted at the end of the chapters, and the Glossary and Index appended at the end of the text are multifaceted approaches to motivating and enriching the students' learning repertoire—to help student readers seek better answers to many more questions about HMIS—as new knowledge and technological breakthroughs in HMIS-related fields continue to emerge in a rapidly changing world.

Notes

1. Retrieved from www.samsung.com/us/ssic/press/philips-and-samsungteam-to-expandconnected-health-ecosystem/ (August 2018).
2. Tan, J. (2003). Information systems (IS) in health care, peer-reviewed article by special invitation. In H. Bidgoli (Eds.), *Encyclopedia of information systems* (Vol. 2, pp. 519–536). San Diego, CA: Academic Press.
3. Tan, J. (with F.C. Payton). (2010). *Adaptive health management information system* (3rd ed.). Sudbury, MA: Jones & Bartlett Learning.
4. Digital Health Ecosystem for African Countries: A Guide for Public and Private Actors for establishing holistic Digital Health Ecosystems in Africa. Retrieved from www.bmz.de/en/publications/topics/health

/Materilie345_digital_health_africa.pdf (*BMZ Report,* August 2018).

5. *BMZ Report, ibid.*, p. 9.
6. *Connecting health and care for the nation: A 10-year vision to achieve an interoperable health IT infrastructure.* Report of the Office of the National Coordinator for Health Information Technology, Department of Health & Human Services (HHS), Washington: DC, 2015. Retrieved from www.healthit.gov/sites/default /files/ONC10yearInteroperabilityConceptPaper.pdf (September 2018).
7. *Ibid.*
8. Stroetmann, K. (2014). Health system efficiency and eHealth interoperability—How much interoperability do we need? In Á. Rocha, A. M. Correia, F. B. Tan, & K. A. Stroetmann (Eds.), *New perspectives in information systems and technologies—Volume 2. Advances in intelligent systems and computing* (Vol. 276, pp. 394–406). Heidelberg: Springer.
9. Greer, S. L., Wismar, M., & Figueras, J. (Eds.). (2016). *Strengthening health system governance—Better policies, stronger performance.* WHO European Observatory on Health Systems and Policies, Maidenhead, England: Open University Press.

10. *BMZ Report, ibid.*
11. Sheikh, A., Cresswell, K. M., Wright, A., & Bates, D. W. (2017). *Key advances in clinical informatics: Transforming health care through health information technology.* London, UK: Academic Press.
12. Retrieved from https://acumenmd.com/blog/the -anatomy-of-a-certified-ehr-what-to-expect-in-2018/ (August 2018).
13. Tan, (2010), *ibid.*
14. Lincoln, T. L., & Korpman, R. A. (1980). Computers, healthcare, and medical information science. *Science, 210*(4467), 257–263.
15. Booz Allen Hamilton, Inc. (2006). *Information sharing.* New York, NY: HarperCollins. Retrieved from www.boozallen.com

Chapter Questions

1-1 What are emergent perspectives of health IS/IT?

1-2 Why is it difficult to integrate IT and medicine? Discuss the need for an integrative perspective for managing health IS/IT.

1-3 List the five major components of a health IS/IT system. Discuss which component deserves the most attention in today's health IS/IT environment and why. Provide specific examples of each component in the context of your work.

1-4 If you were the Chief Information Officer, which of the four types of health IS/IT cultures would you pursue and why?

1-5 What is the concept of a digital health ecosystem? What significance and impact does such a concept have on the transformation of healthcare services delivery systems in the United States, and other developed and developing countries?

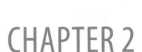

CHAPTER 2

Precision Medicine: Decoding the Biology of Health and Disease

James M. Snyder with case scenario by Joseph Tan

LEARNING OBJECTIVES

- Define Precision Medicine (PM) and showcase how PM transforms traditional healthcare thinking and services
- Articulate underlying concepts and principles of PM, especially in cancer care
- Highlight key discoveries and events leading to PM
- Detail key barriers and challenges in implementing PM

CHAPTER OUTLINE

Scenario: Origo—Crafting a Precision Medicine Platform for Cancer Patients on a Global Scale[1]

In 2017, Genotech Matrix, a New Haven, Connecticut, biotech company, partnered with Vishuo Biomedical, a Singapore healthcare technology company, to advance cancer care on a global scale. Together, these companies have developed an award-winning Precision Medicine Platform to resolve challenges for the need of personalized cancer care faced by a leading Manhattan hospital group that wanted to implement their own precision medicine initiative. This hospital group was not prepared to have their patient database management and cancer genetic sequencing process, including secured information sharing and management, outsourced when the viability of their *Origo* Clinical Cancer Genome (CCG) Platform solution was successfully demonstrated.

According to cancer researchers working in these biotechnology companies,[2](p. 1) "advancements in genetic testing have allowed clinicians and researchers to better characterize types of tumor, specific mutations and then tailor treatment regimens to save time and money. Simultaneously, genetic sequencing costs have decreased significantly, while the speed of analysis and generating results has increased. With this alignment, academic and healthcare organizations have been migrating quickly into the arena of **precision medicine**... Cancer continues to bewilder even the best clinicians. While there are more than 100 types of cancer, we are learning that there are many more genetic mutations that cause one person's tumor to be unique and respond differently to treatments that may work for others with the same type of cancer."

As shown in **FIGURE 2-1**, the proposed solution involves implementing the Genotech Matrix *Precision Medicine Platform* in

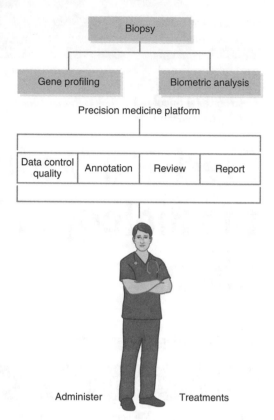

FIGURE 2-1 Precision medicine workflow pipeline.[2](p. 2)

Data from genotechmatrix.com/wp-content/uploads/2017/05/Case-Study.pdf

combination with *iCMDB*® (*intelligence in Clinical Medicine for Decision-Making and Best Practices*), a core product of Vishuo Biomedical. This combination advances the manipulation of a globally enriched knowledge base for automating sequencing and analysis of variants of gene expressions to support personalized treatment by clinicians based on the genetic and histologic pathology profiles of patients.

Aside from integrating *iCMDB* into the Manhattan hospital group's database, a personalized workflow pipeline that supports report generation to meet the specific needs of caring oncologists within the organization's setting has also been developed. For secured patient data management, an on-site server installed with the *Origo* platform has been deployed, and the analysis pipelines have been customized to protect and encrypt any confidential personal information used in generating automated personalized reports that support clinical decision-making. In aiming to provide a more efficient and effective (personalized) approach to cancer care, it is purported that to date over 2000 oncology patient samples have been sequenced and their respective reports have been generated via the *Origo* platform since its 2016 implementation.

Watch the YouTube video about the power of the *Origo* platform.[3] Think about how this new Genotech–Vishuo collaboration will impact the future of global cancer care delivery in light of the rapidly increasing mobility of patients. Additionally, reflect upon why and how precision medicine may now be redefining health care and fulfilling the potential to minimize side effects from traditional cancer treatments as cancer care moves toward more personalized treatment. What other innovative biotechnological services might potentially be supported on the *Origo* platform, and how will such collaborative efforts usher in a new era of precision medicine?

▶ I. Introduction

This chapter introduces the readers to an emerging healthcare model known as Precision Medicine (PM). PM is an approach to health care that is largely dependent on the *digitization of health data and bioinformatics,* a field of study intersecting key areas of computer science and biology. PM attempts to improve health outcomes by refining diagnosis, treatment, and disease prevention through understanding of the many factors that can contribute to the intrinsic biology of disease.

A core principle of PM is that by decoding the genetic and molecular changes that lead to the development of disease, we can alter the course of disease and preserve health. The technology used to analyze someone's genetic sequences and other molecular events is now readily available and may be clinically utilized. Molecular data provide perspective as to how a

disease develops or how someone may respond to treatment. New technologies are creating a wealth of health-related data that will offer additional insight into behavioral and environmental influences on molecular biology and genetic changes that cause specific disease(s). Harnessing the power of computer science to create big data knowledge networks that connect the intrinsic biology of disease with other health-related factors, such as behavior, exposures, and environment, is central to PM.[4]

In this chapter, we review advances in the scientific understanding of the intrinsic biology of disease with an emphasis on genomics, introduce the utilization of large-scale molecular testing in health care, survey barriers to implementing PM, and discuss the future of this new approach.

"And that's the promise of precision medicine – delivering the right treatments, at the right time, every time to the right person. And for a small but growing number of patients, that future is already here." - President Barack Obama[5]

▶ II. Background: What Is PM?

PM is an emergent healthcare perspective focused on the prevention, diagnosis, and treatment of disease based on an individual's unique health features, with an emphasis on the molecular underpinnings of health and disease.[6,7]

In the last several years, there has been a tremendous increase in available healthcare information, including genetic analysis, environment, and behavior. Molecular data, which include information about an individual's genes, gene activity, proteins, epigenome, and cellular activity, have entered everyday clinical care and disease management. There is great optimism that this influx of molecular and other health data into medical management (specifically, PM) will accelerate our understanding of disease and dramatically improve treatment outcomes and disease prevention. This is a progression from Western medicine's current approach of guideline-modeled care where therapeutic regimens are intended to be applicable to large groups of people.

Importantly, advances in computer science and bioinformatics have ushered in PM through the ability to process large amounts of data from many data sources so as to identify new factors in the development, prevention, and treatment of disease. PM attempts to answer why some people with similar risk factors develop an illness and others do not and why a therapeutic strategy is curative in only select cohorts of people, and, ultimately, illustrate how an illness can be prevented from occurring in the first place. The PM community is confident that the answer to these questions is hidden in the subcellular molecular data that we are beginning to understand. Most cancers, for example, are thought to occur due to genetic instability. Three common explanations for the genetic instability include inherited mutations that we are born with, somatic mutations that occur in cells during development or throughout life, and deviations in the regulatory mechanisms that maintain genetic integrity.[8] Science has made great strides in understanding the genetic and genomic features of cancer and noncancerous conditions. Efforts are underway to create networks of knowledge that connect the molecular and genetic building blocks of disease with other health data at a population and individual level.

As an example, we will review a standard patient presentation and physician evaluation in our current model of care. A 52-year-old woman presents to her doctor with symptoms of weight loss and a progressive cough over the last 3 months. The doctor asks a litany of symptom-based questions, performs a clinical exam, and orders additional testing to help make a diagnosis, such as chest X-ray and blood work. The chest X-ray reveals a mass.

The patient undergoes a biopsy of the mass, which shows a type of lung cancer called adenocarcinoma. The cancer is identified by histologic diagnosis (how the cells look under a microscope), and the patient is treated per the national guidelines for that type of cancer. In recent years, we have seen tremendous developments in our understanding of the molecular drivers of disease and have another layer of clinically relevant diagnostic and therapeutic information to add to this patient's diagnosis and treatment decision-making. Through molecular information, we are finding similarities between cancer types that were previously thought to be unrelated. In this example, the patient was identified to have a gene mutation called anaplastic lymphoma kinase (ALK), which is also seen in a type of brain tumor called neuroblastoma. As the network of knowledge matures, advances in treating ALK-mutant lung cancer may shed light on neuroblastoma brain tumors, two diseases that present very differently in the body. The lung cancer patient is started on an approved drug that targets this ALK pathway. Specific treatment recommendations based on molecular information is slowly being integrated into guideline-based care recommendations.

Considerable overlap exists between PM and other approaches to health care, including our current symptom-driven model. P4 medicine stands for *predictive, preventive, personalized, and participatory* health care.[9] P4 medicine approaches health care with a broad view spanning population health to subcellular science and molecular medicine. P4 medicine, developed by the Institute for Systems Biology in Seattle, Washington, attempts to bring together system-based biology with patient-provided data generation and advanced technology through the use of digital tools that aggregate multidimensional patient-health-experience data, which they call the "networks of networks" (see **FIGURE 2-2**).[10]

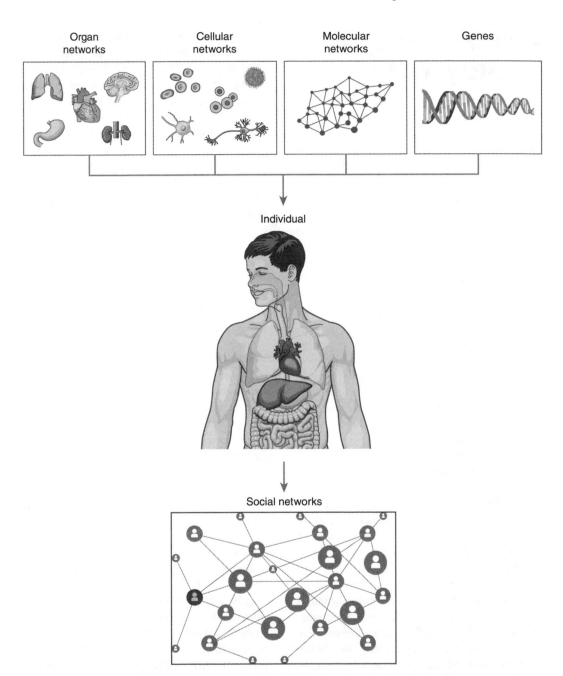

FIGURE 2-2 The "Network of Networks" aggregated health data foundation of the P4 medicine approach.

From http://future.psjhealth.org/scientific-wellness/about-the-institute-for-systems-biology?utm_source=TWITTER&utm_medium=social_organic&utm_term=-–&utm_content=psjh
-1773051757-&utm_campaign=evergreenContent+Type+%28Secondary%29?

▶ III. Key Events in the History of PM

The opportunity to implement PM has occurred due to simultaneous milestones in our understanding and access to molecular data, advances in computer science that can curate and analyze large multivariate datasets, and routine use of molecular testing, which has dramatically reduced cost while increasing efficiency. This has ignited an interdisciplinary effort with cross-training in many disciplines, the most notable being bioinformatics, which is the combination of biology and computer science. In the "omics" research lab, I observe and participate in many biologists and computer scientists work side by side with overlapping educational paths and research skills. "Omics" refers to scientific disciplines that end in the suffix "-ome," which implies large-scale study of the subject field, such as gene(omics).[11] Leading omics disciplines include genomics, proteomics, transcriptomics, epigenomics, metabolomics, radiomics, and others.

Survey of Human Genetics in Health Care

Early understanding of genetics is attributed to Gregor Mendel's work in the 1860s describing the inheritance of traits in pea plants. In the 1950s, the structure of deoxyribonucleic acid (DNA) was identified. DNA is the hereditary chemical code made up of adenine, guanine, cytosine, and thymine base pairs that create a structure called a double helix. The sequence of DNA base pair combinations directs how cells are formed and maintained. A practical method of DNA sequencing was published in 1977, ushering in an era of genomic medicine.[12]

Conceptualized in 1990 and completed in 2002, the Human Genome Project courageously mapped the complete human genome, providing the world with "the structure, organization and function of the complete set of human genes."[13] In 2006, the National Cancer Institute (NCI) launched The Cancer Genome Atlas (TCGA) characterizing the genetic and molecular features of 33 tumor types. Massively Parallel Sequencing (MPS), which is also called Next Generation Sequencing, performs many sequencing tests at once. MPS was introduced in the academic literature in 2008 and dramatically changed the landscape of genetic testing by reducing costs 100-fold and reducing the time to completion of sequencing to just 8 weeks (it can now be done in matter of few days).[14]

Prior to MPS, each exon, which is a segment of DNA that codes for a corresponding segment of ribonucleic acid (RNA) and, ultimately, a protein, had to be sequenced and amplified individually, requiring considerable time and resources. The 2011 report by the National Research Council (NRC) laid out the framework for a molecular taxonomy of disease and implementation of PM, and in the United States in 2015 President Barack Obama committed $215 million to funding a national PM effort. Only recently has genetic sequencing entered routine clinical care, as previously this testing was cost prohibitive.

In 2001, the cost to sequence one entire human genome was estimated at $95 million.[15] Sequencing costs continued to drop, and in 2007 the estimated cost for the sequencing of a single human genome was approximately $10 million.[16] In 2011, the cost was $21,000, and in 2018 whole genome sequencing was obtained for less than $3000.[17] This reduction in cost coupled with the availability of results in less than 2 weeks has brought molecular medicine into clinical practice for a growing list of health conditions.

Now that molecular data are approaching a cost-effective and actionable timeline, efforts are underway to include these data into routine clinical practice. The point of obtaining genetic data is to identify the cellular blueprints of health and disease. In understanding the building blocks of disease, we can better categorize conditions and hopefully reveal why some patients respond to treatment and others do not. The goal is to prevent disease before it occurs, but to do so we must also understand how and why deviations from health develop. Cancer is particularly ripe for a PM approach as most cancers are thought to occur due to a complex relationship between genetic instability and environment at the cellular, individual, and population level.

A brief discussion of genetics and molecular anatomy is helpful to understand the molecular aspects of PM. DNA is the building block of proteins in our body. DNA is the cellular template that undergoes a process called transcription to create precise sequences of ribonucleic acid (RNA). During translation, this code of RNA is the blueprint used to build defined amino acids with which proteins are formed. The epigenome refers to the chemical compounds and proteins that package and control access to the genetic code and cellular functions, controlling how the genetic code is implemented.[18] As one can imagine, environmental factors such as smoking, age, or disease can impact this process. There are many additional factors that contribute to the development of disease and disruption of "normal" molecular pathways. Phenotype refers to the observable characteristics or expression from the genetic code,[19] which can be thought of as the manifestation of the genetic code. The relationship between the genetic code and an individual's phenotype is also complex, with each interconnected layer of biologic information harboring tremendous potential insight into health and disease.

"Variant calling" is the identification of molecular deviations from the expected genetic code, which are also called mutations. There is no consensus definition of the "normal" genetic code in humans, as existing data are based on small sample sizes that may not reflect the general population. Prospective efforts are underway to characterize the genomic and health data of large groups of people, numbering from 500,000 to more than 1 million people. Many existing molecularly characterized datasets are based on retrospective data, or data obtained in isolation that may not include other relevant attributes such as someone's activities, quality of life, geographic location, comorbidities, environmental exposures, or family history. Large prospective studies that track participants longitudinally over a number of years with cross platform data collection, including Electronic Health Records (EHR), and personal health data like the All of Us project and others have the potential to illuminate the complex factors that contribute to disease development and, ultimately, prevention.[20]

Research to characterize the nearly 3 billion units of DNA across 23,000 DNA base pairs has made tremendous progress over the last several years. Similar research in other omics disciplines has also shown progress. The magnitude, specificity, and types of testing available in health care are evolving rapidly as is our insight into the relationships between this data and health. Some diseases may reveal direct variants in DNA or RNA that can be successfully targeted with PM therapies; however, it is more likely that there is a complex relationship between many factors, including environment, molecular events, and other attributes that contribute to the development of disease.

In 2011, the NRC laid out the framework for a molecular taxonomy of disease summarizing the state of molecular medicine and presenting an action plan to implement PM. Implementing PM requires a profound change to clinical practice, including how data are recorded, what data are recorded, how clinicians analyze and process vast quantities of data, how patients participate in healthcare data, the medical decision-making process, access to molecular testing, access to targeted therapies, approval and safety process for drug development, and many other aspects of our current care model, in addition to new technologies that will develop.

▶ IV. Current Perspective

Over the last few years, we have seen the availability and commercialization of high-throughput sequencing flood oncology clinics with real-time genetic data, including hundreds (and soon thousands) of anticipated genetic variants that may have clinical significance, as well as new biomarkers that can be used to measure health or disease. These genetic data are typically reported within 2 weeks of sending out the bio-specimen and are therefore clinically actionable. Molecular testing is usually requested to subclassify a diagnosis, refine therapeutic options, or fulfill claims of PM. Oncology centers are racing to utilize these data through molecular tumor boards (MTBs) and third-party data navigation platforms provided by academic institutions, non-profit organizations, and for-profit companies.

In addition, new realms of data such as digital phenotyping, wearable devices, Internet of Things (IoT) medical devices, smart phones, patient self-reporting, social media inputs, and beyond are being generated for the healthcare sector at a rapid pace, leaving clinical teams scrambling to digest all of these data. Curating medical data for security and meaningful use is necessary to maximize this opportunity and ensure the safety of potentially vulnerable patient health information (PHI). At the time of this publication, there is no publicly available standard tool to view these data in concert and leverage their collective value. To accomplish this task, advancements in healthcare genetics education, health data curation, and technology implementation in clinical practice will have to occur.

This volume of genetic and molecular testing available in clinical care and the commercialization of this data production process through large third-party providers that aggregate test results into large privately held or public datasets is a paradigm shift in medicine. Our current use of molecular data is built upon the groundbreaking work of expansive genome atlases, such as TCGA and others. Whereas participation in foundational genomics studies like the TCGA was primarily performed at large academic medical institutions, the utilization of MPS through commercial platforms and regional labs is available through any provider with access to a tissue sample. This testing, which typically investigates a panel of known genetic variants, is now commonly performed in academic and community centers alike. This is a critical shift—placing volumes of genetic medical data into public registries and private companies. Both private and academic bodies offer genetic testing using MPS methods, retaining data in functional databases that hold great intellectual and financial value. Increasingly, these groups are partnering with private and for-profit entities to harvest the data for research and discovery such as drug development or academic consortia. Prior collaborative academic efforts (like TCGA) have generated this data for public utility, fueling countless research efforts, and are available in searchable formats through web interfaces such as the NCI genomic data commons portal, the open source Clinical Interpretation of Variants in Cancer (CIViC) dataset, Cbioportal, and others.[21-23] Of note, most federally funded research efforts are required to provide the molecular data in a publicly accessible format after publication. Owing to the escalating financial and intellectual value of healthcare data, new paradigms of data protection and monetization have evolved.

Molecular data are increasingly integrated with routine cancer care. Many cancer types use some molecular or genetic data for diagnosis or to define disease subtypes. Multiple cancers have guidelines that use molecular data for treatment decisions that are oftentimes also supported by dramatically improved patient outcomes, such as those seen in melanoma and lung cancer. Many major cancer centers are in the early phases or have recently created dedicated molecular tumor boards. A few cancer centers have had dedicated MTBs for several years. A MTB or PM tumor board typically refers to a multidisciplinary team of healthcare professionals who prospectively review a patient's molecular testing in the context of their disease and treatment plan. An MTB often discusses treatment options when: (1) a possible drug target is present; (2) associated conditions require further testing (i.e., concern for a germline mutation); and (3) the molecular variant may impact health outcomes. Most MTBs are restricted to cases with actionable genetic variants but are not restrictive to any disease or histologic type. At larger tertiary centers, specialized tumor boards, which are also called prospective multidisciplinary cancer meetings, are organized by disease site such as a lung cancer tumor board or a nervous system tumor board. Tumor boards at dedicated cancer centers typically consist of a medical oncologist, disease-specific surgeon, radiation oncologist, radiologist, pathologist, nurses, and other healthcare providers, such as genetic counselors, social workers, and clinical trial experts.[24]

There are several barriers to implementing a PM recommendation, such as identification of a targeted therapy that disrupts a critical tumor growth pathway, access to the desired drug or therapy, and safety of administration. A PM-targeted therapy must disrupt the identified molecular pathway, and the tumor must be dependent on the specific pathway.[25] Some variants that are identified may not be the primary driver of the disease and are less likely to have a clinical impact if targeted. The goal is to identify molecular variants that are thought of as driver mutations or master regulators that may have great impact on disease development. The process

to bring a new drug into clinical practice requires tremendous regulatory oversight that should be followed in the interests of patient safety and scientific advancement. Investigational therapies should be administered through a clinical trial with extensive safety monitoring.

Clinical trials are historically organized by disease, organ involved, and histology (the cellular features seen under a microscope). Only recently have molecularly driven clinical trials become available. Scientists have postulated for many years that the specific molecular features of a disease likely contribute to therapeutic response but have lacked tools of scale to prospectively investigate and quantify these features. PM and the addition of molecular taxonomy to histologic diagnosis have changed the way diseases are categorized and also impacted the way clinical trials are designed. Clinical trials are historically described in phases, with different questions being asked at each phase. Phase 1 trials primarily research safety and the tolerated dosing of a new therapy. Phase 2 and 3 trials investigate if the intervention has an impact on the disease as well as associated adverse events.[26]

Two newer types of clinical trials designed for PM are "basket" trials (treatment cohorts are based on a shared mechanism of action across multiple histologic tumor types) and "umbrella" trials (which may include multiple molecular pathways and corresponding investigational drugs in the same trial designed for one histologic cancer type).[27] Several other innovative clinical trial designs are being explored.

In addition to refining histologic diagnosis with molecular subclassification, we must also decipher the variation of molecular and genetic expression both spatially within a tumor and as time progresses. This variation likely contributes to treatment resistance. Some healthcare clinics are attempting to obtain longitudinal genetic testing at multiple points in a person's disease course or samples from multiple locations within a tumor. As the cost of testing decreases and the insights provided by the test increase, we will undoubtedly see the utilization of molecular testing for cancer throughout a disease course as a monitoring tool. As the knowledge networks mature, we anticipate increased use of PM-driven informatics in disease prevention programs. If a person is identified to have known risk factors for disease, they may undergo periodic molecular screening tests to measure their risk of developing the disease and to hopefully reduce known risk factors. To accomplish this, the medical community must understand the many factors that contribute to disease development, identify a way to measure these factors, and then implement an intervention process.

Several technology platforms exist with the purpose of curating molecular and healthcare data. Major U.S. hospitals often use some form of EHR to curate healthcare data. In the PM space, there are specific technologies designed to organize and help clinical teams interpret genetic and other molecular data, facilitate PM MTBs, aggregate clinical data, and navigate clinical trial opportunities. Some of these platforms are open source, while others are proprietary. Through multisite PM applications, large databases are created that hold immense monetary and intellectual value. The opportunity to impact health care through big data analysis with machine learning and other analytic approaches in medicine is currently underutilized. The bulk of existing healthcare systems have not capitalized on big data; however, many are showing greater interest, which may be in response to the avidity with which private companies are trying to accomplish this task. To maximize this opportunity, healthcare data will need to evolve and solve concerns over semantic heterogeneity, technical heterogeneity, patient data security, financial limitations, and the resulting impact on clinician workflows.

Genetic Data

In the clinical practice of oncology, physicians use genetic panels to look for known cancer variants to fuel PM. Many of these panels test for changes at specific areas of DNA but may also include other molecular investigations, such as RNA or whole genome sequencing. Clinically available sequencing tests look at DNA for base pair substitutions, deletions, insertions, and fusions that have been shown to be relevant in cancer.[28] In some cases, investigators will look for only a few specific pertinent mutations or genetic aberrations that are important for a type of disease. For example, in neuro-oncology, which is the field of medicine focused on cancer and the nervous system, the molecular features of brain tumors have only been included in the World Health Organization's pathologic diagnosis recommendations since 2016.[29]

Prior to 2016, a brain tumor diagnosis was made solely on histologic review despite the availability, clinical utility, and known importance of molecular data in the classification of brain tumors. When someone is diagnosed with a brain tumor, it is standard practice for the pathologist to report select mutations such as IDH1 mutation, which conveys information on tumor development and prognosis; MGMT promoter hypermethylation, which provides insight into treatment response with certain types of chemotherapy; and genetic deletions on the 1p arm and the 19q arm, which are a diagnostic requirement for a tumor type called oligodendroglioma.[30] This is an example of PM in current practice. The clinical team may elect to investigate these tests as part of a broader panel or they may test individually. There are many ways to perform these tests; however, some centers may not have the needed equipment or expertise and elect to send the tissue to a qualified testing center.

In this chapter, we have focused on known variants of DNA used in the clinical management of someone diagnosed with cancer, although there is a wealth of additional molecular testing available. Many other pertinent investigations into molecular data are evolving at a rapid pace. RNA, protein expression, genetic fragments found in blood, whole genome sequencing, tests that investigate the accessibility of DNA, and the characterization of the tumor microenvironment are other areas of research. Nonetheless, a detailed discussion is beyond the scope of this chapter. Some molecular tests are only used in preclinical research, while others have met requirements that permit use in clinical care. Historically, research and clinical testing have been performed and analyzed separately, but with the development of PM and the reduced cost of testing, we hope to see hybrid research and clinical molecular investigations.

In summary, genetics is the study of how specific traits are inherited. This differs from genomics, which is the study of large-scale genetic data, such as the entirety of the human genome. "Omics" refers to scientific disciplines in biology that end in the suffix "-ome," which implies large-scale study of the subject field, such as gene(omics). Genomics is generally considered the first of the omics disciplines—but now there are many. The omics disciplines were ignited by advancements in computer processing that now allow scientist to analyze large quantities of biologic data. A driving message of PM, and the root of the omics disciplines, is that through processing large multivariate datasets, we can unlock the keys of health and disease. The emphasis on connecting data from many different sources by removing barriers across research disciplines and data silos is a tremendous undertaking and a rate-limiting factor for PM, as well as health informatics.

▶ V. Future Trends

In 2013, the NRC laid out the framework for a molecular taxonomy of disease summarizing the state of molecular medicine and presenting an action plan to implement PM.[31] Most of the issues, objectives, and solutions outlined in this landmark publication are still relevant and can be applied toward curating and accessing the data and implementation of findings. As discussed, PM has existed in health care for many years and has made significant progress toward a mechanism-based classification of disease and treatment decision-making. Large-scale efforts to understand human genomics across populations (a) in the pre-disease state, (b) as disease develops, and (c) during treatment, are now underway. In cancer and other disease states, molecular-derived classification and treatment protocols are becoming routine clinical practice; still, much work is needed to fully support a paradigm shift toward PM.

Curating the Data

Only recently has western medicine recorded healthcare data in digital formats through adoption of an EHR. While EHRs are relatively similar in concept to Electronic Medical Records (EMRs), an EHR is meant to encompass more data and extend beyond the health system or an individual doctor's office. In the United States, a handful of large commercial EHR services dominate the market. It is possible that separate institutions or hospitals that use the same EHR software can link medical records for an individual patient. By reducing institutional barriers and promotion of data aggregation, PM efforts may also be strengthened; however, this may require aggregating the data to some level of uniform reporting and analysis.

The power in PM stems from connecting many data types into a larger knowledge network so that subgroups and patterns can be identified. For an individual healthcare dataset to contribute to a larger knowledge network, the descriptors and attributes that describe the same value must use the same language. In medicine, there are many ways to say the same thing. A common data model should be implemented across healthcare sectors to permit data aggregation and sharing. A common data model uses a defined dictionary of terms. If care teams are not recording data using a common language, then a solution is required to convert the recorded information into the common data model while maintaining the integrity or value of the data. For example, a devastating brain tumor that affects people of all ages may be referred to as a glioblastoma, glioblastoma multiforme, astrocytoma grade IV, or GBM; despite these four names, the clinical diagnosis is the same. If the cohort is reduced by "fragmented naming," then the power of the sample size may not be sufficient to reveal disease subtypes and associations needed to power PM.

With developing technology comes renewed questions of ethics and barriers to implementation. PM is limited by a litany of regulatory hurdles that are designed to protect patient safety and security. Smartphone navigation platforms and wearable devices provide a wealth of available environmental and behavioral data that until recently was too complicated to record and aggregate. Collecting healthcare data while maintaining privacy and adherence to strict regulatory policy as required by the Health Insurance Portability and Accountability Act (HIPAA) remains a challenge. Digital phenotyping, as defined by Dr. John Touros et al., is the use of digital devices to provide health data through "moment-by-moment quantification of the individual-level human phenotype in-situ".[32] Digital phenotyping holds tremendous potential to identify modifiable disease risk factors and environmental association with molecular data and health outcomes. Best practice in aligning these data sources while respecting privacy is unclear. One solution is that patient groups opt in and provide their own digital phenotyping data and connect this with their health history or molecular testing. But can this solution provide the volume required to power analysis and what bias does this introduce?

How can science be representative when segments of the population do not have access to molecular data or digital phenotyping devices? Implementing PM requires thoughtful review of regulatory and ethical concerns as each new technology enters the knowledge network and clinical arena.

PM is dependent on the merger of clinical and research data from across the spectrum of health and disease. Clinical medicine in cancer requires multidisciplinary collaborative teams of clinicians to adequately care for patients with complex disease. Cancer-based PM research may benefit from a similar approach of multidisciplinary teams to connect disparate data sources and fuel collaborative research. Open data networks can compromise intellectual property housed in the data and devalue individual or institutional contributions, which are critical aspects of research funding. A shift in how research is being organized and approached is needed. Only laboratory tests that meet strict requirements can be used in patient care. There is clearly opportunity to learn from preclinical work and research-level investigations. New policies of preclinical research investigation of molecular mechanisms and targeted therapies that support clinically approved molecular testing and PM treatment access are needed. PM and the enormity of new health data sources pose unique challenges to health informatics, requiring collaboration and data fluidity across traditionally isolated clinical and research efforts. Research and clinical care should be a connected, closed-loop system in the interest of delivering on PM for improved health outcomes.

The data commons needed for promoting PM will have data inputs from many different sources. A knowledge network will require data inputs from technically heterogeneous sources into a shared data commons. The days of a medical record coming solely from the doctor's scribbles and notes are gone. A patient may have a histology report from proprietary software, DNA methylation analysis from another software type, nutrition data from a phone app, and environmental data from a smartwatch that must all connect in a central repository. The opportunity for new streams of healthcare data is endless. A PM solution will need to address how to connect technical heterogeneous information so that the data commons can access and support data from many sources.

Informatics and computational science play a huge role in processing this vast quantity of information so that it can be digested and harvested for scientific discovery and improvement in human health. With this explosion in innovation and opportunity comes a never-ending stream of questions. How are the individual patient's rights protected in this age of mass data collection? The patient always "owns" their health record, but when this data is monetized who is the beneficiary? How can healthcare systems pay for the considerable resources needed to execute PM? How do we safeguard this data against irresponsible use and prevent harm to those who agree to share their personal health data?

Access to the Data

In a PM-optimized healthcare environment, all data would be uploaded into a large, publicly accessible, international, pan socioeconomic, anonymized knowledge network that shares the common data model with uniform definitions and testing assays connected to a wealth of multi-dimensional omics data, powered to decode the molecular mechanisms of disease and therapeutic discovery. In the United States, private companies, hospitals, government organizations, consortiums, and other healthcare groups are racing to develop large interdisciplinary datasets to power PM discovery. Such datasets are extremely valuable and require considerable resources to manage.

In oncology, a basic knowledge network includes patient demographics, genetic or molecular test results, chemotherapy history, and imaging, with the opportunity for so much more. PM informatics platforms require access to health data, analytics to process the data, regular updating to reflect advancing knowledge, and at least one user interface to facilitate use of the data by clinicians and researchers. There are public and private PM platforms that can provide a user or health system with the tools needed to participate in PM. It is possible that individual repositories fragment the data to the point that discoveries in rare diseases or infrequent health attributes no longer have the sample size to be found. On the other hand, curation of an information commons requires considerable resources that could potentially be funded through monetizing the healthcare data that many companies are racing to obtain. A mechanism is required to support this infrastructure for a large cross-sectional PM network and provide the resources needed to achieve data aggregation across health systems and populations. These datasets harbor valuable intellectual property, which may need to be protected so researchers can invest in new discoveries that enrich the information commons. The bottom line is that these data belong to the patients, something institutions and companies often lose sight of.

Rare diseases and molecular aberrations may require extremely large datasets to achieve the volume required to draw conclusions. Others have identified this concern and started independent repositories of information, either for rare disease types or for rare mutations. One such effort is the NCI-backed Rare Diseases Registry (RaDaR) Program that connects investigators of rare diseases to a common data management center utilizing shared data practices and resources harnessed from public–private partnerships to collectively progress our understanding of rare diseases.[33]

Although there are strict rules and regulations safeguarding patient data, new solutions are needed to protect patient privacy in the age of PM and digital phenotyping.

As our healthcare data evolve, so must the conversation regarding data privacy and security. Individual health data now include second-by-second data points from smart devices that track behaviors, actions, and locations—information that could help determine modifiable risk factors. This level of monitoring, however, comes with additional ethical and data management concerns. Increasingly, genetic testing and healthcare data are bypassing the clinical team and being delivered directly to the patient. Two examples include My Family Health Portrait by the Surgeon General, where individuals can input family history to learn about disease risk factors, and home genetic testing kits that provide a window into genetic risk factors that predispose people to different diseases.[34,35]

Largely due to opportunities to improve care through advancing technology, physicians and health systems have loosened their grip on healthcare data, increasingly using third-party services, such as genetic testing that harbor large aggregate patient-derived datasets and patient-centered health registries. Applications exist that store useable personal EMR data on cell phones and provide ways to connect with your own EHR. Patients with rare diseases are coming together through social media and creating dedicated data repositories, tissue banks of pathologic specimens, and clinical trials for their rare conditions.[36] Patient advocacy groups are creating apps to chronicle patient-reported symptoms and outcomes. In the United States, the Patient Centered Outcome Research Institute (PCORI) is driving structured inclusion of the patient perspective into healthcare delivery models and research implementation to enhance value and improve patient trust.[37] Investment by patients in personal health data when applied to molecular and clinical information may lead to new discoveries of environmental or behavioral influence on health and individualized quality of life metrics. Patient-led participation in healthcare research beyond traditional institutional or geographic boundaries has also led to increased enrollment in clinical trials, as well as other advances that are yet unseen.[38]

Implementation of PM Findings

The impetus for PM is anchored in the hope of drastic improvements in health outcomes for all people through continuing advances in biology and computer science. The addition of a molecular taxonomy and subclassification of disease is the first stage of PM implementation; it is already well underway. PM has helped to identify subsets within a histologic diagnosis that harbor distinct subcellular molecular disease development pathways that result in an altered response to therapy and outcomes when compared with the general disease cohort. These molecular subsets help explain response variability among people who carry the same diagnosis and eventually will decode why some people respond to a drug and others do not. For some conditions, targetable genetic variants have been identified that respond to pathway-disrupting therapies, whereas other subclassifications reveal less malignant conditions that may not require as aggressive therapies. These discoveries have ushered in new perspectives into clinical care and research. To fully implement PM, considerable work is required to change how health information is recorded, collected, aggregated, and analyzed. Incorporating molecular data into the current diagnostic process and treatment algorithms has proved to be a challenging albeit solvable problem. Connecting data in a useable way across health systems or from sources that are not routinely integrated into clinical care (diet and activity) will be an important milestone toward delivering on PM.

Many contemporary clinical trials are designed to disrupt the molecular and genetic events that drive disease development. For the last few decades, clinical trials have used agents that target critical molecular pathways, but the investigators may not have had the data or computational power to prospectively stratify treatment groups based on a molecular feature or genetic biomarker. Examples of contemporary clinical trials that assign treatment cohorts based on shared biomarkers or key genetic variants as a key to trial design include basket and umbrella trials. Completed biomarker-driven clinical trials have shown feasibility and promise with this scientific approach.[39,40]

A developing treatment design referred to as N-of-1 trials asks clinical trial questions of efficacy; side effect profiles are at an individual level, using a person's own genetic and health data.[41] N-of-1 trials in PM oncology require considerable data resources and have many design concerns; however, the meta-analysis from individualized studies, if done in a controlled and reproducible manner, may reveal generalizable data and identify new disease or treatment subsets. Another nuanced trial design often referred to as "personalized medicine" is when an individual's genetic profile or other features are used to determine the optimal dose of a medication or predict an individual response to an intervention. Of note, there is ambiguity in the terms "precision" and "personalized" medicine in the medical community. Increasingly, health care is seeing the use of commercially provided screening panels as a navigational tool for participation in a clinical trial or as a deciding factor in assigning a specific therapy in a multi-arm trial. This is largely because such panels are common in clinical care and provide verified central testing sites and assays, which are important to maintain research quality. The molecular investigations of interest that define disease subgroups or treatment regimens are also evolving. Science is identifying ways that global changes to DNA, modification of tumor suppressor signals, cellular access to the genetic code, and other molecular events impact cancer and clinical outcomes in addition to the identified genetic

variants that are commonly investigated. Next-generation clinical trials and other means of using PM to deliver treatments and impact patient care will need to adapt and capitalize on evolving technology and scientific discovery.

Developing a high-quality integrated multivariate knowledge network was the foundation of the U.S. NRC's landmark 2011 publication that outlined a vision for PM.[42] Delivering on PM requires a large comprehensive knowledge network capable of fueling big data analysis with sufficient volume and quality to tease out molecular subgroups and associations with other health features. National, academic, and commercial PM efforts are underway, with nearly all participants utilizing a cross-sectional data repository connected to molecular and genetic testing. This knowledge network is anchored to the intrinsic biology of disease but must also continue to evolve and add new pertinent data sources that may shed light on modifiable factors in disease development.[43]

The success of PM will depend on the quality and volume of data that is aggregated in the knowledge network. Transitioning health data into a searchable structured format is a critical step that many health systems are finding difficult. To maximize adoption, PM platforms should be designed to augment existing healthcare operations and understanding of disease. PM can only change the healthcare landscape if it is adopted into clinical care and research. The transition to indexed healthcare data where clinical and other data sources are easily aggregated in a uniform and structured way may be the Achilles heel of implementing PM.

PM principles are already integrated into the clinical care of cancer patients. Many cancer types have established molecular subclassifications that are used to subtype a diagnosis or refine disease-specific treatment options. In some settings when a patient has failed standard therapies or if no standard therapy exists, a provider may pursue a molecularly targeted

PM approach. In this scenario, the patient's cancer specimen is investigated with a cancer genetic variant panel, or test of specific actionable variants, in hopes of identifying a growth-dependent tumor-driving mutation that can be targeted by an approved drug that is typically used in other conditions or cancer types. Ideally, this patient would qualify for, and have access to, a clinical trial that targets the pathway of interest. Unfortunately, in many cases, a clinical trial or standard option is not available. Outside of a clinical trial, a molecularly targeted approach is best facilitated through an MTB with multidisciplinary review by a dedicated team of experts, including oncologists, pharmacists, other specialized providers, geneticists, and drug procurement specialists.

For patients who fall outside of the structure of a clinical trial, a dedicated and systematic process should occur that emphasizes patient safety. The first step is to identify if the genetic variant of interest is a driver of the cancer type and not a passenger mutation. Hopefully, safety data exist for use with this agent in the organ system being treated and information is available as to whether or not the drug reaches the cancer site. Typically, this information would come from a previously completed early phase clinical trial, which in many instances may not have been performed with knowledge of whether patients harbored the mutation of interest. Once these requirements have been satisfied, then an effort can be made with the support of the MTB to procure the drug. Obtaining and paying for the drug is often met by resistance from insurance providers, as there is often not an approved indication to use this agent for the patient's disease. When a treatment plan is derived in this way, a rigorous standardized process emulating an early phase clinical trial is advised. Contemporary clinical trials, such as basket and umbrella trials, often include multiple treatment arms enrolling patients in parallel based on molecular targeting of

specific pathways identified in the tumor. Clinical trials for rare conditions, such as cancers that harbor rare genetic variants, are often delivered across many institutions to achieve recruitment goals needed to statistically power research questions and justify the resources needed to implement the trial. Clinical trials are the best method to deliver PM when safety, efficacy, and side effects of a treatment plan are not known. Medicine marches forward through clinical trials that validate new treatments and interventions in a rigorous and scientifically reproducible manner.

This chapter attempts to show how advances in the life sciences and informatics have ushered in PM and the molecular taxonomy of diseases and how this information is currently used in clinical care of patients with cancer. The next steps needed are: (a) to implement this change at a larger scale and (b) the creation of a robust knowledge network that has the potential to decode contributors to health and disease. It is my hope that large-scale, population-based genetic and environmental research efforts to catalog millions of people representative of the population at large will reveal modifiable risk factors and intricate associations that lead to disease development—so that we can change these factors and prevent illness. Imagine if you could identify when an individual's modifiable risk factors for a disease, such as smoking, diet, or toxin exposure, are approaching a critical threshold that escalates risk for genetic instability and a resultant cancer or disease. Technology exists that can edit the intrinsic biologic processes that occur during disease formation. It is only a matter of time before this technology is refined to the point that editing a biologic process in humans is a realistic opportunity. Herein lies the excitement behind CRISPR, an acronym that stands for Clustered Regulatory Interspersed Short Palindromic Repeats. CRISPR technology has the power to edit DNA in a precise manner.[44]

At the time of this publication, CRISPR is in its infancy, but the implications of this technology are tremendous as are the associated ethical concerns.[45]

▶ VI. Conclusion

The availability and routine application of vast new realms of health information has ushered in an era in health care referred to as PM. This paradigm shift has occurred due to advancements in molecular analysis using high-throughput sequencing, new ways of recording biologic and environmental data across populations, and large-scale data repositories of genetic and health data, coupled with advancement in informatics to support interdisciplinary health data aggregation and real-time analyses. Understanding disease at a genetic level has become the standard of care for many conditions and has changed how we view disease. Molecular profiling has provided insight into disease development and resulted in new treatment approaches that were previously limited in histology and symptom-based diagnosis. This molecular taxonomy of PM has revealed similarities across conditions previously thought unrelated and identified profound distinctions within conditions that share a histologic diagnosis. To deliver on PM, health care must utilize an interdisciplinary approach, develop systematic ways of recording information, and change current policy to support a new healthcare perspective. Moving forward with PM requires system-wide adjustments in how health data are recorded and delivered. The medical community is only beginning to embrace PM concepts and initiate the changes required to deliver PM, which has the capacity to dramatically improve health outcomes and prevent disease.

Notes

1. *Origo.* Retrieved from www.youtube.com/watch?v=qOhUz9FtdVE
2. *Case study: Developing a precision medicine platform solution for cancer patients at a World-Renowned Hospital.* Retrieved from http://genotechmatrix.com/wp-content/uploads/2017/05/Case-Study.pdf
3. *Origo: YouTube, ibid.*
4. *Toward precision medicine: Building a knowledge network for biomedical research and a new taxonomy of disease.* (2011). Washington, D.C.: National Academies Press. Retrieved from www.ucsf.edu/sites/default/files/legacy_files/documents/new-taxonomy.pdf
5. *Remarks by the President on Precision Medicine.* (2015, January 30). Retrieved from https://obamawhitehouse.archives.gov/the-press-office/2015/01/30/remarks-president-precision-medicine
6. G. H. (n.d.). *What is DNA?* Retrieved from https://ghr.nlm.nih.gov/primer/basics/dna
7. NCI Dictionary of Cancer Terms. (n.d.) [nciAppModulePage]. Retrieved from www.cancer.gov/publications/dictionaries/genetics-dictionary
8. *The genetics and genomics of cancer | Nature Genetics* (n.d.). Retrieved from www.nature.com/articles/ng1107
9. Flores, M., Glusman, G., Brogaard, K., Price, N. D., & Hood, L. (2013). P4 medicine: How systems medicine will transform the healthcare sector and society. *Personalized Medicine, 10*(6), 565–576. doi:10.2217/PME.13.57
10. *Network of networks.* Retrieved from http://future.psjhealth.org/scientific-wellness/about-the-institute-for-systems-biology?utm_source=TWITTER&utm_medium=social_organic&utm_term=--&utm_content=psjh-1773051757-&utm_campaign=evergreenContent+Type+%28Secondary%29
11. Yadav, S. P. (2007). The wholeness in Suffix -omics, -omes, and the Word Om. *Journal of Biomolecular Techniques: JBT, 18*(5), 277.
12. Heather, J. M., & Chain, B. (2016). The sequence of sequencers: The history of sequencing DNA. *Genomics, 107*(1), 1–8. doi:10.1016/j.ygeno.2015.11.003
13. Quoted from https://www.genome.gov/12011238/an-overview-of-the-human-genome-project/
14. Wheeler, D. A., Srinivasan, M., Egholm, M., Shen, Y., Chen, L., McGuire, A., ... Rothberg, J. M. (2008). The complete genome of an individual by massively parallel DNA sequencing. *Nature, 452*(7189), 872–876. doi:10.1038/nature06884
15. Toward Precision Medicine, *ibid.*
16. *DNA Sequencing Costs: Data.* (n.d.). Retrieved from www.genome.gov/27541954/dna-sequencing-costs-data/
17. Toward Precision Medicine, *ibid.*

18. *Epigenomics Fact Sheet.* (n.d.). Retrieved from www
.genome.gov/27532724/epigenomics-fact-sheet/

19. Definition of phenotype—NCI Dictionary of Cancer
Terms. (n.d.), *ibid.*

20. National Institutes of Health (NIH)—*All of Us.* (n.d.).
Retrieved from https://allofus-nih-gov.sladenlibrary
.hfhs.org/

21. Gao, J., Aksoy, B. A., Dogrusoz, U., Dresdner,
G., Gross, B., Sumer, S. O., ... Schultz, N. (2013).
Integrative analysis of complex cancer genomics
and clinical profiles using the cBioPortal. *Science
Signaling*, 6(269), pl1. doi:10.1126/scisignal.2004088

22. Griffith, M., Spies, N. C., Krysiak, K., McMichael, J.
F., Coffman, A. C., Danos, A. M., ... Griffith, O. L.
(2017). *CIViC* is a community knowledgebase for
expert crowdsourcing the clinical interpretation of
variants in cancer. *Nature Genetics*, 49(2), 170–174.
doi:10.1038/ng.3774

23. Grossman, R. L., Heath, A. P., Ferretti, V., Varmus,
H. E., Lowy, D. R., Kibbe, W. A., & Staudt, L. M.
(2016). Toward a shared vision for cancer genomic
data. *The New England Journal of Medicine*, 375(12),
1109–1112. doi:10.1056/NEJMp1607591

24. Snyder, J., Schultz, L., & Walbert, T. (2017).
The role of tumor board conferences in neuro-
oncology: A nationwide provider survey. *Journal of
Neuro-Oncology*, 133(1), 1–7. doi:10.1007/s11060
-017-2416-x

25. Redig, A. J., & Jänne, P. A. (2015). Basket trials and the
evolution of clinical trial design in an era of genomic
medicine. *Journal of Clinical Oncology*, 33(9), 975–
977. doi:10.1200/JCO.2014.59.8433.

26. *NCI Dictionary of Cancer Terms.* (n.d.).
[nciAppModulePage]. Retrieved from www.cancer
.gov/publications/dictionaries/cancer-terms

27. Redig & Jänne, (2015) *ibid.*

28. Frampton, G. M., Fichtenholtz, A., Otto, G. A., Wang,
K., Downing, S. R., He, J., ... Yelensky, R. (2013).
Development and validation of a clinical cancer
genomic profiling test based on massively parallel
DNA sequencing. *Nature Biotechnology*, 31(11),
1023–1031. doi:10.1038/nbt.2696.

29. Louis, D. N., Perry, A., Reifenberger, G., von Deimling,
A., Figarella-Branger, D., Cavenee, W. K., ... Ellison,
D. W. (2016). The 2016 World Health Organization
classification of tumors of the central nervous system:
A summary. *Acta Neuropathologica*, 131(6), 803–820.
doi:10.1007/s00401-016-1545-1.

30. Louis et al., (2016) *ibid.*

31. Toward Precision Medicine, *ibid.*

32. Torous, J., Kiang, M. V., Lorme, J., & Onnela, J.-P.
(2016). New tools for new research in psychiatry: A
scalable and customizable platform to empower data
driven smartphone research. *JMIR Mental Health*,
3(2). doi:10.2196/mental.5165

33. Groft, S. C., & Rubinstein, Y. R. (2013). New and
evolving rare diseases research programs at the
National Institutes of Health. *Public Health Genomics*,
16(6), 259–267. doi:10.1159/000355929

34. Gill, J., Obley, A. J., & Prasad, V. (2018). Direct-to-
consumer genetic testing: The implications of the
US FDA's first marketing authorization for BRCA
mutation testing. *JAMA*, 319(23), 2377–2378.
doi:10.1001/jama.2018.5330

35. My Family Health Portrait. (n.d.). Retrieved from
https://familyhistory.hhs.gov/FHH/html/index.html

36. Gallin, E. K., Bond, E., Califf, R. M., Crowley, W. F.
J., Davis, P., Galbraith, R., & Reece, E. A. (2013).
Forging stronger partnerships between academic
health centers and patient-driven organizations.
Academic Medicine, 88(9), 1220. doi:10.1097/ACM
.0b013e31829ed2a7

37. Frank, L., Basch, E., & Selby, J. V. (2014). The
PCORI perspective on patient-centered outcomes
research. *JAMA*, 312(15), 1513–1514. doi:10.1001
/jama.2014.11100

38. Gallin, et al., (2013) *ibid.*

39. McNeil, C. (2015). NCI-MATCH launch highlights
new trial design in precision-medicine era. *JNCI:
Journal of the National Cancer Institute*, 107(7).
doi:10.1093/jnci/djv193

40. Redig & Jänne, (2015) *ibid.*

41. Lillie, E. O., Patay, B., Diamant, J., Issell, B., Topol,
E. J., & Schork, N. J. (2011). The n-of-1 clinical trial:
The ultimate strategy for individualizing medicine?
Personalized Medicine, 8(2), 161–173. doi:10.2217
/pme.11.7

42. Toward Precision Medicine, *ibid.*

43. Toward Precision Medicine, *ibid.*

44. Cyranoski, D. (2016). CRISPR gene-editing tested in a
person for the first time. *Nature News*, 539(7630), 479.
doi:10.1038/nature.2016.20988

45. Luscombe, N. M., Greenbaum, D., & Gerstein, M.
(2001). What is bioinformatics? A proposed definition
and overview of the field. *Methods of Information in
Medicine*, 40(4), 346–358.

Chapter Questions

2-1 What key events trigger PM?

2-2 What are the underlying principles of PM? Discuss the appeal and challenges of adopting PM principles for patients as well as care providers.

2-3 What drives PM's success or failure? How is PM changing the practice of traditional medicine?

2-4 What significance does PM have on personalizing cancer treatments for cancer patients?

Biography

Dr. Snyder is a board-certified Neurologist and fellowship-trained Neuro-oncologist. His practice is focused on neuro-oncologic conditions, including primary brain tumors and cancer involving the nervous system, with an emphasis on clinical trials and translational research. He received his medical degree from Michigan State University College of Osteopathic Medicine and completed post graduate education at Huron Valley-Sinai Hospital, St. John Providence Health System, and Henry Ford Hospital.

TECHNOLOGY REVIEW I

Review on Big Data Analytics in Health Care

Abir Belaala, Labib Sadek Terrissa, Noureddine Zerhouni, Christine Devalland, and Joshia Tan

Abstract

Owing to the recent digitization of medical services with tools, such as electronic health records, mobile health apps, wearable sensors, and smart fitness devices, huge amounts of medical and healthcare data have been generated and collected at an unprecedented volume, velocity, and variety. Traditional limits in handling these massive and heterogeneous datasets create the need for insights into the latest research on Big Data and Big Data techniques in health care. This review surveys the basic concepts, sources, and types of Big Data applications; the most popular analytical techniques; and tools used in the medical-Big Data field appearing in the extant literature between 2015 and 2018.

CHAPTER OUTLINE

▶ Introduction

With massive amounts of heterogeneous data emerging from various sources,[1] such as patient information, biomarkers (e.g., genomic, proteomic, metabolomic), and diagnosis results (radiology, blood test, etc.), as well as pharmacy (e.g., prescriptions, medications), administrative (e.g., cost and claims data, population, and public health data) and behavior data (e.g., those from mobile apps, social media, sensors, wearable devices, and fitness monitors), the shift from paper-based patient records to electronic health records (EHR) represents a necessary digitalization in today's healthcare systems. With fast growth, increased complexity, heterogeneity, and size of these accumulated data, the big challenge now is how to collect, store, analyze, and manage these Big Data in healthcare systems to improve the quality of care delivery, including the move toward personalized medicine, the sharing of real-time decisions in diagnosis and treatments, and the prediction of treatment outcomes at earlier stages, as well as the understanding of new diseases and therapies.

Traditional data analysis cannot adequately handle Big Data processing. New approaches that can analyze a wide variety of complex data and generate valuable insights are needed.[2] When applied to healthcare Big Data, these tools will have the potential to identify patterns, improve care quality, reduce costs, and enhance real-time decision-making. Big Data analytics integrate machine learning and statistical analysis. They include a set of tools and techniques, such as classification, clustering, regression, and association,[3] each serving a distinct purpose depending on the modeling objective. Often, the choice of the right technique depends on the problem at hand and how the data are represented and stored.

This review encompasses Big Data in health care. It explains the processing of Big Data in health care from collection to decision-making, citing and classifying the sources of Big Data, and illustrating the tools and technologies used to handle Big Data, for example, the *Hadoop* ecosystem. Additionally, the review covers the applied analytical techniques, such as machine learning algorithms, and sheds light on the potential benefits of Big Data to health care. Finally, it highlights some challenges of Big Data analytics and discusses potential future developments in the related areas.

▶ Background

The review process starts with searching information databases, such as *ScienceDirect*, *PubMed*, *IEEE Xplore*, and other electronic databases, with keywords, such as "Big Data" OR "Big Data analytics" AND "Healthcare" OR "Medicine" OR "Biomedicine" OR "Medical" OR "Bioinformatics". As **FIGURE TR1-1** noted, the review covers 76 identified articles that deal with Big Data in health care published between 2015 and 2018. Six main categories emerged from an analysis of these selected

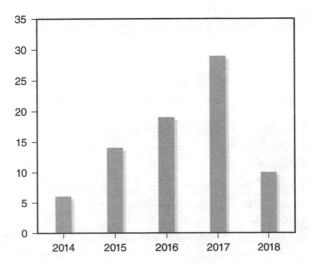

FIGURE TR1-1 Distribution of identified articles by year (76 articles).

papers: (a) Big Data definition and basic concepts; (b) Big Data sources; (c) Big Data tools and technologies; (d) Big Data analytical techniques; and, finally, (e) Big Data challenges and opportunities. These various subtopics are elaborated next.

Definition and Basic Concepts

Big Data have been defined variously in the literature. Bellazzi, et al.[4] cited Haper[5] as viewing Big Data to have "scale, diversity, and complexity," requiring "new architecture, techniques, algorithms, and analytics to manage it and extract value and hidden knowledge from it." Hemingway, et al.[6] alluded to Big Data as high volume, velocity, and variety information assets demanding new forms of processing to drive enhanced decision-making, insight discovery, and process optimization. More simply, Big Data are very large datasets, structured or unstructured, static or dynamic, simple or complex, that may be gathered, stored, processed, and analyzed using different advanced techniques. **FIGURE TR1-2** contrasts between traditional versus Big Data according to *4Vs*: *Volume, Variety, Velocity,* and *Value*.

In biomedical informatics, Luo, et al.[7] and Mathew, et al.[8] define Big Data in health

care according to its *Vs*: first is the exponential growth in the *Volume* of data in biomedical informatics from real-time health monitoring systems, EHRs, electronic patient records (EPRs), labs, sensor devices, and more. In fact, the U.S. healthcare system alone already reached 150 exabytes (10^{18}) of data 5 years ago.[9] Second is *Variety* of data types and structures, that is, the ecosystem of biomedical data can be structured, semi-structured, or unstructured, collected from different sources, such as wearable sensors, health community blogs, social media, and more (often in numerous formats, such as relational tables, flat files, and comma separated values or comma-separated values [CSV] files). Third is *Velocity*, which is the need to process the data in real-time, whether it is coming from streaming data, such as remote patient monitoring, from sensor devices or telemedicine servicing (e.g., the new generation of sequencing technologies that enables the production of billions of DNA sequence data each day at a relatively low cost). Fourth is *Veracity,* which deals with the quality of data being captured. Here, the truthfulness of data, or how certain we are about these data, matters. The last, and most important, *V* is *Value*. Unlike other *Vs*, this *V* is the desired outcome of processing Big Data in health care as we are

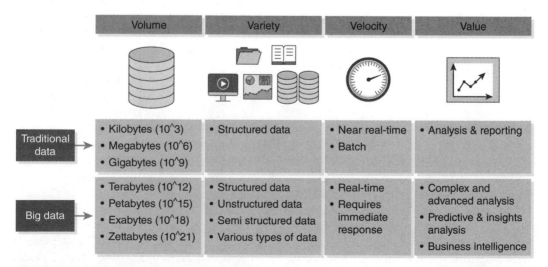

	Volume	Variety	Velocity	Value
Traditional data	• Kilobytes (10^3) • Megabytes (10^6) • Gigabytes (10^9)	• Structured data	• Near real-time • Batch	• Analysis & reporting
Big data	• Terabytes (10^12) • Petabytes (10^15) • Exabytes (10^18) • Zettabytes (10^21)	• Structured data • Unstructured data • Semi structured data • Various types of data	• Real-time • Requires immediate response	• Complex and advanced analysis • Predictive & insights analysis • Business intelligence

FIGURE TR1-2 Traditional Data vs. Big Data.

primarily interested in extracting maximum value and generating insights from Big Data so as to improve the quality of health care.

Sources

In health care, data heterogeneity and the variety of structured, semi-structured, and unstructured data are derived from diverse biomedical data sources. These include physiological, behavioral, molecular, clinical, environmental exposure, medical imaging, disease management, medication prescription history, nutrition, exercise parameters, and more.[10]

Big Data sources have been classified in various ways in the literature. Stokes, et al.[11] divide data sources into two general classes: Administrative (Government [CMS], National surveys [Medical Expenditure Panel Survey], commercial vendors [health plans, PBMs]) versus Clinical (Hospital EMR, Physician EMR, Integrated delivery network EMR, Clinical database). Hemingway, et al.[12] simply suggest a classification using structured versus unstructured data in clinical care: *Structured EHR* data are recorded using controlled clinical terminologies, such as Systematized Nomenclature of Medicine Clinical terms (SMOMED-CT) or statistical classification systems, such as ICD-9, ICD-9-CM, or ICD-10, while *unstructured clinical data* can be patient medical histories, discharge summaries, handover notes, and imaging reports. These data are often captured and recorded in patient's health records as raw unformatted text.

In Mathew & Pillai,[13] Big Data sources may come from: (a) Providers: medical data (EHRs, EPRs); (b) Payers: claims and cost data; (c) Researchers: academic or independent; (d) Consumers and Marketers: patient behavior and sentiment data; (e) Government: population and public health data; and/or (f) Developers: pharmacy and medical device research and development (R&D). Briefly, two underlying types of sources emerged here: internal sources, such as EMRs, computerized provider orders entry (CPOE), imaging data, and others versus

external data sources, such as government, insurance (e.g., claims, billing), and social media. Andreu-Perez, et al.[14] also focused on two clusters: quantitative (e.g., sensor data, images, gene arrays, laboratory tests) versus qualitative (e.g., free text, demographics). However, Ma, et al.[15] identified four major sources of pharmacy Big Data: (a) Pharmaceutical research and development from pharmaceutical companies and academia, clinical trials, and high-throughput screening libraries; (b) Claims and cost data from payers and providers that contain utilization of care and cost estimates; (c) Clinical data provided by the EMR that contain patient-specific data on treatment outcomes; and (d) Patient behavior and sentiment data that come from consumers and stakeholders outside of health care (for instance, from retail exercise apparel and exercise monitoring equipment). Finally, Fang, et al.[16] classify healthcare Big Data differently with categories ranging from: (a) Human-generated data: physicians' notes, email, and paper documents; (b) Machine-generated data: readings from diverse health monitoring devices; (c) Transaction data: billing records and healthcare claims; (d) Biometric data: genomics, genetics, heart rate, blood pressure, X-ray, fingerprints; (e) Social media data: interaction data from social websites; to (f) Publications: clinical research and medical reference material.

The large variety of Big Data in health care sources and their corresponding classifications inspired from aforementioned authors are summarized in **FIGURE TR1-3**, showcasing prominent taxonomies of Big Data sources in health care.

FIGURE TR1-4 offers another proposed classification which adds more details about data types including their format (text or ASCII, image, and video) and sources (internal, external). This domain-based classification is constructed according to three specialized areas in health care: cardiology, diabetes, and oncology. **TABLE TR1-1** presents various data types used in the selected papers being reviewed.

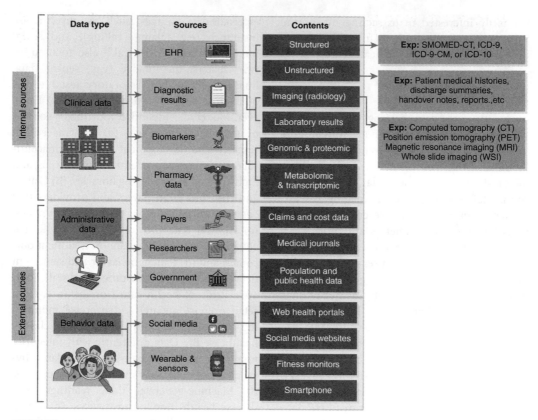

FIGURE TR1-3 Main sources of Big Data in health care.

Tools

Big Data in health care, which are difficult to store and process via traditional methods, require the use of new technological tools for their capture from different sources and systems, their transformation, storage, analysis, and visualization. Mathew & Pillai[17] classify tools of Big Data into two options: open source versus available commercial solutions. Here, some key products include Hadoop-based analytics, data warehouse for operational insights, stream computing software for real time analysis of streaming data, and NoSQL databases such as Cassandra, MongoDB, and DynamoDB.

We start with Apache Hadoop open source platform as it is among the earliest tool successfully applied in different Big Data specialized software projects. Hadoop supports the processing and storage of extremely large

datasets in a distributed computing environment. Data in a Hadoop cluster is divided into small pieces and stored throughout a computer cluster with thousands of nodes. Hadoop uses two main components, MapReduce and Hadoop Distributed File System (HDFS). Closely related software tools include NoSQL databases such as MongoDB, Cassandra, and HBase, which are basically an open source version of BigTable.[18]

Vijayarani & Sharmila[19] classify Big Data tools vis-à-vis Big Data phases:

- In Big Data storage, three types of storage (in memory, in the cloud, and hard disk storage) are noted;
- In Big Data processing, we have real-time processing using Storm, Spark, S4, and more versus batch processing (Hadoop); and

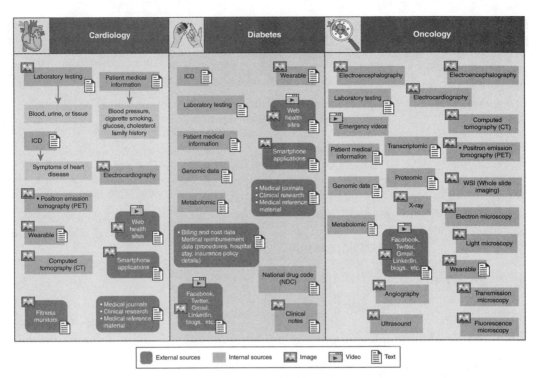

FIGURE TR1-4 Domain-based classification of Big Data in health care.

- In Big Data technologies, we have many successful applications in biomedicine,[20] including four types of tools used in bioinformatics, clinical informatics, and imaging informatics:
  - Tools used in data storage and retrieval;
  - Error identification;
  - Data analysis; and
  - Platform integration deployment.

Bellazzi, et al.[21] highlighted the main types of Big-Data tools oriented solutions in health care as comprising of: cloud computing, parallel programming, and NoSQL databases.

TABLE TR1-2 (adapted from Lourenço, et al.[22]) shows the existing Big Data platforms and tools for storing Big Data, with the advantages and disadvantages of each technique. NoSQL databases (i.e., nontraditional relational databases) are becoming the core technology for Big Data. Here, we examine the following three main NoSQL databases:

key-value databases, column-oriented databases, and document-oriented databases, each based on certain data models.

Sharing and storing data over the cloud plays a key role in providing flexible, reliable, and cost-effective solutions to users.[23–25] Despite advantages of a cloud-based healthcare system, privacy of data is a major problem.[26] **TABLE TR1-3** highlights the existing Big Data platforms and tools for batch and real-time processing. As shown, there are three main types of Big data processing tools: (i) batch-only tools, (ii) stream-only tools, and (iii) hybrid tools (see also **FIGURE TR1-5**).

▶ Analytical Techniques

The literature on Big Data techniques in health care is broad. Alonso, et al.[27] highlighted the most popular techniques of machine learning and Big Data classification (decision tree, Naïve Bayes, Artificial Neural Network

TABLE TR1-1   Types of Data Used in Literature

Data Type	Reviewed Papers
Genomic data	Turgut, et al.[89]; Xiao, et al.[96]; Su, et al.[84]; Hinkson, et al.[24]; Maia, et al.[62]; Morovvat, et al.[67]; Shah, et al.[78]; Ding, et al.[46]; Zheng & Zhang[97]
Imaging	Volynskaya, al.[92]; Nawaz, et al.[68]; Kurc, et al.[60]; Shah, et al.[78]; Margolies, et al.[65]; Albarqouni, et al.[37]; Wang, et al.[2]; Silva, et al.[81]; Panayides, et al.[69]; Kovalev, et al.[59]; Alickovic & Subasi[38]; Ivanova[56]; Hinkson, et al.[24]
Biomedical data	Asri, et al.[41]; Shen, et al.[79]
Behavior data	Asri, et al.[41]; Shen, et al.[79]
Pharmaceutical data	Choi, et al.[43]; Ma, et al.[15]; Walczak & Okuboyejo[93]
Billing data	Erekson & Iglesia[49]
Clinical notes	Forsyth, et al.[50]
Lab tests	Miranda, et al.[66]
CDI_9	Choi, et al.[43]; Forsyth, et al.[50]

[ANN]) to bundle the objects or data into groups. Clustering and search optimization are also applied as data mining strategies, such as self-organization map; vector quantization; and genetic algorithm, regression, association, and prediction. Bachiller, et al.[28] showed the various computational methods applied in health care and classified them into two clusters: machine learning (Support Vector Machines or SVM, Naïve Bayes, ANN, Auto-encoders); and deep learning (Convolutional Neural Networks, Recurrent Neural Network, Restricted Boltzmann Method). Mathew & Pillai[29] showed that analytics can be classified into three major types: predictive, descriptive, and prescriptive analytics. Mehta & Pandit[30] reviewed some of the Big Data analytical techniques across various healthcare applications including cluster analysis, data mining, graph analytics, machine learning,

natural language processing (NLP), neural networks (NNs), pattern recognition, spatial analysis, and more to argue that the choice among techniques really depends on the problem at hand and the nature of the stored datasets.

As shown in Table TR1-3, there is a large variety of techniques for Big Data in health analytics. Each technique serves a different purpose depending on the modeling objective, with some techniques applicable to more than one modeling objectives (e.g., classification, regression, clustering, and more). **FIGURE TR1-6** maps out the existing analytical techniques vis-à-vis their utilizations whereas **TABLE TR1-4** defines existing computational algorithms popularly used in the medical field.

As noted previously, there are three main types of analysis: (a) Diagnostic analytics are used to answer what happened and why it happened; (b) Predictive analytics cater to

TABLE TR1-2 NoSQL Databases Comparison

Big Data Storage Platforms	Store Type	Cons	Pros
Cassandra	Column oriented data stores	Recovery Time Read Performance	Write-Performance Multi data center replication High scalability Supports rich data structure and Powerful query language (CQL). Availability Consistency
HBase		Availability Read Performance Robustness	Consistency Partition tolerance Scalability
BigTable		Availability Read Performance	Consistency Partition tolerance
MongoDB	Document data stores	Availability Scalability Write-Performance Stabilization Time	Support complex data types Consistency Partition tolerance Powerful query language High-speed access Reliability
CouchDB		Consistency Write-Performance Scalability	Flexible Availability Partition tolerance (AP)
DynamoDB	Key-value stores	Unable to do complex queries Latency in read/write	High expandability and smaller query response time Consistency Automatic data replication
Voldemort		Consistency	Availability Partition tolerance Write-Performance
Redis		Availability	Consistency Partition tolerance
OrientDB	Graph oriented data stores	Requires more schema design up front	Useful in dealing with data where relationships play an important role Easy to query Robust
Neo4j			

Data from Lourenço, J. R., Cabral, B., Carreiro, P., Vieira, M., & Bernardino, J. (2015). Choosing the right NoSQL database for the job: a quality attribute evaluation. *Journal of Big Data, 2*(1), 18.[22]

TABLE TR1-3   Big Data Processing Tools

Processing Type	Big Data Platform	Definition
Batch processing	Hadoop MapReduce	The MapReduce is a parallel programming model that enables many of the most common calculations on large scale data to be performed on computing clusters containing a large number of computing nodes efficiently using two functions: Map and Reduce (Rahim, et al.[74]).
	Oozie	Oozie is a workflow processing method that allows users to define a series of jobs written in different languages (e.g., Pig, Hive, and MapReduce) and then logically links them with each another (Raghupathi & Raghupathi[73]).
	Mahout	Mahout is another Apache project; it enables the generation of free applications of distributed and scalable machine learning algorithms that support big data analytics on the Hadoop platform (Landset, et al.[61]).
	Hive	Hive is a runtime Hadoop support architecture that supports Structure Query Language (SQL) with the Hadoop platform. It permits SQL programmers to develop Hive Query Language (HQL) statements similar to SQL statements (Raghupathi & Raghupathi[73]).
Batch processing	Pig	Apache Pig is a high-level platform for creating programs that run on Apache Hadoop. The language for this platform is called Pig Latin. Pig programming language is configured to assimilate all types of data (structured/unstructured, etc.) (Singh & Reddy[82]).
Stream processing	Spark	Apache Spark is a next generation batch processing framework with stream processing capabilities. On the speed side, Spark extends the popular MapReduce model to efficiently support more types of computations, including interactive queries and stream processing (Singh & Reddy[82]).
	Storm	Apache Storm is an open-source Apache tool; its scalable and fast distributed framework has a special focus on stream processing. Storm provides a topology to control data transfers, which is a critical part of routing data where it needs to go for analytics and other operations (Fang, et al.[16]).
	Flink	Apache Flink is a tool for supporting Hadoop project structures and processing real-time data. Its stream processing framework can also handle batch tasks. As a type of batch processor, Flink contends with the traditional MapReduce and new Spark options (Gurusamy, et al.[53]).

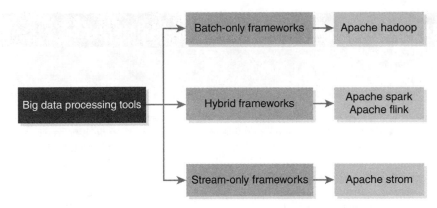

FIGURE TR1-5 Types of Big Data processing tools.

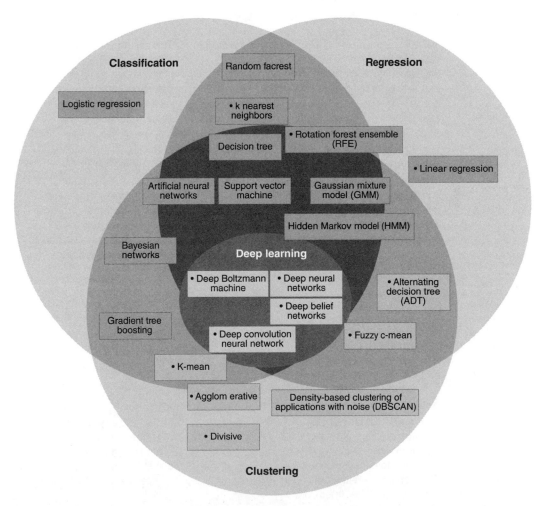

FIGURE TR1-6 Mapping out the classification of existing analytical techniques.

TABLE TR1-4 Analytical Techniques and Their Application in Health Care

Technique	Definition	Application Area	Description
Decision Tree (DT)	DT is a most popular and powerful classification technique. It classifies instances by sorting them in a tree, where each internal node denotes a test on an attribute, each branch represents an outcome of the test, and each leaf node holds a class label. (Sivakami & Saraswathi[83]).	Oncology	This publication presents a decision tree based data mining technique for early detection of breast cancer. This is helpful because early detection of breast cancer makes it far easier to cure (Sumbaly, et al.[85]).
Naïve Bayes	Naïve Bayes are probabilistic classifiers based on applying Bayes theorem with strong independence hypothesis between the features (Prerana, et al.[71]).	Cardiology	This paper proposes a mining model using a naïve Bayes classifier that could detect cardiovascular disease and identify its risk level for adults (Miranda, et al.[66]).
Logistic regression	Logistic regression is a statistic model where the log-odds of the probability of an event are a linear combination of independent or predictor variables (Alickovic & Subasi[38]).	Oncology	This work aims to predict grad 2 acute radiation-induced dermatitis after hybrid intensity modulation radiotherapy for breast cancer using a logistic regression normal tissue complication probability model (Sung, et al.[87]).
Artificial Neural Network (ANN)	ANNs are a family of computational models based on biological neural networks, which are used to estimate complex relationships between inputs and outputs (Wu, et al.[95]).	Cardiology	They use decision support systems based on artificial neural networks to predict heart failure risks (Samuel, et al.[75]).
Support Vector Machines (SVM)	SVM is an example of supervised learning. Known labels help indicate whether the system is performing the right way or not. This information points to a desired response, either validating the accuracy of the system, or to help the system learn to act correctly (Sivakami & Saraswathi[83]).	Diabetes	The paper explores the hybrid of SVM and a system of ANN as the finest binary classification system for calculating the diabetic nature of people in comparison to SVM (Aliwadi, et al.[39]).

Random forest	Random forest is one type of ensemble learning algorithm that constructs multiple trees at training time. This algorithm overlaps the over fitting problem of decision trees by averaging multiple deep decision trees (Fang, et al.[16]).	Genomics	Identify variables correlated with a diagnosis of diabetic peripheral neuropathy (DPN) using random forest modeling applied to EHR (DuBrava, et al.[47]).
Hierarchical clustering	In data mining and statistics, hierarchical clustering (also called hierarchical cluster analysis or HCA) is a method of cluster analysis which seeks to build a hierarchy of clusters (Ding, et al.[46]).	Genomics	This work aims, to find differentially expressed genes rather than directly de-noise the single cell data. They present a method to remove technical noise. These cells use these genes to cluster by hierarchical clustering (Ding, et al.[46]).
K-means	K-means is a known partitioning clustering algorithm. It partitions objects into k clusters, computes centroids (mean points) of the clusters, and assigns every object to the cluster that has the nearest mean in an Expectation-Maximization fashion (Fang, et al.[16]).	Cardiology	In this work they use medical terms, such as age, weight, gender, blood pressure, and cholesterol rate, for prediction. To perform grouping of various attributes, it uses a k-means algorithm and for predicting it uses the Back propagation technique in neural networks (Malav, et al.[63]).
Hidden Markov Model (HMM)	HMM is a statistical model representing probability distribution over the sequences of observations. This model uses a Markov chain to model signals in order to calculate the occurrence probability of states (Fang, et al.[16]).	Oncology	They use a Bayesian HMM with Gaussian Mixture (GM) clustering approach to model the DNA copy number change across the genome for cancer diagnosis (Manogaran, et al.[64]).
Gaussian Mixture Model (GMM)	GMM is a statistical model widely used as a classifier in pattern recognition tasks. It consists of a number of Gaussian distributions in the linear way (Fang, et al.[16]).	Oncology	This paper proposes a framework using voice pathology assessment as a case study. The machine learning algorithms in the form of a support vector machine, an extreme learning machine, and a GMM are used as the classifier (Hossain & Muhammad[55]).

(continues)

TABLE TR1-4 Analytical Techniques and Their Application in Health Care *(continued)*			
Deep learning	The success of deep learning for big data is the use of a large number of hidden neurons and parameters such as deep neural networks, deep convolution neural network, and deep belief networks (Remadna, et al.[98]).	Oncology (Breast cancer)	This paper presents results of the use of the deep learning approach and Convolutional Neural Networks (CNN) for the problem of breast cancer diagnosis (Kovalev, et al.[59]).

knowing what will happen; and (c) Prescriptive analytics are used to find the best course of actions by providing decision support for specific scenarios or situations. **TABLES TR1-5A** and **5B** classify papers in the extant literature according to the type of analysis and summarize which machine learning techniques have been used.

By combining big data and machine learning, the knowledge and information hidden in Big Data can be uncovered to improve the quality of healthcare delivery. As shown in **FIGURE TR1-7**, key benefits are allowing diseases to be detected at earlier stages; making the right treatment decisions at the right time; identifying new diseases, new therapies, and new approaches for health care; and reducing costs.

Figure TR1-7 concludes by showing the high complexity of the big health data processing steps, which transforms the raw big health data into valuable insights. This is due to the difficulty faced in each step, with the large variety of data types and a range of competing choices in selecting the best tools and techniques to store and analyze these datasets. **TABLE TR1-6** shows the distribution of identified papers in this review (76 articles) according to the application domains.

Big Data Challenges

Despite the large potential benefits of exploring big data uses in health care, challenges and problems remain to be resolved if outcomes are to be improved. Hemingway, et al.[31] highlighted several formidable challenges: data quality; knowing what data exist; the legal–ethical dimension for their use; data sharing; building and maintaining public trust; developing standards for defining disease; developing tools for scalable, replicable science; and equipping the clinical and scientific work force with new interdisciplinary skills. Other challenges identified by Mathew & Pillai[32] include the lack of standards for representing and sharing of healthcare data, the complication in integrating heterogeneous data sources, the need for skilled resources, attention to privacy, security and infrastructure issues, the need for quality control of the acquired and input data, the demand on real-time processing, and the interpretation of the analytical results.

More challenges are identified by Cyganek, et al.[33] These include the understanding of doctors' notes (unstructured text analysis); the handling of huge volumes of medical images that are part of the EHR, which increase storage requirements; and the need to backtrack the effect of medical decisions. In pharmacy, Ma, et al.[34] noted several challenges for big data: (a) a storage challenge on the size scale of petabytes, for secure data transmission and continued development of tools to analyze the data; (b) a variety challenge and the issue of data integrity and validity; (c) a patient confidentiality challenge where Big data also raises issues regarding how to keep the information safe; and (d) a physician prescribing patterns challenge; here, the issue at hand is whether detailed information about prescriptions written by doctors (with the doctor identified) can be bought and sold.

TABLE TR1-5A The Utilization of Machine Learning Technique by Type of Analysis

	K-means	SVM	DT	ANN	CNN	RF1	RF2	LR	NB	RVM	MLP	KNN	GBM	Ada Boost	Others
Chen, et al.[25]		✓	✓	✓	✓										
Zheng & Zhang[97]						✓		✓						✓	
Sundara-sekar[86]		✓	✓									✓			
Ivanova[56], Miranda, et al.[66]									✓		✓				
Alickovic & Subasi[38]		✓	✓				✓	✓	✓						
Asri, et al.[41]		✓	✓						✓			✓			
Wang, et al.[2]		✓													✓
Shen, et al.[79]					✓										
Albarqouni, et al.[37]					✓										
Silva, et al.[81]	✓	✓	✓	✓	✓	✓	✓		✓						
Turgut, et al.[89]											✓	✓	✓	✓	
Forsyth, et al.[50]										✓					✓
Gambhir, et al.[51]			✓	✓											

TABLE TR1-5B Prognostic

	K-means	SVM	DT	ANN	CNN	RF1	RF2	LR	NB	RVM	MLP	KNN	GBM	Ada Boost	Others
Kalyankar, et al.[57], Prasad, et al.[70], Brims, et al.[42], Shah, et al.[78]															
Kourou, et al.[58]		✓	✓	✓					✓						
Sivakami & Saraswathi[83]		✓	✓												
Nawaz, et al.[68], Hernandez, et al.[54], Amirian, et al.[40], Choi, et al.[43]															✓
Asri, et al.[41]		✓	✓						✓			✓			
Morovvat, et al.[67]		✓	✓						✓						
Xiao, et al.[96]		✓	✓			✓						✓			
Forsyth, et al.[50]															✓
Walczak & Okuboyejo[93]				✓											
Priyanga, et al.[72]		✓		✓								✓			

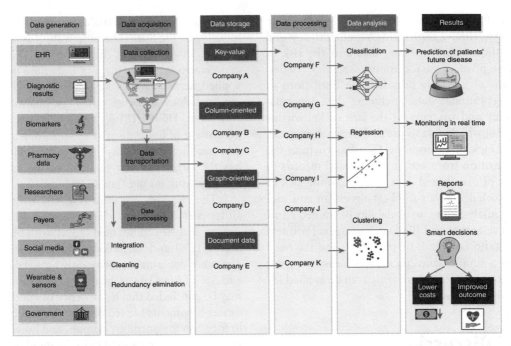

FIGURE TR1-7 Big Health Data Process.

TABLE TR1-6 Distribution of Selected Papers by Application Domains

Big Health Data Application Areas	Reviewed Papers
Ophthalmology	Clark, et al.[44]
Alzheimer	Geerts, et al.[52]; Varatharajan, et al.[90]; Aramendi, et al.[36]
Oncology	Turgut, et al.[89]; Xiao, et al.[96]; Forsyth, et al.[50]; Albarqouni, et al.[37]; Asri, et al.[41]; Margolies, et al.[65]; Shah, et al.[78]; Kurc, et al.[60]; Nawaz, et al.[68]; Brims, et al.[42]; Thiebaut, et al.[23]; Su, et al.[84]; Hinkson, et al.[24]; Ivanova[56]; Alickovic & Subasi[38]; Maia, et al.[62]; Kovalev, et al.[59]; Taglang & Jackson[88]; Wang, et al.[2]; Silva, et al.[81]; Volynskaya, et al.[92]
Pharmacy	Hernandez & Zhang[54]; Ma, et al.[15]; Geerts, et al.[52]; Taglang & Jackson[88]
Diabetes	Prasad, et al.[70]; Kalyankar, et al.[57]; Bellazzi, et al.[4]; Zheng & Zhang[97]; Chen, et al.[25]; Miranda, et al.[66]; Eljil,et al.[48]; Saravana, et al.[76]; Aliwadi, et al.[39]
Cardiology	Miranda, et al.[66]; Hemingway, et al.[6]; Choi, et al.[43]; Priyanga & Naveen[72]
Personalized medicine	Daniel, et al.[45]; Viceconti, et al.[91]

Finally, Mehta & Pandit[35] argued that major challenges include patient privacy and confidentiality; missing data and the risk of false-positive associations; security issues, such as Big Data breaches; the limitations of observational data, including data inconsistency and inaccuracy; the lack of knowledge about which data to use and for what purpose; the lack of appropriate IT infrastructure; the transition from use of paper-based records to use of distributed data processing; the lack of knowledge about the best algorithm and tool for analysis; the unavailability of trained clinical scientists and Big Data managers for interpretation of Big Data outcomes; and the need for a simple, convenient, and transparent Big Data analytics system which can be applied for real-time cases.

▶ Discussion

This review highlights the role of Big Data in enhancing care quality. Specifically, it identified the latest findings on Big Data in health research between 2015 and 2018. Evidently,

there is a variety of Big Data definitions largely focusing on Big Data's characterization as large volume, high velocity, huge variety, value, and veracity. In medicine, Big Data have been applied across various key domains including cardiology, diabetes, oncology, pharmacy, and more. **FIGURE TR1-8**, which displays the percentage of Big Data articles applied in specific healthcare domains, shows that oncology has the largest interest in most of the latest research work on Big Data (53%).

The oncology Big Data research includes all types of cancer, especially breast and lung cancer. Diabetes comes next (13%), with pharmacy (11%) and cardiology (9%) following. The other domains comprise only between 2% and 5% of Big Data in health applications. It may be concluded that the absence of effective cancer treatments has led Big Data researchers to focus on the oncology domain and how Big Data analytics can be used to understand these very complex diseases.

The medical field is considered among the most important sources of Big Data. In gathering Big Data in health care (see Figure TR1-3), we notice varied sources such as:

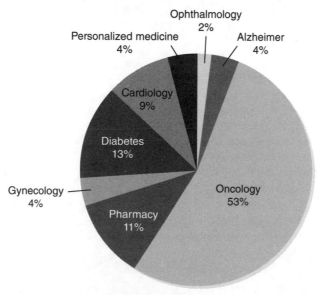

FIGURE TR1-8 Percentage of medical domains applied in big data research papers.

healthcare providers, laboratories, diagnostic companies, insurance companies, pharmaceutical firms, fitness devices and wearable sensors, government, and Web-health portals. These diverse sources generate data in various types and formats: structured, unstructured, and semi-structured data in the form of text, image, video, audio, ASCII characters, and so on. **FIGURE TR1-9** shows the results of Table TR1-1 that presents data type used in the papers we reviewed. Here, four main types were identified: genomic, behavior, imaging, and pharmaceutical data. The other EHR data involve clinical notes, International Classification of Disease or International Classification of Disease (ICD) codes, blood tests, and more. As shown in the histogram, it is clear that the majority of papers use imaging data (16 articles), including Whole Slide Imaging (WSI), Computed Tomography (CT), Positron Emission Tomography (PET), Magnetic Resonance Imaging (MRI), X-ray, infrared thermographs, and more. As expected, genomic data represent the second most dominant type.

Altogether, the Big Data heterogeneity led to the issue of data integrity and validity. Vendors offer a variety of extract transform load (ETL) and data integration tools designed to make the process easier, but many researchers believe that they have yet to solve the data integration problem. The collected data from care monitoring devices vary with respect to noise, redundancy, consistency, and more. The challenge here is to improve the data quality so as to get accurate analytics (**FIGURE TR1-10**).

In the storage and processing of big health data, the extant literature on Big Data tools and techniques is broad and largely varied (see Table TR1-2). But we still have the problem of infrastructure, cost, security, corruption, scalability, user interface (UI), and accessibility. The latest research has identified that the Hadoop ecosystem is the most common adopted family of software tools used for storage and processing big health data, but since they are batch-processing tools, developers have created new tools for streaming and real-time data; for example, Spark, Storm, and GraphLab. Cloud computing has also increased our attention on accessing and storing Big Data. In health care, to share and store data over the cloud plays a key role in offering flexible, reliable, and cost-effective solution to users. Despite many advantages of a cloud-based healthcare system, security and privacy of data remain a major cause for concerns,

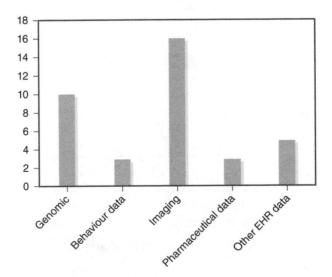

FIGURE TR1-9 Data Type used in the Extant Literature.

which have restricted the acceptance of the cloud-based model.

Various analytical techniques have been applied in health care. Currently, the most popular one is machine learning, such as NNs and SVM, decision tree, deep learning, k-means, random forest, rotation forest, conventional NN, and more. **FIGURE TR1-11** presents the machine-learning techniques most cited in the literature according to analysis type (diagnosis, predictive, prescriptive).

Overall, we notice that SVM is the most used technique in diagnosis analytics. However, in predictive analysis, decision tree dominates. All in all, SVM appears to be the most accurate compared to other techniques. Despite this large advanced analytics, we still have some critical questions in this phase; for example: Does all data need to be analyzed? How does one go about finding out which data points are really important? How can the data be used to the best advantage? Which technique is more accurate? As the accuracy of medical analysis is critical, any mistake in diagnosis or prediction puts the patient's life at risk. So, the huge volume of data poses technological challenges not only for storage on the size scale of petabytes but for continued development of tools to analyze the data

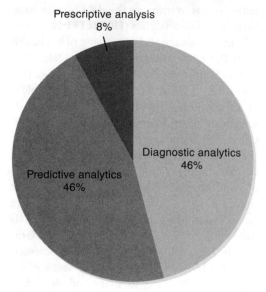

FIGURE TR1-10 Percentage of papers utilized each type of analysis.

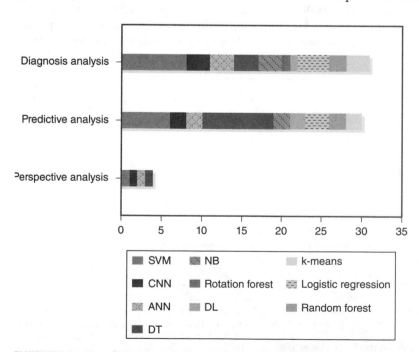

FIGURE TR1-11 Use of Machine Learning Technique vis-à-vis Major Type of Analysis.

properly, for knowing what has happened, why it happened (diagnostic), what will happen (predictive) and how we can make it happen (prescriptive). The target here is to find how to choose the right technique with the right data, to make the right decision at the right time, at the lowest cost.

Data analysis is the final and the most important phase in the processing of Big Data in health care. It has three main types:

- Diagnosis analytics is usually used to answer the question what happened and why it happened? It uses the past and current healthcare data to make quality healthcare decisions.
- Predictive analytics can be used to forecast what might happen in the future. It uses statistical approaches to search through large patient datasets and analyzes those data to predict individual patient outcomes.
- Prescriptive analytics is a type of analytics used to prescribe actions for the decision makers to act upon. In health care, prescriptive analytics is used in evidence-based medicine to improve patient care and to prescribe better business practices.

The graph in Figure TR1-10 shows results adapted from Table TR1-5, which illustrates the distributed percentages of papers that deal with diagnosis, prognosis, and perspective analyses. From the pie chart, it is clear that the majority of papers focus on diagnosis and prediction using big data in health care with equal percentage (46%); only a small minority falls in the domain of prescriptive analysis.

▶ Conclusion

This work overviews Big Data analysis to improve health sector performance. It has focused on the newer scientific research published between 2015 and 2018 to identify the latest trends and direction of researchers in this field. The review affords a comprehensive picture of how Big Data analysis can impact medicine. Yet challenges abound, the most prominent of which is the nature and integrity of the Big Datasets serving as input to the analysis. On account of the strong relationship between quality of data and accuracy of analysis results that led to the decision taken, in addition to the sensibility of working on human lives, researchers should concentrate on this problem, as any mistake can have critical consequences.

The future of Big Data health analytics sees rapid advances in more empowering tools and technologies, incorporating greater intelligence, more user-friendliness, and other optimization features so as to ease users in making the appropriate choice when choosing among the various techniques applicable to particular dataset(s). With Big Data analytics exhibiting greater success in improving care quality, effectiveness and cost, a deeper understanding of patients, a more personalized treatment, as well as a great help for doctors to make the right decisions, there is hope for greater longevity among humankind.

Notes

1. Mehta, N., & Pandit, A. (2018). Concurrence of big data analytics and healthcare: A systematic review. *International Journal of Medical Informatics, 114,* 57–65.
2. Wang, D., Khosla, A., Gargeya, R., Irshad, H., & Beck, A. H. (2016). Deep learning for identifying metastatic breast cancer. arXiv preprint arXiv:1606.05718.
3. Alonso, S. G., de la Torre Díez, I., Rodrigues, J. J. P. C., Hamrioui, S., & López-Coronado, M. (2017). systematic review of techniques and sources of big data in the Healthcare Sector. *Journal of Medical Systems, 41*(11), 183.
4. Bellazzi, R., Dagliati, A., Sacchi, L., & Segagni, D. (2015). Big data technologies: New opportunities for diabetes management. *Journal of Diabetes Science and Technology, 9*(5), 1119–1125.
5. Haper, E. (2014). Can big data transform electronic health records into learning health systems? *Studies Health Technology Informatics, 2014*(201), 470–475.

6. Hemingway, H., Asselbergs, F. W., Danesh, J., Dobson, R., Maniadakis, N., Maggioni, A., & Anker, S. D. (2018). Big data from electronic health records for early and late translational cardiovascular research: Challenges and potential. *European Heart Journal, 39*(16), 1481–1495.

7. Luo, J., Wu, M., Gopukumar, D., & Zhao, Y. (2016). Big data application in biomedical research and health care: A literature review. *Biomedical Informatics Insights, 8*, BII-S31559.

8. Mathew, P. S., & Pillai, A. S. (2015, March). *Big data solutions in healthcare: Problems and perspectives.* 2015 International Conference on Innovations in Information, Embedded and Communication Systems (ICIIECS) (pp. 1–6), IEEE, Coimbatore, India, 19–20 March 2015.

9. Andreu-Perez, J., Poon, C. C. Y., Merrifield, R. D., Wong, S. T. C., & Yang, G. Z. (2015). Big data for health. *IEEE Journal of Biomedical and Health Informatics, 19*(4), 1193–1208.

10. Mehta & Pandit, (2018), *ibid.*

11. Stokes, L. B., Rogers, J. W., Hertig, J. B., & Weber, R. J. (2016). Big data: Implications for health system pharmacy. *Hospital Pharmacy, 51*(7), 599–603.

12. Hemingway et al., (2018), *ibid.*

13. Mathew & Pillai, (2015), *ibid.*

14. Andreu-Perez et al., (2015), *ibid.*

15. Ma, C., Smith, H. W., Chu, C., & Juarez, D. T. (2015). Big data in pharmacy practice: Current use, challenges, and the future. *Integrated Pharmacy Research & Practice, 4*, 91.

16. Fang, R., Pouyanfar, S., Yang, Y., Chen, S. C., & Iyengar, S. S. (2016). Computational health informatics in the big data age: A survey. *ACM Computing Surveys (CSUR), 49*(1), 12.

17. Mathew & Pillai, (2015), *ibid.*

18. Huang, T., Lan, L., Fang, X., An, P., Min, J., & Wang, F. (2015). Promises and challenges of big data computing in health sciences. *Big Data Research, 2*(1), 2–11.

19. Vijayarani, S., & Sharmila, M. S. (2016). Research in big data—An overview. *Informatics Engineering, an International Journal (IEIJ), 4*(3), 19–23.

20. Luo et al., (2016), *ibid.*

21. Bellazzi et al., (2015), *ibid.*

22. Lourenço, J. R., Cabral, B., Carreiro, P., Vieira, M., & Bernardino, J. (2015). Choosing the right NoSQL database for the job: A quality attribute evaluation. *Journal of Big Data, 2*(1), 18.

23. Thiebaut, N., Simoulin, A., Neuberger, K., Ibnouhsein, I., Bousquet, N., Reix, N., & Mathelin, C. (2017). An innovative solution for breast cancer textual big data analysis. arXiv preprint arXiv:1712.02259.

24. Hinkson, I. V., Davidsen, T. M., Klemm, J. D., Chandramouliswaran, I., Kerlavage, A. R., & Kibbe, W. A. (2017). A comprehensive infrastructure for big data in cancer research: Accelerating cancer research and precision medicine. *Frontiers in Cell and Developmental Biology, 5*, 83.

25. Chen, M., Yang, J., Zhou, J., Hao, Y., Zhang, J., & Youn, C. (2018). 5G-Smart Diabetes: Toward personalized diabetes diagnosis with healthcare big data clouds. *IEEE Communications Magazine, 56*, 16–23.

26. Bouzidi, Z., Terrissa, L. S., Zerhouni, N., & Ayad, S. (2018). An efficient cloud prognostic approach for aircraft engines fleet trending. *International Journal of Computers and Applications*, 1–16.

27. Alonso et al., (2017), *ibid.*

28. Bachiller, Y., & Busch, P. (2018). *Survey: Big data application in biomedical research.* ICCAE 2018 Proceedings of the 2018 10th International Conference on Computer and Automation Engineering.

29. Mathew & Pillai, (2015), *ibid.*

30. Mehta & Pandit, (2018), *ibid.*

31. Hemingway et al., (2018), *ibid.*

32. Mathew & Pillai, (2015), *ibid.*

33. Cyganek, B., Graña, M., Krawczyk, B., Kasprzak, A., Porwik, P., Walkowiak, K., & Woźniak, M. (2016). A survey of big data issues in electronic health record analysis. *Applied Artificial Intelligence, 30*(6), 497–520.

34. Ma et al., (2015), *ibid.*

35. Mehta & Pandit, (2018), *ibid.*

36. Alberdi, A. A., Weakley, A., Schmitter-Edgecombe, M., Cook, D. J., Aztiria, A., Basarab, A., & Barrenechea, M. (2018). Smart home-based prediction of multi-domain symptoms related to Alzheimer's Disease. *IEEE Journal of Biomedical and Health Informatics, 22*(6), 1720–1731.

37. Albarqouni, S., Baur, C., Achilles, F., Belagiannis, V., Demirci, S., & Navab, N. (2016). AggNet: Deep learning from crowds for mitosis detection in breast cancer histology images. *IEEE Transactions on Medical Imaging, 35*(5), 1313–1321.

38. Alickovic, E., & Subasi, A. (2017). Breast cancer diagnosis using GA feature selection and Rotation Forest. *Neural Computing and Applications, 28*(4), 753–763.

39. Aliwadi, S., Shandila, V., Gahlawat, T., Kalra, P., & Mehrotra, D. (2017, September). *Diagnosis of diabetic nature of a person using SVM and ANN approach.* 2017 6th International Conference on Reliability, Infocom Technologies and Optimization (Trends and Future Directions) (ICRITO) (pp. 338–342), IEEE, Amity University Uttar Pradesh (AUUP), Noida, India.

40. Amirian, P., van Loggerenberg, F., Lang, T., Thomas, A., Peeling, R., Basiri, A., & Goodman, S. N. (2017). Using big data analytics to extract disease surveillance information from point of care diagnostic machines. *Pervasive and Mobile Computing, 42*, 470–486.

41. Asri, H., Mousannif, H., Al, H., & Noel, T. (2016). Using machine learning algorithms for breast cancer risk prediction and diagnosis. *Procedia—Procedia Computer Science, 83*(Fams), 1064–1069.

42. Brims, F. J., Meniawy, T. M., Duffus, I., de Fonseka, D., Segal, A., Creaney, J., & Nowak, A. K. (2016). A novel clinical prediction model for prognosis in malignant pleural mesothelioma using decision tree analysis. *Journal of Thoracic Oncology, 11*(4), 573–582.

43. Choi, J. Y., Cho, E. Y., Choi, Y. J., Lee, J. H., Jung, S. P., Cho, K. R., & Park, K. H. (2018). Incidence and risk factors for congestive heart failure in patients with early breast cancer who received anthracycline and/or trastuzumab: A big data analysis of the Korean Health Insurance Review and Assessment service database. *Breast Cancer Research and Treatment, 171*(1), 181–188.

44. Clark, A., Ng, J. Q., Morlet, N., & Semmens, J. B. (2016). Big data and ophthalmic research. *Survey of Ophthalmology, 61*(4), 443–465.

45. Daniel, B., Leff, R., & Yang, G. (2015). Views & comments big data for precision medicine. *Engineering, 1*(3), 277–279.

46. Ding, B., Zheng, L., Zhu, Y., Li, N., Jia, H., Ai, R., & Wang, W. (2015). Normalization and noise reduction for single cell RNA-seq experiments. *Bioinformatics, 31*(13), 2225–2227.

47. DuBrava, S., Mardekian, J., Sadosky, A., Bienen, E. J., Parsons, B., Hopps, M., & Markman, J. (2017). Using random forest models to identify correlates of a diabetic peripheral neuropathy diagnosis from electronic health record data. *Pain Medicine, 18*(1), 107–115.

48. Eljil, K. S., Qadah, G., & Pasquier, M. (2016). Predicting hypoglycemia in diabetic patients using time-sensitive artificial neural networks. *International Journal of Healthcare Information Systems and Informatics (IJHISI), 11*(4), 70–88.

49. Erekson, E. A., & Iglesia, C. B. (2015). Improving patient outcomes in gynecology: The role of large data registries and big data analytics. *Journal of Minimally Invasive Gynecology, 22*(7), 1124–1129.

50. Forsyth, A. W., Barzilay, R., Hughes, K. S., Lui, D., Lorenz, K. A., Enzinger, A., & Lindvall, C. (2018). Machine learning methods to extract documentation of breast cancer symptoms from electronic health records. *Journal of Pain and Symptom Management, 55*(6), 1492–1499.

51. Gambhir, S., Malik, S. K., & Kumar, Y. (2018). The diagnosis of dengue disease: An evaluation of three machine learning approaches. *International Journal of Healthcare Information Systems and Informatics (IJHISI), 13*(3), 1–19.

52. Geerts, H., Dacks, P. A., Devanarayan, V., Haas, M., Khachaturian, Z. S., Gordon, M. F., & Brain Health Modeling Initiative. (2016). Big data to smart data in Alzheimer's disease: The brain health modeling initiative to foster actionable knowledge. *Alzheimer's & Dementia, 12*(9), 1014–1021.

53. Gurusamy, V., Kannan, S., & Nandhini, K. (2017). The real time big data processing framework advantages and limitations. *International Journal of Computer Sciences and Engineering, 5*(12), 305–312.

54. Hernandez, I., & Zhang, Y. (2017). Using predictive analytics and big data to optimize pharmaceutical outcomes. *American Journal of Health-System Pharmacy, 74*(18), 1494–1500.

55. Hossain, M. S., & Muhammad, G. (2016). Healthcare big data voice pathology assessment framework. *IEEE Access, 4*, 7806–7815.

56. Ivanova, D. (2017, December). *Big data analytics for early detection of breast cancer based on machine learning.* AIP Conference Proceedings (Vol. 1910, No. 1, p. 060016), AIP Publishing.

57. Kalyankar, G. D., Poojara, S. R., & Dharwadkar, N. V. (2017). *Predictive analysis of diabetic patient data using machine learning and Hadoop.* 2017 International Conference on I-SMAC (IoT in Social, Mobile, Analytics and Cloud) (I-SMAC) (pp. 619–624), Palladam, India.

58. Kourou, K., Exarchos, T. P., Exarchos, K. P., Karamouzis, M. V., & Fotiadis, D. I. (2015). Machine learning applications in cancer prognosis and prediction. *Computational and Structural Biotechnology Journal, 13*, 8–17.

59. Kovalev, V., Kalinovsky, A., & Liauchuk, V. (2016, June). *Deep learning in big image data: Histology image classification for breast cancer diagnosis.* Proceedings of 2nd International Conference Big Data and Advanced Analytics (pp. 44–53), BSUIR, Minsk.

60. Kurc, T., Qi, X., Wang, D., Wang, F., Teodoro, G., Cooper, L., & Foran, D. J. (2015). Scalable analysis of big pathology image data cohorts using efficient methods and high-performance computing strategies. *BMC Bioinformatics, 16*(1), 399.

61. Landset, S., Khoshgoftaar, T. M., Richter, A. N., & Hasanin, T. (2015). A survey of open source tools for machine learning with big data in the Hadoop ecosystem. *Journal of Big Data, 2*(1), 24.

62. Maia, A., Sammut, S., Jacinta-fernandes, A., & Chin, S. (2017). ScienceDirect big data in cancer genomics. *Current Opinion in Systems Biology, 4*, 78–84.

63. Malav, A., Kadam, K., & Kamat, P. (2017). Prediction of heart disease using K-means and artificial neural network as hybrid approach to improve accuracy. *International Journal of Engineering and Technology, 9*(4), 3081–3085.

64. Manogaran, G., Vijayakumar, V., Varatharajan, R., Malarvizhi Kumar, P., Sundarasekar, R., & Hsu, C. H. (2018, October). Machine learning based big data processing framework for cancer diagnosis using hidden Markov model and GM clustering. *Wireless Personal Communications, 102*(3), 2099–2116.

65. Margolies, L. R., Pandey, G., Horowitz, E. R., & Mendelson, D. S. (2016). Breast imaging in the era of big data: Structured reporting and data mining. *American Journal of Roentgenology, 206*(2), 259–264.

66. Miranda, E., Irwansyah, E., Amelga, A. Y., Maribondang, M. M., & Salim, M. (2016). Detection of cardiovascular disease risk's level for adults using naive Bayes classifier. *Healthcare Informatics Research, 22*(3), 196–205.

67. Morovvat, M., & Osareh, A. (2016). An ensemble of filters and wrappers for microarray data classification. *Machine Learning and Applications: An International Journal, 3*(2), 01–17.

68. Nawaz, S., Heindl, A., Koelble, K., & Yuan, Y. (2015). Beyond immune density: Critical role of spatial heterogeneity in estrogen receptor-negative breast cancer. *Modern Pathology, 28*(6), 766–777.

69. Panayides, A. S., Pattichis, C. S., & Pattichis, M. S. (2016, November). *The promise of big data technologies and challenges for image and video analytics in healthcare.* 2016 50th Asilomar Conference on Signals, Systems and Computers (pp. 1278–1282), IEEE, Pacific Grove, CA.

70. Prasad, S. T., Sangavi, S., Deepa, A., Sairabanu, F., & Ragasudha, R. (2017). *Diabetic data analysis in big data with predictive method.* International Conference on Algorithms, Methodology, Models and Applications in Emerging Technologies (ICAMMAET) (pp. 1–4), Chennai, India.

71. Prerana, T. H. M., Shivaprakash, N. C., & Swetha, N. (2015). Prediction of heart disease using machine learning algorithms-Naïve Bayes, Introduction to PAC Algorithm, Comparison of Algorithms and HDPS. *International Journal of Science and Engineering, 3,* 90–99.

72. Priyanga, P., & Naveen, N. C. (2018). Analysis of machine learning algorithms in health care to predict heart disease. *International Journal of Healthcare Information Systems and Informatics (IJHISI), 13*(4), 82–97.

73. Raghupathi, W., & Raghupathi, V. (2014). Big data analytics in healthcare: Promise and potential. *Health Information Science and Systems, 2*(1), 3.

74. Rahim, A., Forkan, M., Khalil, I., & Atiquzzaman, M. (2017). ViSiBiD : A learning model for early discovery and real-time prediction of severe clinical events using vital signs as big data. *Computer Networks, 113,* 244–257.

75. Samuel, O. W., Asogbon, G. M., Sangaiah, A. K., Fang, P., & Li, G. (2017). An integrated decision support system based on ANN and Fuzzy_AHP for heart failure risk prediction. *Expert Systems with Applications, 68,* 163–172.

76. Saravana, N. M., Eswari, T., Sampath, P., & Lavanya, S. (2015). Predictive methodology for diabetic data analysis in big data. *Procedia—Procedia Computer Science, 50,* 203–208.

77. Schatz, B. R. (2015). National Surveys of population health: Big data analytics for mobile health monitors. *Big Data, 3*(4), 219–229.

78. Shah, M., Wang, D., Rubadue, C., Suster, D., & Beck, A. (2017, November). *Deep learning assessment of tumor proliferation in breast cancer histological images.* 2017 IEEE International Conference on Bioinformatics and Biomedicine (BIBM) (pp. 600–603), IEEE, Kansas City, MO.

79. Shen, L., Chen, H., Yu, Z., Kang, W., Zhang, B., Li, H., & Liu, D. (2016). Evolving support vector machines using fruit fly optimization for medical data classification. *Knowledge-Based Systems, 96,* 61–75.

80. Sherri, L., & Zhangxi, C. (2016). Accepted Manuscript, 0–67. Morovvat, M. & Osareh, A. (2016). An ensemble of filters and wrappers for microarray data classification. *Machine Learning and Applications: An International Journal, 3*(2), 01–17.

81. Silva, L. F., Santos, A. A. S., Bravo, R. S., Silva, A. C., Muchaluat-Saade, D. C., & Conci, A. (2016). Hybrid analysis for indicating patients with breast cancer using temperature time series. *Computer Methods and Programs in Biomedicine, 130,* 142–141.

82. Singh, D., & Reddy, C. K. (2015). A survey on platforms for big data analytics. *Journal of Big Data, 2*(1), 8.

83. Sivakami, K., & Saraswathi, N. (2015). Mining big data: Breast cancer prediction using DT-SVM hybrid model. *International Journal of Scientific Engineering and Applied Science (IJSEAS), 1*(5), 418–429.

84. Su, Q., Wang, Y., Jiang, X., Chen, F., & Lu, W. C. (2017). A cancer gene selection algorithm based on the K-S test and CFS. *BioMed Research International, 2017,* 1–7.

85. Sumbaly, R., Vishnusri, N., & Jeyalatha, S. (2014). Diagnosis of breast cancer using decision tree data mining technique. *International Journal of Computer Applications, 98*(10), 16–24.

86. Varatharajan, R., Gunasekaran, M., Priyan, M. K., & Sundarasekar, R. (2018, March). Wearable sensor devices for early detection of Alzheimer disease using dynamic time warping algorithm. *Cluster Computing, 21*(1), 681–690.

87. Sung, K. C., Ting, H. M., Chao, P. J., Guo, S. S., Tran, C. K., Huang, Y. J., & Lee, T. F. (2016). Predicting grade 2 acute radiation-induced dermatitis after hybrid intensity modulation radiotherapy for breast cancer using a logistic regression normal tissue complication probability model. *European Journal of Cancer, 60,* e4.

88. Taglang, G., & Jackson, D. B. (2016). Gynecologic oncology use of "big data" in drug discovery and clinical trials. *Gynecologic Oncology, 141*(1), 17–23.

89. Turgut, M., Turgut, A.T., & Kosar, U. (2006, October). Spinal brucellosis: Turkish experience based on 452 cases published during the last century. *Acta Neurochirurgica, 148*(10), 1033–1044.

90. Varatharajan, R., Manogaran, G., Priyan, M. K., & Sundarasekar, R. (2017). Wearable sensor devices for

early detection of Alzheimer disease using dynamic time warping algorithm. *Cluster Computing*, 1–10.

91. Viceconti, M., Hunter, P. J., & Hose, R. D. (2015). Big data, big knowledge: Big data for personalized healthcare. *IEEE Journal of Biomedical and Health Informatics, 19*(4), 1209–1215.

92. Volynskaya, Z., Chow, H., Evans, A., Wolff, A., Lagmay-Traya, C., & Asa, S. L. (2017). Integrated pathology informatics enables high-quality personalized and precision medicine: Digital pathology and beyond. *Archives of Pathology & Laboratory Medicine, 142*(3), 369–382.

93. Walczak, S., & Okuboyejo, S. R. (2017). An artificial neural network classification of prescription nonadherence. *International Journal of Healthcare Information Systems and Informatics (IJHISI), 12*(1), 1–13.

94. Wang, Y., & Hajli, N. (2017). Exploring the path to big data analytics success in healthcare. *Journal of Business Research, 70*, 287–299.

95. Wu, D., Jennings, C., Terpenny, J., & Kumara, S. (2016). *Cloud-based machine learning for predictive analytics: Tool wear prediction in milling.* Proceedings—2016 IEEE International Conference on Big Data (pp. 2062–2029), Big Data, Washington, DC.

96. Xiao, Y., Wu, J., Lin, Z., & Zhao, X. (2018). A deep learning-based multi-model ensemble method for cancer prediction. *Computer Methods and Programs in Biomedicine, 153*, 1–9.

97. Zheng, T., & Zhang, Y. (2017, August). *A big data application of machine learning-based framework to identify type 2 diabetes through electronic health records.* International Conference on Knowledge Management in Organizations, Beijing, China.

98. Remadna, I., Terrissa, S. L., Zemouri, R., & Ayad, S. (2018, March). *An overview on the deep learning based prognostic.* 2018 International Conference on Advanced Systems and Electric Technologies (IC_ASET) (pp. 196–200), IEEE, Hammamet, Tunisia.

Biographies

Abir Belaala is presently a PhD student in computer science, with a specialty in Artificial Intelligence. She received a master's degree in Computer Science in 2015 from Biskra University, Algeria. Her current research interest is Big Data Analytics and Machine Learning in the medical field.

Labib Sadek Terrissa is an Associate Professor in Computer Science at Biskra University, Algeria. He is the intelligent systems and networking team head within the smart computer science Laboratory (LINFI), where he conducts his research activities. After receiving an engineering degree in electronics, he received a postgraduate degree (DEA) and a PhD in computer engineering in 2006 from LeHavre University, France. He received the first award in the national exhibition of research and development in 2017 and the best paper award in IEEE-Cist's 2016 conference. His current research interests include Cloud Computing, Cloud Robotics, Machine learning, Medical Big Data, Smart maintenance, and Prognostic and Health Management.

Zerhouni Noureddine is a full professor at École Nationale Supérieure de Mécanique et des Microtechniques. He is a member of PHM team of Automatic Control and Micro-Mechatronic Systems department within FEMTO-ST Institute. He has worked since 1999 on modeling, analysis, and control of production systems. His specializations include system modeling, artificial intelligence techniques for diagnostic and prognostics, and machine learning.

Devalland Christine is head of the Department of Pathology, specializing in breast pathology. Her current research interest is the indication of neural network in pathology.

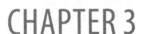

CHAPTER 3

Adoption and Commercialization of Digital Health

Greg Moon and Phillip Olla

LEARNING OBJECTIVES

- Define digital health and rationalize the need for digital health commercialization
- Understand the investments in digital health
- Comprehend the challenges of digital health commercialization
- Understand the leading causes of the digital health commercialization gap
- Create awareness of future trends that may impact the kinetics of digital health adoption

CHAPTER OUTLINE

Scenario: Accenture: Adding AI Bots to Enhance Digital Health Solution

- I. Introduction
- II. Background
- III. Current Perspective
  - *Current Challenges: Origins of the Commercialization Gap*

- IV. Future Directions
- V. Conclusion

Notes
Chapter Questions
Biography

Scenario: Accenture: Adding AI Bots to Enhance Digital Health Solution[1]

In September 2018, Accenture released news on the addition of interactive AI bots to the Accenture Intelligent Patient Platform for enhancing overall patient care-seeking experience. Fueled by artificial intelligence (AI), these virtual-assistant bots (Ella and Ethan) are expected to support shared decision-making and interactions among the Platform users such as patients, care providers, clinicians, and life sciences companies. Apparently, these bots will be learning continually while offering recommendations intelligently when requested. The ultimate goal is to enhance the overall patient health- and wellness-seeking experience, beginning from clinical trial participation to ongoing treatment management.

According to the news release, Ella and Ethan are part of Accenture's "Patient Engagement Support solution in the Accenture Intelligent Patient Platform"; in this sense, they are also part of "Salesforce Fullforce Solutions that are powered by Salesforce Health Cloud and Einstein AI and Amazon's Alexa." Specifically, these bots are designed to aid patients throughout their complete healthcare-seeking experience by providing high-level personalized attention as well as enhanced patient support. As Managing Director of Accenture Life Sciences, Tony Romito, noted: "With the inclusion of these new AI capabilities, the Accenture Intelligent Patient Platform continues to expand the value of using analytics and collaborative technologies to support the healthcare industry's goal to deliver better outcomes."

Ella—the virtual care assistant for patients—comes with a suite of multiple services such as medication reminders, vitals tracking, and appointment scheduling. Ethan is the virtual service assistant for healthcare providers (HCPs). It enables life sciences companies to help HCPs easily work with patients, manage their health activities, and coordinate with other care team members to offer critical services in a comprehensive manner.

To augment the user experience, Accenture's Patient Engagement solution has also been empowered with additional AI and other processing capabilities, such as Onboarding Contact Center (to ease treatment accessibility for patients), Adherence and Care Management Contact Center (to ensure patient adherence to a treatment protocol by personalizing services and experience and providing timely recommendations as needed), and Provider Portal and Mobile Application (to ensure the right information is given at the right time to the right physician who is serving a particular individual patient).

Imagine you were hired to promote investments in Accenture with these newly added AI-featured solutions. How would you articulate Accenture's future ability to further transform traditional healthcare services delivery vis-à-vis its growing use of analytics and collaborative technologies within the competitive healthcare marketplace? Why do you think Accenture's recent move will continue to grow its Health and Public Service and Products segments even further, given that both these segments have already thrived in the last reporting period? Is the healthcare marketplace ready for Accenture's innovations? Why or why not?

▶ I. Introduction

Based on the positive impact of digital transformation on nearly all other industry sectors, digital health solutions hold the promise to redefine health care, by dramatically enhancing the care experience, improving clinical outcomes, and reducing costs. There have been significant investments into digital health over the years. Startup Health has been tracking the Digital Health investments since 2010 when investments hit at $1.2 billion. In 2018, the digital health market had reached extraordinary growth, reaching $11.1 billion.[2]

At present, however, the industry is beset by a significant "digital health commercialization gap," meaning the large differential between the potential value of digital health and actual clinical and commercial adoption by healthcare delivery systems to date. The cause of the gap is multifactorial, due to fundamental disconnects between digital health innovator companies and healthcare delivery systems on cultural, technological, operational, and business levels. These disconnects lead to long, frequently unsuccessful sales cycles, which present major business challenges to innovator companies and ultimately threaten the full potential of digital health.

This chapter examines the origins of the digital health commercialization gap and explores solutions to help bridge this gap.

▶ II. Background

The tectonic power of digital transformation cannot be overemphasized, with information-based technologies upending business and society on a global basis. Every sector has been affected to some degree or another—including banking, retail, transportation, manufacturing, logistics, food production, education, and government—with profound gains in customer experience, operational efficiency, and cost reductions. The World Economic Forum (WEF) estimates that digital transformation could unlock $100 trillion of value over the next decade,[3] and the phenomenon appears to be an enduring force for the foreseeable future.

"Digital health" has been defined in many ways. For the purpose of this analysis, it will be defined very broadly as the use of intelligent, connected hardware- and software-based systems to enhance health and wellness. In this context, digital health can be viewed as health care's version of digital transformation, with the promise of analogous benefits—increased patient engagement, satisfaction, and empowerment; improved clinical outcomes; improved efficiency and quality; and lower healthcare costs. Unsurprisingly, then, digital health has captured the keen interest of every healthcare stakeholder, including patients, providers, health systems, traditional payers, employer payers, pharmaceutical and medical device vendors, technology vendors, regulators, policymakers, and investors. Accordingly, the digital health space has attracted significant investment; in 2017, venture funding hit $5.8 billion, which included seven deals over $100 million.[4] This investment has powered the development of myriad solutions for diagnosing and monitoring of disease, population health management, patient education and empowerment, decision support, precision medicine and genomics, fitness and wellness, telemedicine, and operations surrounding care delivery—all of which are in various stages of development, validation, and use. The rapid pace of innovation has been enabled by the convergence of requisite technologies in the areas of connectivity (a mature internet and mobile ubiquity), data capture mechanisms (patient self-reporting tools, scalable biometric sensors, and the electronic health record [EHR]), and data processing capabilities (Big Data and AI).

Despite all this excitement, digital health's clinical and commercial adoption by health systems—the current epicenter of healthcare delivery—has been anemic to date. This differential between the perceived value of digital health and actual paid adoption presents a commercialization gap. Slow digital technology adoption is nothing new in health care, which has traditionally lagged far behind other sectors such as banking and retail.[5,6] This inertia has been the case even when there is universal consensus regarding a technology's value, with the most glaring example being the EHR. Despite being in existence since the 1960s, by 2009, only 9.1% of hospitals had at least a basic EHR.[7] Unfortunately, similar inertia has plagued the uptake of digital health solutions, resulting in a situation wherein the supply of new solutions has far outstripped demand.[8]

This is not to say that there is insufficient interest and will to move to a digital future. Rather, the digital health commercialization gap results more from a current lack of capacity to get from here to there. We focus next on an analysis of this phenomenon, as well as a summary of proven and potential solutions.

▶ III. Current Perspective

Current Challenges: Origins of the Commercialization Gap

The origin of the digital health commercialization gap is multifactorial, due to characteristics inherent to digital health innovator companies and health systems, as well as dramatic disconnects between these two parties. These factors are detailed as follows:

- Cultural disconnects
- Reimbursement ignorance
- Health Systems Priorities
- Customers' needs
- Integration
- Business Models
- Data and Information Overload
- Levels of Evidence

(a) Cultural disconnects and mismatched expectations. Digital health innovator companies and health systems have emerged from two very different cultural traditions, which have hampered alignment. On the one hand, innovators come from a technology tradition, in which constant change is expected and disruption is a prized endpoint. Although from a different industry vertical, Mark Zuckerberg's infamous directive to "Move fast and break things" represents the iconoclastic ethos that pervades the technology industry, with an overt disregard for existing processes and norms. By contrast, health system customers come from a medical tradition, which, by nature, is much more conservative; change comes slowly and disruption is viewed much more as a threat. As Buzz Stewart, Chief Research Officer at Sutter

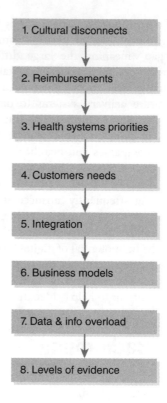

1. Cultural disconnects

2. Reimbursements

3. Health systems priorities

4. Customers needs

5. Integration

6. Business models

7. Data & info overload

8. Levels of evidence

Health, a large, distributed healthcare system, puts it, "For every $100 million that start-ups spend to create innovative health solutions, the health systems are spending $100 million to keep everything exactly the same."[9]

These divergent philosophies play out as different work styles, which, in turn, set up very different expectations around the pace of change. Innovator companies often comprise small, nimble teams, operating on short time horizons. Many digital health solutions are software-based, which are typically created and iterated rapidly through an "agile" development process; that is, entirely new features can be created in "sprints" lasting 1–4 weeks, driven by ad hoc cross-functional project teams. These companies have often embraced the "lean" approach, whereby a "minimum viable product" is purposefully released, intended to be further shaped by user actions and feedback, in an iterative, hypothesis-driven manner.[10] In this structure, decision-making is centralized and therefore very efficient. On the other hand, healthcare systems tend to be much larger organizations, employing well-honed operations, built on predictability. Multiple, tribal power centers exist within these organizations (e.g., clinicians, staff, and administrators), leading to a slower, more deliberative decision-making style, all of which contributes to institutional inertia. When change does come, it is carefully planned, well in advance, and is usually implemented through a traditional "waterfall" project management approach. As an example, the recommended EHR implementation plan from the Office of the National Coordinator (ONC) for Health Information Technology (HIT) calls for a multi-stakeholder project plan,[11] which often takes over 1 year to execute, especially for larger organizations.[12] As a result of these differences, there can be considerable mismatch in expectations regarding timeframes for decision-making and implementation. For these reasons, healthcare enterprise sales cycles are notoriously long, on the order of 12–18 months.[13] While health systems have the luxury of time, such timelines can pose an existential threat to an innovator company, for which operational bandwidth and financing are usually in short supply. Hence, these profound cultural differences and the practical implications thereof set the stage for rocky engagements between digital health vendors and their customers.

(b) Insufficient understanding of reimbursement trends. Many digital health companies do not grasp the ongoing, fundamental shift in the healthcare reimbursement landscape, which can lead to widely mis-targeted offerings. The macro trend, which will likely unfold fitfully and asynchronously across the industry over the next several years, is a move from *volume-based* (i.e., traditional fee-for-service-based) reimbursement to *value-based* reimbursement. Under a fee-for-service (FFS) scheme, health systems are paid for each service performed. Most of the cost liability therefore sits with the payer, with the rational result that FFS organizations focus heavily on

driving top-line revenue by maximizing volume and billing and pay much less attention to cost containment. Value-based payment (VBP) models, in contrast, reward or penalize health systems based upon the quality and cost of care that is provided[14]; for Medicare payments, the Medicare Access and CHIP Reauthorization Act (MACRA) of 2015 formalized and established timelines for the implementation of these models.[15] As a result, cost liability is shifted in varying degrees to the healthcare system, which incentivizes greater attention to cost reduction.

VBP programs exist on a continuum, defined by the level of cost risk that is shifted to the health system. On one end of the spectrum, the pay-for-performance (P4P) model uses a backbone of FFS reimbursement, which is adjusted based upon quality indices; in such a model, no added cost risk is incurred by a health system. On the opposite end of the spectrum is the global capitation model, in which a health system is paid a fixed amount per patient, per unit of time, reimbursed prospectively to the health system for furnishing all services. In a capitated model, the health system takes full financial risk for quality and cost; traditional health maintenance organizations (HMOs) like Kaiser Permanente, Medicare Advantage plans, and national health systems in other countries are the most obvious examples of entities using this model. In between these two extremes, other VBP paradigms exist, such as shared savings and bundled payment models, shared risk models, and accountable care organization (ACO) programs.

Put simply, a health system's primary reimbursement model determines the organization's level of cost liability, which defines whether it focuses more on revenue expansion or cost containment. This strategic emphasis, in turn, shapes the type of innovation that will be of interest to the organization. Bob Rebitzer, a seasoned expert in healthcare transformation and digital health, explains the dynamic as follows: "It is very straightforward. If you want to sell a digital health solution to a fee-for-service organization, make sure it can increase billing. If your customer is operating under value-based model, sell something that improves efficiency and reduces costs."[16] For the value-based systems, Sutter Health's Buzz Stewart summarized similar success factors for a sale. "A winning combination is that your digital health solution leads to better outcomes, allows providers to get more done, preferably with fewer resources, and leaves them more delighted than the standard process."[17]

(c) Limited health system mindshare. Health systems juggle competing priorities that have crowded out their receptivity to digital health. During the last 5–10 years, two interrelated priorities have consumed health systems' attention: EHR implementation and healthcare payment reform. The Health Information Technology for Economic and Clinical Health (HITECH) Act established a set of incentives and penalties to accelerate the rate of EHR adoption and promote meaningful use of this fundamental technology. The result is that by 2015, 87% of U.S. office-based physicians used an EHR.[18] Implicit in this impressive statistic are the herculean planning, implementation, and training efforts undertaken by health systems in recent years.

With a functioning EHR as a cornerstone, health systems have turned their attention to building out the technical and human infrastructure to address the new payment models dictated by MACRA. Value-based care models require considerable reporting around utilization, costs, and outcomes. Underlying this reporting is the ability to capture and analyze the appropriate data, which requires the development or sourcing of software-based tools, as well as teams to handle and interpret the data, all of which are new to most organizations. Furthermore, the cost reduction initiatives incentivized under these new payment models have pushed organizations to adopt new care paradigms that emphasize much greater coordination. One paradigm being widely implemented is the Patient-Centered

Medical Home (PCMH). This care delivery model uses a multidisciplinary, team-based approach to provide high-quality, accessible, patient-centered, tightly coordinated, end-to-end care.[19] The PCMH requires radically new workflows, provider communication processes, and technology solutions, such as decision support tools, telehealth capabilities, and patient registries.[20,21]

As can be seen, health systems have had their hands full adapting to new technical, economic, and operational realities necessitated by the ongoing transformation of health care. It should therefore be no surprise that companies have found it difficult to capture the level of health system mindshare suitable for the buy-in of digital health offerings. The silver lining is that the earlier activities, which have so consumed health systems' attention to date, have created technical environments and business conditions that are now ripe for accelerated digital health uptake.

(d) Misapprehension of specific customer business needs. Most innovator companies confidently believe that they understand health systems' business needs, but they often widely miss the mark. One common mistake is to rely on a top-down business needs analysis, based on conclusions from the literature, to assess demand for a product or service. For instance, because heart disease is a leading cause of death and currently leads to $500 billion in annual costs, a company might conclude that a large, easily accessed market exists for a digital heart disease solution. While this may be true, a greater understanding of health system customers' perceived needs, pressures, and priorities might have driven to an entirely different conclusion. Innovator companies tend not to seek this critical input before embarking in development. Don Turner, Global Head of Commercialization at IBM's Watson Health, who works with many early-stage digital health companies, noted: "One time I was addressing a room full of founders, and I asked them to raise their hands if they had spoken to

potential customers to validate demand. Not a single hand went up."

(e) Integration challenges. Another major barrier to digital health adoption is that the technical infrastructure does not yet exist for seamless, plug-and-play use of digital health offerings. "The big problem is that everybody is developing point solutions—here's something for diabetes, here's another thing for depression, each with a different interface and data format," explains Dr. Krishna Udaykumar, Director of the Duke Global Health Innovation Center. "We need a unifying platform and coordinated set of solutions to truly move things forward."[22] Theoretically, the EHR should be the unifying platform, yet EHR integration is typically a costly and time-consuming task. Health systems, having just sunk hundreds of millions of dollars into EHR implementation, fear a massive data dump from third-party vendors. They are also generally disinclined to commit resource for a more intelligent integration that would properly visualize just the right information from a digital health solution to make an informed decision (a so-called "wrap-around" integration).[23] Furthermore, a handful of vendors dominate the EHR, and these systems generally use "closed" application program interfaces (APIs), so that they can gate-keep integration of functionality from third-party developers. This centralized integration paradigm helps EHR vendors to ensure data integrity and control of the user experience, but at the same time, they throttle the development of interoperable systems.[24]

Perhaps more challenging is clinical workflow integration, which digital health companies tend to woefully underestimate. Digital Health applications can impact multiple parties in the chain of care—patients, providers, nurses, case managers, and support staff—all of whom may have competing agendas and differential receptivity to a new procedure. An example of the difficulties involved with workflow integration comes from the author's personal experience at Proteus Digital Health.

The company was collaborating with two U.S. health systems to implement a solution to help prevent hospital readmission for heart failure. The platform used sensor-enabled medications to monitor adherence and a telemetric weight scale. Leading up to "going live," strong clinical, strategic, and operational support was built around the solution, and multiple training sessions were conducted with relevant personnel. Thereafter, one customer achieved brisk clinical use in the clinic, while the other ultimately managed zero patients with the system. The latter customer, an integrated health system in the Pacific Northwest, explained, "We learned from this experience that we are not organizationally prepared to innovate. It was simply too hard to change standard operating procedure, even for this valuable new patient management approach."

(f) Data and Information overload. A recent survey by the American Medical Association (AMA) found that while nearly half of providers are enthusiastic about new digital health solutions, they also have significant concerns regarding effectiveness, data overload, professional liability, and financial remuneration related to new digital health solutions.[25] Busy clinicians are notoriously unwilling to actively seek patient data if opening a new user interface (website or app) outside of the primary EHR application is required; such an interaction model is typical for digital health offerings which have not yet been integrated into the EHR. Another common interaction model, which is problematic for different reasons, is the use of alerts to advise providers of abnormal data, potentially worrisome trends, or reminders for care-related actions. If not properly designed, alerts are perceived as annoying and disruptive to workflow.[26] Too many alerts can also result in "alert fatigue," wherein physicians and staff become desensitized and begin to ignore or fail to respond appropriately to the incoming information.[27] Sutter's Stewart relates the following from when he was previously at Geisinger: "One analysis we performed revealed that we were

generating 7 million alerts per year. How is any system going to absorb that kind of volume on a practical basis?"[28] As can be seen, until a more seamless interface exists between information systems (IS) and cognitive and practical workflow, integration will be an ongoing headwind to the adoption of digital health.

(g) Mismatched perspectives on levels of evidence. Even if there is agreement on the potential utility of a solution, innovator companies and health system customers often have different expectations of evidence required to drive a purchase decision. Innovator companies often suffer from being overly enamored with their solutions, expecting the elegance of the technology and its capabilities to be self-evident to all and sufficient to sell the product. While this factor may open the door for a business conversation, it is almost never sufficient to result in a sale. Furthermore, innovators often conflate the data package required for regulatory approval with the evidence needed to drive a sale with a health system customer. To place a product on the market, lower bars of evidence—safety, efficacy, and frequently, human factors data—are required; in the case of many digital health solutions, "efficacy" often requires demonstration of measurement performance alone. The health system customer, however, views safety and technical performance merely as one prerequisite. In order to expend resource on assessment, purchase, and implementation, they much prefer higher-level evidence upfront, such as data from a trial that demonstrate positive clinical, productivity, or economic outcomes. Again, based on the author's personal experience at Proteus, a frequent refrain from potential customers in the early days of commercialization went something like this: "I know that adherence is essential to the effectiveness of medications, your technology is elegant, and it can measure medication taking events very well [>98% accuracy]. However, how do I know if it will improve adherence or clinical outcomes?" Proteus went on to develop these types of proof points, but

such evidence requires considerable time and expense, neither of which are in abundant supply in a typical innovator company. As a result, the evidence expectations divide can be difficult to bridge, potentially thwarting valuable collaboration at an early stage.

(h) Inadequate business models. Existing business models are in many ways unsuitable for digital health. Most, but not all, digital health offerings are fundamentally services, albeit enabled by technology. Although deployed to impact health or wellness directly, analogous to a medicine or a device, they usually do not fit into pharmaceutical or medical device spending buckets. Digital health also does not map well to an encounter-based model, given longitudinal, continuous use of many offerings.

One relevant business framework, familiar to both innovator companies and health systems alike, is an enterprise solutions contract. Digital health companies typically come from a software tradition, where subscription and Software as a Service (SaaS) business models are the norm, and health systems already buy solutions from vendors on a volume-based SaaS model (e.g., the EHR). Unfortunately, this model is challenging for a couple of key reasons. First, in the absence of strong health economics data, systems have trouble placing an economic value on digital health offerings, usually to the detriment of the innovator company. Second, enterprise sales involve multi-stakeholder purchasing decisions, which leads to the highly protracted sales cycles noted earlier. Julie Papanek Grant, a healthcare-focused partner at Canaan Partners, summarizes a common investor belief in this regard: "I am very bullish on digital health, but I am highly skeptical of businesses based upon enterprise purchases by healthcare systems."[29]

▶ IV. Future Directions

At the ecosystem level, a multi-stakeholder approach and aligned incentives are required for the successful digital transformation of health care. Key stakeholders include patients, providers and staff, health system administrators, digital health innovator companies, major technology companies, payers, investors, regulators, and policy makers. The "triple aim of health care" is a powerful, unifying framework for all these stakeholders: improved patient care experience, improved health of populations, and reduced per capita costs.[30] To rally the ecosystem around these aims, though, economic forces—more so than any philanthropic impetus—will be the determinant factor, if history is any guide. Healthcare actors ultimately tend to make decisions based upon financial incentives—with the possible exception of patients, although this is changing as they are bearing greater financial responsibilities for an increasing share of their healthcare costs. For this reason, recent policies and related reimbursement paradigms that target *value* will be a potent tool for aligning incentives and actions across this ecosystem.

Given the tremendous market forces at work, digital health adoption should accelerate significantly. Based upon experience to date, health systems will not be the proactive change agents; rather, digital transformation will ultimately be imposed upon providers and health systems. First, ongoing reimbursement trends will force health systems to assume much more liability for healthcare costs and quality, as the payment paradigm shifts from FFS to VBP models. The increased focus on cost will, in turn, open the door to technology-based solutions. Second, self-insured employers will flex their market power and squeeze health systems to deliver cheaper, higher-value care. Coupled with SIEs' openness to technologic solutions, it is not unreasonable to imagine that they could mandate the use of effective digital health solutions. Finally, in light of emerging care delivery competition from unexpected quarters (i.e., payers, technology companies, and retailers), health systems will need to innovate, or they will perish. These new competitors have embraced digital health, and to compete effectively, health systems will be pressed to follow suit.

At the tactical level, intermediaries have begun to establish forums and frameworks to more efficiently match health system needs with digital health solutions. Doing so front-loads into the design and development process, a clearer understanding of the specific clinical and business needs being solved, as well as knowledge of integration constraints. Some well-known examples have an academic affiliation, such as Harvard/Partners HealthCare's Center for Connected Health and the Biodesign program at Stanford University. Other intermediary organizations have emerged from the accelerator tradition, serving as matchmakers with industry stakeholders, including health systems; prominent examples are Rock Health in San Francisco and Startup Health in New York City. In addition, Avia, a Chicago digital health consulting firm, has created a consortium of digital health innovators and 29 prominent health systems. These members pool resources to identify unmet needs and pressure test the suitability of digital solutions from clinical, operational, and financial perspectives. The end result of these collective efforts will hopefully be a common, more rational framework for the design, development, adoption, implementation, evaluation and dissemination of valuable digital health solutions.

Technical integration will require tremendous work in the near-term. Interoperability issues will need to be solved as data capture devices proliferate and the volume of input datasets grow exponentially, which will require intelligent synthesis to be of any utility. As in other industries, technical standards and APIs (preferably "open") will likely expand and solidify to facilitate this requisite integration. EHR companies will need to become more open and proactive around this issue. Additionally, new companies have also emerged to focus exclusively on this issue. For example, Validic's platform enables continuous access to data from nearly 400 in home and wearable devices and serves as a single, regulatory-compliant point of integration for health systems' IT systems.

The challenge of clinical integration will likely reveal itself as the critical path for the digital transformation of health care. The state-of-the-art digital health solutions that currently exist aim to *support* clinical decision-making by supplying providers with more complete and timely information. The resulting integration challenge is fairly circumscribed and mainly requires considerable work: development of technical solutions to process, synthesize, and visualize data, plus the revision of workflow to present and act upon the data surrounding an episode of care. The rapidly approaching next frontier, however, involves the incorporation of AI into clinical care, at which point integration becomes infinitely more complex. For all intents and purposes, digital health solutions will have the capacity to *directly effectuate* clinical decision-making. This new capacity will unleash a torrent of new issues, which we have only begun to imagine: a radical redefinition of the provider's role; a disruption of the patient–doctor relationship; an emergence of new and profound ethical considerations; a medicolegal paradigm shift; and an intensified debate around data ownership, stewardship, and privacy, to name but a few. The future of digital health should be very interesting, indeed.

▶ V. Conclusion

Despite enormous clinical and business promise, digital health solutions have been very difficult to commercialize to date, especially via health systems as customers. These challenges have resulted in a substantial digital health commercialization gap. Standout companies have been able to bridge this gap successfully by selling more intelligently to health system customers; among other things, this entails targeting alternative customers like consumers, self-insured employers, traditional payers, and life science companies; or becoming vertically integrated HCPs themselves.

The coming decade will be a period of tremendous change in the healthcare market. It is hypothesized that employers, traditional payers, and non-medical technology giants will likely drive the adoption of digital health solutions, rather than providers and health systems. In any case, the digital transformation of health care is likely inevitable so opportunities will be significant for digital health companies, health systems, providers, and patients alike—even if the exact path is only now coming into focus.

Notes

1. Accenture adds two AI bots to its digital health solution for better healthcare by *The RIQ News Desk*. (September 24, 2018). Retrieved from www.readitquik.com/news/digital-transformation/accenture-adds-two-ai-bots-to-its-digital-health-solution-for-better-healthcare/

2. Retrieved from https://hq.startuphealth.com/posts/startup-health-insights-q3-2018-global-digital-health-funding-report NY, 2018

3. World Economic Forum. (2017). Digital transformation initiative: Unlocking $100 trillion for business and society from digital transformation. Retrieved from www.accenture.com/t20170116T084450__w__/us-en/_acnmedia/Accenture/Conversion-Assets/WEF/PDF/Accenture-DTI-executive-summary.pdf

4. Rock Health. (2018). Digital health funding: 2017 year in review. Retrieved from https://rockhealth.com /reports/2017-year-end-funding-report-the-end-of-the-begining-of-digital-health/

5. Currie, W. L., & Seddon, J. J. M. (2016). Health organizations' adoption and use of mobile technology in France, the USA and UK. *Procedia Computer Science, 98*, 413–418.

6. Gandhi, P., Khanna, S., & Ramaswamy, S. (2016). Which industries are the most digital (and why)? *Harvard Business Review*, online edition. Retrieved from https://hbr.org/2016/04/a-chart-that-shows-which-industries-are-the-most-digital-and-why

7. Jha, A. K., DesRoches, C. M., Campbell, E. G., Donelan, K., Rao, S. R., Ferris, T. G., … Blumenthal, D. (2009). Use of electronic health records in U.S. hospitals. *New England Journal of Medicine, 360*(16), 1628–1638.

8. Bhavani, S. P., Parakh, K., Atreja, A., Druz, R., Graham, G. N., Hayek, S. S., … Shah, B. R. (2017).

2017 Roadmap for innovation—ACC health policy statement on healthcare transformation in the era of digital health, big data, and precision health. *Journal of the American College of Cardiology, 70*(21), 2696–2718.

9. Buzz Stewart, personal communication.
10. Ries, E. (2011). *The lean startup: How today's entrepreneurs use continuous innovation to create radically successful businesses.* New York, NY: Crown Business.
11. The Office of the National Coordinator for Health Information Technology. (2017). Health IT playbook. Retrieved from www.healthit.gov/playbook/electronic-health-records
12. Shalger, A. (2009). *An EHR checklist: A process checklist for planning your EHR purchase, installation, and implementation.* Waltham, MA: Massachusetts Medical Society.
13. Coppedge, R. (2017). Digital health is dead, says this health-tech investor. *CNBC.* Retrieved from www.cnbc.com/2017/09/06/digital-health-is-dead-says-this-health-tech-investor-rob-coppedge.html
14. Center for Medicare and Medicaid Services. (2017). What are the value-based programs? Retrieved from www.cms.gov/Medicare/Quality-Initiatives-Patient-Assessment-Instruments/Value-Based-Programs/Value-Based-Programs.html
15. Center for Medicare and Medicaid Services. (2018). Quality payment program. Retrieved from www.cms.gov/Medicare/Quality-Payment-Program/Quality-Payment-Program.html
16. Bob Rebitzer, personal communication.
17. Buzz Stewart, personal communication.
18. The Office of the National Coordinator for Health Information Technology. (2017). Health IT dashboard. Retrieved from https://dashboard.healthit.gov/quickstats/pages/physician-ehr-adoption-trends.php
19. Rich, E. C., Lipson, D., Libersky, J., Peikes, D. N., & Parchman, M. L. (2012). Organizing care for complex patients in the patient-centered medical home. *Annals of Family Medicine, 10*(1), 60–62.
20. Kraschnewski, J. L., & Gabbay, R. A. (2013). Role of health information technologies in the patient-centered medical home. *Journal of Diabetes Science and Technology, 7*(5), 1376–1385.
21. Bates, D. W., & Bitton, A. (2010). The future of health information technology in the Patient-Centered Medical Home. *Health Affairs, 29*(4), 614–621.
22. Krishna Udaykumar, personal communication.
23. Wu, A. W., Jensen, R. E., Salzberg, C., & Snyder, C. (2013). *Advances in the use of patient reported outcome measures in electronic health records.* Washington, DC: Patient Centered Outcomes Research Institute (PCORI).
24. Sheikh, A., Sood, H. S., & Bates, D. W. (2015). Leveraging health information technology to achieve the "triple aim" of healthcare reform. *Journal of the American Medical Informatics Association, 22,* 849–856.
25. American Medical Association. (2016). Digital health study: Physicians' motivations and requirements for adopting digital clinical tools. Retrieved from www.ama-assn.org/sites/default/files/media-browser/specialty%20group/washington/ama-digital-health-report923.pdf.
26. Wright, A., Phansalkar, S., Bloomrosen, M., Jenders, R. A., Bobb, A. M., Halamka, J. D., ... Bates, D. W. (2010). Best practices in clinical decision support: The case of preventive care reminders. *Applied Clinical Informatics, 1,* 331–345.
27. Agency for Healthcare Research and Quality. (2017). Alert fatigue. US Department for Health and Human Services. Retrieved from https://psnet.ahrq.gov/primers/primer/28/alert-fatigue
28. Buzz Stewart, personal communication.
29. Julie Papanek Grant, personal communication.
30. Berwick, D. M., Nolan, T. W., & Whittington, J. (2008). The Triple Aim: Care, health, and cost. *Health Affairs, 27*(3), 759–769.

Chapter Questions

3-1 Why are health systems likely to resist digital innovations?

3-2 What are ways to reduce the communication barriers between health systems and digital health innovators?

3-3 What are some of the good business practices and proven strategies for selling innovations to health systems? Provide specific examples to support your arguments.

3-4 What types of innovations will thrive in today's digital health ecosystem?

Biography

Greg Moon is a physician-entrepreneur and digital health expert. He is deeply committed to the digital transformation of health care as a means to improve quality and outcomes, increase patient engagement, and deliver higher-value care. Board-certified in Internal Medicine, Dr. Moon is a graduate of Stanford University, Stanford School of Medicine, and UC Berkeley's Haas School of Business. His experience spans medical care, technology, clinical product development, strategic marketing, and regulatory affairs. At Proteus Digital Health, he was a key pioneer of "digital medicines," where he drove scientific validation, foundational regulatory approvals, clinical product definition, and workflow integration for Proteus' system of ingestible and wearable sensors to promote medication adherence. At Medibio LTD, an AI-based mental health company, he served as Chief Medical Officer, where he charted the company's clinical, regulatory, and quality strategy, culminating in the first-ever approval of an objective, biomarker-based depression diagnostic. He was previously cofounder and Chief Marketing Officer of a consumer electronic start-up, where he led marketing, sales, and distribution of a first-in-class mobile accessory. He currently leads the creation of Blue Cross North Carolina's value-based analytics platform to streamline engagements with health systems around advanced payment models. Synthesizing these experiences, Dr. Moon helps companies navigate the practical and business challenges of commercializing device, software, and analytics-based solutions amidst the rapidly changing healthcare landscape.

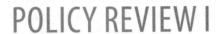

POLICY REVIEW I

Online Health Information Seeking: Recasting Access and Digital Equity

Fay Cobb Payton and Lynette Yarger

Abstract

Information and communities technologies (ICTs) are ubiquitous, and are playing a more significant role in the delivery, utilization and creation of health care services and content. Consumers are increasingly engaging in online health information seeking behaviors – as both nagivators and diagnosers. These roles are continuing to challenge longstanding forms of content creation, meaning and effectiveness among underrepresented populations. This policy review highlights data on who and why groups engage in health information seeking, and discusses the myHealthImpact platform which used a participatory design approach to counter digital inequity.

POLICY REVIEW OUTLINE

▶ I. Introduction

Information and communications technologies (ICTs) have enabled the digitalization of many industries and play a significant mechanism in health information dissemination. In the healthcare domain, ICTs have enabled disruptive change with regard to processes, people, and patients.[1] Namely, this change has resulted in access to real-time clinical and financial patient data, advances in personalized medicine and health, population health monitoring, minimal time and spatial barriers, innovation and diffusion of medical research, and improved patient empowerment. These advances, however, are not void of counter (often negative) narratives, including health information fragmentation, continual digital and health inequities among underrepresented populations, data quality limitations and lack of interdisciplinary approaches to health information, and inappropriate access to third parties.[2,3]

The Web and online platforms continue to be a key source of health information among health seekers and provide an increasingly social experience for users. Specifically, the Pew Research Center reports "that seven-in-ten (72%) adult Internet users say they have searched online for information about a range of health issues, the most popular being specific diseases and treatments. One-in-four (26%) adult Internet users say they have read or watched someone else's health experience about health or medical issues in the past 12 months. Yet, 16% of adult Internet users in the United States have gone online in the past 12 months to find others who share the same health concerns."[4]

To reduce social isolation, increase emotional support, and improve health information seeking, ICTs facilitate micro-blogging, care coordination, social media, patient–patient communication, and patient support channels to sustain patients with a variety of illnesses,[5-7] such as epilepsy,[8] smoking cessation,[9] and HIV.[10] While earlier studies implemented home-care health information networks to meet the needs of patients via decision support, nurse moderation, email, and discussion functionality, these studies have some observable distinctions. Current health information seeking tools are (1) widely enabled by social media and (2) created to support online communities though diffuse to shape offline experiences. Hence, health information seeking can inform those both infected by a given disease as well as those affected.

For instance, among cancer patients, the Internet has proven to be a communication source for patients infected and their affected families. Researchers concluded that computer-mediated communities supporting cancer patients fosters emotional support and empowerment,[11] in addition to providing a vehicle by which patients and family members can acquire familiarity with the disease and its stages.[12] Computer-mediated communities are even more critical as the number of worldwide cancer death rates has escalated to 7.6 million people.[13] Moreover, researchers[14,15] have determined that breast cancer patients have distinct needs for care and coping, engage in online and personal support groups, and seek information regarding treatment plans and medical progress. Differences in race and ethnicity, education level, and cultural backgrounds are significant and can impact the prospective psychological benefits as a result of Internet use and other modes of communication among women with breast cancer.

Profiling Health Seekers

While Internet use has increased among all demographic groups, access is greatest among those most educated with higher incomes. Per earlier reports, access was least significant among African Americans and Hispanics who trailed whites and Asian Americans.[16] This phenomenon contributes to the digital divide or exclusion and stands to impact education and health quality, access, and availability.[17-20] According to the National Telecommunications and Information Association,[21] Internet use and online activities have significantly increased in more recent years. More recent reporting by Statista indicates that "roughly 76.2% of the U.S. population accessed the Internet as of 2016. While Internet adoption in the United States is equal amongst both genders, online usage increases among demographic groups with higher levels of education and income,"[22] Statista data shows that 2018 Internet use by race and/or ethnicity for whites, Hispanics, and African Americans was 89%, 88%, and 87%, respectively.[23]

While the primary use of the Internet is email, users tend to engage in a myriad of online activities, such as email, use of search engine, finding health information, getting news updates, and purchasing products, as shown in **TABLE PR-1**.

Table PR-1 indicates that the percentage of users seeking health information is roughly 80% for all U.S. adults Internet users. Generation X (age 35–46) showed the highest use of health information, and this is followed by Older Boomers (age 57–65), while the G.I. Generation (over age 75) showed the lowest percentage at 73%. Internet use, however, was highest among millennials (age 18–34), and this figure declines by generation. Despite these numbers, a recent Michigan State University Extension briefing reported (based on a 2018 Pew Internet and American Life Project) that 80% of Internet users, or about 93 million Americans, say they have looked online for health-related information within the last year. This is an increase of 18% from 2001, when only 62% of Internet users went online to research health-related topics.[24]

TABLE PR-1 Online Activities (Percent of Internet By Generation/Age)

Activity	Millennials Ages 18–34 (%)	Gen X Ages 35–46 (%)	Younger Boomers Ages 47–56 (%)	Older Boomers Ages 57–65 (%)	Silent Gen. Ages 66–74 (%)	G.I.Gen. Age 75+ (%)	All Online Adults Age 18+ (%)
Go online	95	86	81	76	58	30	79
For the following activities, the youngest and oldest cohorts may differ, but there is less variation between generations overall:							
E-mail	96	94	91	93	90	88	94
Use search engine	92	97	86	87	82	72	87
Look for health info	78	84	80	83	73	69	80
Get news	76	79	76	76	67	54	75
Buy a product	68	66	64	69	59	57	66

Pew Internet and American Life Project (2011). Findings for individual activities are based on adult internet users. For survey dates of all activities citied, please see the Methodology section at the end of the Generations 2010 report: http://pewinternet.org/Reports/2010/Generations-2010/Methodology/Note-on-survey-dates.aspx

A survey conducted by the Pew Internet and American Life Project[21] indicated that 8 of 10 Internet users seek health information online. Eighty-two percent of the women and 75% of the men surveyed by Pew indicated that they sought health information online. **TABLE PR-2** offers a profile of the health information seekers as informed by the Pew survey. Seventy-eight percent of the samples were between ages 50 and 64 while 71% had a high school education or less.

Using Pew Internet and American Life data from 2006, several key observations can be observed using the Internet for health information (**TABLE PR-3**):

■ Of the 537 survey participants in the study, 79% of Internet users investigated at least 1 of 16 health topics.
■ In comparison to 60% of the men surveyed, 71% of the women participants searched for a specific disease or medical problem.

TABLE PR-2 Health Seekers from Pew Internet and American Life Project

Demographic Group	Percent Who Have Looked for Health Information Online
Online women	82
Online men	77
Internet users ages 18–29	79
Internet users ages 30–49	84
Internet users ages 50–64	78
Internet users ages 65+	68
Internet users with a high school diploma or less	71
Internet users with some college education	80
Internet users with a college degree	89
Internet users with 2–3 years of online experience	62
Internet users with 6+ years of online experience	86
Internet users with a dial-up connection at home	75
Internet users with a broadband connection at home	86

Pew Internet and American Life Project, August 2006 survey ($n = 1990$). Margin of error for the entire sample of Internet users is ±3%. Margins of error for comparison of subgroups are higher.

TABLE PR-3   Health Topics Searches from the 2006 Pew Internet and American Life Project

In all, 80 percent of Internet users have looked online for at least 1 of 17 health topics. Certain subgroups reported significantly higher interest in some topics and are marked in bold type. For example, when compared with online men, online women reported significantly more interest in information about specific diseases, certain treatments, diet, and mental health.

Health Topic	All Internet Users (n = 1990) %	Online Women (n = 1116) %	Online Men (n = 874) %	Ages 18–29 (n = 333) %	Ages 30–49 (n = 751) %	Ages 50–64 (n = 579) %	Ages 65+ (n = 277) %	High School or Less (n = 614) %	Some College (n = 510) %	College Graduates (n = 853) %
Specific disease or medical problem	64	**69**	58	61	67	64	54	52	**65**	**74**
Certain medical treatment	51	**54**	47	45	**56**	51	40	41	**51**	**62**
Diet, nutrition, vitamins	49	**53**	45	45	**55**	19	29	40	**52**	**56**
Exercise or fitness	44	46	41	**55**	**47**	35	24	35	**47**	**51**
Prescription or over-the-counter drugs	37	39	35	29	**42**	**40**	30	29	**38**	**45**

(continues)

TABLE PR-3   Health Topics Searches from the 2006 Pew Internet and American Life Project   *(continued)*

In all, 80 percent of Internet users have looked online for at least 1 of 17 health topics. Certain subgroups reported significantly higher interest in some topics and are marked in bold type. For example, when compared with online men, online women reported significantly more interest in information about specific diseases, certain treatments, diet, and mental health.

Health Topic	All Internet Users (n = 1990) %	Online Women (n = 1116) %	Online Men (n = 874) %	Ages 18–29 (n = 333) %	Ages 30–49 (n = 751) %	Ages 50–64 (n = 579) %	Ages 65+ (n = 277) %	High School or Less (n = 614) %	Some College (n = 510) %	College Graduates (n = 853) %
A particular doctor or hospital	29	31	27	27	**33**	26	18	21	**25**	**40**
Health insurance	28	27	29	23	**34**	27	12	20	**28**	**37**
Alternative treatments or medicines	27	29	25	25	29	29	14	22	**29**	**31**
Depression, anxiety, stress, or mental health issues	22	**26**	17	25	24	20	7	21	24	22
Environmental health hazards	22	21	22	25	23	22	10	16	**23**	**26**

Experimental treatments or medicines	18	19	18	19	18	14	15	**21**	**20**
Immunizations or vaccinations	16	17	**18**	**18**	12	7	13	15	**19**
Dental health information	15	15	17	16	12	6	13	14	**16**
Medicare or Medicaid	13	13	10	11	15	22	12	14	13
Sexual health information	11	12	**21**	10	7	2	10	**15**	10
How to quit smoking	9	8	**13**	8	9	3	11	10	7
Problems with drugs or alcohol	8	8	**14**	6	7	2	8	**10**	7

Margin of error for the entire sample of Internet users is ±3%. Margins of error for comparison of subgroups are higher. Significant differences between demographic groups are in **bold** type.
Pew Internet and American Life Project, August 2006 survey ($n = 1990$).

■ Women sought more information related to depression/stress/mental illness and smoking than did men.

■ Internet searches on a specific disease or medical condition were significant and comparable among those with some college education and those who have completed college.

Table PR-3 highlights additional significant differences among demographic groups (noted in blue).

While these data highlight consumer behaviors, recent findings by Fox and Duggan (2013) of the Pew Internet Project suggest that there is a shift from health seeking to self-diagnosis modalities.[25] Pew considers this diagnostic behavior and characterizes these users as "online diagnosers." Via online information seeking, diagnosers often determine if they will utilize health services as well as the point of care. Diagnosers tend to be white, female, younger, earn more than $75,000 annually, and are college graduates with undergraduate or graduate degrees. The Internet and ICTs provide the tool to facilitate these online to offline health behaviors, and lead 53% of all surveyed diagnosers to seek the clinical expertise of physicians.

▶ II. Accessing Health Information Beyond the Internet

While the Internet has proven to be a means of health information dissemination and a commonly used tool among health seekers and diagnosers, there are populations that are best reached via other communication modalities or that chose not to engage in online use. While issues associated with digital divide, divide inequity, and social exclusion[26,27] have been used to rationalize the resistance among non-Internet users for going online, interesting

facts exist to demonstrate the need for targeted strategies.

Research[28] has shown that health divides are not limited to technology access. Rather, cultural, racial, and gender intersections can allow user identities to be encapsulated into online artifacts to improve online health information seeking. As Kvasny and Payton[29] delineated, this encapsulation requires details of and attention to platform design, privacy, relatability, respectability politics, and environmental context (referred to as "silence on campus" in their study).

▶ III. Alternative Means of Accessing Health Information

Interesting enough, alternative communication modes and health information dissemination can capture the diversity of social, economic, ethnic, racial, gender, and educational backgrounds of the healthcare populations in a specific region or community. For instance, the MyHealthImpact Project[30] has targeted African American college students to create sexual and mental health awareness. Starting with HIV awareness, the project initially focused on African American females and evolved to include issues around mental health. MyHealthImpact was created using participatory design with the intention of providing the target population with both consumption and creation roles. **FIGURES PR-1** and **PR-2** are MyHealthImpact screen captures which highlight the blog, health facts, social media, and video content.

In a survey of 327 Hispanics alongside a series of planned focus group interviews, the researchers determined the top 10 ways the targeted Los Angeles Hispanic community seeks health information. From these data,

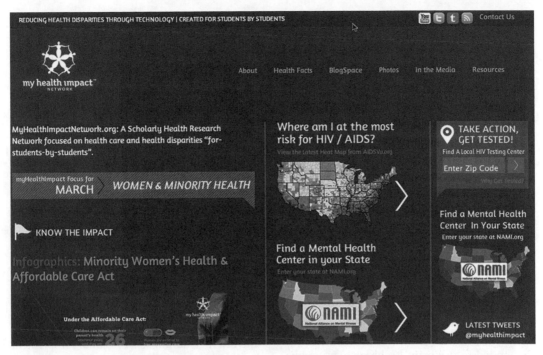

FIGURE PR-1 MyHealthImpact Screen Capture 1.

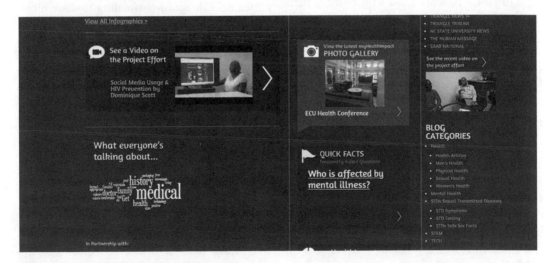

FIGURE PR-2 MyHealthImpact Screen Capture 2.

they also determined the most cited referral sources. They found that: (1) over a third (35%) of the Hispanics in the study received their health and medical care information via television; (2) discussions with friends and family on the telephone are pivotal (slightly over 30%); (3) a smaller sample (about 22%) consulted with care providers;

and (4) radio and print media (newspapers, books, magazines, leaflets, folders) should not be ignored. More importantly, Latino men play a pivotal role as influencers in women's lives and should not be ignored. Accordingly, the researchers concluded, "increased education while maintaining control by the men may influence increased support of early detection and medical care of Latina women."[31(p. 375)]

Others[32] have investigated the relationship between race and use of health information resources. In a random-digit dialed survey of 509 women (341 white, 135 African American, and 33 of other races), Nicholson et al.[33] investigated the independent effect of race on women's use of health information resources. Print, news, broadcast media, Internet, health organizations, and organized health events were among the sources of information in their study. Women with higher education levels tended to use print health or news media, broadcast media, health policy organizations, and organized events 2.0–2.4 times more than less educated women (high school education or less); these findings, however, were not statistically significant. Increasingly, more than 40% of white women used the Internet compared to 20% of African American women. Whites, however, used health policy and other organizations three times more than African Americans.

▶ IV. Future Directions

The literature demonstrates that implementation of multiple access points to health information is critical. The profile of the information seeker/participant in medical studies, particularly longitudinal investigations, has an essential role in the interpretation of health outcomes, reducing disparities, and health dissemination. A single communication mode or approach will and does not attract diverse populations to medical studies, clinical trials, or sites intended to disseminate online health information. Digital equity is pivotal to this notion along with awareness of cultural-competent and relevance approaches to healthcare delivery. Social networking among online healthcare support groups continues to proliferate and often drives offline behaviors and care services utilization. Despite the proliferation of the Internet, administrators should implement multiple communication modalities (mobile phones, television, print media, and radio) and then provide multi-channeling to disseminate the information, reaching out to diverse socioeconomic, cultural, and global populations. As our prior work[34,35] concluded, web designers and content creators are encouraged to engage communities, think and do inclusive computing, and assess equity in your healthcare online seeking applications. The MyHealthImpact network offers a starting point to do so.

Notes

1. Payton, F., Pare, G., LeRouge, C., & Reddy, M. (2011). Health care IT: Process, people and patients and interdisciplinary considerations. *Journal of the Association of Information Systems—Special Issues on Health Care IT, 12,* 2.
2. *Ibid.*
3. Mureo, M., & Rice, R. E. (2006). *The internet and health care: Theory, research and practice.* Mahwah, NJ: Lawrence Erlbaum Associates.
4. Pew Research Center—FactTank. (2014). The social life of health information. Retrieved from www.pewresearch.org/fact-tank/2014/01/15/the-social-life-of-health-information/
5. *Ibid.*
6. Paek, H. J., Bae, B. J., Hove, T., & Yu, H. (2011). Theories into practice: A content analysis of anti-smoking websites. *Internet Research, 21*(1), 5–25.
7. Payton, F. C., & Kvasny, L. (2016). Technology affordance–Maybe Not: The case of stigmatized health conditions. *Journal of the American Medical Informatics Association,* 1–6. doi:10.1093/jamia/ocw017
8. Pew Research Center—FactTank, (2014), *ibid.*
9. Paek et al., (2011), *ibid.*
10. Payton & Kvasny, (2016), *ibid.*
11. Turner, J. W., Grube, J. A., & Meyers, J. (2001). Developing an optimal match within online

communities: An exploration of CMC support communities and traditional support. *Journal of Communication, 51*, 231–251.

12. Ziebland, S., Chapple, A., Dumelow, C., Evans, J., Prinjha, S., & Rozmovitis, L. (2004). How the internet affects patients' experience of cancer: A qualitative study. *BMJ*. Retrieved from www.bmj.com /content/328/7439/564

13. World Health Organization. (2006). Retrieved from www.who.int/mediacentre/news/releases/2006/pr06 /en/

14. Fogel, J., Albert, S. M., Schnabel, F., Ditokk, B. A., & Neugut, A. I. (2003). Racial/ethnic differences and potential psychological benefits in use of the internet by women with breast cancer. *Psycho-Oncology, 12*, 107–117.

15. Barnett, G. A., & Hwang, J. M. (2006). The use of the internet for health information and social support: A content analysis of online breast cancer discussion groups. In M. Mureo & R. E. Rice (Eds.), *The internet and health care: Theory, research and practice.* Mahwah, NJ: Lawrence Erlbaum Associates.

16. National Science Board. (2006). *Science and engineering indicators.* Arlington, VA: National Science Foundation.

17. Zarcadoolas, C., Pleasant, A., & Greer, D. S. (2006). *Advancing health literacy: A framework for understanding and action.* San Francisco, CA: Jossey-Bass.

18. Payton, F. C. (2008). Digital divide or digital equity: Other considerations? In W. A. Darity Jr. (Eds.), *International encyclopedia of the social sciences* (2nd ed., vol. 9). Detroit, MI: Macmillan Reference USA.

19. Kvasny, L., & Payton, F. C. (2007). Minorities and information technology: Critical issues and trends in digital divide research. In M. Khosrow-Pour (Eds.), *Encyclopedia of information science and technology* (2nd ed.). Hershey, PA: IGI Publisher.

20. Pew Internet & American Life Project. (2006). Online Health Search 2006. Retrieved from www .pewInternet.org/pdfs/PIP_Online_Health_2006 .pdf

21. Internet usage in the United States—Statistics and facts. Retrieved from www.statista.com/topics/2237 /Internet-usage-in-the-united-states/

22. *Ibid.*

23. Share of adults in the United States who use the Internet in 2018, by ethnicity. Retrieved from www.statista .com/statistics/327134/Internet-usage-usa-ethnicity/

24. Demitz, C., & Beyer, M. (2018). Health information on the Internet. Retrieved from www.canr.msu.edu /news/health_information_on_the_Internet

25. Fox, S., & Duggan, M. (2013). Health Online 2013. Retrieved from www.pewInternet.org/2013/01/15 /health-online-2013/

26. *Ibid.*

27. Kvasny, L., & Payton, F. C. (2018). Managing hypervisibility in the HIV prevention information seeking practices of black female college students. *Journal of the Association for Information Science and Technology, 69*(6), 798–806.

28. Kvasny & Payton, (2018), *ibid.*

29. *Ibid.*

30. Kvasny & Payton, (2018), *ibid*, 5.

31. Erwin, D. O., Johnson, V. A., Trevino, M., Duke, K., Feliciano, L., & Jandorf, L. (2006). A comparison of African American and Latina social networks as indicators for culturally tailoring a breast and cervical cancer education intervention. *Cancer Supplement, 109*(2), 368–377.

32. Nicholson, W. K., Grason, H. A., & Powe, N. R. (2003). The relationship of race to women's use of health information resources. *American Journal of Obstetrics and Gynecology, 188*(2), 580–585.

33. Nicholson et al., *ibid.*

34. Payton & Kvasny, (2016), *ibid.*

35. Kvasny & Payton, (2018), *ibid.*

Biographies

Fay Cobb Payton, PhD, is Full Professor of Information Technology at North Carolina State University. She is a named University Faculty Scholar for her leadership in turning research into solutions to society's most pressing issues. The *National Science Foundation, National Institutes of Health, AT&T, Kenan Institute*, and others have supported her research and teaching. Her research focuses on the social and technical impacts of technology innovations, particularly on health care, STEM workforce, the arts, and education domains. Payton earned a PhD in Information and Decision Systems from Case Western Reserve University.

Lynette Yarger, PhD, is an associate professor in the College of Information Sciences and Technology at the Pennsylvania State University. She is also the 2018–2019

Administrative Fellow in the Office of the Vice President for Information Technology/CIO. Her research program, supported by the *National Science Foundation,* examines how underserved groups utilize information and communication technologies to improve their quality of life. Yarger earned a PhD in Computer Information Systems from the Robinson College of Business at Georgia State University.

MINI-CASE (PART I)

Ginger.io: Mental Health Behavioral Analytics

Phillip Olla and Greg Moon

▶ I. Introduction

Ginger.io was launched in 2011 as a behavioral health analytics startup, incorporating the features of a smartphone as *automated diaries,* to provide critical insight into a person's mental wellbeing. Smartphones generate substantial data that could help interpret our behavior, including locations visited, calling patterns, and texting frequency, as well as actual applications used. Collectively, these activities plot out a user's daily patterns.[1]

▶ II. Commercialization

In 2014, Ginger.io launched a commercial app, which was an accumulation of research from the MIT Media Lab. The app could passively analyze the mobile data to detect if a patient with mental illness, such as depression, anxiety and bipolar disorders, or schizophrenia, was symptomatic. Importantly, having the capability to discover meaningful deviations from anticipated behaviors in the user's daily patterns could be an indication that something may be wrong.

The symptoms the Ginger.io commercial app detected included lethargy, which was captured by motion sensors, accelerometers, or intermittent texting. If the app detects an unusual pattern, it sends a text to both the patient and the care provider, who can keep tabs and intervene if necessary. The app was implemented as a pilot in multiple settings for a variety of health conditions. Some of the sites included:

- University of California at San Francisco (UCSF), for exploring the role behavioral data plays in heart disease.
- Forsyth Medical Center in North Carolina, for studying how data could help to determine the behavioral differences in diabetes patients.
- University of California at Davis (UCD), as a low-cost method of monitoring psychosis.

▶ III. Moving Forward

Today, Ginger.io is a very successful pioneer of digital mental health, having raised over $20 million in 2015 to launch a commercial offering of the platform. But in the early days, they encountered challenges understanding the *customer business needs.* Digital health innovators believe they understand health systems' business needs; however, they are not always on track.

A greater understanding of health system customers' perceived needs, pressures, and priorities might have driven Ginger.io to an entirely different conclusion. Innovator companies tend not to seek this critical input before embarking on development. Ginger.io embarked on the UCD-based development journey, concluding that the solution needed to embody three core elements:

   i.   a completely passive use model,
   ii. trustable privacy and security, and
   iii. a means of effectuating follow-up.[2]

Armed with a solution designed to meet patients' needs, plus health economic data indicating that their approach could increase quality and decrease costs, the company was able to secure commercial engagements with leading health systems. However, they soon discovered that their product was *too* effective at identifying potentially depressed individuals, and that case managers and behavioral health services were overwhelmed with new cases that could not be absorbed.

"We learned a lot in the early days and have the scars to prove it," says Karan Singh, Ginger.io cofounder. "The actual problem facing patients and the health systems turned out to be *care access,* not a lack of depression identification." Fortunately for the company, this hard-won epiphany also fueled a critical business evolution, resulting in their becoming the network for providing care.

▶ IV. Takeaway

The lesson from the Giner.io's initial experiences was that a well-informed solution for a compelling user need automatically translates into a salable product. This outcome is often not the case in the world of health care as the end-user(s) and the paying customer are usually not the same stakeholder, and the first-order analysis of the paying stakeholder's pain points—most often financial and operational—has been neglected in the ideation and development process.

In order to create a market niche for Ginger.io's innovative app across different care institutions to improve monitoring of mental health patients, the stage is now set to challenge conventional approaches in the care of these patients. What directions and potential marketing options would Ginger.io have to take in the coming years to best ensure the startup app that the steps it had nurtured to date will continue to grow meaningfully, especially amidst rapid competition from major technology companies trying to enter the mental health patient analytics market?

Notes

1. Retrieved from www.ginger.io/
2. Madala, S., McCutcheon, S., Denend, L., & Zanchi, M. G. (2017). *User-focused ideation and design: Ginger.io.* (Case BIOE273-3). Stanford, CA: Stanford University, Byers Center for BioDesign.

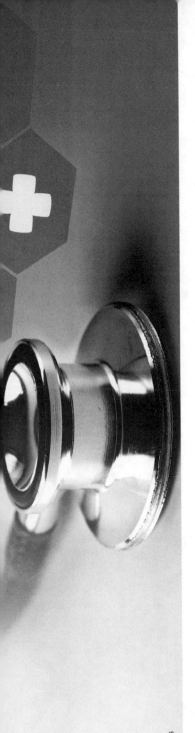

PART II

HMIS Technology and Applications

CHAPTER 4

Data in Digital Health Systems

Siti A. Arshad-Snyder

Scenario: Network Connectivity for Connected Health in U.S. Health System[1]

Network connectivity is transforming healthcare services delivery in today's U.S. health systems. With a secure, 24/7 network, medical devices and other health IT tools can remain connected to their digital environments so that care providers can access, interact, and share relevant health data and information more safely, efficiently, and ubiquitously. In turn, this will afford caregivers more time to spend interacting with patients and their extended family members.

Based on 2016 statistics released by John Hopkins' researchers, medical errors, including errors with technology, digital tools, and connectivity, now stand as the third leading cause of death in the United States, just behind heart disease and cancer. Health systems organizations should therefore work with their IT department to ensure availability of digital tools 24/7 and that the entire team is working toward removing errors from the systems in order to protect patients from poorly functioning equipment.

Over the past few years, connected health conceptualization has grown to include tablets, smartphones, Internet of Things (IoT) devices, and an increasing host of health monitors. All of these devices are continually linked and can constantly deliver timely information into the electronic health records (EHR), other administrative software, and health IT tools that are also connected to the network, ensuring that all pertinent information are available, accessible, and meaningfully used by clinical caregivers and other care specialists as and when needed.

The fact that appropriate and necessary care can only be provided based on timely information transmitted from connected devices makes the connectivity of health networks a critical component in any health IT infrastructure. Shafiq Rab, Senior Vice President and CIO of Rush University Medical Center, noted to HITInfrastructure.com.

"Information is liquid gold . . . Getting the right information at the right time for the right person in the right format, securely, every time is very important … . In the world of healthcare, the choices we need to make can be critical life and death decisions."

Often, all of such health information exchange is delivered in packets that travel over the network, whether via hardwired connections or Wi-Fi. "A reliable network needs to work 100% of the time. Not 99.99% of the time - all the time," Rab continued. "In the world of health care, information has become part of the standard of care." Wireless is becoming ubiquitous; sensor-based and cellular devices are also rapidly advancing. If organizations want timely information delivered without any latency, a reliable network is a must. Patients rely on the network and also use "connected tools to learn how to navigate their stay, such as learning when the cafeteria is open, or even to check their email to keep in touch with home."

Imagine you are asked to survey caregivers, as well as patients, on what their needs are, and to then work with the IT department on specifying the requirements for such a 24/7 network-connected infrastructure which would support modern care delivery. Speculate on the type of answers you believe you would hear from the different stakeholders and who or what you think should or might be blamed if the different stakeholders were faced with any shortcomings or delays after the IT department implemented such a network infrastructure?

▶ I. Introduction

The Office of the National Coordinator (ONC) of Health Information Technology (HIT) reported that the percentage of hospitals in the United States that allow patients to access their medical records online went up from 10% in 2013 to 69% in 2015.[2] This multi-fold increase is a manifestation of the significant change that has occurred in the nation's healthcare delivery system. This change has been made possible by the use of EHR as a mechanism for the collection and storage of digital healthcare data. This chapter provides an overview on healthcare data, the sources of such data, and the use as a primary and secondary data sources, as well as issues and trends related to it.

▶ II. Background

The push for EHR in health care has been a driver behind the vast accumulation of electronic data. Further, the massive accumulation of health data and the recent shift to value-care in health care have intensified the need for quality data in health systems organizations. Health systems organizations are relying more on data in their efforts to improve patient care outcomes, increase patient satisfaction, manage community health, and reduce healthcare costs. Industry experts predict that data and

data analytics will play a bigger role in influencing healthcare outcomes, particularly in disease prevention and population health.[3,4]

Understandably, the amount of data that will be amassed by health systems will continue to grow. In fact, for the period of between 2013 and 2020, health data are expected to grow at the rate of 48%. This represents an increase of 8% higher than the overall data growth in other industries, which thus makes it one of the fastest growing industries in terms of data collection and accumulation.[5] Considering the predicted growth rate, the volume of health data accumulated by the year 2020 will be about 2314 exabytes—a massive increase from 153 exabytes amassed in 2013.[6]

Just how much is an exabyte? **TABLE 4-1** shows the units of digital storage size capacity.

This growth prediction of healthcare data suggests that data will continue to be a critical element of healthcare data analytics and

TABLE 4-1 Units of Digital Storage Size Capacity

Unit	Symbol Designation	Size
bit	b	1 bit
byte	B	1 byte
kilobyte	KB	1,000 bytes = 1000^1 bytes
megabyte	MB	1,000,000 bytes = 1000^2 bytes
gigabyte	GB	1,000,000,000 bytes = 1000^3 bytes
terabyte	TB	1,000,000,000,000 bytes = 1000^4 bytes
petabyte	PB	1,000,000,000,000,000 bytes = 1000^5 bytes
exabyte	EB	1,000,000,000,000,000,000 bytes = 1000^6 bytes
zettabyte	ZB	1,000,000,000,000,000,000,000 bytes = 1000^7 bytes
yottabyte	YB	1,000,000,000,000,000,000,000,000 bytes = 1000^8 bytes

informatics. Data analytics is concerned with "... the analysis of large volumes of data and/or high-velocity data."[7] Clinicians rely on patient data to develop, execute, monitor, and evaluate treatment plans; healthcare administrators and managers make administrative and operational decisions based on the information derived from data; and public health specialists use data to manage community health. Altogether, health data allow clinicians, administrators, and researchers to transform these data into information that is valuable for many uses and purposes within the healthcare services delivery system, such as patient outcome optimization, healthcare cost management, operational efficiencies, and public health.

▶ III. Healthcare Data

In health care, data are collected from various sources for various purposes. Naturally, health data are collected for patient care. Beyond patient care, data are used for other purposes that benefit patients, organizations, and communities. Primarily, health data are used to:

- Improve the quality of patient care
- Improve clinical outcomes
- Receive financial payments
- Analyze care delivery costs
- Identify unmet health needs in communities
- Assess and monitor public health
- Plan use of healthcare resources for workflow optimization, staffing, and strategic planning

In health informatics, data serve as input for various capabilities of data analytics. As informatics continue to be embraced by, and incorporated into, the health services delivery system, data will not only be an essential asset in health systems organizations but will also be a leveraged resource to meet organizations' operational and strategic objectives, including clinical–administrative outcomes.

Data v. Information

It is not uncommon for some people to use the terms *data* and *information* interchangeably. Notwithstanding, these terms are not interchangeable and do not mean the same thing. Indeed, healthcare data do not equate to healthcare information.

Healthcare data refer to individual pieces of fact. In health systems organizations, electronic data are stored in databases. Each datum may be in the form of alphabets, numbers, images, signs, and so on. Some examples of health data are patient last name, temperature, and date of admission. In and of themselves, data offer little or no meaning; they must have context to be meaningful. A collection of data is called a *dataset*. Consider the following text in **EXHIBIT 4-1**.

As is, it would be difficult to determine what these data represent. Now, consider the following information presented in **TABLE 4-2**.

The same data has now been contextualized, and the association between these data has been established. It could be determined that Mary John who is 6 years old, 41 inches tall, and weighs 79 pounds is a patient of Dr. William Smith and has a temperature of 102.2°F. When the temperature of the patient is compared to a normal body temperature, it is determined that the patient has a fever. This, in essence, is information. *Information* is conceived by processing raw data to give meaning and context for the given data. Data are the building blocks or inputs for information.

EXHIBIT 4-1 Sample Textual Data

John Mary 6 41 79 102.2 William Smith White Chris 2 36 32 98.4 Johnson Gary

TABLE 4-2 Contextualized Information of Exhibit 4-1

Last Name	First Name	Age	Height (in Inches)	Weight (in Pounds)	Temperature (in Fahrenheit)	Physician
John	Mary	6	41	79	102.2	William Smith
White	Chris	2	36	32	98.4	Gary Johnson

TABLE 4-3 A Summary of Types and Sources of Data for Each Data Type

Sources	Data Types
Handwritten notes and drawings; signed patient consent form	Document image data
Laboratory orders/results; medication orders/medication administration records; online charting and documentation, detailed charges	Discrete structured data
Digital radiography (DR); computerized radiography (CR), computerized axial tomography (CT); magnetic resonance imaging (MRI); pathology images	Diagnostic image data
EKG/EEG/fetal signal tracings	Vector graphic data
Heart sound; voice annotations	Audio data
Ultrasound; cardiac catheterization examinations	Video data
Transcribed radiology and pathology reports; itemized bills other transcribed reports	Unstructured text data

Data from Kohn, D. (2010). The role of content management in electronic health records. Presentation presented at the AIIM Golden Gate Chapter Meeting, San Francisco, CA. Retrieved October 2017 from http://daksystemsconsulting.com/html/webArchive/AIIMGG2010-05-25EHR.pdf

Data Sources

In health care, patients are the source of data. Data about patients are often collected by health systems organizations or care providers. Healthcare data can be categorized into seven data types. **TABLE 4-3** summarizes types and sources of data for each type.

Therefore, a patient's health data can be in any form; for example, patient history and lab result data are more likely to be in the form of discrete data, whereas physician's transcribed notes from a patient consultation are stored as *unstructured* text data. *Discrete data* are structured data that are in the most basic form; specifically, in a database, discrete data are stored at the lowest level of granularity. At this level, data cannot be broken down into further detail. For instance, the data, "*46-year-old female*" are not at the lowest level of granularity because the data may be broken down into *age* (46), and *gender* (female). Discrete data are clearly defined, searchable, and readily available for analysis. *Unstructured text* data, on the other hand, are freeform, undefined data—usually in text format, and contain alphabetic, numeric, and other special characters. This type of data is not searchable and may require extensive processing before it can be used for analysis.

In contrast, X-rays, voice recordings, and recordings of an ultrasound procedure are stored in multimedia formats, such as audio, video, vector graphic, or image format. Prior to the implementation of EHR, patient records were stored in paper format. When these paper records are digitized by means of scanning, the records are converted into digital image format, therefore making it possible to store the data in a computer database instead of physically stored paper records. Nevertheless, the contents of the digitized files are not in discrete format and are therefore not readily available for analysis.

Regardless of the format of data, health data are typically about patients, such as patient illness history, patient demographics, patient insurance, inpatient data, patient's physician, and more. Thus, patients are the sources of data in healthcare services. Patient data are mostly collected and generated during patient registration, consultation with clinicians, diagnostic lab and radiology procedures, and during inpatient stays. The data are stored in various data repositories and are used for a variety of purposes.

- *Primary and Secondary Data*: Data that are used for the purpose related to the original reason for why they were collected are considered as *primary data*. In health care, patient-level data are collected for medical care services in clinical settings. Data may be classified as: (1) clinical data; (2) administration data; and (3) financial data. Clinical data are those data relating to patient health and care, for example, patient billing, insurance, and payment data. Administrative data are those collected and used by the administration to

make decisions about the overall operation of the organization; for instance, when a patient fills out a survey following an inpatient stay, the patient will essentially be providing feedback to the hospital administration regarding the patient's experience during that stay. This type of survey will most likely be used by the hospital to collect data about patient satisfaction and will not be used by clinical staff in making decisions related to the patient treatment; nor will the billing department use these data to bill the patients. Instead, the data will most likely be used for quality improvement initiatives.

The use of patient data is not restricted to medical treatments or other administrative decisions that may pertain to individual patients. De-identified patient data can be used for other purposes, such as research, disease monitoring, public health, benchmarking, and marketing. The National Institute of Standards and Technology (NIST) defines identifiers as "information used to claim an identity, before a potential corroboration by a corresponding authenticator",[8] while indirect identifier is defined as "information that can be used to identify an individual through association".[9] The removal of identifiers from patient data can safeguard patient privacy and confidentiality, which can therefore allow the data to be stored in various data warehouses, registries, and other databases in the public domain as *secondary data* sources.

- *Secondary Data*: These are data used for purposes other than the original reason(s) for their collection. In addition to having identifiers removed, this type of data source may also be stored in aggregate format where individual data are compiled, consolidated, and summarized, which makes associating such data with a specific patient impossible. A registry is a type of secondary data source that comprises of a collection of health data related to a specific medical procedure or health condition. Clinical registries are repositories that typically contain non-identifiable patient data that have been grouped by certain medical conditions (such as breast cancer) or procedures (such as bypass surgery). Examples of registries are the National and State Cancer Registries, Alzheimer's Prevention Registry, and Development of a National Incompatible Kidney Transplant Registry.[10] The availability of data from these registries lends itself greatly to evidence-based clinical practice, improvement of patient care, quality improvement initiatives, and research projects.

Many aggregated state-level healthcare data—another variation of secondary data—can also be accessed online. Most of the state data are presented in high-level summary and/or in visual format, such as graph or charts. The U.S. National Library of Medicine website (https://www.nlm.nih.gov) provides a compilation of various data repositories, including those containing state data.

- Secondary Data for Public Use: HealthData.gov is a data-sharing platform that offers an extensive collection of data to the public. Data are linked to various sources, such as Centers for Medicare and Medicaid (CMM), Centers for Disease Control and Prevention (CDC), Food and Drug Administration (FDA), and National Institute of Health (NIH). The goal of this governmental organization is to make ". . . high value health data more accessible to entrepreneurs, researchers, and policy makers in the hopes of better health outcomes for all".[11] Datasets are organized by topics related to health, community, public safety, finance, business, and others. With respect to health care, almost 2000

datasets can be found, covering, among others, chronic diseases, nutrition, drug use, life expectancy, mortality rates, and hospital quality of care data.

• *The Value of Data in Non-Clinical Setting*: EHR adoption has transformed the delivery of health care. Although the main benefit associated with the use of electronic data is in the context of clinical care, many potential benefits exist beyond clinical settings.

- Data for Fraud Detection & Controls: The role of data in intercepting and detecting healthcare frauds as well as improper practices is evident. In 2016, the Department of Health and Human Services (DHHS) joined forces with state and federal agencies in an operation known as the National Health Care Fraud Takedown that brought to justice about 300 individuals who filed $900 million worth of fraudulent Medicare and Medicaid claims.[12] One of the factors that contributed to the success of this operation was the availability of data from the CMM. Additionally, the U.S. Department of Justice reported that the government successfully litigated and ordered pharmaceutical company Wyeth and Pfizer Inc. to pay around $785 to the federal government and Medicaid for alleged deceitful business practices.[13] These cases demonstrated the value of data in verifying transactions and ensuring compliance.

In 2017, the National Health Care Anti-Fraud Association (NHCAA) launched an online database that ". . .allows authorized users to effectively share critical information about suspected fraudulent activity throughout the country".[14(p. 5)] This aspect of information sharing can accelerate the speed of information dispersion and anti-fraud efforts, which indirectly helps control healthcare expenditures and, to some degree, ensures patient safety.[15]

- *Data for Quality Improvement*: As healthcare delivery places emphasis on value-based care, it is important for health systems organizations to be able to assess the care they provide by accurately and meaningfully measuring various outcome levels, such as safety, patient-centeredness, timeliness of care, and efficiency. Equally important is the assessment of the organization's operational efficiency. In the context of health systems organization operations, some of the common categories with respect to quality projects that involve data are benchmarking, cost reduction, revenue optimization, and facility management.[16] Data allow organizations to measure their performance, identify areas where they excel and fall short, and make informed decisions about how to capitalize their strengths and/or to make systematic improvements on their weaknesses.

▶ ## IV. Issues and Problems Related to Health Data

As more health data are being collected and stored, greater dependency is placed on the quality of these data in many aspects of healthcare services delivery. Unfortunately, digital data that are meant to enhance the quality and cost efficiency of care have also posed many challenges.

Data Errors and Quality Issues

As health systems organizations embrace the notion of health care as a data-driven industry, they are actively and rapidly collecting data as part of their daily operations. The EHR systems are all intended to provide an effective and efficient way to collect data. Even so, despite the most carefully designed EHR systems and the best efforts of those who enter data, no EHR system can guarantee error-free data. Errors found in health data, such as erroneous patient identifiers, spelling errors, and missing data, degrade the overall quality of data, in turn affecting the quality and safety of care services delivery.

The quality of data may be reduced by a number of factors. Some of the common contributing factors include:

- *Data Entry Errors*: This type of error is generally a result of human errors, and may be caused by typographical errors or by clicking on incorrect checkbox options or buttons. Some systems have a default value for a certain data field, which is intended to speed up data entry. However, this may also cause erroneous data entry if the default value does not reflect the correct data to be entered and if the person who enters the data does not change the default value.
- *Incomplete Data*: Missing data in a dataset may result in flawed data. For example, a patient data that includes some, but not all, of the patient's medications is considered an incomplete dataset.
- *Incorrect Input*: Miscommunication between a patient and healthcare provider may contribute to unreliable data. Clinicians might not ask the right questions and thus fail to get the right information. Additionally, patients may either misinterpret questions or not fully understand the question and inadvertently provide an unexpected answer. Patients may also offer only partial information. Cultural and language differences may play a role in poor communication.
- *Data Omission*: Whether intentional or unintentional, data omission results from not entering required data for a variety of reasons. For instance, a patient may not have certain information available at the time when patient data are being recorded, which may result in the person entering the patient's data to skip the data

entry for that particular data item. It is also possible for a user to accidentally skip a data entry item when navigating the data entry screen. Fatigue and time pressure are a couple of factors that can contribute to unintentional data omission.

- *Poorly Designed System*: A convoluted user interface screen design may frustrate and confuse physicians, nurses, and other users of a system. Likewise, data entry text fields that are not clearly labeled may be confusing to users and thus may result in incorrect data entry.

The quality of data can directly impact the value of information derived from it, which can ultimately affect the quality of patient care, as well as healthcare operational efficiency and success. Clinical practitioners rely on patient data to make patient treatment plan decisions, while health systems organization administrators rely on data for strategic and tactical decisions. If data are erroneous, they may lead to flawed conclusions, decisions, and/or actions—any or all of which may bring about unintended negative consequences.

Data Privacy and Security Issues

Human errors could not only compromise the quality of data, as discussed earlier, but could also jeopardize the security and privacy of data. An employee might forget to log out and accidentally leave the system and its data accessible to those without system access authorization. This may lead to a *data breach*, which occurs when private and confidential patient information is viewed and accessed by an unauthorized individual. It could be merely curious eyes looking at patient information; however, in more serious cases, it could involve those with malicious intent to steal patient information and then use it for personal or financial gain. The fraudulent use of other people's personal information is a crime known as *identity theft*. Regardless of the intent and severity—that is, simply looking vs. stealing information—the

intentional or unintentional exposure of identifiable patient health data constitutes a legal violation of the Health Insurance Portability and Accountability Act (HIPAA) of 1996.[17]

Notably, unauthorized access to data is not always due to an employee's failure to exercise proper procedures in safeguarding patient data. Many persistent and ominous risks of data security and privacy are imposed by external threats. Hackers—individuals who find security flaws and vulnerabilities of a system and exploit them to gain unauthorized access to the system—actively attempt to access and acquire patient data. Despite security measures put in place by health systems organizations, hackers seem to somehow be able to find ways to exploit system shortcomings and thereby access patient data.

The more recent data breaches are in the form of ransomware attacks. Attackers use sophisticated malicious computer programs, known as a virus or malware, to gain control to a system or, more specifically, the data stored in the system. An attacker can block access to the system and data (known as ransomware) and demand a ransom payment. Until payment is made, the attacker will prevent the victim organization from accessing its data. In health systems organizations, inaccessible data could severely affect their ability to provide life-saving care and treatments to their patients. CryptoniteNXT reported that incidents of ransomware attacks increased by 89% from 2016 to 2017[18]; this upward trend is expected to continue to affect all types of healthcare organizations, including hospitals, physician clinics, skilled nursing facilities, and stand-alone diagnostic facilities.

Lack of Experts in Data Analytics and Informatics

Despite the increasing amount of accumulated healthcare data, health systems organizations may not be maximizing the potential value of their data due to their inability to transform data into valuable, actionable information. Limited human expertise and technical resources to process and interpret data so as to generate meaningful and useful information remains a constraint to effective data-information conversion.[19] One of the major challenges in working with *big data*—characterized by extremely large datasets—is related to the existence of unstructured data. Unstructured data are freeform data that do not have pre-defined form, format, and categories and are not readily available for analysis. Email content, physician notes, video content, and scanned documents are a few examples of unstructured data. Although this type of data is a rich source of information, they must be processed to transform them into structured data before they can be analyzed. The transformation of unstructured to structured data can be extremely time consuming and technically cumbersome. This ultimately adds another challenging layer in data analysis.

▶ V. Addressing Issues and Problems Related to Data

Issues related to data in the healthcare environment must be managed and risks associated with data-related issues to patients must also be mitigated. As the quality of information is directly determined by the quality of data used in the analysis, health provider organizations must not only diligently ensure that proper processes, policies, and procedures are in place to promote accurate and dependable data but that the requisite human skills and technologies needed to facilitate activities related to data analysis are also in place.

AHIMA's Data Quality Measures

Data quality is a challenge that will continue to affect health systems organizations.

Accordingly, these organizations must continually evaluate the accuracy of data and the overall relevance of data to the organization.[20]

The American Health Information Management Association (AHIMA) developed a model for data quality that can be used as a framework to define the functions of the system for data collection, data collection process, data archiving and warehousing, and data analysis for health systems organizations. As shown in **TABLE 4-4** the AHIMA model includes 10 distinct characteristics that must be present to ensure the quality of data.[21]

Data Governance

As the quality and proper use of data matter greatly in health systems organizations, certain measures must be put in place to provide specific policies and guidelines for the collection, use, and management of data. The Data Governance Institute (DGI) has established a data governance framework that can be adopted by health systems organizations. The institute defines data governance as ". . . a system of decision rights and accountabilities for information-related processes, executed according to agreed-upon models which describes who can take what actions with what information and under circumstances, using what methods".[22(p. 3)]

The DGI's data governance comprises of three groups of components. The first group contains components related to "rules and rules of engagement of the organization".[23(p. 15)] Specifically, it incorporates components related to the mission and vision of the organization; goals, data governance outcomes measurements, and funding strategies; data definitions and data rules; data decision rights; data accountabilities; and data controls. The second group in the DGI's data governance framework includes components that "deal with people and organizational bodies".[24(p. 17)] This component of data governance is intended to establish policies for all stakeholders who affect and/or are affected by data. The framework

TABLE 4-4 Source from AHIMA, 2015 for Definitions of Data Characteristics

Data accuracy	Data that are clean and accurate and without any discernible flaws.
Data accessibility	The ability to access data in the most efficacious manner possible while maintaining physical and electronic security safeguards with respect to their legitimate access.
Data complehensiveness	Data that are gathered for a specific range of requirements by an organization are complete and satisfy those requirements. Any gaps in, or omission of, data must be documented in accordance with the policies as prescribed by the organization.
Data consistency	The assurance that the type, size, format, and other characteristics of health related data that exist across all systems are the same and are in sync with each other.
Data currency	Data points are up-to-date and reflect the current status of the event or concept that they represent; differ from data points that have become anachronous and thus erroneous.
Data definition	A detailed description of all captured health-data elements.
Data granularity	The depth or the scale of detail of health-related data. Data with a high level of granularity are considered to be more intricate or more detailed.
Data precision	With respect to data, the level of measurement utilized to achieve a defined objective or to delineate the nearness of two related measurements.
Data relevancy	Health data offer utility or benefit with respect to the reason or objective for their collection.
Data timeliness	Accurate and timely data are made available when needed.

also advocates for the establishment of a data governance office (DGO) to promote the progress of data governance activities, including communication and support; additionally, the framework also calls for instituting a *Data Stewardship Council*. Data stewards are most likely employees who have in-depth knowledge about data in their specific functional area. Data stewardship ensures compliance to policies and processes with respect to data-related activities.

The remaining group of components in DGI's data governance framework deals with data governance processes. DGI's framework calls for well-documented sustainable processes to support data governance activities.

Information Governance

Regardless of the specific design of data governance at any organization, it is imperative that the goals and objectives of data governance are aligned with and support the organization's information governance. Information governance, which is defined as "an organization wide framework for managing information throughout its lifecycle and for supporting the organization's strategy, operations, regulatory, legal, risk, and environmental requirements"[25(para 1)] is the overarching domain for data governance. The AHIMA Information Governance Adoption Model (IGAM) consists of 10 subdomains: data governance, information governance structure, strategic alignment, privacy and security, legal and regulatory, information technology governance, analytics, information governance performance, enterprise information management, and awareness and adherence.

Employee Education and Training

Education for healthcare employees will continue to be the ongoing focus of health systems organizations in mitigating risks associated with data security and confidentiality. Besides bolstering their system network and keeping up-to-date with appropriate technologies[26] to minimize external attacks, health systems organizations will need to provide an enterprise-wide education to all employees regarding the organization's policies and procedures related to system access and security in order to defend their system and data internally.

Specific to value maximization of data, data analysts with advanced skills are needed to work with the increasing volume of digital healthcare data. The Bureau of Labor Statistics[27] estimated that between the years 2016 and 2026, jobs related to data analysis and the application of "mathematical and statistical techniques to help solve real-word problem in business, engineering, healthcare, or other fields" will experience a growth that is much higher than the average growth of all jobs. This anticipated demand of human skill may be met by proper education and trainings.

▶ VI. Future Trends of Data and Data Analytics

The application of data analytics will continue to be both a challenge and opportunity in health informatics. Advanced data processing technologies and algorithms utilized in data analytics promise great potential to enhance evidence-based practice. Data analytics can be used to discover patterns and associations that exist in data to offer new information to health practitioners.[28] This information will inform and assist health practitioners in making decisions about treatment efficacies and disease prevention. Real-time data processing can offer various benefits to health care in various settings. In public health, real-time data processing can promote early detection of infectious diseases and support more rapid containment efforts. The World Health Organization (WHO) stresses the importance of information sharing as a tool in the monitoring and controlling of communicable diseases.[29] The combination of human expertise in data analytics and the availability of technological capabilities to process data promises the potential for early detection, effective treatment, and imperative prevention of disease transmission at the local, national, and international level.

Related to the business side of health care, Wang and Hajli[30] contended that the application of healthcare analytics in the financial and administrative domains of healthcare operations is yet to be optimized. This is due to the focus of health data applications on the clinical side. Adequate investments in human skills and data processing technologies can contribute greatly to the capitalization of healthcare data, all of which can advance operational and administrative efficiencies to more effectively augment a healthcare organization's financial performance.

Additionally, the use of healthcare data will extend beyond patient care, population health, and a healthcare organization's daily operations. Considering the pervasive nature and the massive amounts attributed to healthcare fraud, surveillance efforts will need to be amplified to prevent and detect frauds and to recover payments related to fraudulent and improper billing practices. While the actual dollar amount related to fraudulent billing activities is unknown, the estimated amounts are staggering. The Institute of Medicine of National Academies estimates $75 billion a year[31]; other estimate ranges from $90 billion to $300 billion.[32] Additionally, according to the Department of Human Health Services, Medicare and Medicaid improperly paid out almost $90 billion to various healthcare providers in 2015.[33] Healthcare data will serve an important role in future fraud detection and financial recovery efforts. In fact, the Health Care Fraud and Abuse Control Program of the Department of Health and Human Services and The Department of Justice acknowledge the need for enhanced information technologies and data analysis to assist with tracking payment trends and utilization patterns, and with fraud detection.[34]

The ethical aspect of healthcare data use will unceasingly be scrutinized and debated. With respect to data quality, the concerns are more about the accuracy of information. Specifically, if data are inaccurate and incomplete, any information derived from that data may be inaccurate. There may be serious ethical implications if any decisions made or actions taken based on flawed information pose harm to patients, the sustainability of healthcare organizations, or to the safety of the public. Naturally, users' trust in data and their confidence in relying on data for decision-making will continue to evolve.

Moreover, data security and confidentiality have remained a challenge and ominous threat. Although various data and information governance frameworks have been widely adopted to mitigate risks associated with security threat, reports on ransomware attacks and security breaches continue to challenge those whose job is to protect health data.

▶ VII. Conclusion

EHR has transformed the delivery of health care by potentially improving all aspects of patient care, including safety, effectiveness, patient-centeredness, communication, education, timeliness of care, and efficiencies as well as equity. Following EHR implementation, a massive amount of data has been collected. Patient data are collected primarily by care providers, and it can be used as a primary data source in clinical settings to provide care to patients. Additionally, patient data can be used as a secondary data source for other purposes, such as quality improvements, organizational planning, fraud detection, and health registries.

Alongside opportunities to improve patient safety, treatment outcomes, effectiveness and efficiency of healthcare delivery, and cost reductions, there also exist some major challenges. One of the biggest challenges is the management of increasingly massive amounts of data, particularly in term of maintaining quality data.[35] End-user errors and system designs can contribute to the overall quality of data. With respect to data analytic optimization, the lack of human skill and appropriate computer technologies remains the biggest factor. Challenges also exist with regard to maintaining the confidentiality and privacy of information. Issues related to lack of data analysis skill in employees as well as lack of computer technologies to process data also prevail in many health systems organizations. These and other potential hurdles are the challenges facing those in the informatics and data analytics fields.

Notes

1. Retrieved from https://hitinfrastructure.com/features /addressing-healthcare-network-connectivity -challenges
2. The Office of the National Coordinator for Health Information Technology. (n.d.). U.S. hospital adoption of patient engagement functionalities. Retrieved from https://dashboard.healthit.gov/quickstats/pages /FIG-Hospital-Adoption-of-Patient-Engagement -Functionalities.php
3. MobiHealthNews. (2018, October). What to expect from digital healthcare in 2018? *British Journal of Healthcare Computing*. Retrieved from www.bj-hc .co.uk/what-expect-digital-healthcare-2018
4. Wills, M. J. (2014). Decisions through data: Analytics in healthcare. *Journal of Healthcare Management, 59*(4), 254–262.
5. EMC. (2014). *The digital universe driving data growth in healthcare: Challenges and opportunities for IT*. Retrieved from www.emc.com/analyst-report /digital-universe-healthcare-vertical-report-ar.pdf
6. The exponential growth of data. (2017, October). InsideBIGDATA. Retrieved from https://insidebigdata .com/2017/02/16/the-exponential-growth-of-data/
7. Informatica. (2018, October). Retrieved from https://kb.informatica.com/proddocs/Product%20 Documentation/6/IN_1021_BigDataManagement UserGuide_en.pdf
8. Garfinkel, S. L. (2015). *De-identification of personal information (NISTIR 8053)* (p. 41). Retrieved from https://nvlpubs.nist.gov/nistpubs/ir/2015/NIST .IR.8053.pdf
9. *Ibid.*
10. NIH—National Cancer Institute. (2018). *List of registries*. Retrieved from www.nih.gov/health -information/nih-clinical-research-trials-you /list-registries
11. HealthData.gov. (2018, October). Retrieved from https://healthdata.gov
12. U.S. Department of Health and Human Services, Office of Inspector General. (n.d.). *Media materials: National health care fraud takedown 2016*. Retrieved from https://oig.hhs.gov/newsroom/media-materials/2016 /takedown.asp
13. U.S. Department of Justice. (2016). *Wyeth and Pfizer agree to pay $784.6 million to resolve lawsuit alleging that Wyeth underpaid drug rebates to Medicaid*. Retrieved from www.justice.gov/opa/pr/wyeth-and -pfizer-agree-pay-7846-million-resolve-lawsuit -alleging-wyeth-underpaid-drug-rebates
14. National Health Care Anti-Fraud Association. (n.d.). *2017 year in review*. Washington, DC: National Health Care Anti-Fraud Association. Retrieved from www .nhcaa.org/media/71683/nhcaa_annualreport_2017 .pdf
15. U.S. Department of Health and Human Services, Office of Inspector General. (2016). *Medicare and Medicaid Program Integrity: Combatting improper payments and ineligible providers, Testimony before the United States House of Representatives Committee on Energy and Commerce: Subcommittee on Oversight and Investigations (Testimony of Ann Maxwell)*. Retrieved from https://oig.hhs.gov/testimony/docs/2016/maxwell -testimony05242016.pdf
16. Shah, A., Aurelio, M., & Fitzgerald, M. (2018). Quality improvement for non-clinical team. *New England Journal of Medicine Catalyst*. Retrieved from https://catalyst .nejm.org/elft-quality-improvement-qi-nonclinical/
17. Health Insurance Portability and Accountability Act of 1996, 42 U.S. Code § 1320d-6.
18. CryptoniteNXT. (2017). *Health care cyber research report for 2017*. Rockville, MD: CryptoniteNXT.
19. Fatt, Q. K., & Ramadas, A. (2018). The usefulness and challenges of big data in healthcare. *Journal of Healthcare Communications, 3*(2), 1–4. doi:10.4172 /2472-1654.100131
20. Whitler, K. (2017, November). *6 data and technology trends for 2018*. Retrieved from www .forbes.com/sites/kimberlywhitler/2017/12/03 /the-top-6-data-and-technology-trends-for-2018 /#8a226b036805
21. AHIMA. (2015). *Data quality management model*. Retrieved from http://library.ahima.org/PB/DataQuality Model#.WrqcMJdrz8A
22. Thomas, G. (n.d.). *The DGI data governance framework*. Retrieved from www.datagovernance.com /the-dgi-framework
23. *Ibid.*
24. *Ibid.*
25. AHIMA. (2018). *Information governance basics: Overview*. Retrieved from www.ahima.org/topics /infogovernance/igbasics
26. Abouelmehdi, K., Beni-Hessane, A., & Khaloufi, H. (2018). Big healthcare data: Preserving security and privacy. *Journal of Big Data, 5*(1), 1–18. doi:10.1186 /s40537-017-0110-7
27. U.S. Department of Labor, Bureau of Labor Statistics. (2018, October). *Occupational outlook handbook*. Retrieved from www.bls.gov/ooh/math /mathematicians-and-statisticians.htm
28. Wang, Y., Kung, L., & Byrd, T. A. (2018). Big data analytics: Understanding its capabilities and potential benefits for healthcare organizations. *Technological Forecasting & Social Change, 126*, 3–13. doi:10.1016 /j.techfore.2015.12.019

29. World Health Organization. (2018, October). *Surveillance, forecasting and response.* Retrieved from www.emro.who.int/surveillance-forecasting-response/emerging-diseases/public-health-measures.html
30. Wang, Y., & Hajli, N. (2017). Exploring the path to big data analytics success in healthcare. *Journal of Business Research, 70,* 287–299. doi:10.1016/j.jbusres.2016.08.002
31. Institute of Medicine of the National Academies. (2013). *Best care at lower cost.* Washington, DC: The National Academies Press.
32. Blue Cross Blue Sheild. (2017). *Higmark's Inc's anti-fraud programs continue to see results.* Retrieved from www.bcbs.com/news/press-releases/highmark-incs-anti-fraud-programs-continue-see-results
33. U.S. Department of Health and Human Services, Office of Inspector General. (n.d.). *Media materials: National health care fraud takedown 2016.* Retrieved from https://oig.hhs.gov/newsroom/media-materials/2016/takedown.asp
34. National Health Care Anti-Fraud Association. (n.d.). *2017 year in review.* Washington, DC: National Health Care Anti-Fraud Association. Retrieved from www.nhcaa.org/media/71683/nhcaa_annualreport_2017.pdf
35. Kohn, D. (2010). The role of content management in electronic health records. Presentation presented at the *AIIM Golden Gate Chapter Meeting,* San Francisco, CA. Retrieved from http://daksystemsconsulting.com/html/webArchive/AIIMGG2010-05-25EHR.pdf

Chapter Questions

4-1   What are some possible sources of low-quality data? Why is it important to keep erroneous data minimized?

4-2   Data stored in EHR systems are almost always reduced to the simplest form. What is this type of data called, and why is this done?

4-3   Why does the DGI's data governance framework exist, and what role does it play in EHR?

4-4   What is the primary difference between data and information? What purpose does each serve in an EHR system?

4-5   Consider the implications of EHR systems in health care. Is it feasible for a healthcare provider to use the data they collect to discover health risks in a city or community?

4-6   What sort of contribution can secondary data provide beyond that of registries to improve healthcare delivery in general?

4-7   In considering the issues surrounding data errors and quality issues, what would be considered the common underlying component driving its cause?

4-8   What do you see as the trend of healthcare big data analytics? Why do you think proper analysis of data can aid in the prevention of healthcare frauds?

Biography

Dr. Siti Arshad-Snyder currently serves as a Professor at Clarkson College in Omaha, NE, where she regularly teaches courses in computer applications, healthcare information systems, healthcare informatics, and healthcare data analytics. She has 16 years of teaching experience in higher education and 10 years of business/healthcare working experience.

Dr. Arshad-Snyder holds a bachelor's degree in Business Administration with double majors in Finance and Economics, a master's degree in Computer Systems Management, and a doctoral degree in Interdisciplinary Leadership in Education. She is also a Certified Professional in Health Information and Management Systems (CPHIMS). Her research interests include healthcare education, computer technologies in health care, leadership, student retention, student persistence, teaching pedagogy, and social responsibility education.

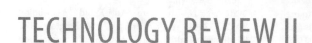

TECHNOLOGY REVIEW II

Big Data, Geospatial Technology, IoT, and Cloud Computing for Health Systems

Prabha Susy Mathew, Anitha S. Pillai, and Joseph Tan

TECHNOLOGY REVIEW OUTLINE

▶ I. Introduction

With the adoption of health information technologies (IT), particularly big data analytics on data extracted from electronic health records (EHRs) and sensors, to improve care, adding location-based spatial information would enable caregivers to further visualize patterns and trends in health care. Geospatial data, combined with data available from other sources, will significantly aid in epidemiological investigations including the detection of disease clusters, influence of environmental factors on patients across geographical regions, and population health and wellbeing. This brief overviews the connectivity of various health IT and shows their combined impact on health care, for example, how the Internet of Things (IoT) and cloud computing can improve insights from geospatial big data analytics.

Internet of Things

In 1999, Kevin Ashton, cofounder of MIT's Auto-ID Center, coined the term "Internet of Things" (IoT) based on radio frequency identification (RFID)-usage concept. By June 2000, the world's first Internet-connected refrigerator, the LG Internet Digital DIOS emerged. Soon, with enabling technologies, such as wireless technology, sensors, and cloud computing,[1] IoT embodies an ecosystem of connected ubiquitous IP-enabled devices and objects that are able to sense and collect surrounding data and transfer these over the network for further processing without human intervention. Essentially, IoT use enables the healthcare industry to remotely monitor a patient's condition. By tracking hospital assets to improve the quality of patient care, IoT use not only saves time but eliminates wastes via a continuum of devices-objects cleverly interconnected through Bluetooth, Wi-Fi, ZigBee, and Global System for Mobile Communications (GSM) to transmit data and receive commands from remotely controlled devices.[2] IoT can function via: (a) Internet-oriented (middleware); (b) things-oriented (sensors); and (c) semantic-oriented (knowledge).

Big Data

In today's interconnected world, the structured, semi-structured, or unstructured data from multiple devices (e.g., sensors, smartphones, social media, medical devices, satellite, and more) produce a massive amount of data, resulting in big data.[3] In a previous brief, we noted the many *V*'s of big data, namely, Volume, Velocity, Variety, Variability, Veracity, Validity, Vulnerability, Volatility, Visualization, and Value.[4,5] As data are diverse in types, volume, and formats, the traditional systems lack the ability to gather data from multiple sources and to effectively analyze the massive data to produce valuable and actionable insights. Several issues remain unresolved, such as what and how data are to be collected from multiple sources, the storage of massive and diverse data, the privacy of the data, and the need to perform analytics on these data. Increased demands for IoT and big data soon led to cloud computing diffusion.

Cloud Computing

Realizing the aforementioned big data challenges, more and more organizations are turning to cloud computing, a technology that provides the scalability needed for storing the big data, as well as to provide processing power and resources required to deal with the massive datasets. The cloud provides pay-per-use model, which allows organizations to pay only for resources used, resulting in the reduction of their operational and investment costs. Three most commonly deployed models of cloud computing are private cloud, public cloud, and hybrid cloud,[6] which are defined in the *Glossary* appended to the end of this text.

Spatial Big Data

Spatial big data (SBD), similarly characterized as that of the many *V's* of big data, have grown exponentially with the growing popularity of geographic information system (GIS), geo-social media, geo-sensor network, and geo-images from satellite, mobile devices, drones, cameras, and more. Indeed, a significant portion of big data comes from spatial information; for instance, location-based services have contributed to a significant amount of geospatial data. These huge spatial datasets often cannot be stored/processed via traditional means but will have to rely on technologies, such as cloud computing, big data technologies, and special data mining techniques, as existing open-source distributed systems, such as *Hadoop, HBase, Hive, Spark,* and *Impala,* are already lacking in support for efficient spatial data analytics.[7,8] The *Hadoop Distributed File system (HDFS)* stores the heterogeneous health data together in a distributed manner by dividing the data into smaller clusters (Hadoop cluster) and distributes them across the various servers and nodes, which perform more efficiently than traditional storage systems. *HBase* works on non-structured query language (non-SQL) approach and is easily able to hold and assimilate heterogeneous data. *Hive, Spark,* and *Impala* support the SQL-like interfaces to Hadoop, but Hive uses Java to permit queries to be easily written in order to obtain results; Impala uses C++, while Spark, which has been proven to be a fast and general engine for big data analytics with built-in modules for streaming, SQL, machine learning, and graph processing, uses a variety of languages.

▸ II. Geospatial Data and Technologies in Health Care

Today, the healthcare industry is deploying geospatial data with advancing technologies to strategize treatment, prevention, and control of infectious disease as well as optimize the allocation of public health resources, coordination, and policy recommendations.[9,10] Mobile applications along with sensors, IoT, and cloud computing allow seamless collection, storage and management, of spatial data to provide care services in rural areas. Conclusive results from the data can be obtained from heat map visualization.[11] Examples of geospatial data and technologies include: (a) cancer tracking in specific locations, such as evidence of increased prostate cancer levels in communities close to heavily pesticides-treated crops; (b) infectious disease spread analysis to monitor and control the disease in high-risk communities; (c) identifying location details to explore the prevalence of childhood obesity in a specific region; and (d) using location data by health insurance companies to understand a patient's locality so as to command a higher insurance premium for polluted locations.[12]

Geospatial Data

Geospatial data, also generally termed as geographic information, spatial information or data, geo-data, or spatial datasets, are used to locate the geographic positioning on coordinates that may be mapped. Geospatial data allow one to make better decisions, analyze spatial connections, and identify location-related patterns that were previously undetected.[13]

SBD sources include: (a) activity data, such as records/documents, phone data, keyboarding, optical character recognition (OCR) scanning, interviews, field surveys, and paper files; (b) conversation data, such as digitizing maps and drawings, emails, phone conversations, GIS, and CAD databases as well as data on social media platforms (e.g., Facebook, Twitter, and Instagram); (c) visual data, such as pictures on smartphones or digital cameras, CCTV videos, satellite imagery, aerial photography, and images captured by unmanned aerial vehicles (UAVs); and (d) sensor data, such as GPS-enabled devices, satellite sensors, mobile mapping.[14,15] The nature of spatial data may be characterized by: (a) spatial component, which represents relative position among objects like location, size, and shape of object on earth via the geographic coordinate system; (b) attribute component, which provides more information about the entity represented and describes characteristics of the spatial features; and (c) time component, which has a temporal element in it; as well as (d) spatial relationship, which specifies the relationship between objects.[16]

Dimensionality of spatial data goes from zero (0-D), where point pattern analysis is often used for identifying if occurrences (events) are interrelated; to one dimension (1D), where lines are used to represent linear entities such as roads, pipelines, and cables, which frequently build together into networks; to two dimension (2D), where area objects are used to represent natural objects; to three dimension (3D), where volume objects are used to represent natural objects, such as river basins, or artificial phenomena, such as the population potential of shopping centers and so on; to four dimension (4D), where time is often viewed as the fourth dimension of spatial objects.[17] Finally, GIS-represented spatial data models (data types) include vector data or raster data model. Three basic primitives of vector data are point, line, and polygon, whereas in raster data, grid cells or an array of cells or pixels are used to represent an object.[18]

Geospatial Technology

A field focusing on geographic, spatial, and temporal data, geospatial technology[19] includes: (a) Global Positioning System (GPS); (b) Remote Sensing; (c) Geographic Information Systems (GIS); and (d) Internet Mapping Technologies.

GPS is deployed in many health-monitoring systems to offer precise coordinate location details. An example in navigational bronchoscopy is the LungGPS technology, a diagnostic tool employing virtual reality and a GPS-guided system to precisely guide physicians to the lesion, expediting treatment and improving the outcome.[20] Geo-location tracking and monitoring services are often used as a solution for those suffering from Alzheimer's, Dementia, or other cognitive disabilities.[21] Wearable technology paired with a GPS-enabled smartphone can provide data regarding a patient's health parameters to alert family members of the wearer's status and respond quickly in emergencies.[22]

Remote sensing acquires information about an object or earth's phenomenon without directly making any physical contact. It is used in disease study and control to improve public health.[23] Remote sensing of Ebola-affected patients coupled with analytics can offer alerts on critical changes in patients' health to give them lifesaving, timely medical support without risking care providers.[24] GIS is considered to be a powerful tool for addressing healthcare issues, such as tracking communicable and/or non-communicable diseases, identifying health trends, and improving care services. Data gathered from GIS can aid toward enhancing healthcare outcomes[25] with incidence, mortality rate, and risk factors associated with effectively and efficiently identifying chronic diseases, such as cancer, cardiovascular disease, obesity, and so on. Internet mapping technologies, such as ArcGIS Earth, Nokia HERE, Bing maps by Microsoft, MapQuest, and OpenStreetMap, are changing the way geospatial data are viewed and shared on the World Wide Web.[26] ArcGis is a dengue surveillance system that used a combination of Google earth and GIS mapping; it was successfully implemented for dengue control.[27]

▶ III. Geospatial Analytics

Today, with IoT-based applications, location-based services, smartphones, and medical devices, among others, geospatial data volume has surged. As well, queries against geospatial big data have grown, resulting in the failures of the traditional database, query processing, and algorithms to adapt well. Accordingly, researchers have come up with new frameworks.

Zhou Huang[28] advocated an effective GeoSpark SQL framework to enable spatial query processing with Spark. They compared PostGis, PostgreSQL, GeoSpark SQL, and Environmental Systems Research Institute (ESRI) framework for Hadoop and found relatively low efficiency of ESRI framework for Hadoop, which is more suited for offline batch processing of massive spatial data. For some spatial queries, PostGIS and PostgreSQL traditional databases perform better than GeoSpark SQL and ESRI, but efficiencies fell for spatial join queries; here, GeoSpark SQL attains a 2.6 times speedup due to Sparks' memory computing characteristics. GeoSpark SQL efficiency is greater when processing compute-intensive spatial queries, such as the K-Nearest Neighbor (kNN) query and the spatial join query. Also, Spark-based spatial database (GeoSpark SQL) is user friendly and relatively easy to deploy.[29]

HadoopViz, a MapReduce-based framework, supports SBD visualization in gigapixels. HadoopViz has been shown to be scalable, extensible, and efficient in handling complex spatial data.[30] When comparing Spatial Hadoop v. GeoSpark, both are efficient in real-time SBD processing; however, GeoSpark comes out much faster. GeoSpark also supports Java and Scala and has limited community support.[31]

Physical Analytics Integrated Repository and Services (PAIRS), a newly developed platform on top of open source big data technologies, such as Hadoop and Hbase, is designed to accelerate real-time geospatial analytics by providing features such as automatic data download, data curation, scalable storage, and homogenized data layers in space and time.[32] IBM PAIRS Geoscope, a cloud-based platform, is designed to handle massive geospatial-temporal data. Apart from the big data analytics service, it handles ingesting, integration, and management of data.[33]

Spatial in-memory big data Analytics (Simba)[34] offers in-memory spatial query processing and analytics through SQL and the Data-Frame API on Spark will support runs over a cluster of commodity machines. Simba is a full-fledged query engine, supporting query planning, optimization, and concurrent query processing through thread pooling. While GeoSpark and SpatialSpark are user programs that run on top of Spark libraries, Simba offers better throughput and latency than other existing cluster-based spatial analytics such as GeoSpark, Hadoop-GIS, SpatialSpark, DBMSX, and Voronoi-based kNN jointly implemented on Hadoop (denoted as VKJHadoop). Fog computing-based framework, FogGIS[35], is proposed for improved throughput and reduced latency for transmitting geospatial data and analytics in geospatial cloud environment. Efficiency of SoA-Mist, a Mist-based framework for enhanced geospatial health data analytics, is better than cloud and/or fog computing. In assisting the fog and cloud computing, Mist computing can benefit big data analytics in geospatial applications.[36] Knowledge discovery in large spatial database is very complex, so compression algorithms and clustering tools are needed in order to extract precise geographic information. Modified Density-Based Spatial Clustering of Applications with Noise (MDBSCAN) algorithm[37] can be used for discovery of clusters in large spatial datasets. It modifies the density-based spatial clustering of applications with noise (DBSCAN) algorithm. MDBSCAN includes consideration of spatial and non-spatial variables and uses the Lagrange-Chebyshev metric instead of the usual Euclidean. The algorithm can correctly locate clusters of arbitrary shape in the presence of noise.

▶ IV. SBD Unique Security Requirements

Attention is called to the unique security requirements for SBD, including access control and privilege, copyright protection, security, role-based access controls for interoperable GIS repositories, and privacy of geospatial data at different levels while storing, distributing, and retrieving SBD.

Zope-Chaudhari and Venkatachalam[38] proposed a conceptual framework to provide security at the storage level using an authorization model and distribution level via cryptographic algorithms, use of digital signature, and data watermarking algorithms. Rajpoot[39] offers a location-based access control mechanism that restricts access to spatial data at two levels. First, users are categorized into different groups based on their authority, having views of data in certain formats. Next, based on user-specified location information provided during the registration process, only images from that location can be accessed, which increases the speed, while reducing time to locate the image of interest to the respective user(s).

Cloud-Based IoT Security-Privacy Requirements

IoT interconnects devices (e.g., remote health monitoring, wearable fitness, network-enabled medical devices) to share data without human intervention. It applies data analytics to gain insights, transforming patient care delivery, especially for the disabled and the elderly, leading to improved quality of life at low costs. While IoT benefits from the scalability, processing, and pay-as-you use model of the cloud infrastructure, it is still challenged with technological convergence, privacy, and security concerns.[40–42]

Identity-Location and Query Privacy

Identity-location privacy is very critical to users of mobile IoT as it would disclose the users' living habits and real identities. Pseudonym technique can preserve such privacy. Queries also pose a threat on location

privacy of users by revealing sensitive information about users via tracked IP source addresses. An approximate (KNN) query built on the Paillier public key cryptosystem can preserve both location and query privacy.[43]

Privacy-by-Design and Transparency-Privacy Aware Development

In a privacy-by-design solution, users can use tools to manage their own data. They can use a dynamic consent tool every time a data fragment is produced to limit access by certain services according to their wish. To achieve transparency-privacy awareness, the service developer integrates documentation of detailed usage of data during the development of a cloud service. Here, the users gain full and fine-grained transparency by design over the usage of their data before they permit the use of a specific service with their sensitive data. Such an approach for monitoring and auditing the usage of data allows the user and the auditors to check at any time adherence to the actual implementation of a cloud service's functionality.

Forward-Backward security

In forward security, the newly joined IoT users can only decipher the encrypted messages received after, but not before, they join the cluster; while in backward security, IoT users can only decipher the encrypted messages before, but not after, leaving the clusters. Yong-Yuan Deng et al.[44] proposed a secure and lightweight body-sensor network based on the IoT for cloud healthcare environment to achieve forward-backward security. In their framework, the session key is randomly chosen by the parties in communication and is used only during that communication. The attacker cannot use the same session key for future communication.

Secure Packet Forwarding in Cloud-Based IoT

Secure packet forwarding network focuses on: (a) the node compromise issue, where a new threshold credit-based incentive mechanism is proposed to stimulate packet transmission cooperation, optimizing IoT users' utility, and achieving fairness among them; and (b) layer adding-removing attack, where an aggregated transmission evidence generation algorithm is proposed that uses a new technique of secure outsourced data aggregation without public key homomorphic encryption.

Several other secure cloud-based IoT applications should be noted. These include: (a) secure device booting by the use of cryptographically generated signature to validate the authenticity of the digitally signed software in the device while first booting; (b) threat mitigation of sensors for secure smart applications; (c) role-based access control; (d) timely encrypted security updates and remote device attestations to confirm integrity and authenticate remote devices; and (e) use of standard security techniques, such as Secure Socket Layer (SSL)/Transport Layer Security (TLS), cryptographic algorithms, and firewalls, to ensure basic functional safety of the device and establish a secured data communication channels. Finally, application level security can be attained via secure coding practices, scanning tools to remain secured from attacks and account lockouts, password protection, and recovery mechanisms for building a secure foundation for IoT.

▶ V. Geospatial Technology, Big Data, IoT, and Cloud Convergence

Like other industries, the healthcare industry benefits from technological innovations.

IoT-led health care is being realized through converging geospatial technology, mobile, big data, cloud, and IoT to enhance the quality of patient care by fostering real-time engagement with patients, providing assisted-living options to disabled patients, monitoring patients' essential vitals, offering personalized reminders and alerts, and quickly dispatching emergency medical assistance following the occurrence of any patient injury.

Issues in Healthcare Geospatial Data, Cloud, and IoT Convergence

Although technological convergence provides cost-effective and quality solutions, several issues need to be addressed. The convergence of emerging technologies is often more complex than what it appears to be, with opportunities for research to streamline and optimize applications which has a blend of various technologies.[45] Key issues include:

a. *Security and Privacy*: Security of IoT devices, communication channels, and cloud applications remain a top priority; as newer solutions for security are being devised, the growth of new security challenges continues. While prior security measures worked fine with cloud computing, these no longer adapt well to its extensions, such as fog, edge, and mist computing.[46] Malicious code can be injected into sensors to tamper the data, data on the cloud is at a risk of being stolen or tampered, and gateways and communication channels can be compromised and may cause security breaches in a cloud-based IoT system. Considering the fact that health care deals with sensitive patient data, ensuring privacy by role-based authorization and transparency in data management as well as privacy policy is often always a challenge, especially when there are multiple entities involved.

b. *Interoperability*: The true potential of IoT-based applications can be achieved only once the interoperability issue is sorted out. With the inclusion of modern techniques, frameworks, and platforms like IoT, cloud-based solutions, SBD technologies will result in different devices that need to communicate in order to store, disseminate, and process diverse datasets that are not interoperable. Solutions to the interoperability challenge lie in unifying the diverse platforms via standard protocols to communicate with diverse devices and services and developing an interoperable programming interface. Real-time interactions between user and computing platform often gets disrupted due to the multi-hop from different IoT data sources. For cloud-based IoT-enabled healthcare systems, failures of real-time interactions may lead to life-threatening incidents for patients. To tackle the limitations of cloud computing, fog-based solutions have been developed. Interoperable fog-based IoT-healthcare solutions with some additional features will extend the capabilities of cloud-based IoT-healthcare solutions in that fog-based solutions have managed to tackle issues related to latency, energy usage, cost, and service distribution.[47]

c. *Standardization and Scalability*: The lack of standards to support diverse platforms, APIs, operating systems (OS), and open-source frameworks needed to facilitate the interconnectivity of heterogeneous devices and services will limit the uniformity among IoT medical devices for the scaling of integrated solutions. With a growing number of devices for connected health, efficient mechanisms are needed to provide scalable solutions. While traditional relational database management systems (RDBMS) can give results for geospatial queries, scalability is an ongoing challenge. New database engines, such as SQream DB and GPUdb, specifically designed for geospatial queries use the supercomputer power of the GPU in order to compute the complex geospatial functions and provide fast responses.[48] IoT often follows cloud-centric IoT (CIoT) architecture where cloud takes care of storage, processing, and management of data collected from the connected devices in the IoT architecture. CIoT generally faces challenges in BLURS (Bandwidth, Latency, Uninterrupted network connection, Resource-constraint, and Security). Fog and edge computing (FEC) has been successful in filling the gaps between cloud and IoT and offers advantages, namely Security, Cognition, Agility, Latency, and Efficiency (SCALE).[49]

d. *Energy Efficiency*: In a cloud-based IoT, there is a constant exchange of data between the IoT devices, gateways, and cloud. In such healthcare systems where the patient's vital status is being sent continuously to the physician for monitoring and real-time diagnostics, a continuous supply of battery and energy for efficient transmission is needed. Energy consumption in a mobile device can be reduced by up to 42% through off-loading to cloudlets compared to cloud offloading. Fog computing is considered to be faster and more energy efficient than cloud-only approaches.[50] More energy efficient schemes and algorithms used to minimize energy consumption at network and device level must now be devised.

e. At this point, the public-private healthcare sectors are using cutting edge technologies to curtail cost and improve efficiency. The boon of technology ranges from those that improve the comfort of patients to those that save their lives. In this sense, both benefits and challenges abound, which are discussed in the following sections.

Benefits in SBD Technological Convergence

Benefits of geospatial data coupled with IoT and cloud include[51]:

a. Identifying health trends in different locations—where doctors and specialists can view the locations and identify regions prone to specific diseases and the probable reasons;

b. Identifying the spread of infectious diseases—will allow preliminary disaster preparation and intervention activities to be planned prior to the outbreak of these diseases;

c. Utilizing personal data—data collected from individuals through wearable devices (e.g., eating habits, average heart rate, sleeping patterns, and exposure to the sun) can be used to identify patterns and predict diseases associated with the personal data trends;

d. Using social media—social media can also play a key role in identifying geographic locations where a particular disease is emerging; social media content with disease-related terms and the origin from where it was sent have aided in identifying or predicting various epidemic disease outbreaks, such as mapping of the Zika virus spread in some regions[52]; and

e. Improving services—GIS technology use has enabled community leaders and developers to work more closely with hospitals in taking larger steps to address national healthcare needs and also help in identifying which neighborhoods are in greater need of specific healthcare services, such as more rehab centers or senior care facilities. The use of geospatial data and analysis provides impact and benefits to the healthcare industry daily. Geospatial tools are able to visualize and inform service providers about changes in patterns, environmental impacts, identification of and changes within high-risk areas, and where the greatest need for resources providing the greatest benefit should be deployed.[53]

Challenges in SBD Technological Convergence

Some of the challenges faced by Geospatial big data include[54]:

a. Rapid growth of geospatial data leading to increased demands for potentially costly high-speed devices to capture, store, and analyze these data;

b. Lack of specialized skillset and knowledge in privacy policy when gathering high-resolution geospatial data;

c. Lack of specialized skillset and knowledge about protecting privacy rights when handling geospatial datasets by organizations without the appropriate know-how and experiences;

d. Lack of specialized skillset and knowledge among most organizations for handling the complexities of geospatial technology;

e. Awareness of the risk in compromising the anonymity of geospatial data linked to other public databases;

f. The need to ascertain the validity of spatial data as a representation of the real world, which is often imperfect;

g. Limited processing power, making it difficult to fully exploit the high volume and exponential growth of geospatial data.

In summary, the main challenges dealing with geospatial big data are the need for specialized skilled labor, followed by high costs and a lack of awareness.

▶ VI. Use Cases of Healthcare IoT, Cloud, and Geospatial Data

Increasingly, care providers are using GIS, IoT, and cloud-based platforms to integrate and analyze clinical records, such as health information of patients, their lifestyle habits, activities, and changing environments, to gain a more holistic understanding of the needs of their patients, as well as the non-medical factors affecting them and leading to poor health outcomes.

GIS technology from Esri is collecting and mapping geographic data points related to the Zika Virus and other emergencies to identify the location of the problem and strategically target resources to restore the public's health and wellness. In another example, people suffering from Alzheimer's often progressively lose their cognitive abilities and wandering is a high-risk behavior for such patients; fortunately, geo fencing software based on GPS technology can now be used to track patients with such a condition. A sensor device sends messages to caregivers if the patient leaves the geofencing boundary. Such systems give caregivers the precise patient location, which can be life-saving information.[55]

One such work that exemplifies the convergence of GIS, cloud, and IoT is GeoBlood[56]— a Web-based system for the analysis of biological data. For each patient, blood analysis, disease information, vital details via connected devices (IoT), and geographical data (GIS) are collected and stored on the cloud and analyzed on a geographical perspective to identify correlations between environment vis-à-vis the state of health. The inference from this work was the identification of a correlation between the geographical location of individual patients and their glycemic value. A narrow-band IoT hyper-connected asthma inhaler uses technologies such as narrow-band IoT, cloud, big data, and security to reduce the occurrence of asthma, hospitalization, and death.[57]

▶ VII. Conclusion

The growing popularity of wearable devices has increasingly driven demands for self-care management as well as remote monitoring of patients, especially for those who are also aging with critical ailments. Moreover, many communities are becoming more health conscious and looking for advances in smart technologies to revolutionize the healthcare industry.

Location-based information provided by GIS alongside technologies such as cloud, IoT, artificial intelligence (AI), machine learning, and big data can aid the healthcare industry by providing insights to enhance patient care, design better clinical trials, track complex problems related to infectious diseases, provide personalized medicine, improve one's quality of life, and reduce costs. Fog and mist computing, which extends cloud computing, can be used to improve efficiency of the health systems, reducing latency and increasing throughput, while analyzing big data in geospatial healthcare applications.

For future researchers, more focus on further development of open-source platforms will help in achieving interoperable and seamless integration of devices, while providing end-to-end solutions to address the emerging needs of the IoT ecosystem. Even though the convergence of tools and technologies brings a whole new range of opportunities, new challenges arise for which more intelligent and groundbreaking solutions must now be devised.

Notes

1. Tozzi, C. (2016, May 25). Retrieved from www.channelfutures.com/msp-501/iot-past-and-present-history-iot-and-where-its-headed-today
2. Marjani, M., Nasaruddin, F., Gani, A., Karim, A., Abaker, I., Hashem, T., & Siddiqa, A. (2017, March 29). *Big IoT data analytics: Architecture, opportunities, and open research challenges.* Retrieved from https://ieeexplore.ieee.org/document/7888916
3. *Ibid.*
4. Firican, G. (2017). Retrieved from https://tdwi.org/articles/2017/02/08/10-vs-of-big-data.aspx
5. *Technology Review I. (In Part I of this same textbook)*
6. Zanoon, N., Al-Haj, A., & Khwaldeh, S. M. (2017). Cloud computing and big data is there a relation between the two: A study. *International Journal of Applied Engineering Research, 12*(17), 6970–6982. Retrieved from www.ripublication.com/ijaer17/ijaerv12n17_89.pdf
7. Eldawy, A., & Mokbel, M. F. (2017). The era of big spatial data. *Proceedings of the VLDB Endowment, 10*(12), 1992–1995. Retrieved from www.vldb.org/pvldb/vol10/p1992-eldawy.pdf
8. Deshmukh, A. G. Retrieved from http://omangeospatialforum.org/presentation/spatial-big-data.pdf
9. Lopez, D., Gunasekaran, M., & Murugan, B. S., Kaur, H., & Abbas, K. M. (2014, October). Spatial big data analytics of influenza epidemic in Vellore, India. *Proceedings of the 2017 IEEE International Conference on Big Data.* 19–24. doi:10.1109/BigData.2014.7004422
10. Lee, E. C., Asher, J. M., Goldlust, S., Kraemer, J. D., Lawson, A. B., & Bansal, S. (2016). Mind the scales: Harnessing spatial big data for infectious disease surveillance and inference. *The Journal of Infectious Diseases, 214*(Suppl 4): S409–S413. doi:10.1093/infdis/jiw344
11. Praveenkumar, B. A., Suresh, K., Nikhil, A., Rohan, M., Nikhila, B. S., & Rohit, C. K. (2014). *Geospatial technology in disease mapping, E-Surveillance and health care for rural population in South India.* International Archives of the Photogrammetry, Remote Sensing and Spatial Information Sciences, SPRS Technical Commission VIII Symposium (Vol. XL-8, pp. 221–225), Hyderabad, India.
12. Willis, J. (2017). GIS in healthcare.
13. Deshmukh, *ibid.*
14. Murack, J. (2016, January). *MIT Libraries.* Retrieved from ocw.mit.edu/resources/res-str-001-geographic-information-system-gis-tutorial-january-iap-2016/spatial-data/MITRES_STR_001IAP16_Intro.pdf
15. Deshmukh, *ibid.*
16. Retrieved from www.gislounge.com/data/
17. Longley, P., Goodchild, M., Maguire, D., & Rhind, D. (2005). *Geographical Information Systems and Science* (2nd ed.). John Wiley & Sons, Ltd. ISBNs: 0-470-87000-1 (HB); 0-470-87001-X (PB). Retrieved from www.scribd.com/document/406409694/Paul-A-Longley-Michael-F-Goodchild-David-J-Maguire-David-W-Rhind-Geographic-Information-Systems-and-Science-Wiley-2005-1-doc
18. Dempsey, C. (2017, May). *Types of GIS data explored: Vector and raster.* Retrieved from www.gislounge.com/geodatabases-explored-vector-and-raster-data/
19. American Association for the Advancement of Science. (2018). Retrieved from www.aaas.org/content/what-are-geospatial-technologies
20. Raffaella Nathan Charles. (2017, December). *Safer lung cancer diagnosis with first VR and GPS-guided procedure in Singapore.* Retrieved from www.straitstimes.com/singapore/health/safer-lung-cancer-diagnosis-with-first-vr-and-gps-guided-procedure-in-singapore
21. Gilani, K. (n.d.) *Integration of heterogeneous motion sensors and GPS in healthcare oriented body sensor networks.* Berkeley: University of California. Retrieved from https://people.eecs.berkeley.edu/~yang/software/WAR/MobileBSNandGPS.pdf

22. Aziz, K., Tarapiah, S., Ismail, S. H., & Atalla, S. (2016). Smart real-time healthcare monitoring and tracking system using GSM/GPS technologies. *IEEE.* doi:10.1109/ICBDSC.2016.7460394

23. Zhang, Z., Ward, M., Gao, J., Wang, Z., Yao, B., Zhang, T., & Jiang, Q. (2013). Remote sensing and disease control in China: Past, present and future. *Parasites & Vectors, 6*, 11.

24. Steinhubl, S. R., Marriott, M. P., & Wegerich, S. W. (2015, September). Remote sensing of vital signs: A wearable, wireless "Band-Aid" sensor with personalized analytics for improved ebola patient care and worker safety. *Global Health: Science and Practice, 3*(3). doi:10.9745/GHSP-D-15-00189

25. MJ Scott D.O. Associates. (2016). Retrieved from www.occdocnj.com/using-gis-to-track-and-prevent -cardiovascular-disease/

26. Salminen, J. (2015). *Visualizing location based data on an HTML platform.* Retrieved from www.theseus.fi/bitstream/handle/10024/92405 /thesisjannesalminen.pdf?sequence=1&isAllowed=y

27. Chang, A. Y., Parrales, M. E., Jimenez, J., Sobieszczyk, M. E., Hammer, S. M., Copenhaver, D. J., & Kulkarni, R. P. (2009, July). Combining Google Earth and GIS mapping technologies in a dengue surveillance system for developing countries. *International Journal of Health Geographics, 8*, 49. doi:10.1186/1476-072X-8-49

28. Huang, Z. (2017). GeoSpark SQL: An effective framework enabling spatial queries on SparkISPRS. *ISPRS International Journal of Geo-Information, 6*(9), 285. doi:10.3390/ijgi6090285

29. *Ibid.*

30. Eldawy, A., Mokbel, M., & Jonathan, C. (2016). Hadoopviz: A mapreduce framework for extensible visualization of big spatial data. *IEEE International Conference on Data Engineering (ICDE)* (pp. 601–612). Helsinki, Finland.

31. Lenka, R. K., Barik, R. B., Gupta, N., Ali, S. M., Rath, A., & Dubey, H. (2017). *Comparative analysis of SpatialHadoop and GeoSpark for geospatial big data analytics, India.* Retrieved from https://arxiv.org /pdf/1612.07433.pdf

32. Klein, L. J., Marianno, F. J., Albrecht, C. M., Freitag, M., Lu, S., Hinds, N., ... Hamann, H. F. (2015). PAIRS: A scalable geo-spatial data analytics platform, Big Data'15. *Proceedings of the 2015 IEEE International Conference on Big Data*, 1290–1298.

33. Lardinois, F. (2018). *IBM's PAIRS Geo-scope helps developers wrangle geospatial data.* Retrieved from https://techcrunch.com/2018/03/06/ibms-pairs -geoscope-helps-developers-wrangle-geospatial-data/

34. Xie, D., Li, F., Yao, B., Li, G., Zhou, L., & Guo, M. (2016, June-July). *Simba: Efficient in-memory spatial analytics, SIGMOD'16.* San Francisco, CA: ACM. doi:10.1145/2882903.2915237

35. Barik, R. K., Dubey, H., Samaddar, A. B., Gupta, R. D., & Ray, P. K. (2016). *Foggis: Fog computing for geospatial big data analytics.* In 3rd IEEE Uttar Pradesh Section International Conference on Electrical, Computer and Electronics, India Institute of Technology (Banaras Hindu University), Varanasi, India.

36. Barika, R. K., Dubeyb, A. C., Tripathic, A., Pratikd, T., Sasanee, S., Lenkad, R. K., ... Kumarh, V. (2018). Mist data: Leveraging mist computing for secure and scalable architecture for smart and connected health. *Procedia Computer Science, 125*, 647–653.

37. Schoier, G., & Borruso, G. (2016). A methodology for dealing with spatial big data. *International Journal of Business Intelligence and Data Mining, 1*(1), 1.

38. Zope-Chaudhari, S., & Venkatachalam, P. (2013). Conceptual framework for geospatial data security. *International Journal of Database Management Systems (IJDMS), 5*(5), 29–35.Retrieved from www.academia.edu/13018237/CONCEPTUAL _FRAMEWORK_FOR_GEOSPATIAL_DATA _SECURITY

39. Rajpoot M, S. (2013, October). A location-based secure access control mechanism for geospatial data. *International Journal of Computer Applications, 79*(11), 28–32.

40. Henze, M., Hermerschmidt, L., Kerpen, D., Hau-ling, R., Rumpe, B., & Wehrle, K. (2015). A comprehensive approach to privacy in the cloud-based internet of things: A comprehensive approach to privacy in the cloud-based Internet of Things. *Future Generation Computer Systems, 56*, 701–718.

41. Zhou, J., Cao, Z., Dong, X., & Vasilakos, A. V. (2017, January). Security and privacy for cloud-based IoT: Challenges, countermeasures, and future directions. *IEEE Communications Magazine, 55*(1), 26–33.

42. Krishan, S., Sharma, V., & Dubey, P. (2017). IoT connected world: Security and Privacy. *White Paper, Infosys.* Retrieved from www.infosys.com /industries/communication-services/white-papers /Documents/IoT-connected-world.pdf

43. VARADAN. (2016, December). Practical approximate k nearest neighbor queries with location and query privacy, *IEEE, 28*(6), 1546–1559.

44. Deng, Y. Y., Chen, C. L., Tsaur, W. J., Tang, Y. W., & Chen, J. H. (2017). Internet of Things (IoT) based design of a secure and lightweight body area network (BAN) healthcare system. *Sensors (Based), 17*, 2919; doi:10.3390/s17122919

45. Botta, A., de Donato, W., Persico, V., & Pescap´e, A., (2015, September). Integration of cloud computing and internet of things: A survey. *Journal of Future Generation Computer Systems, 56*, 684–700.

46. Wang, S., Zhang, X., Zhang, Y., Wang, L., Yang, J., & Wang, W. (2017). A survey on mobile edge networks: Convergence of computing, caching and

communications. *IEEE, 5,* 6757–6779. doi:10.1109/ACCESS.2017.2685434

47. Mahmud, R., Koch, F. L., & Buyya, R. (2018). *Cloud-fog interoperability in IoT-enabled healthcare solutions.* In ICDCN '18: 19th International Conference on Distributed Computing and Networking (10 pages), January 4–7, 2018, Varanasi, India ACM, New York, NY. doi:10.1145/3154273.3154347.

48. SQREAM. (2015). Geospatial big data analysis opens up new opportunities for Homeland Security. Retrieved from https://sqream.com/geospatial-big-data-analysis-opens-new-opportunities-homeland-security

49. Chang, C., Srirama, S. N., & Buyya, R. (2019). *Internet of things (IoT) and new computing paradigms.* In R. Buyya & S. N. Srirama (Eds.), *Fog and edge computing: Principles and paradigms,* Chapter 1/Internet of Things (IoT) and New Computing Paradigms (pp. 3–21). Hoboken, NJ: John Wiley & Sons, Inc.

50. Wang, et al., (2017), *ibid.*

51. Pennic, F. (2015). Retrieved from https://hitconsultant.net/2015/02/16/8-millennials-trends-shaping-the-future-of-digital-health/#.XQbq-a0VRE4

52. Abouzhara, M., & Tan, J. (2016, September). *Twitter vs. Zika: The role of social media in epidemic outbreaks surveillance.* Presented Paper in Yuan Ze University, Taiwan.

53. Behm, D., Bryan, T., Lordemann, J., & Thomas, S. R. (2018). The past, present, and future of geospatial data use. Retrieved from http://trajectorymagazine.com/past-present-future-geospatial-data-use

54. Joshi, N. (2018). The challenges and opportunities that follow Geospatial Big Data. Retrieved from www.allerin.com/blog/the-challenges-and-opportunities-that-follow-geospatial-big-data

55. week. Retrieved from www.geospatialworld.net/article/application-gis-iot-private-healthcare-2/

56. Canino, G., Scarpino, M., Cristiano, F., Mirarchi, D., Tradigo, G., Guzzi, P. H., … Veltri, P. (2016). Geoblood: A web based tool for geo-analysis of biological data, International Workshop on Data Mining on IoT Systems (DaMIS16). *Procedia Computer Science, 98,* 473–478.

57. Thuemmler, C., & Bai, C. (2017, pp. 23-37). Health 4.0: Application of industry 4.0 design principal in future asthma management. In C. Thuemmler & C. Bai (, Eds.), Health 4.0: *How virtualization and big data are revolutionizing healthcare.* Cham, Switzerland: Springer International Publishing. doi:10.1007/978-3-319-47617-9_2

Biographies

Prabha Susy Mathew has a master's degree in computer science. She has over 10 years of academic experience and industry experience as Test Engineer. She is currently serving as a Guest Lecturer at Bishop Cottons Women's Christian College, Bangalore, India. Her research interests include data mining, big data, and IoT.

Anitha S. Pillai has a PhD in Computer Science in the area of Natural Language Processing. She has over 23 years of academic and research experience. She is working as a professor in the School of Computing Sciences, Hindustan Institute of Technology and Science, Chennai. Her research interests include AI, NLP, big data, Machine Learning, and Healthcare Analytics. She has published over 50 papers in national and international journals and books. She has also served as a reviewer for various journals and international conferences.

CHAPTER 5

Digital Health Enterprise Software: SCM, CRM, and ERP

Joshia Tan with Joseph Tan

LEARNING OBJECTIVES

- Overview Health Management Information Systems (HMIS) Enterprise Software
- Identify Supply Chain Management (SCM) Software
- Review Customer Relationship Management (CRM) Software
- Recognize Enterprise Resource Planning (ERP) Software

CHAPTER OUTLINE

Scenario: Customer Relationship Management with Blue Cross Blue Shield of Minnesota[1]

In 2001, Blue Cross Blue Shield (BCBS) of Minnesota sought to persuade executives at the consumer goods giant General Mills to join its regional health plan. These executives decided they would switch health plans on one condition: BCBS of Minnesota needed to install a Web-based customer service system that would allow subscribers to manage their health profiles and benefits online. BCBS of Minnesota consented, and the task of building a customer relationship management (CRM) system that would live up to General Mills' standards fell upon John Ounjian, then senior vice president and CIO of BCBS of Minnesota.

From the very beginning, Ounjian clearly understood the requirements imposed by General Mills: to give subscribers the ability to select health plans tailored to their individual needs and budgets, to calculate their own contributions to their coverage, to research information on prescription drugs and other treatments, to locate nearby participating physicians, and to check the status of their claims at any time of the year. Prior to developing and/or installing such a system, however, Ounjian needed to create a brand new infrastructure that linked website and call center operations with timely, accurate, and relevant information. Additionally, he needed to transfer terabytes of data from back-end data warehouses to the Web or Cloud so that it could be accessible and meaningful to consumers directly. During the early years of health digitalization and health data digitization, this was indeed a very challenging assignment with limited time and budget.

In the end, Ounjian pulled it off. But how did he do it? The difference, Ounjian liked to think, was in the planning. From the outset, Ounjian had a data management strategy. He likened constructing an online customer self-service system without this type of strategy to building a bridge without support. "If you don't have a data management strategy, then you're only building half the bridge," he reasoned. Thus, he and his staff began the project by attempting to develop a new infrastructure to record, over the Internet, automated interactions that had previously taken place over the phone. They then proceeded to pursue a strategy that would overcome many of the problems that could arise from converting raw data from back-end systems to consumer-accessible information on the Web and/or the Cloud. Had Ounjian been restricted to moving data back and forth, customers would end up looking at information that was essentially outdated, inaccurate, or unsynchronized with other company information channels.

Once its website platform was ready for beta testing, Ounjian and his staff invited a focus group of customers to evaluate it. The customers were initially unimpressed, mainly because they found the platform interface to be lacking consumer-friendliness. Specifically, BCBS-hired engineers discovered that they needed to redesign the layout of pull-down menus that guided viewers around the site. The interface was eventually improved with added features; as a result, customers were able to access information in a more efficient, productive, and relaxed manner.

Today, the aforementioned platform or similar systems are widely used by employees to track their insurance benefits and claims. Ounjian used a car metaphor to describe the flexibility of this new system: "We have the chassis on which to build our investments from year to year. If my transmission needs to move from a three-speed to a five-speed, I don't have to redesign the whole car."

Now, imagine you are hired to be the next CEO of General Mills and would like to build a strong in-house IS/IT department to do systems development with the criteria of these systems being even more cost-effective and engaging, having AI-empowered interfaces for all end users. What types of integrative software systems beyond just an isolated CRM should be included in the General Mills' IS/IT portfolio? What would be some key challenges and/or must-have features for these systems? Would Ounjian be a person you may want to consider hiring to be in charge of General Mills IS/IT department? If so, why? Otherwise, why not?

▶ I. Introduction

In Part I, we learned that a health management information system (HMIS) comprises people, data, workflow processes, and health information technologies to collect, process, store, and provide needed results—all in support of unit functions and task activities within an evolving digital health ecosystem. This is the foundational knowledge to prepare us for how to go about managing HMIS as complex, adaptive systems within health learning systems so that different parts throughout these systems can thrive in an intensely competitive and increasingly digitalized marketplace.

Part II of this text covers HMIS technology and applications. At this point, we need to specify the type of corporate HMIS applications in an increasingly digital health environment in which strategic and operational initiatives may be championed to yield competitive advantages. Our focus in this chapter will therefore be on HMIS administrative applications at the enterprise level. At this level, the performance of the overall health system depends on the building of an interoperable, integrated HMIS infrastructure; instilling effective communications among its connecting members; and, finally, the implementation of effectively integrated enterprise software to up-scale existing legacy administrative systems that go beyond just supporting the routine workflows and activities within the learning system, but having every connecting parts of the system to be able to engage, interact, and improve the overall user digital experience and/or journey.

As we move steadily toward globalization; e-commerce; knowledge asset management; collaborative partnerships; total quality management; and greater expectations for the security, privacy, and confidentiality of patient data, HMIS must evolve into an integral part of any health learning systems. To sustain an intense competitive edge and promote strategic initiatives, several high-profile enterprise software systems have emerged in the HMIS landscape. Key among these include:

- Supply chain management (SCM)
- Customer relationship management (CRM)
- Enterprise resource planning (ERP)

These key enterprise software play numerous important roles, including supporting and enhancing communication, coordination, collaboration, information exchange, and resource management sharing among key stakeholders inside and outside of the networked enterprise. The successful implementation of these systems will also ensure that every internal enterprise unit is somehow interrelated and interoperable and, furthermore, able to link with external support infrastructure systems. Just as a jigsaw puzzle, comprised of a mass of irregularly shaped pieces, forms a total picture

when fitted together, these strategic HMIS initiatives combine effectively to help integrate the enterprising functions and task demands arising from interactions among the various constituencies while improving the overall user digital journey and experience. SCM, CRM, and ERP are thus designed to link both internal and external entities so as to provide seamless high-quality healthcare administrative services, as are expected in an increasing digitalized care services delivery environment.

While these enterprise software systems often target the large-scale health maintenance organizations (HMOs) and integrated health delivery systems in light of the continuing trend toward increased growth, acquisitions and merger arrangements, and globalization within the healthcare sector industry, with the rapid drop in the cost of computing power and devices, these systems are finally scalable to smaller and/or newer forms of care provider organizations, such as self-insured employers (SIEs), patient-centered medical home (PCMH), and shared clinics. Today, the increased volume of daily purchasing, claims, and information exchange transactions faced by care providers can often be more efficiently supported. Therefore, discussion of these systems takes center stage in this text, rather than the disparate legacy administrative systems, such as hospital financial systems, material purchasing systems, nursing scheduling systems, facilities management systems, and many other systems that are typically covered in most published standardized and more traditionally oriented HMIS texts.[2-4] We believe that the major HMIS enterprise applications presented here are already in place as the new generation administrative applications for most, if not all, healthcare services organizations.

▶ II. Supply Chain Management

Owing to rapid advances in medical devices, innovations in health technology, new discoveries in prescription drugs, and increasing demand for quality services in the U.S. healthcare marketplace, large-scale HMO, and multi-provider healthcare organizations must now begin to evaluate their SCM.

The design of an effective SCM essentially involves an understanding of how to manage the information flow throughout a supply chain (SC) so that the total SC effectiveness is maximized.[5-7] Generally, the primary goals of SCM are: (1) to optimize service quality in terms of an organization's internal, as well as *inbound* information flow processes, while reducing costs and delivery time and (2) to achieve increased efficiencies with regard to information flows and exchanges between the organization and its external parties (*outbound* information flow and processes), including all its vendors and suppliers.

Take the case of the materials purchasing and handling department of an HMO that oversees, on a daily basis, the purchasing and inventory of supplies from a multitude of suppliers for several HMO-affiliated hospitals. First, it is almost always a challenge to predict, at any one time, the composition of patients in the different affiliated hospitals and, ultimately, their supply consumption of medical equipment or devices, prescriptions, ambulances, and office supplies, such as computer hardware and software. Second, different vendors and suppliers may behave very differently with differing systems, policies, and procedures for fulfilling orders. These vendors and suppliers can change from time to time, and depending on their efficiencies, some orders may be misfiled, shipped to the wrong places, or even lost in the process—any of which would lead to unsatisfactory backlogs and further logistical delays. Poor inventory management and inadequate quality control on the part of any of the suppliers, as well as on the part of the materials purchasing and handling department of the HMO, will also significantly affect subsequent costing and budgeting, as well as delivery time or recalls of these supplies. Many of these events will, in turn, affect the availability and eventual pricing of certain products and,

ultimately, the customers' perceived product and service quality.

The deployments of e-commerce enterprise-wide software, such as electronic data interchange (EDI) and/or Web facing services to such management of inventory controls, are examples of SCM solutions. Having the materials purchasing and handling department set up and send electronic orders to all the vendors and suppliers in a preauthorized, standardized format not only reduces errors in manual paperwork, lessens inconsistencies among disparate legacy systems, minimizes mail order delays, lowers costs, and increases the overall efficiency achieved in order procedures, but it also reduces the need to spend time chasing unfilled orders or canceling orders. Moreover, information flows among manufacturing, purchasing, and acquiring parties on quality control can easily be an added component in the SCM.

SCM also ensures readily available access to electronic order information, such as order tracking and block chaining, anytime and anywhere the e-commerce application is operable. It even grants the materials purchasing and handling department the ability to confirm approximate delivery time and availability of products—such as the type, number, and functionalities of wheelchairs at order placement. Moreover, staffing in the materials purchasing and handling department may also be reduced. Electronic healthcare requisition, or e-procurement, therefore, saves tremendous logistics costs, with the added possibility of instituting just-in-time (JIT) inventory. JIT is a strategy used by many businesses to improve the return on investment (ROI) by reducing in-process inventory and its associated costs. Demand printing, such as the publication of required health information brochures, is an example of JIT because only the number of ordered brochures is printed for delivery as orders are received. It is expected that the HMO's process efficiencies, service quality, and performance effectiveness will dramatically improve if JIT inventory can also be implemented as part of the SCM strategy.

Over the years, the healthcare industry has lagged in terms of innovative HMIS implementations and IT applications compared with banking, manufacturing, retail, and many other service industries. As HMIS enterprise software strategy begins to gain strategic emphasis, SCM provides the healthcare industry with an opportunity to systematize materials purchasing and handling processes, among other possibilities. For example, there is the possibility that globalization will soon transform SCM for healthcare supply purchasing into global sourcing.

With an increasing mobile population, healthcare services organizations—although long recognized to have thrived as one of the most established industries—are also now predicted to become the world's fastest growing industry sector. Medical tourism, for example, is touted to become a ballooning industry. Because the SC is being identified as a means of equating supply and demand in terms of the high daily volumes of information that are exchanged between suppliers and customers, the management of healthcare services organizations should not analyze just a single department, or even a single enterprise. Instead, these organizations should collaborate and, perhaps, integrate purchases by applying SCM philosophy for networks of healthcare services organizations and partnering care providers in today's sharing economy. Not only will this lower the cost of SCM investments, it will also increase SCM efficiencies and promote cost-effectiveness in the building of supplier–customer relationships. As a result, both the primary and support activities levels will see greater competitive advantages among the partners with shared, innovative infrastructure investments. To this end, it could be demonstrated that outsourcing may be the next growth-strategic initiative for many health systems (individuals, groups, or organizations), so that the current borders in the relationship between suppliers and customers are expanded. Evidently, the traditional approach of "make or buy" is rapidly approaching extinction, yielding to transformational outsourcing as an SCM

strategy in redesigning traditional links. This would allow healthcare services organizations to focus on their core businesses and core competencies, which are, essentially, patient care.

To further illustrate the SCM concepts for health systems, we present two relevant cases drawn from different vendor-published websites. The first is Marion Area Health System (MAHS) of north-central Ohio's Caduceus Material Management Information System (Caduceus MMIS)[8]; the second is a press release of Andersen's pharmaceutical, biomedical, and health services (PBH) SC practice on its attempt to project, in the IT industry, the valuation of future, achievable, e-commerce benefits.[9]

MAHS, whose affiliates include the Marion Area Health Center, Smith Clinic, and Marion Ancillary Services, recently licensed the Caduceus MMIS for implementation throughout its system. The Caduceus MMIS involves more than 70 physicians, whose specialties range from minor illnesses to full-blown surgery. Because of its sheer size, a new technological approach to managing its inventory and records was needed. Rick Brunswick, the director of materials management at MAHS, believes the system will fill this need by "automat[ing] a wide range of supply-related processes and eliminat[ing] a series of manual tasks." Such processes and tasks include the ability of electronically managing purchasing contracts, invoices, and financial records.

Using wireless technology and automatic updates, Caduceus MMIS seeks to cut costs by managing inventory and finances in a comprehensive manner. This extinguishes any superfluous or redundant practices and diminishes the risks associated with human error and safety hazards. MAHS physicians and clinicians will then have more time to personally care for patients without having to worry about locating and correcting misplaced or mislabeled supplies. As the system is developed with a scalable and receptive architecture, existing systems can be incorporated into Caduceus MMIS. Not only will this reduce the funding needed to replace existing systems, but it will also save implementation time.

Ed Lane, the president and CEO of Caduceus Systems, has faith that "the Caduceus MMIS will equip MAHS with the capabilities to realize significant efficiency improvements, cost savings, accurate charge generation, and improve communication with their suppliers and trading partners while positioning MAHS with a strategic software platform for managing their internal supply chain operations."

A study by Andersen's PBH SC practice found that the future value of e-commerce is predicted to fall between 2% and 10% of total benefits for members of the healthcare industry supply chain. Providers would receive 1% or 2% of the benefit, while suppliers would obtain the remainder. These values were calculated from interviews and activity-based costing methods, involving both tangible and intangible future values of e-commerce. These included improvements in procuring products, managing orders, invoice processing, integrating systems, managing contracts, and operational efficiency.

However, the largest benefit has been purported to be from controlling redundancy, such as overpayment and rework. Furthermore, as administrative issues can now be handled with less effort through e-commerce, and real-time information is easily accessible and available, salespeople now have more time to focus on completing sales transactions and acquiring new clients. "This study quantifies the future state of the healthcare industry through the use of e-commerce," said Ramona Lacy, partner with Andersen's PBH SC practice. "It will be a roadmap for all parties involved in the supply chain."

▶ III. Customer Relationship Management

Customer relationship management (CRM) is another major HMIS enterprise software system that is emerging in the healthcare IT marketplace. As noted in the scenario at the beginning of this chapter, the responsibility eventually rests on BCBS of Minnesota's CIO, John Ounjian, to implement Web-based CRM software so that executives at General Mills are convinced to join BCBS of Minnesota's health plan. Such software would permit subscribers to manage and personalize their healthcare services' benefits online. Essentially, the CRM will empower its users to customize their own plans to their individual needs and budgets, locate and select highly recommended participating physicians and specialists, decide on their own coverage contributions, check on the status of their submitted claims, and uncover the research information on prescription drugs and/or other recommended treatments at their own convenience.

How, then, would having CRM software distinguish BCBS of Minnesota from its competitors? Although CRM applies to organizations of every market, John Ounjian claimed that healthcare organizations, such as BCBS, are ready for such a system and would find it extremely beneficial in retaining its customers. Evidently, in order to maximize revenue generation and maintain customer loyalty, BCBS of Minnesota, as a leading-edge HMO, must be ready to implement such a solution and use it to carefully manage all of the customers' associations with the organization—this is exactly what CRM is all about, and what BCBS of Minnesota's competitors have now discovered.

With CRM, BCBS of Minnesota customers can now communicate with the HMO through numerous means and at different times. An archetypal CRM scheme would record each interaction a customer has had with the HMO and allow all the different departments of BCBS of Minnesota to access this record. In so doing, the HMO can garner valuable perspectives on both the effectiveness of its current systems and the preferences of any individual customer. Furthermore, with this knowledge, BCBS of Minnesota can save considerable costs by eliminating corporate-wide inefficiencies. Customer satisfaction will also be improved, because the treatment of each individual client can be further personalized, given that BCBS of Minnesota can access the record of interactions the customer has had with it, and then offer, accordingly, only the services and information that the customer seeks. Targeted e-mailing of information will also reduce waste. With reduced inefficiencies leading to reduced costs, and increasing customer loyalty leading to augmented sales, BCBS of Minnesota can then, as a result of implementing powerful and unique CRM software, maximize its revenue generation.

Still, in order to design the most appropriate CRM software, the health systems member organization must have an in-depth recognition of its customers' specific needs. Accordingly, Shams and Farishta[10] argue that the application of CRM philosophy is based on understanding the communications architecture of the healthcare services organization. The communications architecture should include a center core communications piece, augmented by branding and strategic communications. In terms of core communications, the patient's profile, which includes a synopsis of his or her physical demographics and other treatment-specific information (such as gender, age, allergies, and so forth) would be used to further trigger event-specific communications. In terms of branding communications, the messages will be used to distinguish the type and quality of products, programs, and services that the health organization in question is able to offer from its competitors in the regional, or even global, healthcare marketplace. Finally, strategic communications refer to the enhancement of existing programs and services, as well as to the development of new programs and creative services that would progress and fulfill the organizational long-term goals.[11,12]

Ultimately, the CRM being designed should first capture and generate customer profile data. With the core communications architecture in place, it should then allow an authorized employee or affiliate of the healthcare organization to offer, at the patient's convenience, appropriate information on treatments in a relatively shorter span of time. With the additional branding and strategic communications layers implemented, CRM would further allow the healthcare organization to reach its target audience for specific programs, such as immunizations, by contacting only those patients whose profiles suited the need. The CRM would also be able to communicate to the selected customers specifically why these services or programs are unique and competitively desirable, compare these services and programs to other apparently similar programs and services available in the regional healthcare marketplace, and offer special and personalized packages to the customers. Not only would such a system save the healthcare organization significant funds from general advertising and marketing costs, but it would also, indubitably, recover the cost of its implementation over the long run. Moreover, it will increase patient retention by offering customers a personalized relationship with tailored suggestions that other health organizations are not yet able to offer.

Finally, the CRM can also be used as a marketing and sales mechanism, for example, increasing patient referrals of other patients who may be interested in these services or even targeting them just for information sharing and marketing purpose. Reviews of services may also be implemented within the CRM to provide the health systems insight into relatively important feedback for future systems and services delivery improvements.

▶ IV. Enterprise Resource Planning

ERP is the final, major, enterprise-wide software system to be covered in this chapter. As with many businesses, legacy systems in healthcare services organizations require employees to post different departmental financial, purchasing, and other service-oriented data in separate systems. These siloed systems may not be consistent with each other, thereby encouraging the proliferation of islands of HMIS. Posting is the essence of manual operations. In an integrated environment, all that is needed is a "view." For instance, a patient's claims and claims reimbursement filing forms are just different views of the same data set in different order.

In this regard, Duncan et al.[13] observe that the integration of intraorganizational processes can significantly affect strategic management. Linked inventory control, if it exists, can be updated every time a drug, special diet, medical device, or other item is ordered; the cost of the item can then be added electronically to the patient's claims and claims reimbursement filing forms, thereby improving efficiency and reducing costs. Extending this linkage externally, the process of reordering items from designated suppliers, so that sufficient safety stock is maintained, can also be automated. With SCM, suppliers can be linked to customers in real-time for electronic order processing, third-party payers can be linked to health providers for billing and claims reimbursement procedures, government regulators can be linked to providers for documentation, and researchers can be linked to all of the various stakeholders for the purpose of conducting studies.

In essence, the ERP philosophy is an attempt to integrate all departmental and functional processes throughout the enterprise into a single, integrated HMIS, enabling enterprise-wide information management and decision-making on all organizational operations. If the entire organization is not sold on the philosophy of change accompanied by the use of ERP applications, for example, unintended and highly disruptive consequences may result. Existing ERP packages include SAP, R/3, Baan, PeopleSoft, and Oracle.[14]

In the same context as the assembly of isolated legacy systems into an integrated system with real-time access of different views (allowing decisions to be made intelligently across the enterprise) is the idea of reducing, or possibly eliminating, all paper-based forms. If all

transactions between customers and providers can be captured online and directly shared (where authorized, needed, and permitted) via CRM, SCM, and ERP, then all the troubles of any manual follow-up that may be needed could be avoided. With CRM and SCM in place, ERP can provide management quick access to enterprise-wide resource planning summaries, such as the generation of enterprise-wide purchasing aggregate reports, shipping status reports, and revenue-generation reports from all related services, programs, and investments.

Yamanouchi Pharmaceutical Co. Ltd. and Fujisawa Pharmaceutical Co. Ltd. merged in April 2005 to form Astellas Pharma Inc., ranking among the top 20 global pharmaceutical companies. Astellas Pharma US Inc., headquartered in Deerfield, Illinois, represents the U.S.-based Astellas operation.[15] Previously, Yamanouchi Pharmaceuticals, with sales at $3.9 billion, was also the third-largest pharmaceutical company in Japan. It has made information systems the key component in improving the timeliness and quality of answers to customers' tough questions. Product support personnel at Yamanouchi can immediately answer most of the questions that come in from the doctors or pharmacists. To find answers to more difficult questions, they have access to Yamanouchi's Web-based PRoduct INformation CEnter Supporting System (PRINCESS).[16] With the help of JRI Consulting, Astellas Pharma was able to further integrate both Yamanouchi's and Fujisawa's systems to quickly achieve stable operations within a short period of time. The Astellas ERP system is based on SAP R/3 products, integrating the business processes in accounting, production, sales and distribution, purchasing, and personnel from both companies.[17]

Still, ERP is not a panacea. Take, for instance, a typical healthcare services organization today, where management, employees, or customers need specific answers to important product order or service information. There are also the related questions about suppliers, shipping status, and sales status, causing the front offices of these healthcare services organizations to typically scramble behind the scenes for answers. The inconsistency across disparate databases and business operations in legacy systems often make it difficult for conflicting data sets to be reconciled. These cannot be used to provide straight answers, either, to many of the questions pertaining to the provided services. Moreover, it will always be complicated to provide straight answers for questions such as, "How long does it take to perform a knee replacement operation today?" or "How much does it cost the HMO to schedule a knee replacement operation today?" The members of the health systems can generate the answers only after that knee replacement operation is completed—its expenses depend on, among other things, who performs the surgery, how is it performed, when is it performed, the patient's insurance subscription and the extent of its coverage, the length of the patient's post-operation stay in the hospital, and any complications arising from the operation(s). Administrators of healthcare services organizations cannot provide specific answers until their employees and subordinates have had sufficient time to deal with addressing many of these questions. Operational practices within health systems and organizations, as well as subcomponents, are as diverse and sometimes unique as anyone can imagine. Software development has to be done on a project-by-project basis, because the service processes are often non-standardized. Developing ERP software, or even customizing and implementing some off-the-shelf packages, is, therefore, a very lengthy, risky, and difficult venture. In this sense, the information architecture that can be achieved through the integration of core business processes and requirements will sometimes be limited, complex, and expensive.

The goal for ERP, then, is to achieve single data-entry points throughout the organization so that the goal of enterprise data modeling can be realized wherever possible. Today, this has been proven to be an attainable goal with more and more members of large health systems ready and willing to adopt health data and process standardization, advances in business process reengineering, and the willingness of healthcare professionals and employees to streamline processes and operations. When standardization goes beyond the basic data levels to a service process level via the blockchain conceptualization, invoices and paper-based orders can be eliminated, and payments or services can be made without the need for a paper trail. Often, the major issues are not technical, but process reconceptualization and educational issues. Overcoming these issues is key to making intra- and interorganizational systems work together. Simply put, ERP software can be used to facilitate data integration by amalgamating existing business processes in an organization via blockchain. ERP implementation for an integrated delivery system (IDS) essentially connects the different pieces of existing HMIS applications in the system to fit into the ERP centerpiece software.

FIGURE 5-1 shows how the ERP replaces the existing islands of HMIS for an IDS with a resulting centerpiece ERP application, which allows sharing of core administrative data. It is important to note that not all services and functions currently performed in healthcare services organizations can be easily integrated and/or are interoperable.

The service process model for healthcare services proposed in the previous editions of this text is the beginning of an ERP conceptualization for healthcare services organizations. It is an attempt to re-conceptualize and streamline all services and processes transpiring within these organizations into an integrated model. We briefly summarize the approach here; those who are enthusiastically interested can seek out further details by consulting the previous editions of this text, as referenced.[18]

All organizations, including healthcare services organizations, provide services. The service process is therefore a common link among organizations, subsets of organizations, and various people who work for these

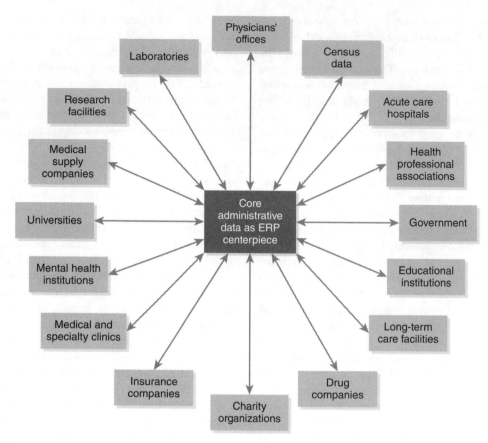

FIGURE 5-1 The Enterprise Resource Planning (ERP) conceptualization.

organizations. All service processes have three common basic elements: a customer, a service that is provided, and a provider. Information pertaining to these elements may be maintained as servicing records in master tables. Service processes are simple and very consistent; in general, most organizational services can be classified into three levels, each having a few major types. Uniformity in service processes is essential because it shortens the customization and implementation time for an integrated ERP application.

Service transactions occur at three levels within a unit: (1) external services, (2) internal services, and (3) procured services. *External services* are services provided by the unit or persons to external units or persons. *Internal services* are services provided within the unit

by one person or unit to another person or unit. *Procured services* are services procured by units or persons from external units or persons. Within each of these three levels, service processes of (or for) units or individuals can be classified as consultative, procedural, material (consumable), facility (use of hard or soft assets), monetary, or information (maintenance). In healthcare services organizations, *consultative services* involve logical interactions between customers and providers; these include services provided by doctors, management consultants, and clinical specialists. *Procedural services* involve physical interactions between customers and providers. This type of service may also involve the use of equipment, such as a hard or soft instrument. *Material services* transfer the ownership of hardware or software from providers to customers. Such services can result in debits or credits to the material accounts of providers and customers. *Facility services* involve the blocking and releasing of assets used. In this case, the service providers typically limit the use of their hardware or software to the customers. Examples are use of hospital beds (hard assets) or Internet services (soft assets). *Monetary services* are either independent or reciprocal of other service types; for example, money is transferred from customers to providers by various negotiable instruments, resulting in debits and credits to monetary accounts of customers and providers, respectively. *Information services* merely involve updating the service master tables after transactions. The customer, provider, and service master tables are the result of such service transactions, and the structure of these service master tables depends on the type of the service provided.

IDS can easily customize the layout of data on these services into service master tables, depending on their needs and information requirements. Services of all types within each level are processed with multiple steps. At

least four of these steps are common to most service processes: request for service, acknowledgment of request, service delivery, and confirmation of service delivery. **FIGURE 5-2** shows how these steps can be sequenced and analyzed along a value-chain or blockchain, resulting in a service outcome. Services can sometimes, alternatively, be processed with a single step, or multiple steps can be merged into a single step. It is also possible for these steps to take place all at the same time. First, a service process is initiated through a request for service. Numerous forms have been used in the manual process for making requests (e.g., drug prescriptions and test orders). Apart from other attributes, these service request forms commonly identify the customer, the service to be provided, and the provider—that is, the basic elements of the service process. The manual forms necessitated a docket number (header) and a detailed type of reference system, which are not necessary in our standardized model. Abolishing this concept of header and details requires a change of the old mind-set for many health professionals. This also means abolishing the names used for identifying all the different request forms. In the integrated,

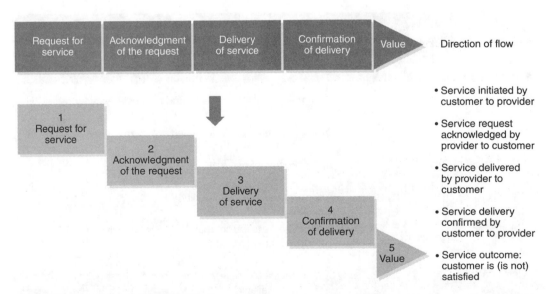

FIGURE 5-2 The Service Model Value Chain.

computerized model, each record consists only of one customer, one deliverable item of service, and one provider.

In general, requests are generated one at a time. However, it is possible for group requests to be made for several services linked together. Moreover, requests may also be prescheduled with a start time, end time, and follow-up periods. Requests for a particular service may also be automatically generated for a predefined condition by activating it through a triggered built-in logic when a change in certain fields is registered. For example, a purchase request for an item can be generated automatically when the reorder level is reached. This type of request is unnecessary in an integrated environment, because the provider who is sharing the data will supply the item with an automated built-in request. In this case, what should have been a reorder level would now become a supply level. Also note that requests and services flow in opposite directions between the various request levels and that external and procured services are usually accompanied by reciprocal monetary transactions.

Following the service request, the acknowledgment screen of the service provider is updated with the new request. The service provider then acknowledges the request by some preliminary action. For example, in the case of a laboratory test request arising within a hospital, the phlebotomist will have to collect the required blood sample. In the case of a machinery breakdown, the request is made to the service engineer to carry out a preliminary inspection of the equipment. **TABLE 5-1** shows the "acknowledgment actions" of the different requests, as noted on the system by the provider. The system also notes the user identity of the person acknowledging the request and the date and time of acknowledgment. After the acknowledgment is registered, the person actually responsible for delivering the service is notified through an automatic update of this person's pending actions list. Services are then delivered and the records of "delivery actions" are updated electronically by the providers or, subsequently, by individuals acting on their behalf, as shown in **TABLE 5-2**. Again, the identity of the person updating the records and the date and time are noted by the system.

The last step is confirmation of the service provided, that is, an acceptance or approval of the service by the customer. As noted, all

TABLE 5-1 Services Processes and Acknowledgment Actions Taxonomy	
Types of Service Processes	**Acknowledgment Actions**
Consultative	Confirmation that the provider and the customer are both ready
Procedural	Pre-procedure preparation carried out by the system
Material (consumable)	Transportation of material
Facility (use of hard or soft asset)	Reservation/allotment of facility
Monetary	System checks to ensure that the service is deliverable and instruments are acceptable
Information	System checks to ensure that all information required for master updating is available

TABLE 5-2 Services Processes and Delivery Actions Taxonomy	
Types of Service Processes	**Acknowledgment Actions**
Consultative	Recording the outcome parameters
Procedural	Recording the procedure outcomes
Material (consumable)	Transfer of ownership of material to the customer; stock records update
Facility (use of hard or soft asset)	Physical occupation of the facility
Monetary	Transfer of money to the customer; financial records update
Information	Master update

services have outcomes; for example, a service may be completed to satisfaction or below satisfaction. The consultative and procedural services may have outcome values for various parameters, as recorded by their providers. An outcome may also be the identity of another service request. Moreover, a service may be canceled or rolled back at any stage. Hence, if the service is accepted, the system merely updates the acknowledgment; otherwise, a feedback occurs, and the "chain" of service activities is repeated accordingly. Following the service delivery, the transaction data are archived into a service data archival table or the service database.

It is possible that services may be grouped and ordered together by a group name, and a hierarchy pattern of multiple levels of groups thus enables rapid ordering of related services.

▶ V. Conclusion

Only the primary features underlying the service process model have been presented so far to give the reader a sense of the benefits of what process standardization can provide. In other words, standardization can incur benefits at levels beyond data codes, data schema, and data exchange formats; in fact, significant efficiencies can be recovered from standardizing the service processes. Standardization of all these levels, if pursued appropriately and vigorously, holds great potential for reduced costs, diminished complexity, greater security control, and better data management—a systems philosophy that prepares the organization to move into an SCM, CRM, and ERP environment. Adoption of HMIS standards is discussed elsewhere in this text and the previous editions of this text.

In closing, here are some pointers toward achieving HMIS integration in an IDS context. The first significant change, as was noted throughout many of the illustrations covered in this chapter, is increasing awareness of the organization to reconceptualize its business and services processes in the form of digitalization as well as the need to adopt a new corporate culture of data sharing in a sharing economy. This cultural change needs to be supported across all organizational units and departments. In this light, SCM, CRM, and ERP play key roles in supporting meaningful sharing, integration, and exchange of data; such software systems allow enterprise-wide views of the organization, thereby ensuring efficient and effective interorganizational cooperation and intraorganizational collaborations. For such inter- and intraorganizational linkages to succeed, Sprague and McNurlin[19] note that all linked programs and processes should be expandable to other links in the future, whether these are at community, regional, state, national, or international levels. This can only be possible if an enterprise view, process standardization, and a data-sharing culture are upheld and if stakeholders and users are educated about the significance of the standardization process. In an IDS context, the more technologically advanced partners will typically have to pull the others along, whether it is through education or some other means. Standardization also requires the cooperating organizations to be involved in the ongoing development of standards. Government agencies, regulators, and third parties are often also involved. Standards task forces can be formed to operate as electronic intermediaries, facilitating the flow of information. In hammering out a consensus among the stakeholders involved in a standardization process, a change in one of the co-operating systems often must be coordinated with all others.

Finally, as illustrated by the Yamanouchi–Fujisawa case, applications of the HMIS enterprise software will, sooner or later, allow individual organizations to go beyond their limitations as such software systems require the participation of other organizations before total efficiencies and effectiveness can be achieved. As long as organizational employees and staff are ready to share views, and management is open to high-performance changes, new enterprise software can be instituted to add value to the organization's growth and development. Along this line, we close this chapter by summarizing a press release on the combination of ERP and SCM solutions for pharmaceutical distribution channels across Europe.

Frost and Sullivan[20]—a global innovative growth strategies consulting company—proposes, in one of its press releases through its London office, the use of ERP and SCM solutions to ease the flow of pharmaceutical distribution channels across Europe. The company argues that ERP and SCM solutions will ease integration of processes across various functional areas and streamline related functions of key stakeholders in the pharmaceutical distribution channel, resulting in rapid and secure delivery of pharmaceutical products. Rahul Philip Mampallil, a Frost and Sullivan research analyst, claims that "with these IT solutions, manufacturers and other participants in the distribution channel can track the flow of drugs from pharmacy shelves and replenish accordingly to avoid stock outs…. Moreover, companies can monitor the movement of stocks and detect the illegal intrusion of batches into the distribution channel." The challenge, he believes, lies in correcting the current lack of understanding about specific business requirements that organizations have when implementing particular add-on ERP modules, and when these modules do not support those requirements. Accenture[21] projected, given the high market potential, that adding AI (machine learning) to managing drug inventory and SC management, such solutions will generate revenues in the European pharmaceutical sector far in excess of the current amounts if these newer technologies became widespread. Put simply, the application of IT solutions, such as SCM, CRM, and ERP, will translate into new efficiencies, new boundaries, and new possibilities.

Notes

1. Levinson, M. (2003). Blue Cross and Blue Shield of Minnesota's success with CRM. *CIO.* Retrieved from www.cio.com/article/31903/Blue_Cross_and_Blue_Shield_of_Minnesota_s_Success_With_CRM/4

2. Tan, J. (2001). *Health management information systems: Methods and practical applications* (2nd ed.). Gaithersburg, MD: Aspen Publishers.

3. Austin, C. J., & Boxerman, S. B. (1998). *Information systems for health services administration* (5th ed.). Chicago, IL: AUPHA/Health Administration Press.

4. LaTour, K., & Eichenwald Maki, S. (2006). *Health information management: Concepts, principles, and practice* (2nd ed.). Chicago, IL: AHIMA.

5. Lee, H. L., Padmanabhan, V., & Whang, S. (1997). Information distortion in a supply chain: The bullwhip effect. *Management Science, 43*(4), 546–558.

6. Forrester, J. W. (1958, July–August). Industrial dynamics: A major breakthrough for decision makers. *Harvard Business Review, 38,* 37–66.

7. Bechtel, C., & Jayaram, J. (1997). Supply chain management: A strategic perspective. *International Journal of Logistics Management, 8*(1), 15–34.

8. Retrieved from www.caduceussystems.com/news-marion-selects-caduceus-systems.html

9. Pastore, M. (2001, June 27). *The ClickZ Network.* Retrieved from www.clickz.com/showPage.html?page=792781

10. Shams, K., & Farishta, M. (2006). Knowledge management. In K. LaTour & S. Eichenwald Maki (Eds.), *Health information management: Concepts, principles, and practice* (2nd ed.). Chicago, IL: AHIMA.

11. Paddison, N. (2001, January 26). Benefits of Event-Driven CRM in Healthcare, Part 1, *DM Review.*

12. Paddison, N. (2001, February 2). Benefits of Event-Driven CRM in Healthcare, Part 2, *DM Review.*

13. Duncan, W. J., Ginter, P. M., & Swayne, L. E. (1996). *Strategic management of health care organizations* (2nd ed.). Cambridge, Massachusetts: Blackwell Business Publications.

14. Koch, G., & Loney, K. (1996). *Oracle: The complete reference.* New York, NY: McGraw-Hill.

15. Retrieved from www.astellas.com/us/

16. Gates, B. (1999). *Business at the Speed of Thoughts.* New York, NY: Time Warner.

17. Retrieved from www.jri-america.com/aboutus_corp.htm

18. Tan, (2001), *ibid.*

19. McNurlin, B. C., & Sprague, R. H., Jr. (1989). *Information systems management in practice* (2nd ed.). Englewood Cliffs, NJ: Prentice-Hall.

20. Retrieved from ww3.frost.com/files/4115/4702/8528/Frost__Sullivan_Weekly_Analyst_Insight_Issue_1_EDT_AG_SS.pdf

21. Retrieved from https://emerj.com/ai-sector-overviews/ai-machine-learning-european-pharmaceuticals-current-applications/

Chapter Questions

5-1 What are some of the major HMIS enterprise software systems? Discuss the need for a data-sharing culture in implementing the various HMIS enterprise software systems.

5-2 Why would it be (or not be) beneficial to combine SCM and CRM into a single system for healthcare services organizations? What about combining SCM with ERP, or other combinations of HMIS enterprise software systems for healthcare services organizations?

5-3 How should one go about standardizing service nomenclature, such as the process service names and outcomes, in order to achieve a level of ease with implementing enterprise-wide software? Why must people be sold on the software and be ready to change before moving ahead with a large-scale implementation, such as ERP?

5-4 What do you see as the trend of healthcare services organizations with the applications of HMIS enterprise software?

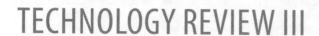

© phasin/Getty Images

TECHNOLOGY REVIEW III

Supply Chain Management (SCM) for Health Systems

Matilda Isaac Mustapha and Joseph Tan

Abstract

Healthcare Supply Chain Management (SCM) involves allocating limited resources and supplies, delivering goods and services effectively between providers and patients. To date, four innovative platforms (Environmental Improvements, Pharmaceuticals/Chemicals, Diagnostic Technologies, and Medical Devices) have been proposed in healthcare SCM. These platforms create standards that would ensure quality care by continuously contributing excellent practices within the industry. To ensure safe and high quality care, hospitals are finding ways for care practitioners to make accurate decisions in patient care, none of which can be accomplished without smart resource allocation. To this end, hospitals are innovatively using automated point units to track some of their medical and pharmaceutical products. The Omni Cell PAR Excellence-closed cabinet systems are one such innovative system. Managing healthcare SCM also requires leaders who would facilitate team collaborative efforts, unifying care practitioners and other stakeholders in the design and implementation of standardized care. Strong leadership involves the know-how in formulating various strategies, recognizing the intricacies of its corporate culture and assessing its impact on patient-related variables such as care, performance, integration and quality implementation. Conceptual Value Framework (CVF) is one of the most extended and comprehensive models used to foster cohesiveness and cooperation and prevent patient care interruption. For successful CVF, a healthcare industry must allocate resources for technology orientation for the development of exploratory, and exploitative innovative competence. While the idea of healthcare SCM is still in its infancy, some drivers for optimized care include a rapid response time, minimized cost and data accumulation and leaders that maintain a culture of excellence.

TECHNOLOGY REVIEW OUTLINE

▶ Introduction

Over the years, innovative measures to implement best practices for health systems have resulted in both improved efficiencies and cost effectiveness. In the current global economy, managing care processes via supply chain management (SCM) is one measure for health care to remain sustainable. Given that medical supplies account for 30%–40% of hospitals' operating cost, researchers have suggested that a network of value chain partners in patient treatment is needed to realize efficiencies such as better inventory control to enhance patient identity management, increase safety, reduce human errors, improve the rate of delivery, and optimize outcomes.

Notwithstanding, SCM is a shift from commercial settings to the health systems. Noting that the value chain from commercial industries may be transferred to hospitals as it links several infrastructures and management processes for effective outcomes, Johnson et al.[1] propose four taxonomies to revamp hospital operational thinking: (a) firm hospital infrastructure; (b) human resources-hospital staff management; (c) technology growth-research; and (d) development and procurement of medical supplies. These infrastructures form a linkage from the goods and services to the customer. One fact remains; in health care, product availability is a matter of life and death. Hence, emerging technology is crucial in implementing SCM in health care. To date, several studies have highlighted SCM benefits in health care.[2–4]

▶ Innovative Standard of Care

Meeting patient (customer) expectations safely and with assurance is a recognized standard of care in hospitals. It can be effectively achieved via a proper SCM implementation by fitting patients with the right products and services as provided in the admission diagnosis; otherwise, such a fitting process will be more an art than an exact science. Accordingly, advances in health systems methods are just as important as those in the drugs and medical devices. Four innovative SCM platforms are environmental improvements, pharmaceuticals and chemicals, diagnostic technologies, and medical devices.

Environmental Improvements

Broadly, these encompass: (a) a clean, healthy space to support patient treatments, thereby minimizing the spread of disease; (b) basic hygiene and sanitary conditions as a safeguard to prevent patient relapse; (c) constant monitoring of surroundings to prepare for floods and other emergencies that could breed infection; and (d) use of biological–clinical treatments, if needed, to circumvent over-dependency on advanced technologies.

Pharmaceuticals and Chemicals

These are: (a) pharmaceutical advances, vaccines, bio-pharmaceuticals, and chemicals needed to treat and prevent disease; (b) an emphasis on postoperative health after surgical procedures and the operation itself; and (c) the use of effective treatment options such as cholesterol-reducing drugs, HIV control, penicillin, antidepressants, and anti-rejection drugs.

Diagnostic Technologies

Specifically, these include: (a) diagnostics tools to help with disease treatment; (b) X-ray technologies to improve treatment diagnosis; and (c) blood-analyzers to generate measures of oxygen levels, blood sugar levels, and blood tests across the charts.

Medical Devices

These are: (a) drug delivery devices such as "micro-fine" needles which have the ability to deliver necessary drugs to places such as the brain; (b) medical devices that are used to enhance medical procedures such as prosthetics and the replacement of body parts; and (c) implantable delivery devices alongside painless delivery devices to help negate previous traumatic experience.

Combining these SCM elements will allow a hospital to better understand what types of supplies are needed for particular patients. It is argued, for example, that technological innovation is key to transforming the health systems. Here, Van and Szymanski[5] addressed the utilization of SCM on Clinical Units by highlighting the technological innovation of PAR Excellence system, a system comprising a control wand associated with touch buttons for different supply items. The Omni cell PAR Excellence (closed-cabinet system) and Cardinal Health Pyxis products were also developed with prompts, allowing members of the nursing staff to identify themselves, state the patient in need of the supply, and a final prompt to extract the supply. Healthcare Purchasing News Senior Editor Rick Dana Barlow asked Joe Dattilo, president of PAR Excellence Systems Inc., if hospitals already struggling with cost associated with enterprise resource planning or ERP systems, upgraded material management information systems (MMIS) or Internet e-commerce technologies, would find justification in automated supply cabinets? Joe Dattilo responded:

> For many hospitals, the addition of a point-of-use system might be all that is necessary to, in effect, upgrade their present MMIS. We typically control all the various PAR Location inventories throughout the organization. We automatically create orders/requisitions for both stock and non-stock items and forward these to the hospitals ERP systems. The ERP system may be interfaced to the e-commerce systems; however, we can also directly interface with vendors, if desired. We can foresee that sometime in the future, point-of-use systems may work in tandem with e-commerce technologies to provide all of the functionality required in a streamlined supply chain.[6]

Dattilo further noted that although many organizations may not be able to justify a shift to the PAR system, they needed to consider prioritizing the automated point-of-use system. An open cabinet system is a good way to manage supply within an organization; in a high traffic area, a closed cabinet system (as depicted) may be better served (**FIGURES TR3-1** and **TR3-2**).

A more recent innovative SCM is the Chain-analytics, a cost-to-serve model in healthcare inventory management. This system allows the emergence of internal process capabilities with high volume product while increasing analytical capabilities in decision-making. The key is a continuous link between the inventory cost, the inventory target location, and the level of products. For a single product-line, this SCM model has generated a total cost savings of $2M with the manufacturer of this model rating itself as a global multi-billion high medical product manufacturer. Here, big data accessibility works to enhance workflow by helping clinicians integrate imaging record applications, a development that sets forth a shift from single care area of digital imagining to other areas of neurology.

▶ Resource Optimizing

Application Infrastructure Provider (AIP) focuses on maximizing profits related to selling capacity whereas Application Service Provider (ASP) focuses on the determination of optimum pricing vis-à-vis optimum volume of purchases. Adjusting capacity of patient orders in the pharmaceutical sector enable the proper inventory flow in SCM. Supply chain (SC) coordination is a vital task directly related to the elements. "Lean production" in multiple industries has been championed by Japanese management practices.[7] In health care, however, lead time inventory management allows for crucial inventory out-preventions. Long hospital wait times in the emergency room (ER) have raised public concern warranting a more strategically placed pattern and structure. Today, hospitals are experiencing shorter wait times with proper patient diagnosis via real-time simulated patient models (e.g., Registration & Categorization-Consultation-Testing & Treatment), reduced product development cycle time, and new product introduction time. Thus, with reduced service capacity delays, healthcare services can become more efficiently delivered, and proper protocols may be administered. This then generates a standard protocol for disease control and prevention.

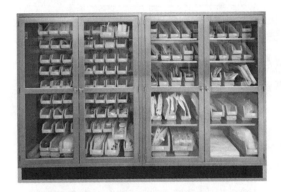

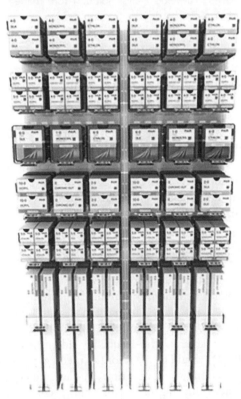

FIGURE TR3-1 Closed cabinet system v. open cabinet system.

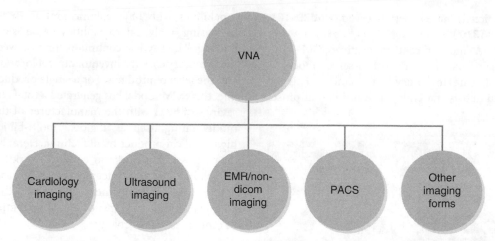

FIGURE TR3-2 Another innovative value chain system is the Vendor Neutral Archive (VNA). VNA consolidates data imaging from different vendors into a user-friendly repository. It is an imaging technology for standardized data storage with interfaces, allowing for easy access in a vendor-neutral fashion by other systems as imagery are increasingly disseminated and shared. A practice embraced by care practitioners is the interoperation or image sharing at a higher application level to develop analysis solution from image storage infrastructure—such an infrastructure is crucial to SCM.

▶ Supply Chain Management and Cost

Total costs for SC in the U.S. healthcare market are about 140 billion dollars; significantly, 25% of pharmaceutical costs and 40% of medical costs are due to SCs. SC delivery spectrum has created a positive impact on cost as the patient gets the appropriate care while the supplier provides the hospital with the right products. Still, a steady increase of drug recalls, which are detrimental to patient safety, has emerged. Another concern is that SCM is not yet a priority for ambulatory surgery, clinics, diagnostic imaging, physician practices, and urgent care. The lack of synergy among these care centers creates difficulties in cost minimization.[8] The health systems lack SC cost-minimization tools as the industry suffers from inefficient capital and resource utilization with a high medical supply turnover rate. Further, the amount of drug shortages has tripled in the United States. Since 2005, inefficiencies in

healthcare services have cost the industry more than half a billion dollars. Recognizing that overall patient safety is the top priority, hospitals are strategizing to help alleviate cost. Some of these strategies include forming smaller sections of operation comprising manufacturers, distributers, hospital, and pharmacies to handle products and delivery. Four SC models (segmentation, agility, measurement, and alignment) have been proposed to optimize performance and reduce cost.

Segmentation

Drug retailers use a one-size-fits-all SC even though profitability might be different if drugs were valued by weight, demand, and/or importance. Kumar et al.[9] opined that supply-chain radio-frequency identification (RFID) would be great for the medical field as the system would save time, money, and effort besides limiting paperwork and record misplacement. Accordingly, the RFID equipment will allow clinicians to more easily manage patient care processes and access patient's files, thereby reducing the overall operational costs.

Agility

Agility speeds up operational functions, ensuring faster responses whenever there are demand emergencies. Quickness is not the only key, but with it comes satiability, replenishment, and visibility—key concepts that will assist with supply issues, customer issues, and impending bottlenecks. Again, Kumar, et.al.[10] observed that the RFID can help with faster patient discharge; for example, the discharge time for new mothers was found to be lengthy with much paperwork. The RFID can create a smoother and more efficient discharge process. Also, allocating funds to better align production will reduce supply shortages and reduce costs due to fluctuation in manufacturing, transport, warehouse, inventory hold, staffing, and obsolescence.

Measurement

Owing to manufacturing, transport, warehouse, inventory hold, staffing, and obsolescence, cost can fluctuate with production change. To stabilize cost, a better production system may be created to minimize supply shortage by incorporating "Kaizen," the Japanese lean production system. "Kaizen" means "improvement" so that in business, "Kaizen" can be applied to processes such as logistics, purchasing, and several organizational SC-related functions. The underlying idea is to properly measure the demand in proportion to the supply so as to minimize costly waste.[11]

Alignment

Properly aligned production occurs in the following six steps: (i) agree on benefiting models; (ii) select collaborative partners; (iii) act as a team; (iv) place resources to help involve leadership; (v) manage and perform as a team; and (vi) look at the long-term perspective to minimize SCM cost. By following these steps, less mistakes and more efficacy will emerge. Key components of collaboration include joint planning, shared problem-solving, and collaborative decision-making.[12] Forming partnerships can help firms to increase competitive advantage, manage knowledge flow, share information, manage inventory levels, align supply chain, manage risk coordination, and enhance firm performance. It is equally important to note that by cutting service time, errors might emerge; hence, to minimize such risks, healthcare institutions need to have a well thought-out plan while looking at the long-term benefits.[13]

▶ Supplier Cost in Supply Chain Management

The cost dilemma for health systems from the supply sector is that data for supply usage and patient information are incongruent. In many hospital systems, specific information relating supply cost to patient care lacks the association needed to effectively serve patients. Supply costs are tracked in financial systems to optimize revenue generated from patients, making it susceptible to vendors–physicians collaboration. Vendors can incentivize physicians to buy specific products for no good reason. Many hospitals are aggressing supply spend and engaging physicians in more disciplined procurement of high-end devices, thereby limiting their potential due to cost manipulation associated with patient discharge information. This concern has compromised the quality of care and cost efficiency[14]. Accordingly, the Food and Drug Administration (FDA) has vowed to establish a unique device identification system to aid hospitals in better tracking and managing medical devices and analyzing their effectiveness.

▶ Optimizing Supply Identifiers

Parkinson[15] identified several strategies for optimizing the utilization of the new supply identifiers as follows:

Fine-Tune the Electronic Health Record (EHR)

Grant access to care providers to use information in EHRs about treatment, variation, or supply use for drug testing modalities and frequencies because such information will be stored in data warehouses that store patient information.

Support Value Analysis with Adequate Data Processes

Perform value analysis in supply-intensive areas (e.g., the operating rooms (OR) and cardiac procedure areas), strategically aligning physician preference to key quality-cost saving targets; also, identify cost deficits in supply data, account for EHR missing data, and establish proper routines to monitor the value analysis process.

Adopt a Unique Device Identification (UDI) to Capture-Evaluate the Effectiveness of Medical Devices

The UDI will assist in tracing medical supplies from purchase to the patient's usage. Hospitals should realize maximum cost savings from their efforts once the identifiers are printed on product labels.

Automation Can Create a Cost-Effective Supply Chain, but Support for Supply Chain Automation Hospitals Is Minimal

As the revenue-focused business in health care has induced an under-investment in technology, support for SC efficiencies is often lacking.

▶ Engineering Approaches to Supply Chain Management

Engineering approaches to prediction control-design have much to offer health care in terms of systemic improvement via cost-quality data modeling and simulations. Liotta[16] observed that suppliers, manufacturers, and retailers linked by material and information as well as financial flows should be used to satisfy patient's demand. Engineering approaches can take advantage of knowledge gained from medical science along with other sources to develop business models. These models must, however, be first mathematically validated over time prior to their applications in practice. Liotta[17] postulated that to reduce healthcare cost, "what if" analysis based on designed experiments can be conducted and that the decision aid may be developed from a hierarchy of strategic, tactical as well as operational standpoints.

▶ Organizational Culture and Supply Chain Management

Cultures ranging from organizational culture, development culture, group culture, rational culture to hierarchical culture will influence healthcare supply chain resilience (HCRES). Organizational culture is defined as a set of shared values, beliefs, or patterns of understanding that underlines the fabric of employees working in the organization. Clan culture, hierarchy culture, adhocracy culture, and market cultures are key enablers of governance and orientation in organizations via routine information acquisition, transmission, and utilization. Studies indicate that hierarchy culture inhibits all phases, but mostly acquisition, transmission, and utilization. Even so, positive influences have been found for development, group, and rational cultures on HCRES. Managers tend to focus more on developing competing values framework (CVF)-based dimensions to provide services in a timely manner. Resilience is an important dynamic capability in healthcare SC as it elicits an uninterrupted treatments and services to patients. SCM success requires managers to: (a) conduct training programs directed to clarifying the importance of organizational climate and its CVF-based dimensions at the employee level; (b) focus on enriching specific cultures in the respective organizations to enhanced HCRES; and (c) encourage healthcare entities to work as cohesive groups to enhance coordination and cooperation. Equally important to recognizing resilience is to understand disruption. In healthcare SCs, context disruption is defined as an unexpected event that can hinder the delivery of care services to patients. While SC resilience is essential, SC capability requires the safeguarding of operations. When disrupted, hospitals must develop risk management strategies—they and their partners in healthcare SC must devise capabilities that can safeguard their operations. Indeed, it is the firm's dynamic capability that will enable it to prepare for uncertainties via adequate planning with SC partners to sustain performance; here, healthcare SC entities must maintain the capability to work in a synchronized manner to provide uninterrupted patient care.

▶ Technology Orientation in Supply Chain Management

Defined as the will and ability to evolve a sound technical background in new product developments, technology orientation (TO) incorporates product, service, production, and innovation orientations. TO in health systems hinges on emerging technology adoption to exchange real-time information with SC partners for services coordination. Studies suggest discoveries and innovations in health systems have a positive influence on TO organizations. For medical entities, service innovation initiatives aided by TO enable hospitals to develop exploratory and exploitative innovation competences. The development culture suggests that firms should have a long-term orientation for sustainability. Higher levels of TO supports culture developments, inspiring employees to accentuate organizational objectives.

▶ Managerial Implications of Supply Chain Management Implementation

A smooth SCM implementation can result in a consistent, easy flow of information with a physical flow of goods-services emphasizing patient outcome. Benefits of an innovative

SCM entail simplifying various interactive and collaborative processes. These include the nurse–physician and the patient–physician interactions as well as collaboration sought among producers, vendors, suppliers, service providers, and financial entities, thereby adding value to the entire SCM process. Health systems leadership arising from improper decision-making will be one of the major flaws; for example, adopting the decisions of clinicians (doctors, nurses, and pharmacists) as the ultimate preference of drugs prescription, leading to overstocking, and waste. Essentially, if all clinical outcomes rest on these entities, does the end user lose autonomy? In an attempt to offer a management solution for cost reduction, a university-based teaching hospital implemented the clinical product value (CPV) or stock keep unit standardization (SKU). The first step was to identify variation in the cost assessment, standardize all care and practice, and, most importantly, the formation of leadership teams (the Analysis Committee) to help facilitate the process. An analysis committee unites health professionals of all departments and medical distribution centers. The committee moderated the process to fill and evaluate new product requests. As a result, this committee reduced hospital medical supply costs while ensuring the products' quality and patient safety.[18] Prior to introducing the analyzing committee, it was common for new products to appear in hospital units without the knowledge and preparatory education of clinicians.

▶ Conclusion

An effective SCM in health care involves defining standards of care, investing in automated systems, and improving ongoing interactions with the SC partners. Key benefits include rapid customer response times, lower inventory costs, and an integrated SC visibility. Management can develop structures and use existing tools to enhance services. Researchers can harvest big data in the SCM. The big data comprises miscellaneous web searches, social media trends, GPS information, texts, blogs, and a multitude of personal information. Some have argued that big data compilations come with several challenges and limitations. The data collected are sometimes immeasurable and too varied or unstructured, which makes it nearly impossible for traditional technology to decipher crucial information.[19] Others have viewed big data as a national weapon developed by the government and large corporations to control purchasing and our livelihood. Whatever side of the argument you may subscribe to, it is important to note that an appropriate handling of such complex data collection and progressive technological innovation will ultimately yield safer, more adaptive, efficient, and cost-effective health learning systems.

Notes

1. Johnson, G., Scholes, K., & Whittington R. (2009). *Exploring corporate strategy* (625 pages). Essex, England: Financial Times (FT) Prentice Hall, An Imprint of Pearson Education Ltd.
2. Hong, P., Dobrzykowski, D., & Won Park, Y. (2012). Challenges and opportunities for supply chains in turbulent times. *Benchmarking: An International Journal*, 19(4/5). doi:10.1108/bij.2012.13119daa.001
3. Soosay, A, C., Hyland, P. W., & Ferrer. M. (2008). Supply chain collaboration: Capabilities for continuous innovation. *Supply Chain Management:* *An International Journal*, 13(2), 160–169. Retrieved from https://doi.org/10.1108/135985408 10860994
4. Van de Castle, B. L., & Szymanski, G. (2008). Supply chain management on clinical units. In: U. Hübner, & M. A. Elmhorst (Eds.), *eBusiness in healthcare* (pp. 197–217). Health Informatics Series (Formerly Computers in Health Care). London: Springer.
5. *Ibid.*
6. Barlow, R. D., & Akridge. J. (2004–2006). *Supply storage systems: Silver bullet or silver lining for Cost*

management? Retrieved from www.hpnonline.com /inside/2004-06/supply_storage_systems.htm

7. Samuel, C., Gonapa, K., Chaudhary, P. K., & Mishra, A., (2010). Supply chain dynamics in healthcare services. *International Journal of Health Care Quality Assurance, 23*(7), 631–642. doi:10.1108/09526861011071562

8. Barlow, C. (2015). Ambulatory surgery centers: A growing trend in healthcare; *Investment Intern Russell Capital Management.* Retrieved from www .russcap.com/a-recent-trend-in-healthcare--chris -barlowpdf/

9. Kumar, S., Swanson, E., & Tran, T. (2009). RFID in the healthcare supply chain: Usage and application. *International Journal of Health Care Quality Assurance, 22*(1), 67–81. doi:10.1108/09526860910927961

10. *Ibid.*

11. Retrieved from https://www.kaizen.com/learn -kaizen/glossary.html

12. Stank, T. P., Keller, S. P., & Daugherty, P. J. (2011). *Supply chain collaboration and logistical service performance.* Retrieved from https://onlinelibrary .wiley.com/doi/abs/10.1002/j.2158-1592.2001 .tb00158.x

13. Ebel, T., Larsen, E., George, L., Shah, K., & Ungerman. D. (2013, September). *Strengthening health care's supply chain: A 5 step plan* (pp. 1–7). Chicago: McKinsey & Company. Retrieved from https://health .economictimes.indiatimes.com/web/files/retail _files/reports/data_file-Building-New-Strenghts-In -Healthcare-Supply-Chain-1421845643.pdf

14. Parkinson, R. C. (2014). Tying supply chain costs to patient care. *Healthcare Financial Management, 68*(5), 42+. *Academic OneFile.* Retrieved from https://link.galegroup.com/apps/doc/A371969492 /AONE?u=googlescholar&sid=AONE&xid =12c9dcc5

15. Johnson et al., (2009), *ibid.*

16. Parkinson, (2014), *ibid.*

17. Liotta, G. (2012). Simulation of supply chain networks: A source of innovation and competitive advantage for small and medium sized enterprises. *Technology Innovation Management Review.* Retrieved from https://timreview.ca/sites/default/files/article_PDF /Liotta_TIMReview_November2012.pdf

18. *Ibid.*

19. Tan, K., Zhan, Y., Ji, G., Ye, F., & Chang, C. (2015). Harvesting big data to enhance supply chain innovation capabilities: An analytic infrastructure based on deduction graph. *International Journal of Production Economics, 165.* doi:10.1016/j.ijpe.2014.12.034

Biography

Dr. Mustapha is an Assistant Professor of Quantitative Systems, Management, and Marketing in the School of Business at Madonna University. She received her bachelor's degree in science, a master's of Science in Business Administration (Quality Management), and a PhD in Technology Management.

Dr. Mustapha focuses on developing research and analytical skills for both graduate and undergraduate students. She has taught a variety of courses ranging from business statistics, strategic management, leadership and ethics, research methodology, computer science, management information systems, and operations management. She has also taught several business management courses for Madonna University programs in Mainland China.

Dr. Mustapha is involved in several research projects including "The Symbolic Interactionist View on Transnational Education, Managing Virtual Teams, Ethical Organizational Climate, Examining the Paradoxical Relation between Socio-Technology Optimization and Marxist Theory of Alienation. She has co-authored in highly referenced scientific and business journals and has presented in both domestic and international conferences. She is a professional chair member of International Economics Development and Research Center (IERDC), a member of Decision Sciences Institute (DSI), and a member of the Society for Collegiate Leadership and Achievement-Honor Society (SCLA-HS). She is also a honorary faculty member of Delta Mu Delta.

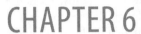

CHAPTER 6

Key Patient-Centric Technologies: EHR, CPOE, CDS, and PP

Joseph Tan with Phillip Olla and Joshia Tan

LEARNING OBJECTIVES

- Understand the Historical Evolution of Patient-Centric Application Systems
- Identify Electronic Health Records (EHR) Application Systems
- Review Computerized Physician Order Entry (CPOE) Application Systems
- Recognize Clinical Decision Support (CDS) Application Systems
- Overview of Patient Portals (PP)

CHAPTER OUTLINE

Scenario: How Samsung Health Redefines Personal Fitness and Beyond

I. Introduction
II. What Are Electronic Health Records, Computerized Physician Order Entry, Clinical Decision Support, and Patient Portals?
III. Historical Evolution of EHR, CPOE, CDS, and PP
IV. Electronic Health Records
V. Computerized Physician Order Entry

VI. Clinical Decision Support
VII. Patient Portals
VIII. Benefits and Challenges of EHR, CPOE, CDS, and PP
  - *Benefits*
  - *Challenges*
IX. Conclusion

Notes
Chapter Questions

Scenario: How Samsung Health Redefines Personal Fitness and Beyond[1-3]

Previously known as S Health, Samsung's popular and well-designed app offers a comprehensive health-and-wellness platform for aiding health consumers and their loved ones in adopting a healthy lifestyle. More specifically, the Samsung mobile app acts as a lifestyle tracker, providing useful health content and connecting health conscious users with lifestyle care management and personal coaching programs. Importantly, these activities are conducted securely within an integrated and easy-to-use mobile phone environment.

More recently, Samsung has also improved its S Health offerings by renaming it as Samsung Health to enable new features for patients to connect with all of their multiple Samsung wearable devices and accessories. Such fitness and medical devices can include glucometers, blood pressure monitors, and heart rate monitors to enable consumers to easily measure and manage on their own a range of health-related and lifestyle metrics. Consumers oftentimes entrust this information to various significant others, such as care providers, pharmacies, insurers, and even laboratories. By taking responsibilities for their own health and lifestyle habits, it is believed that consumers will stay fit longer, eat healthier and more selectively, become more active, lose weight, and better manage their own health conditions. Best of all, these health consumers can complete all such tasks conveniently via a secure mobile app installed on their Samsung Galaxy S8 and/or other Android phones.

Today, Samsung Health has become the forerunner in such self-care management apps because it pays meticulous attention to improving the healthy lifestyle habits of the app users by emphasizing the good lifestyle habits consumers should be adhering to and assisting them in coordinating several key healthy lifestyle habits in the different healthy lifestyle management domains. For instance, the weight management feature automatically computes users' recorded calorie balance, guiding Samsung Health users toward achieving their weight goal. Importantly, users are encouraged to record their daily activities and food consumption meticulously, so that the built-in analytics can get them closer to their health goal. Users are also challenged to walk further and longer, by competing and comparing their own achievements and performance with invited friends, family members, and other Samsung Health users.

At the time of this writing, it is purported that the Samsung Health app already has attracted millions of interested users while supporting its usage in over 70 languages. Most importantly, new features are constantly being added or updated into the earlier version(s). For example, the recent addition of "Ask-an-Expert" capabilities will further allow the smartphone users to conduct tele-medical services via an on-demand, live video consultation with a doctor 24/7. To ease consumers' worries about payments, Samsung has also pre-authorized coverage for such services for selected healthcare plans that are popular with many U.S. health consumers, who can then order these tele-medical services conveniently and as needed. In fact, when thinking about how to make American health care more accessible and more patient-centric to smartphone users, Samsung Health's design team has ensured that the "Ask-an-Expert" feature was fully pilot-tested before implementation, with the aim of enabling users to make low-cost appointments with world-class doctors right from their smartphone. The Samsung design team was able to succeed by having major insurance companies partner with top-tier physicians and leading hospitals across the United States.

Imagine trusting all your personal health data with a third-party platform, such as Samsung Health. Remember that technology giants, such as Apple and Google, are also anticipating future growth potential and profitability, coming up with various innovative products to compete in the health, fitness, and self-care lifestyle management marketplace. The growing number of such offerings can indeed cause quite a bit of confusion and apprehension for some health consumers. As these organizations lack a history of involvement with healthcare services prior to their offering of health and fitness systems, what if the information was sold to, or mined by, people from organizations that are unknown to the health consumers? What is the chance or potential for security breaches and privacy compromises with the consumer health data captured in these various platforms? Take a minute to reflect on these possibilities and debate the various probable scenarios.

▶ I. Introduction

The past few decades have seen continuing cost acceleration, advancing technologies, and growing competition challenging the healthcare marketplace. To adapt, health systems organizations have become increasingly more eager to change from relying on traditional paper-based health data and information processing systems to newer forms of e-health recording practices so as to ensure greater efficiencies in health data management and effectiveness in clinical decision-making. While patients have voiced major concerns over the security, privacy, and confidentiality of their health records being captured electronically, their ultimate objective remains unchanged: to receive high-quality health care, with easily accessible and available records for pre-authorized care providers and referral specialists, especially in emergencies. The Institute of Medicine defines patient-centric care as "providing care that is respectful of and responsive to individual patient preferences, needs and values, ensuring that patient values guide all clinical decisions." "Patient-centric" means that the healthcare provider should be paying attention to the patient's individual needs, and ensuring that the patient is provided with the

tools and opportunity to engage in decisions that impact care, along with the tools needed to comply with treatment recommendations.[4]

Accordingly, the need for electronic data gathering, tracking, and coordinating systems that can provide caregivers with timely, reliable, and secured access to a patient's files—such as his or her complete medical history, laboratory test results, and radiological images—cannot be overly emphasized. An ideal network of health data-entry, storage, and reporting systems should achieve interoperability among themselves, as well as with all of the legacy systems. Such is the concept of electronic health records (EHR), a system that will allow doctors and nurses to access conveniently accurate health records, reduce the need for unnecessary duplication of patient data, and give clarifications to clinicians performing follow-up care, who frequently need a patient's previous treatment or medical information. Without knowing a patient's history, practitioners—especially in the case of an emergency—will have to blindly perform treatments in hope of saving his or her life. It is apparent that the quality and speed of care can be enhanced, in many cases, if only the appropriate and relevant patient information were available, accessible, and verifiable. The role of an electronic medical record is to make all the patient's information available to the clinical staff; typically, this information is not shared with the patients. To alleviate this challenge the concept of a Patient Portal (PP) was conceived. The PP allows patients to access important medical information from the comfort of their homes.

Four major patient-centric management systems have evolved in the healthcare services industry that will continue to affect patient care and the performance of care providers in the coming years: EHR, computerized physician order entry (CPOE), clinical decision support (CDS), and PP. Among these, the EHR system is the most inclusive and important for direct inpatient and outpatient care because it typically also encompasses the other two patient-centric management systems. Therefore, our discussion of CPOE and CDS will be embedded partly in the larger EHR context for delivering error-free and quality patient care. Tan[5] addresses the concerns of those who would like to have a more detailed understanding of these different systems, their historical developments, applications, and cases, especially for EHR and CDS implementations. Meanwhile, a brief review and empirical evidence on the acceptance of CPOE among physicians may be found in Liang, Xue, and Wu.[6]

We begin our limited review by first defining and reviewing the historical evolution of these three patient-centric management systems.

▶ II. What Are Electronic Health Records, Computerized Physician Order Entry, Clinical Decision Support, and Patient Portals?

EHR[7] comprise, essentially, the health information of an individual patient that exists as part of a complete history; such records are, furthermore, designed to provide clinicians with a comprehensive picture of the patient's health status at any time. Today, the term EHR has largely replaced older terms, such as "computerized patient records" and "electronic medical records." Specifically, the U.S. Department of Veterans Affairs defined computer-based patient records (CPR) as records that are stored in decentralized hospital computer software, whereas EMR may be conceived as an enterprise-wide system where patient medical histories are captured in a single repository. The EHR term has taken on an even wider connotation in that these systems are also meant to automate and streamline the clinician's workflow, besides having the ability

to independently generate a complete record of clinical patient encounters, sourcing data from various care episodes over the lifetime of a patient. In other words, these patient-centric, electronic database management systems capture, using all available patient–provider encounters in a longitudinal fashion, both the historic and current records of a patient's health information. Altogether, the system may contain various patient demographics and patient history information, such as progress notes, medical diagnoses, prescriptions, vital signs, immunization records, laboratory test data, and radiology reports.

Closely related to, and often functioning as part of, EHR, a *CPOE*[8] system is basically an automated order-entry system that captures the instructions of physicians with regard to the care of their patients. Physicians enter orders in the EHR using CPOE, which has been shown to increase patient safety and improve the quality of care. The system also provides clinical guidelines for physicians and prints summaries of visits for patients, among other services. CPOE orders are disseminated, via computer networks, throughout various parts of a healthcare services facility, such as pharmacy, laboratory, or radiology, as well as to other care providers, including nurses, therapists, and other consulting medical professional staff, who will then follow up on the orders.

CDS[9] are medical information processing systems that are designed to aid clinicians in making complex and/or less-than-complex clinical-based decisions. CDS provide data banks, alerts and reminders, algorithms, analytic or pathophysiologic models, clinical decision theoretical models, statistical pattern recognition methods, symbolic reasoning, and/or expert knowledge bases to enhance the diagnostic, therapeutic, and prognostic-thinking and cognitive-reasoning strategies of expert and amateur clinicians alike.

Finally, *PP*[10] are online platforms that permit patients to gain remote access to their own digital medical information while performing a multitude of other critical functions, such as allowing patients and their families to become aware of the latest research information pertaining to their specific diseases of interests. In this sense, PP will empower the patients with necessary knowledge on and provide insights into their specific medical conditions and treatment plan so that these patients can play an active role in their own care over the course of the treatment process.

Healthcare managers, administrators, and executives hoping to perform well in complex health systems organizations must therefore become thoroughly familiar with all of these patient-centric management systems. These are four major systems that will drive the majority of diagnostic, therapeutic, and prognostic decisions made for patients attending the different care facilities of a health maintenance organization. These systems have evolved over the years and have drawn significant influence from the early developments and history of computer-based patient records and hospital information systems. We turn now to look briefly at the historical developments of these systems.

▶ III. Historic Evolution of EHR, CPOE, CDS, and PP

Computer-based patient records, according to the 1997 National Academy of Sciences Institute of Medicine (IOM) report,[11] are systems specifically designed to aid clinical users in assessing patient information. Such information typically includes complete and accurate patient history, alerts and reminders, clinical decision support models, guides and links to medical knowledge bases, and other references and informational resources (such as a referencing drug database). The evolution of computer-based patient data systems, such as EHR, CPOE, and CDSS, is best understood in terms of the historic evolution of hospital information systems (HIS), artificial intelligence (AI)

in medicine, health decision aids, and electronic patient records (EPR).

The genesis of HMIS dates back to the early 1950s, when only mainframes were available and when even the processing of a batch of patient-related information required considerable time, knowledge, and expertise. From the 1960s to the 1970s, a new era of HMIS emerged when "pioneering" American and European hospitals joined forces to eventually develop a successful patient information management system prototype, named the Technicon system. It is this prototype that laid the foundation for many of today's working hospital patient information systems throughout North America and Europe. The major lesson learned was the need to focus on users' information needs and the need to change the attitudes of the users, particularly those of physicians, nurses, and other clinicians.

During the early and mid-1970s, computerization was pinpointed as the source of the evident gains in productivity and increased efficiency, prompting the diffusion of large-scale data-processing applications in medicine and health record systems. With the emergence of mini- and micro-computers during the 1980s, physicians and clinical practitioners soon began to realize the speed and astounding harnessing power of computers. During this time, interest in the application of AI in medicine expanded and soon contributed to the development of CDS.

In 1999, the IOM reported a disturbing statistic—each year, in the United States, medical errors were responsible for up to 98,000 unnecessary hospital patient deaths. An urgent call was immediately made for healthcare services organizations to reduce this exorbitant level of medical errors.[12] Several institutions took up the challenge; Palo Alto Medical Foundation (PAMF), for example, became one of the earliest adopters of EHR, replacing paper charts with electronic records, thereby allowing physicians and clinical staff direct and very convenient access to patient information. The adoption not only eliminated the hectic scramble to locate paper records, but also led to a reduction in medical errors. Similarly, in 2004, three suburban Chicago hospitals reported a 20% drop in medication errors and the complete elimination of transcription errors with their EHR implementations. Against this background, Arsala et al.[13] believe that we have undergone four generations in the evolution of computer-based patient records in overcoming the medical error challenge and will soon move into fifth-generation EHR by 2010.

During the first generation of CPR, hospitals relied heavily on the clinical data repository (CDR); in fact, the adoption of a single, comprehensive repository for clinical information during the 1960s–1970s was said to have eliminated about 15% of preventable medical errors in hospital-based patient care. From the 1970s–1980s, the next generation of CPR development was noted to have the added capability of documenting clinical activities, as well as the ability to tailor the IT report for the use and needs of specific caregivers. This resulting improvement was estimated to have garnered up to another 25% reduction in medical errors. Moreover, CDS implementation during this period was thought to have further reduced error rates with their automated intelligence. The combination of these augmented capabilities thus amounted to a 40% level of reduction in preventable errors.

Third-generation CPR/EHR development, during the 1980s–1990s, involved the combination of an improved CDS with the use of a controlled medical vocabulary to standardize medical concepts and the availability of a CPOE system, thus allowing a more effective management of the physician ordering process. It was envisaged that this increased level of automation helped to realize up to a 70% preventable error reduction as compared with the systems capabilities of the previous generations. During this generation, it became progressively critical for workflow capabilities to emerge as tools for supporting the optimal delivery of patient care.

The fourth-generation EHR, which are expected to reduce preventable errors by up to a 90% level, have now been realized. These systems are considered to have an improved CDS function capable of providing a detailed portrait of each patient and automated support for care management protocols. These systems claim to be flexible so that clinician users can tailor them for individual patients; they are also capable of knowledge management so that continual improvement in care delivery can be provided; they are supposedly geared with formal workflow capability so that the consistencies of medical practices can be balanced as needed for optimal care outcomes.

The next-generation EHR are projected to have complex CDS functionalities, to have a networked CPOE, and to be supportive of natural language interfaces. In this sense, EHR software will enable automation of the care processes with preprogrammed alerts and reminders. With CPOE interfacing capability, the future EHR software will not only aid caregivers in obtaining complete, real-time updates of patient information at all times, but also offer caregivers the ability to disseminate their orders efficiently and effectively. As well, with the proliferation of high speed Internet, Web portals such as PPs have become commonplace. These fifth-generation systems are, therefore, expected to aid clinicians intelligently, especially in the caring of patients who may demand real-time monitoring, and even those with multiple, concurrent medical conditions. Finally, with mobile and sensor networks on the rise, all of these systems should also support interfaces to wireless health data networks, enhance mobile healthcare services, and provide secured linkages to sensor-based tracking and health monitoring devices.

▶ IV. Electronic Health Records

For decades, health systems organizations have invested millions of dollars in the research and development of a system that can computerize patient records, thereby satisfying the information needs of care providers who deliver high-quality patient care. Despite the noted progress, some healthcare facilities are still relying on traditional paper-based recordkeeping systems. This may be due, in whole or in part, to the high cost of implementing computerized patient records; the expressed concerns of patients over privacy, confidentiality, and security issues with computerized records; and the lack of government and private funding to support computerized healthcare databases administration, research, and development.

As previously noted, many terms have been used interchangeably to describe how patient records are captured electronically, and these terms have often resulted in some confusion—and a lack of strategic vision alignment and conceptual integration among healthcare administrators and health IT managers. The EHR term has a wider connotation, encompassing automation and streamlining of the clinician's workflow besides being capable of independently generating, by sourcing data from various care episodes throughout a patient's life, a complete record of clinical patient encounters. In addition, EHR will support other care-related activities, including, but not limited to, clinical decision support, care delivery quality management, and clinical reporting.[14] According to Dickinson,[15] the EHR should serve diverse purposes, such as assisting direct patient care, improving routine reporting on the care processes, aiding the processing of claims reimbursement, credentialing care providers, providing an audit trail for care processes, ensuring quality, preventing medical errors, satisfying public health needs, enhancing education, supporting research, and satisfying the legal needs of healthcare services organizations. Ultimately, these incredibly powerful systems are intended to improve physician practices as well as increase health organizational competitiveness and profitability.

An integrated EHR will link all EPR and critical patient care systems so that patient data can be shared and disseminated among authorized clinician users. In general, such an integrated system comprises six primary modules or components working in unison, most of which have already been alluded to in earlier discussions. Specifically, these components include: (1) a CDR, which offers a comprehensive source for storing and retrieving relevant, reliable, and accurate clinical information; (2) a CDS, which provides rule-based alerts, such as warning messages against potential harmful drug interactions when patients are inadvertently placed on two or more potentially interactive medications; (3) a clinical documentation module, which can inform the caring clinician of specific activities taken by other clinicians in managing a particular patient; (4) a CPOE, which will electronically capture the attending physician's instructions so as to help eliminate errors caused by illegible handwritten orders; (5) a controlled medical vocabulary (CMV) module for ensuring that information sourced from various clinical repositories can be easily compared, making it easier to generate proper clinical rules for achieving quality patient care; and (6) a workflow controller module, which manages clinical care processes so that these processes may be sequenced appropriately, executed properly, and executed without omissions.[16]

Other systems that can be integrated with the EHR, but that are discussed later, include laboratory information systems (LIS), pharmacy information systems (PIS), and radiological information systems (RIS).

By implementing an integrated EHR, a healthcare services organization is therefore expected to gain data management speed and accuracy, enhance patient safety and clinical workflow efficiencies, reduce medical errors, and control administrative and medical cost. Not surprisingly, EHR technology is quickly replacing paper-based systems as well as legacy EMR in many healthcare services organizations today.[17]

▶ V. Computerized Physician Order

A CPOE system, as noted in earlier discussions, is often implemented as a component of the EHR. This accompanying system must be able to communicate orders to other connected systems within the EHR. These include ancillary support systems, such as LIS, where laboratory results are captured; PIS, where medication information is captured; RIS, picture archiving and communications systems (PACS), where radiological reports and images are captured; and electronic document/content management (ED/CM) systems, where form documents are captured, streamlined, and managed. Medical records scanning is often a solution when such data are entered manually into forms and need to be archived, stored, and/or shared electronically.

When combined with various other workflow tools, CPOE can also be useful in providing information about patient scheduling, wait times, referral networks, physician work patterns, and disease management. Similarly, the CPOE system may be enabled via PIS for presenting clinical drug choices to the ordering provider. The key success factor for implementing CPOE is overcoming user resistance, particularly the resistance from physicians who may be accustomed to giving verbal or written orders.

Accordingly, acceptance of CPOE by physicians can induce numerous benefits, including decreased delays in order completion and reduced errors from handwritten or transcribed orders. It will also allow order entry at point-of-care or off-site, provide error checking for duplicate or incorrect medication doses or tests, and simplify inventory and posting of charges. A successfully implemented CPOE system can therefore improve the quality of healthcare services delivery and significantly cut healthcare costs.

▶ VI. Clinical Decision Support

At this point, we turn our attention to the last patient-centric systems in the group, the CDS.

In this age of healthcare reform, health administrators and clinicians, with their increasingly complex decision-making activities, are in need of advanced methodological and technological support tools to enhance their effectiveness. CDS are computer-based information-processing and decision support tools that are intended to serve as aids in the rationalization of the clinical decision-making process and justification for the final choices the clinicians have advocated for their patients. Indeed, these systems are not meant to replace the clinical decision-makers. Specifically, if clinicians are armed with CDS containing computerized models, alerts, reminders, and critical sets of data—all of which will contribute in one way or another to analyzing the probability of the onset of certain acute or chronic illnesses for a particular patient—it is anticipated that these clinicians, assisted by the CDS, will exercise better diagnostic, therapeutic, and/or prognostic judgments. In other words, they would not simply jump to conclusions about the complex data set based on the shortsightedness of their self-evaluations, their limited cognitive-reasoning power, or even their intuitive feelings.

Use of CDS interrelates and spans almost every conceivable area of healthcare administrative and clinical decision-making activities. Key components to the building of CDS include database management subsystem, model management subsystem, knowledge bases, inference engine, intelligent graphical interfaces, and any other modules that may enhance the functionalities of the CDS. In this sense, clinicians can use CDS to query general and specific questions about the conditions of their patients based on data that have been collected, stored, organized, manipulated, and retrieved appropriately from its database management subsystem. The model base management component in the CDS permits clinicians to infer and/or forecast resulting outcomes, based on various mathematical computations and analytic model fittings of collected data about the patient's conditions. The knowledgebase component of the CDS typically contains rule-based knowledge, case reasoning, neural networks, artificial intelligence, and/or other expert diagnostic consults for the clinicians. The inference engine component then integrates these different components to arrive at the computed alternatives and/or choice outcomes for the decision makers. It is the intelligent graphical interface that will finally translate and interpret resulting choices in either graphical forms or images to support the decision makers' varying perspectives.

Today, CDS have evolved to support many administrative and medical specialties—examples include nursing decision support systems, pharmacy decision support systems, health executive decision support systems, and specialty medical expert systems. The major cases provided in Part V at the end of this text further discuss the functionalities of many current as well as emerging HMIS technologies, such as EMR, CPOE, devices for tele-home monitoring, virtual reality, 3D printing, and more. For the next part of this chapter, we review the key benefits and challenges of EHR. As previously stated, with CPOE and CDS being typical parts of EHR system installments nowadays, readers can safely assume that the discussion on EHR benefits and challenges apply similarly to the other two patient-centric management systems.

▶ VII. **Patient Portals**

PPs are tools that educate patients about their medical conditions and get them actively involved in their treatment plan, thereby improving their care. PPs perform a multitude of functions.[18] For example, these online platforms allow patients to access their digital personal medical information remotely. Patients can also perform other functions, such as request medication refills, view lab results, and contact physicians. In addition to clinical tasks, patients can also perform administrative tasks, such as pay invoices or schedule appointments. In summary, PPs provide tremendous benefits to patients (some of which are noted in the following bulleted list) while negating the need for patients to be engaged in telephone calls or visit the medical facility in person.[19]

- *PPs reduce incidence of missed appointments*: An unforeseen benefit of PPs is that they significantly reduce no shows, which refers to patients missing a scheduled appointment. The ability to send reminders and connect directly with patients' calendars means people are less likely to forget or double book an appointment. Organizations with patients' portals typically have better quality scores due to the convenience they provide.
- *PPs improve patient engagement*: PPs improve the degree to which patients are more actively engaged with their care as evidenced by patients having better and immediate access to pertinent online information about treatments and medical conditions. Access to important information, such as test results, appointments, and medications, allows patients to stay more informed, knowledgeable, which makes them more engaged in their own care.
- *PPs increase organizational efficiency*: PPs reduce the time needed for administrative staff to complete tedious and consuming daily tasks. Allowing patients access to online tools to book and cancel appointments as their schedules change saves time and reduces costs. Patients having the capability to request medication refills and communicate with their medical team regarding items of concern

also help to streamline and speed up tedious time-consuming tasks.

- *PPs improve communications*: More generally, time spent between the physician and the patient is perceived as being too short and not conducive to a strong relationship between the patient and provider. The added communication via new channels, such as PPs with instant messaging features and secure email facilitates, can improve patients' communication abilities. Patient concerns that would have resulted in an expensive in person office visit can now be avoided by communicating with the medical staff. With the easier and more regular exchange, patients will feel more satisfied with both the care from the physician and the overall healthcare facility.
- *PPs educate the patients*: One of the key benefits of PPs is the ability for the healthcare provider to disseminate relevant, pertinent, and credible health information to patients. As the portal is accessed through the healthcare provider's website, educational material is credible and trustworthy. Examples of formats that can be disseminated are pdfs, photos, videos, and links to other websites, such as "patientslikeme.com" and "dailystrength.org." Material that is relevant to a patient's condition can also be distributed via PPs, such as diabetes information, exercise plans, support smoking cessation advice, and group activity times and dates.

▶ VIII. Benefits and Challenges of EHR, CPOE, CDS, and PP

Health care is an industry that is, apparently, very data intensive; the complexity of healthcare data cannot—and must not—be overlooked.

Imagine what impact human-induced medical errors can wreak on the quality of life and safety of patients and what benefits systems such as EHR, CPOE, CDSS, and PP can have in reversing the adverse effects of these errors.

Paul Tang, the chief medical information officer for the PAMF and chair of the IOM's Committee on Data Standards for Patient Safety,[20] notes that EHRs, such as PAMF's system, can cut healthcare costs, enhance care quality, and significantly lower the risk for medical errors. He believes that providing physicians with convenient and direct access to the information they need for making patient care decisions will automatically raise the bar for ensuring patient safety to a higher level, or "new standard of care."

Aside from the benefits of using EHR and other patient-centric computerized management systems, there are still many challenges in implementing these systems. These benefits and challenges are discussed next.

Benefits

One of several key benefits of using EHR, CPOE, CDSS, and PP is that they allow direct sourcing and capturing of patient data, which, in turn, can be used flexibly for a myriad of purposes. Some of the more important purposes, aside from direct patient care, include continuing patient care, follow-up treatment protocols, medical education for nurses and resident physicians, and research. Many resident physicians, for example, are learning from interacting with these systems on job sites and taking orders when caring for particular patients by automatically extracting captured instructions left for them by mentoring physicians. More importantly, the combined usage of these systems will eventually lead to a noticeable reduction in medical errors, preventing potential patient deaths and possible legal repercussions for clinical malpractices that such mistakes may cause. These systems, therefore, will also assist with legal compliance, cut costs, and improve patient safety by performing such tasks as providing an audit trail for treatment protocols or alerting physicians of potentially adverse drug reactions.

Indeed, the adoption of these systems promises to yield the primary benefit of cost cutting. This will be accomplished through lowering costs related to personnel, paper storage, processing, and treatment delays; enhancing patient safety; reducing medical errors; and controlling quality to eliminate poor or inadequate care. And because patient data and images can be conveniently accessed with the click of a computer mouse via one or more of these systems, physicians and other healthcare providers no longer have to search for misfiled paper charts or wait for another healthcare facility to send duplicate copies of patient records and/or images. Moreover, these systems can even source data from the patient's bedside, if necessary, and furthermore provide a common platform for coordinating patient care across multiple care providers. This provides caregivers a common understanding of a patient's health condition, thereby preventing unnecessary treatments and/or omissions of critical treatments.

Use of these systems will also provide doctors, nurses, and even patients themselves with decision-support capabilities. For example, laboratory and X-ray results can be sent electronically, immediately after completion, to a physician for prioritized interpretation, diagnostic analysis, and decision-making regarding treatment alternatives. The EHR installed at PAMF, for example, enables caregivers to document interactions with patients, improve on physician–patient relationships, ease the charge-capturing process, and eliminate repetitive tests; allows hospital personnel to view patient medical history and insurance information; assists in making referrals; and speeds up prescription orders through electronic requests to pharmacies. PAMF's EHR also incorporated a CPOE system, which provides resident physicians and nurses with clinical guidelines and patients with printed summaries of visits and other services.[21] The

EHR system is also cost-effective, scalable, and flexible in the sense that new security features, improved CDS capabilities, and other ancillary support systems can be added at any time to enhance future healthcare services delivery.

However, the benefits of using an integrated EHR system must be contrasted with the many challenges that also come with its implementation. This topic is discussed in the next section.

Challenges

Several key challenges, with respect to the acceptance and adoption of EHR in health systems organizations, have been noted in the extant literature.[22-26] These include confusion about the concept; the cost of implementing EHR or customizing EHR to a particular healthcare organization; the lack of standardization; and other challenging issues, such as the reliability, privacy, confidentiality, and security of patient data housed by the system. There is also a lack of motivation in creating interoperability among the connected systems of competing care provider organizations until the advent of Health Information Technology for Economic and Clinical Health (HITECH), which was part of the Obamacare initiative to encourage the use of advancing technologies while strengthening the privacy and security protections for health information established under the Health Insurance Portability and Accountability Act of 1996 (HIPAA). Still, the trust between the care providers of one healthcare facility with another facility in coordinating patient care and sharing patient data remains a challenge to be overcome.

Notably, EHR software can be complex— the technology is known by various names, each indicating a specific vision that differs from the others. For example, as previously indicated, the vision of the CPR was popular for a while, albeit a few decades ago. Eventually, the idea of enterprise-wide EMRs replaced the limited CPR concept. Subsequently, a migration to the EHR philosophy seems to have gained worldwide acceptance as the preferred, generic term of use in describing the vision of how the electronic records of a patient should contain information, such that it would allow the trajectory of patient care in the patient's lifetime to be traced. Yet some authors continue to use terms such as CPR, EPR, and EMR interchangeably, which has, inevitably, added to the confusion.[27]

EHR will be one of the costliest project expenditures that a health systems organization will undertake, with regard to the investments of time and money and the resultant challenge of return on investments (ROI). Indeed, the significance of the returns to be realized from an EHR implementation remains a concern for many care executives until the health IT meaningful use initiatives spearheaded by office of the national coordinator for Health IT (ONC) under Obamacare forces them to get it done. Fortunately, the costs of computer hardware and memory chips have also significantly declined over the years so that the initial outlay and challenges can often be justified; however, the costs of software engineers and other experts such as health informaticians who need to do the difficult tasks of customizing the system, linking it with existing legacy systems, and garnering acceptance from the user community have significantly increased. Understanding the needs and wants of healthcare professional users is unlike building an automobile; therefore, drilling into the requirements and specifications for EHR means that either technical people will have to speak a layperson's language, or healthcare professional users must change the way medicine is practiced. Patient examinations and procedures have to be structured differently by the care providers before data can be entered into the EHR, which is completely different from what these professionals practiced when using a paper-based medical record system. Additionally, some familiarity with the EHR procedures is needed; otherwise, the clinical users will soon

become frustrated with using the system, as it certainly does not align easily with what physicians and/or nurses believe to be the typical way of practicing medicine. Hence, continuing educational programs in healthcare informatics is also necessary, as is the training of health IS/IT competencies among care providers. Certainly, the next generation of care providers who are growing up using advanced electronic gadgets and devices will find the health IS/IT transformation of traditional healthcare practices a convenient and welcome change.

Put simply, while the vision of EHR is theoretically possible, it is difficult to realize in current practice until a new generation of care providers can be hired; alternatively, training can be successfully imposed on the more traditionally oriented healthcare workers. EHR would portray a lifetime record of every health encounter between the patient and all of his or her caregivers, regardless of which clinic or hospital the episode was recorded in, and regardless of who the healthcare provider was—a dentist, family physician, physiotherapist, cancer specialist, or nurse. Interestingly, there are good reasons as to why sharing patient data by creating interoperability among systems belonging to competing clinics or hospitals is not practical, even if direct benefits can be obtained with interoperable patient information systems that cut across organizational boundaries. The responsibility of housing patient data in EHR is one that each clinic or hospital would prefer to bear independently. Major gains from implementing EHR are therefore confined within the boundaries of a single enterprise. In this manner, patient safety, care efficiencies, and clinical decision effectiveness can be clearly demonstrated, and the motivation to share patient data among competing health organizations can, as a result, be diminished. Moreover, EHR require practitioners to perform more computer entries and less handwriting, which is often counterintuitive to traditionally trained practitioners in terms of being productive—a computer order entry may, for example, take twice as long as writing or dictating an order, and practitioners who are not familiar with how the EHR-embedded CPOE functions may experience anxiety, thereby finding difficulty in reviewing his or her instructions stored in the system in front of a coworker or patient. Worse still, some practitioners are not in the habit of sharing their analysis of patient data with other practitioners or would prefer to privately review their own notes before distributing them. Such practitioners would not want to see their detailed progress notes automatically stored in a system that other practitioners can freely access.

The lack of standardization has been a major barrier to linking different EHR systems and related components. These standards can range from how patient information is stored, to the terminology used to store the information, to the procedures for exchanging information among different systems. Major areas where the lack of standards prevents interoperability and data sharing include information content (e.g., uniformity or comparability); input procedures (e.g., direct sourcing); representational format (e.g., data coding); clinical practice (e.g., treatment protocols); decision support (e.g., reminders and alerts); performance metrics (e.g., quality assurance); and security, confidentiality, and privacy (e.g., compliance with HIPAA).

Indeed, one of the most formidable challenges for EHR technology adoption involves HIPAA's privacy and security ruling. HIPAA rules prohibit the disclosure of patient health information, except where it is specifically permitted with the patient's consent. HIPAA violations can result in civil sanctions (entailing a limited fine, which varies for individuals and organizations) or criminal liability (entailing fines of \$50,000–\$250,000, or 1–10 years of imprisonment).[28] In any case, training authorized personnel, instituting appropriate organizational policies, and having effective audit processes are all critical factors for properly

securing the EHR information and accomplishing a successful EHR implementation.

▶ VIII. Conclusion

Despite rapid and continuing growth in the healthcare services industry, the application of health IS/IT applications in enhancing organizational efficiency and effectiveness has been slow. Technologies, such as EHR, need to be appreciated (and accepted) by both healthcare administrators and practitioners before EHR can significantly affect the performance of healthcare organizations. As previously discussed, because they will then be made accessible and available to the treating physician and other caregivers, considerable benefits can be gained from the electronic processing of a patient's records. New EHR features will also enable physicians to monitor their patients' responses to treatment interventions quickly and will improve their ability to manage patients with chronic illnesses. Soon, EHR technology will replace many, if not all, of the fragmentary data repositories used in legacy systems throughout the healthcare services industry across the globe. This move will eradicate unnecessary redundancies, unwanted anomalies, and unacceptable errors in patient records, all of which contribute to poor quality in healthcare services.

Upham[29] argues that substantial administrative and clinical benefits can be achieved, and should a universal EHR system finally be realized. His list of benefits include: (1) easy dissemination of critical patient information to other care providers for follow-up assessments; (2) rapid accessibility of patient records universally; (3) fewer documentation errors, less paperwork, and less filing of paperwork; (4) more efficient navigation through patient records; (5) no misfiled or lost charts; (6) standardization of care procedures among providers; (7) ease of clinical data management; (8) shared coding; (9) greater awareness of medical errors, possible drug interactions, and inherent patient allergies; and (10) ease of performing quality, risk, utilization, and ROI analyses due to the improved accessibility and availability of clinical data. Of course, as noted, these benefits must still be weighed against the challenges of implementing EHR.

At present, much of a patient's health information acquired from a specific health-care facility stays within the facility; it is not routinely shared with other clinics or health-care providers. This has been a significant problem, especially for patients who happen to require emergency treatment. To eliminate this predicament, future patient records should use EHR technology and PPs to provide connectivity, reliability, flexibility, efficiency, security, mobility, availability, and accessibility. Ideally, the EHR and PPs should be receptive to continuous updates. Newer functions—such as statistical reporting for varying purposes, wireless links to other databases and systems, and the incorporation of advanced decision support and graphical imaging tools for short-cutting the clinical decision processes—will further enhance the quality of patient care. Other features and connecting devices—such as Web-based personal health records (PHR), radio-frequency identification (RFID), virtual medical patient records (VPR), and smart cards—will combine with EHR and PPs to empower patients and providers. The ultimate aim is to ensure the highest quality of patient care provided anywhere, anytime.

A Web-based PHR system or PP will, for example, empower patients with access to their own records and help them take a more active role in managing their own health. They will be able to check these records, ensuring that they are receiving appropriate care in a safe and effective manner. A PP or Web-based PHR system may also be designed so that it will also organize the patient's private health information, allow them to restrict certain caregivers to particular views, and allow them to efficiently communicate

with their caregivers about test results and follow-up plans. Older patients may be able to add remote patient-monitoring tools so their caregivers are kept abreast of possible warning symptoms, thereby managing their chronic states of health, from anywhere in the world, in a more effective manner.

RFID[30] is an unusual form of health IT; based on the VeriChip system, an RFID microchip can be implanted under the skin, granting instant access to a patient's records. Developed by Applied Digital Solutions Inc. of Delray Beach, Florida, this VeriChip system works by transmitting a unique code to a scanner, permitting caregivers to confirm a patient's identity and extract detailed patient information from a connected database. The implant will only provide the identification so that the system will remain limited to hospitals, doctors, and patients who have access to the scanner.

VPR,[31] another approach to the access of patient medical records (in which data from all the different sources are merely linked electronically as and when needed), allow integration of patient information from all sources, including data from the many ancillary health information systems used in enhancing patient care. VPR are electronically created, edited, and stored in electronic digitized media, just as traditional patient records were done with the medium of ink on paper.

A smart card is an integrated circuit card that can retain a patient's vital medical information. The information can then be easily retrieved, after entering the necessary security information, by swiping the card through a reader. The technology is also compatible with mobile healthcare computing, so that products, medical treatments, or alternative medical therapies can be purchased wherever a card reader is available.

More research and development is needed to ensure that future EHR and other related systems discussed in this chapter meet the needs of patients, providers, administrators, researchers, and policymakers. Pressing issues relating to reliability, privacy, confidentiality, and security also need to be resolved. The need to protect patient privacy must be balanced by the need for efficient access to data from multiple sites. It is therefore necessary to find the solutions that will reduce the barriers in implementing and

developing these patient-centric technologies. If all of the challenges and concerns are resolved, future EHR and other related technologies will quickly propel the health services industry to new heights and possibilities.

Notes

1. *Samsung S Health relaunched as Samsung Health, telemedicine capability added.* (2018, September). Retrieved from www.zdnet.com/article/samsung-s -health-relaunched-as-samsung-health-telemedicine -capability-added/

2. *S Health and Samsung Digital Health SDK.* (2018, September). Retrieved from https://developer.samsung .com/tech-insights/health/shealth-and-samsung -digital-health-sdk

3. *Samsung Health: The beginning of smart health care.* (2018, September). Retrieved from http://health.apps .samsung.com

4. Retrieved from www.nationalacademies.org/hmd/~ /media/Files/Report%20Files/2001/Crossing-the -Quality-Chasm/Quality%20Chasm%202001%20 %20report%20brief.pdf (IOM)

5. Tan, J. (2005). *E-Health care information systems-an introduction for students and professionals.* San Francisco, CA: Jossey-Bass.

6. Liang, H., Xue, Y., & Wu, X. (2006). User acceptance of computerized physician order entry: An empirical investigation. *International Journal of Healthcare Information Systems & Informatics, 1*(2), 39–50.

7. *Wikipedia,* Retrieved from http://en.wikipedia.org /wiki/Electronic_health_record

8. *Wikipedia,* Retrieved from http://en.wikipedia.org /wiki/CPOE

9. Tan, J., & Sheps, S. (1998). *Health decision support systems.* Gaithersburg, MD: Aspen Publishers.

10. Retrieved from www.exscribe.com/orthopedic-e -news/ehremr/4-benefits-of-patient-portals

11. Institute of Medicine. (1997). *The computer-based patient record: An essential technology for health care.* Retrieved from www.nap.edu/openbook.php?isbn =0309055326

12. Arsala, M., Rosenblatt, N., Singer, S., & Slouffman, L. (2008, June 1). *EHR history and technology* (2005). Retrieved from www7.kellogg.northwestern.edu /techconcepts/Winter2005Projects/healthcaresoftware /techhome.htm

13. *Ibid.*

14. HIMSS EHRVA. (2006). *Definitional model and application process.* Retrieved from www .himssehrva.org/docs/EHRVA_application.pdf

15. HL White Paper. (2004). *HL7 EHR system functional model and standard.* Retrieved from www

.hl7.org/documentcenter/public_temp_F85CF62B -1C23-BA17-0C67F8C1D097BA14/wg/ehr/EHR -SWhitePaper.pdf

16. Arsala et al., (2008), *ibid.*

17. CTEC. (2006). *Glossary of telemedicine and eHealth.* Retrieved from www.cteconline.org/terms.html

18. Retrieved from www.exscribe.com/orthopedic-e-news /ehremr/4-benefits-of-patient-portals, *ibid.*

19. *Ibid.*

20. Palo Alto Medical Foundation. (2006). *EHRs revolutionize care for patients, physicians.* Retrieved from www.pamf.org/news/2006/0706ehrs.html

21. *Ibid.*

22. Melczer, A. (2005). *Background on electronic health records.* Retrieved from www.providersedge.com /ehdocs/ehr_articles

23. Electronic Health Record. (2007, June 15). Retrieved from http://findarticles.com/p/articles/mi_hb4365 /is_200602/ai_n18950965

24. Amatayakul, M. (2006). *Electronic health records.* In K. M. LaTour & S. Eichenwald-Maki (Eds.), *Health information management: Concepts, principles, and practice* (2nd ed., pp. 211–237). Chicago, IL: AHIMA.

25. Waegemann, P. (2003). *Healthcare informatics online (EHRs vs. CPRs vs. EMRs).* Retrieved from www.providersedge.com/ehdocs/ehr_articles/EHR _vs_CPR_vs_EMR.pdf

26. Waegemann, P. (2004). *EHR vs CCR: What is the difference between the electronic health record and the continuity of care record?* Retrieved from www .providersedge.com/ehdocs/ehr_articles/EHR _vs_CCR-What_is_the_difference_between_the _EHR_and_the_CCR.pdf

27. Waegemann (2003, 2004), *ibid.*

28. *Wikipedia,* Computer physician order entry.

29. Upham, R. (2004). *The electronic health record: Will it become a reality?* Retrieved from http://www .hipaadvisory.com/action/ehealth/EHR-reality.htm

30. Fuhrer, P., & Guinard, D. (2006). *Building a smart hospital using RFID technologies.* Retrieved from http://diuf.unifr.ch/people/fuhrer/publications /external/RFIDECEH.pdf

31. Malamateniou, F. (2007). *A workflow-based approach to virtual patient record security.* Retrieved from http:// ieeexplore.ieee.org/xpl/freeabs_all.jsp?arnumber =735778

Chapter Questions

6-1   What is the rationale for classifying EHR, CPOE, and CDSS as patient-centric management systems?

6-2   Why might it be important to link EHR to CPOE and/or CDSS? What about linking EHR to LIS, PIS, RIS, and any other clinical-based IS? What about linking it to a physician PDA?

6-3   Why is user resistance—particularly from physicians and nurses—often considered the greatest obstacle to successfully implementing patient-centric management systems?

6-4   What are the benefits for healthcare consumers of PHR versus EHR? Does this imply that EHR can simply be replaced with PHR or that both systems may be necessary? Why or why not?

6-5   Why are patient portals important, and how do they benefit patients?

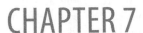

CHAPTER 7

Pharmacy Informatics: Technologies for the Medication Use Process and Professional Education

Misty Jensen and Ping Ye

LEARNING OBJECTIVES

- Analyze current state of informatics technologies in medication use process for various domains in pharmacy informatics
- Explore the interoperability issues in pharmacy informatics
- Identify current competencies in pharmacy informatics education

CHAPTER OUTLINE

Scenario: The SAPHIRE Project[1]

Interoperability is concerned primarily with the challenge of linking software and systems being developed and implemented with diverse platforms and languages when required information has to be shared conveniently and securely among multiple providers and users. For example, it is typical for medical and clinical users to derive information embedded in heterogeneous and independent health management information systems (HMIS), most of which are often supported traditionally with the use of specialized clinical hardware and applications. Briefly, people with varying levels of expertise and needs typically use different parts of a large-scale HMIS supported by different vendors, who will also adopt different standards, technological architecture, and information formats. Once these interoperability problems are tamed, it is believed that large-scale HMIS can be more easily implemented and maintained with the benefits of reusing previously captured data, adopting well-tested programming codes, and diffusing proven and related applications.

In the United States, Europe, and elsewhere, growing demands for health care due to an aging population and the slowing down in mortality rate among older adults over the last few decades have led to further growth and development of wearable medical devices, sensor-based monitoring technology, and mobile health care. Advanced IT, network, and Web technologies must now be combined to offer support to healthcare professionals in delivering healthcare services at a distance. With these advancing HMIS capabilities, it is anticipated that the quality of health care will be further enhanced, whereby people will live longer than they are used to. Owing to the increasing percentage of elderly people in Europe, the SAPHIRE Project was launched.

The aging population trend basically means that a growing number of people will need to become more aware of the basic and clinical research on disease pathophysiology and treatment. Coupled with increased demands on healthcare services delivery systems, this rapid growth has made the future practice of medicine even more complex. Essentially, using an interoperable and integrated platform to connect between the hospital information systems (HIS) and the wireless medical devices, SAPHIRE aims to build an intelligent healthcare monitoring and health decision support system (HDSS) to address the challenge of growing workload intensity in medicine.

Clinical decision support (CDS) systems are used to provide clinicians or patients with clinical knowledge and patient-related information, intelligently filtered and processed to enhance patient care. The healthcare community response to the complex challenge of modern medical practices is through developing clinical practice guidelines to simplify and improve healthcare services delivery. Although there are many clinical standards and practice guidelines, it is easier for healthcare professionals to access and apply these guidelines if computerized CDS (automating these clinical guidelines to support the health professionals) are available readily. When developing computerized CDS, one of the major challenges is to retrieve patient-specific information from the many disparate data sources. There are a large number of legacy clinical systems that have been independently created and administered; they do not, therefore, physically or logically provide support for interoperating and sharing information. Additionally, most of the healthcare systems in Europe are built with various computer technologies (e.g., different system platforms supported by diverse vendors and using various DBMS or database management systems). Moreover, most HMIS applications supplied by local and national service providers are introduced alongside existing departmental applications such as laboratory information systems (LIS) and mental healthcare record systems.

In the SAPHIRE platform, the solution to tackling the interoperability problem is to expose the data coming from sensors as well as the data stored in medical information systems as semantically enriched Web services. Data from both of these sources and their functionalities could then be combined into different Web services through standard-based ontologies. With the support of Web services, different platforms would be enabled to exchange information and share the functions.

Apparently, the interoperability problem is significant and central for the development of an effective intelligent healthcare monitoring tool. The key challenges have to do with the fact that the data coming from the wireless medical sensors are either: (1) in proprietary format or (2) when it conforms to a standard, the interoperability challenge remains or could not be completely solved because there are numerous standards being adopted. For electrocardiogram (ECG) data, the available standards include SCP-ECP, U.S. Food and Drug Administration FDA/HL7 Annotated ECG, I-Med, and ecgML. If these data are to be combined with those stored in electronic health records (EHR), the problem would be compounded due to siloed HIS; even when these systems do conform to an interface standard, there still will be the challenge of different standards (or different versions of the same standards). Specific examples include HL7v2.x, HL7v3 CDA, CEN ENV 13606, EHRExtract, and openEHR archetypes. Therefore, the existence of these differing standards does not achieve the aimed interoperability. Besides, interoperability of data coming from different wireless medical sensors is critical to infer information by integrating data coming from various sensors.

By examining the guideline models that are used in SAPHIRE, an understanding of the interaction with the clinical workflow running in the hospital is necessary. For example, "aspirin should be prescribed to the patient" could be decided on one of the guideline models. For these type of interactions, medical Web services are used to store such medication and procedure orders to the available HIS. These kinds of orders are usually implemented as asynchronous Web services to increase the performance.

As the result of a European commission–funded project, IST-1-002103 Artemis, the SAPHIRE project is being developed. IST-1-002103 Artemis developed a semantic Web service-based peer-to-peer (P2P) infrastructure for the interoperability of medical information systems. With the support of Artemis project, the Healthcare Institutes are able to exchange EHR in an interoperable manner through semantically enriched Web services and semantic mediation. These results are well used by the SAPHIRE project for the integration of the patient data collected through wireless medical sensor devices with HIS. This infrastructure comprises the interoperability base for the intelligent healthcare monitoring system.

Imagine a world where everyone speaks the same language—the international language. How easy would it be for people to exchange ideas—and understand each other? Trading among world partners would occur in a snap, and there would be reduced costs for everything, including paperwork, whether manual or computerized. That, in essence, is interoperability. Why is interoperability an important milestone for HMIS integration in a healthcare services organization? What would be the rationale for some people to be against such an idea?

▶ I. Introduction

Pharmacy is the field of health sciences focusing on patients, medications, diseases, and safe and effective medication use process. One of the fastest growing specialties in pharmacy is informatics. Pharmacy informatics centers on the effective management and delivery of medication-related data, information, and knowledge for the purpose of improving health outcomes.[2] Health information technology (HIT) and pharmacy informatics are intricately linked because technologies provide the framework to support information management in pharmacy. Many pharmacists practice informatics on a daily basis. Some of the technologies used in practice regularly are bar coded medication administration (BCMA), CDS, computerized prescriber or physician order entry (CPOE), and e-prescribing (eRx).[3–5] Importantly, one should be aware that better care does not come solely from the adoption of the technology itself; instead, the exchange and meaningful use of health information with the assistance of technologies improve the quality of health care.

This chapter has three learning objectives: (1) to analyze the current state of informatics technologies in medication use process including prescribing (CPOE, CDS, eRx), dispensing (procurement, packaging, automated dispensing cabinet (ADC), and carousel, compounder, robotics), administrating (electronic medication administration record (eMAR), BCMA, smart pump), and monitoring (surveillance, population health), (2) to describe the interoperability in pharmacy informatics, and (3) to identify current competencies in pharmacy informatics education.

▶ II. Background

In the late 1870s, pharmacists pioneered the modern telemedicine as the first telephone exchange connecting the Capital Avenue Drugstore with 21 local physicians.[6] Since the 1970s, the pharmacy profession has utilized computerized HMIS and automation.[7] Many developments occurred throughout the 1990s in both hospital and outpatient pharmacy information systems (PIS). Core tasks included order entry into the pharmacy IS, online order verification by pharmacists, computer-supported medication supply and distribution, automated label generation, and computerized pharmacy billing. The pharmacy computer systems became more useful and common.[8] The 2007 American Society of Health-System Pharmacists (ASHP) survey found that informatics

technologies are widely present in all steps of the medication-use process.[9] Thus, the profession is well positioned for the implementation of HIT across practice settings.

More recently, the Health Information Technology for Economic and Clinical Health (HITECH) Act of 2009 provided federal funding to encourage the design, development, and operation of a nationwide health information infrastructure that promotes the electronic use and exchange of health information. The pharmacy profession also takes the initiative to integrate pharmacists into the national HIT movement, as evidenced by the Pharmacy e-HIT Collaborative, which released "The Roadmap for Pharmacy Health Information Technology Integration in U.S. Health Care" in 2011.[10]

As a result of the HITECH Act and other strategic plans, significant growth of technology was seen in virtually all areas of pharmacy practice.[11,12] In particular, e-prescribing was often invested as the first step in the adoption of HIT in many states. This was because patient safety is a top priority, and e-prescribing would improve outcomes by significantly reducing medication errors with increased compliance and efficiency. A recent survey found widespread use of pharmacy informatics and technology across the entire medication use process in U.S. hospitals.[13] Based on the adoption rates, CPOE, CDS, eRx, and BCMA are clearly the priorities among all technologies; ADCs are more common in U.S. hospitals than carousels and robots.

▶ III. Current Perspective

Medication Use Process

Pharmacy informatics centers on the steps within the medication use process. The medication use process typically begins with the prescription of a medication from a provider, followed by dispensing from a pharmacy, administration of the medication to a patient, and monitoring for efficacy and potential

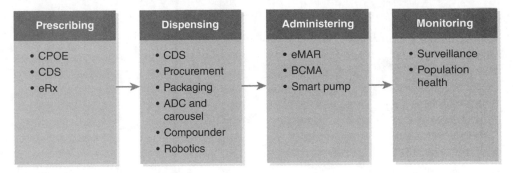

FIGURE 7-1 Steps within the medication use process.

adverse effects as shown in **FIGURE 7-1**. Each of these steps may utilize technology in an effort to increase efficiency and provide the best patient care through enhancing safety and clinical outcomes.

Prescribing

CPOE: CPOE entails the provider's use of computer assistance to directly enter medication orders from a computer or mobile device. The order is also documented or captured in a digital, structured, and computable format for use to improve safety and organization.[14] CPOE has been adopted by over 75% of hospitals. Additionally, more than 20% hospitals plan to adopt this technology within the next few years.[15] Multiple drivers for CPOE implementation exist, including financial, workflow efficiencies, patient safety, and patient outcomes. CPOE offers substantial advantages over the historical prescribing methodology of a handwritten prescription (see **FIGURE 7-2**). Approximately 90% of medication errors occur at either the ordering or transcribing stage. Error causes were identified as poor handwriting, ambiguous abbreviations, or lack of knowledge.[16] CPOE assists with legibility, reduces transcription errors, and reduces incomplete medication orders.

CPOE offers the ability to promote standardization of dosing regimens and eliminate ambiguous abbreviations that have led to medication errors. The usage of CPOE is associated with a greater than 50% decrease in preventable adverse drug events and a similar rate of decline in some medication error types.[17] The likelihood of a prescribing error was reduced by 48% when using CPOE compared to paper orders, which means more than 17 million medication errors are prevented yearly with this technology.[18]

However, as with all new technologies and workflow modifications, unintended consequences of CPOE were discovered. These consequences can undermine patient safety and are broadly attributed to interactions between the healthcare technology and the healthcare organization's sociotechnical systems (i.e., workflow, culture).[19] CPOE systems require clinicians to perform new tasks, which increase cognitive workload and decrease efficiency.[20] Based on these findings, integration of human factors engineering principles is needed to achieve the full potential of CPOE. Human factors engineering accounts for human vulnerabilities and limitations during the design of interactive systems, involving people and technology to ensure safety, effectiveness, and ease of use.[21] This type of engineering has long been used outside of health care. It is also important not to overlook the interplay between new technologies and existing social conditions as well as clinical judgment, teamwork, and direct communication. Moreover, accurate algorithms need to be developed to assess appropriateness of generating alerts or overriding alerts in a CPOE system.[22]

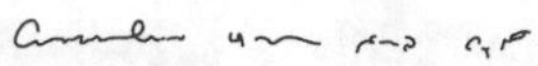

FIGURE 7-2A Handwritten prescription.

Rx Number	New	WARFARIN 4 MG TAB	
*Medication	WRF4T	COUMADIN	
*Order Type	MED	MED	
Clinical Ind} Dosing Wt			
Dose	4	MG	1 TABLET PER DOSE
Rang Dose Low } High			
*Route	PO		ORAL
*Frequency	DAILY@17		
*Schedule } Par Level PRN Reason	SCH		

FIGURE 7-2B Prescription received via CPOE.

CDS: CDS provides clinicians with knowledge and patient specific information, intelligently filtered or presented at appropriate times, to improve health care. CDS encompasses a variety of tools to enhance decision-making in the clinical workflow. These tools may include computerized alerts and reminders, clinical guidelines, condition-specific order sets, focused patient data reports and summaries, documentation templates, reference links, organizational policies, and other tools.[23] Multiple factors are important during prescribing and pharmacist review of medication. The provider must ascertain the diagnosis and decide on the appropriate medication, dose, route, and monitoring parameters. The pharmacist must ensure that the indication for the medication is appropriate for the individual patient. The pharmacist must verify and confirm allergies, dosing, and administration route. The pharmacist must also screen for drug–drug, drug–food, drug–laboratory, and drug–disease interactions with each prescription.

CDS may assist the provider during the prescribing phase of the medication use process. However, CDS is typically more robust in the dispensing phase. CDS enhances the ability of the clinician to detect cross allergenicity, drug interactions, therapeutic duplications, drug compatibilities, and even drug–laboratory or drug–disease interactions. For example, CDS will alert the pharmacist if sulfamethoxazole/trimethoprim is added to warfarin. Concomitant use of these medications will place the patient at significant risk for a severe bleeding event. Thus, CDS enhances the pharmacist's ability to prevent adverse events.

CDS has been available for several decades to assist with clinical decision-making and provide real time alerts for pharmacy specific functions. Despite the longevity of these systems, functionality can still be improved. It has been noted that pharmacy CDS is not fully complete, as gaps related to management of drug interactions, inappropriate dosing, laboratory monitoring, or other issues may yet occur.[24] More recently, CDS has expanded broadly with the adoption of EHR and CPOE. Analysis of decision support systems indicates that clinical practice was significantly improved in ~70% of trials.[25] CDS encompassing computerized alerts and reminders, clinical guidelines and diagnostic support, condition specific order sets, and reference links have been shown to reduce mediation errors, improve adherence to evidence-based guidelines for treatment, increase rates and delivery of preventative care services, and improve prescribing practices.[26] For example, CDS can indicate that typical medication doses must be adjusted due to impaired kidney function as indicated by laboratory results. Some CDS may screen for drug and disease interactions. Parkinson's disease results in a loss of dopamine, which leaves patients with less ability to control movement. Antipsychotics or anti-nausea medications work by depleting dopamine. Should a patient with Parkinson's disease receive these types of medications, their ability to control movement is worsened.

eRx: eRx is the use of electronic tools to prescribe medications. eRx tools can include both software programs and hardware.[27] The provider sends the prescription, and the pharmacy must be able to receive the prescription. This entails a host of technical hoops the information must pass through. Prescribers must meet Drug Enforcement Administration (DEA) requirements for a prescription application, therefore they must be electronic prescriptions for controlled substances (EPCS)-certified, and have identity proofing, local access control, and a two-factor authentication protocol.[28] If a patient has insurance, this information also passes through a pharmacy benefit manager (PBM). The PBM may be able to provide insurance formulary information, cost information, and any preauthorization requirements.

There are significant eRx advantages as compared to the handwritten prescription. Most software systems with eRx also contain CDS. Studies have shown a decrease in medication error rates up to sevenfold for those eRx adopters.[29] Pharmacy personnel prefer eRx to conventional prescriptions related to several outcomes of care.[30] Physicians are positive about general eRx features.[31]

Why doesn't everyone always e-prescribe? Three factors help to explain the gaps: product limitations (i.e., technical interoperability), external implementation challenges (i.e., workflow), and physicians' preferences about using specific product features. Additionally, cultural influences, lack of technical skills, and poor resources must be considered as barriers to the implementation and use of eRx.[32]

Dispensing

Procurement: Nearly all pharmacies order products online from their primary wholesalers. A drug pedigree is an electronic record of each transaction in the ownership of a drug from a manufacturer to a pharmacy. This pedigree is increasingly important due to increased awareness of counterfeit, misbranded, or adulterated medications in the pharmacy supply chain. Approximately 20% of pharmacies reported verification of drug pedigrees.[33] Track-and-trace is the process by which an e-pedigree can be used to track a medication product as it travels from a manufacturer to a patient. Track-and-trace may be accomplished through barcodes or by radio frequency identification (RFID).

Packaging: Hospitals dispense medication in unit doses. Many solid oral dosing forms are available for purchase in unit dose packaging with the appropriate manufacturer barcode. However, not all medications can be purchased in unit dose formulation. Those medications must be repackaged once received. Laws dictate that appropriate information must be included on all repackaged products.

Additionally, for the hospital to implement and maintain barcode medication administration, the re packager must also supply a readable barcode on the individually labeled products[34] (**FIGURE 7-3**).

ADC and carousel: After the prescription is verified, medications must be physically transported to the patient, which can happen in a variety of ways. ADCs are the most common technology for distribution and storage of drugs and used in ~80% of U.S. hospitals.[35] **FIGURE 7-4** is an example of a commonly

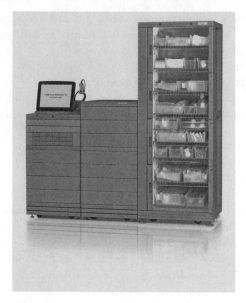

FIGURE 7-4 Automated dispensing cabinets (ADC).
Reproduced from BD Rx Inc.

found ADC in the hospital setting.[36] These cabinets store medication on nursing units in a secure manner and are frequently profiled to the individual patient. Patient profiling limits end user, typically nursing personnel, to access only to medications prescribed and authorized for the administration of a specific patient. Patient-specific profiling of the ADC improves patient safety by limiting access to medications that have been prescribed to that patient only. ADC use can also help to decrease medication access by non-licensed personnel and limit diversion potential in the hospital setting.

Larger hospitals with bed size of >500 are at nearly 90% with implementation of carousels.[37] Carousels are housed in the central pharmacy for dispensing to the nursing units and ADCs[38] (see **FIGURE 7-5**). Carousels allow for a more condensed storage solution and automation of the medication pick process. The users stand in one spot with the lighting to help pick the correct medication bin.

Admixture compounding technology: Technology exists for patient specific compounding

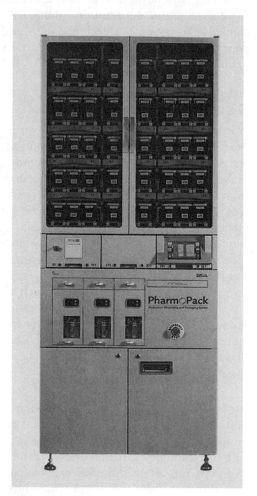

FIGURE 7-3 Readable bar coding on pharmaceutical packed products.
Reproduced from BD Rx Inc.

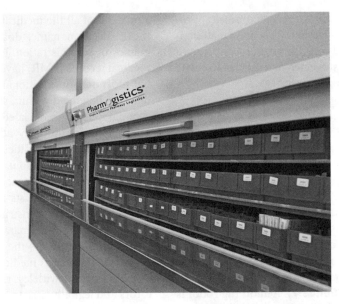

FIGURE 7-5 Carousels housed in the central pharmacy for dispensing to nursing units and ADCs.
Reproduced from BD Rx Inc.

of intravenous admixtures. Software is available for intravenous workflow to manage drug preparation, verification, and dispensing. Pharmacy technicians use barcode scanning to match intravenous components with pharmacist approved compounding recipes to provide medications for patients. Technicians use photographs to document each step of the compounding process. Pharmacists approve after reviewing all documentation. Workflow is designed to enhance safety and ensure compliance with all compounding regulations. **FIGURE 7-6** is an example of intravenous workflow software.[39]

Software and hardware are also available to assist in the ordering, calculation, and labeling process of compounded intravenous medications. Total parenteral nutrition (TPN) admixtures are a nutritional alternative for patients who are unable to receive nutrition via an oral route. The software assists with calculations of admixture amounts and solubility of the final product. For example, the software can calculate the maximum amount of calcium gluconate or potassium phosphate that is permitted in a given volume before precipitation (forming

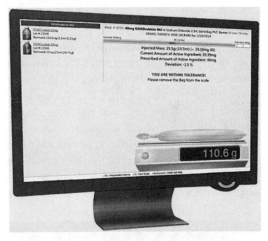

FIGURE 7-6 Example of an intravenous workflow software.

Reproduced from BD Rx Inc. https://www.bd.com/en-us/offerings/capabilities/medication-and-supply-management/medication-and-supply-management-technologies/pyxis-medication-technologies/pyxis-iv-prep

of a solid) occurs. Should even small precipitates occur, the patient is at risk for therapeutic failures due to particulate embolization, which can lead to thrombophlebitis, multi-organ failure, and even death. The pharmacy technician prepares the machine for compounding, again using barcode scanning to ensure appropriate product selection. This information is then transmitted and the appropriate amount of components is injected into the bag to create the final compounded recipe[40].

Robotics: ASHP defines robotics as "mechanical devices that perform programmed, complex, and repetitive manipulations, which mimic human behavior without continuous input from an operator".[41] Many hospital pharmacies use some form of robotics during dispensing. For example, the McKesson robot contains 600 rods that store medications. After receiving medication orders entered by the pharmacist, the robot scans the barcode and then uses electrical power to pick each medication dose[42] (**FIGURE 7-7**). Aethon tug robot is used for automated delivery of medications to nursing units[43].

Administrating

eMAR: Prior to eMAR, there was medication administration record, a handwritten document with medication orders that were transcribed by nursing staff. The orders were initialed and then yellowed out when completed. eMAR is where all documentation of patient medication regimen is stored. eMAR is generated directly from the provider's medication order. The order is then verified by pharmacy. eMAR typically contains the start and stop dates of all the medications, and includes the medication name, dose, route, and frequency of administration. Different electronic medical records (EMR) have different features, but most include additional medication information embedded within, such as medication monographs or associated data needed to safely and appropriately administer medications (e.g., laboratory values, vital signs). Pharmacy personnel can also use eMAR to convey patient or medication specific information to nursing staff. Pharmacists may provide additional administration instructions, such as do not crush, or list other parameters for administration. eMAR offers the advantage of real-time and continuous medication information. eMAR associates with less risk of transcription errors and legibility issues.

BCMA: After the provider has entered an order and the medication order has been verified by pharmacy, the nurse must acknowledge the medication order, retrieve the medication from ADC or elsewhere if needed, administer the medication, and document its administration on the eMAR. BCMA inserts an additional layer of safety in the process between retrieval of the medication and administration. A simplified nursing workflow of administration of medications is shown in **FIGURE 7-8**. The nursing staff follows five rights of administration: right patient, right medication, right dose, right route, and right time.

Patients must always wear a wristband for identification. The wristband includes multiple patient identifiers such as a patient specific barcode. Prior to administration, the nurse must confirm the correct patient for whom the medication is intended. After a verbal or visual confirmation is completed using the information on the wristband, the patient's wristband is scanned. This ensures that the correct patient eMAR is pulled up in the EHR. Once the patient is confirmed, the nurse must scan the medication and then administer and document.

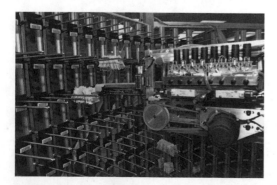

FIGURE 7-7 Robotic dosage scanning.
©ZUMA Press, Inc./Alamy Stock Photo.

Medications supplied by manufacturers do not always arrive with a barcode on unit of use doses. Unit dose is preparing medications in individual doses and individually labeled packets for administration. In 2006, the US Food & Drug Administration (FDA) mandated that manufacturers provide the National Drug Code (NDC) on packaging, including unit dose packaging. Unfortunately, an unintended consequence of this mandate was that many manufacturers decided to opt out of manufacturing unit dose packaging. As a result, pharmacies must repackage a significant percentage of all medications and place a readable barcode to successfully implement BCMA.

A successful BCMA program starts in pharmacy receiving. For all medications, NDC must be scanned into the EHR. Compounded or patient specific products also require readable barcode, which is linked to the patient medication order in the EHR. A readable barcode may be linear or 2D (**FIGURE 7-9**). Scanners must be able to read either format as medications will arrive or be repackaged with either format.

The addition of BCMA into the administration process has multiple benefits for nursing staff and patient safety. The implementation of barcode medication-verification technology embedded in an eMAR was associated with a 41% reduction in administration errors and a 51% reduction in potential adverse drug events from these errors.[44] Given the high number of doses administered and orders transcribed in any acute care hospital, implementation of the barcode eMAR could substantially improve medication safety. The use of BCMA shows an increased rate of error detection because the system is able to capture and record intercepted administration errors.[45] For example, the nurse will receive a pop up alert if a medication that is scanned is not present on the eMAR. This means that the scanned medication is not currently ordered for the patient. Other alerts are warnings of dosing too early or incorrect dose amounts. Each of these alerts allows for nursing review and order clarification before the medication is administered to a patient.

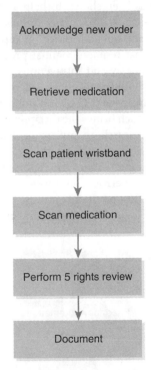

FIGURE 7-8 A simplified nursing workflow of medications administration.

FIGURE 7-9 Linear v. 2D readable barcode.

BCMA is implemented at nearly 75% of hospitals with plans for an additional 15% in a few years.[46] While this technology is being rapidly implemented, warnings of unintended consequences have surfaced. One study discovered 15 workarounds, categorized as omitted steps, steps performed out of sequence, and unauthorized steps. The study further identified 31 causes to these workarounds. Recommendations are provided to focus on improving the design, implementation, and workflow integration of bar coding systems to prevent unsafe workarounds.[47]

Smart infusion pumps: These are used at the bedside to administer intravenous medications to patients. As compared to predecessor pumps, smart pumps allow for the programming of a drug library, which has stricter control over administration. Typically, a pharmacist, in collaboration with nursing, develops the drug library. This library contains the intravenous medication infused in the hospital. The library offers the ability to program medication specific information into the pumps. The medications can be preprogrammed with information such as infusion duration, concentration, and dosing limits. The programming allows for both soft limits, which alert the clinician but may be bypassed, and hard limits, which force reprogramming. If the clinician attempts to enter a value outside of hard limits, they are forced to cancel or reprogram the infusion. For example, dosing limits for a continuous infusion of insulin may be programmed in the drug library between 1 and 50 units/hour. If a clinician inadvertently types 75 instead of 7.5 units/hour, the pump forces a hard stop and the user must reprogram within acceptable dosing ranges.

Data can be examined to better understand the usage of the pumps at an institution. Reports can be run to review distinct types of infusion alerts and corresponding nursing actions. Information derived from these reports enables a closer look at drug library programming to limit nuisance alerts and pinpoint areas of practice improvement. When new clinical evidence becomes available, the drug library must be updated to reflect contemporary standards. Likewise, if the supply changes (e.g., medication shortages, changes in compounding practice), the library must be updated to reflect those changes. Should these edits not occur, the library will be rendered obsolete, and practitioners will be forced to bypass clinical checking, potentially limiting the usefulness of this technology.

While a dose error reduction system (DERS) has been shown to help avert potentially serious errors, many infusion-related errors are still not addressed.[48] A gap remains, however, that requires manual programming between BCMA and intravenous medication infusion (**FIGURE 7-10**). The Emergency Care Research Institute (ECRI) is a nonprofit organization, which brings the discipline of applied scientific research to review devices, drugs, and processes for the best patient care. Its database shows that 75% of the reported infusion programming errors could have been averted with successful pump integration.[49] Next steps are a bidirectional, integrated, and closed-loop

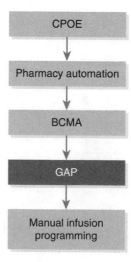

FIGURE 7-10 Gap requiring manual programming between BCMA and intravenous medication infusion.

system pumps to the EHR. Since health IT and infusion pumps were created independently, significant work must be done to synchronize the two systems. For the integration to be successful, infusion pump and health IT vendors must incorporate four foundational strengths: technology infrastructure, pump wireless capability, clinical competency, and ongoing support.[50]

Monitoring

Pharmacy clinical surveillance systems: The volume of individual pieces of data for patients can be overwhelming. Studies have shown that an average of 168 data transactions occur per patient per day.[51] This volume of data creates the chance to miss a potential risk to patient, thereby leading to patient harm. Clinical pharmacy surveillance systems offer the ability to integrate, translate, and provide sense making to data points in real time. Specialized clinical surveillance systems demonstrate the ability to help improve the quality of care, increase efficiency, comply with regulatory pressures, and reduce costs. Specifically, clinical pharmacy surveillance systems provide pharmacy management tools to help ensure the appropriate use of medications, improve stewardship (antibiotics, opioids, etc.), save time, and reduce costs. For example, studies have shown a 32% reduction in inappropriate antibiotic use and the prevention of hundreds of adverse drug events.[52,53]

The surveillance systems use rules created by pharmacists and others to alert when certain parameters are present for a specific patient. Clinical pharmacists care for many patients in a single day. The rules allow for enhanced workflow management, ensuring that critical drug related problems are identified and resolved in a timely manner, thereby enhancing patient care. Depending on the software vendor and EHR compatibility or functionality, rules can be written relating to a variety of factors. For example, rules can be written to identify high risk medications, critical

laboratory values, drug-bug mismatches when the prescribed medication does not have the appropriate antimicrobial spectrum to allow for clinical resolution of the infection, and any other variety of clinically important pharmaceutical monitoring to assist in providing optimal pharmaceutical care.

Big Data and population health: Health care is complex, with multiple treatments and providers. Legislation and payment models are changing, and health information is changing and expanding. Big Data are datasets that are so large and complex that traditional methods for collecting, sharing, and analyzing them are impossible. Data streams that may be included in Big Data sets are claims information, CDS databases, and EHR information including diagnosis, testing, laboratory results, and medications.[54]

Big Data can be used to impact population health metrics by providing insight on indicators such as readmissions, patient triage, adverse drug events, and expensive medications. Big Data can be used to assist in developing clinical workflow. Big Data can also be used to help determine the most effective treatment options by looking at data associated to length of hospital stay, complications, and disease progression[55] (**FIGURE 7-11**). This is an area that is rapidly expanding as we have the ability to collect vast amounts of data.

Pharmacy Interoperability

Interoperability is the ability to exchange health information and, importantly, to meaningfully use the information that has been exchanged. In the context of pharmacy interoperability, the desired exchange is a closed loop medication process between the inpatient and outpatient settings, as well as the inclusion of information generated by patients. Standards used in interoperability and health information exchange (HIE) allow health information to move electronically between different systems to improve patient outcomes. In addition, standardizing data collection on clinical

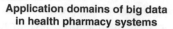

**Application domains of big data
in health pharmacy systems**

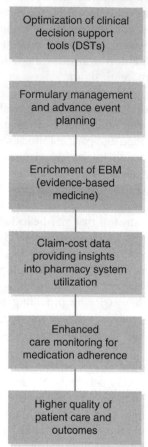

FIGURE 7-11 Big Data analytics to drive complex decision-making.

interventions can be utilized for research as well.

Terminologies specific to the pharmacy industry include SCRIPT, RxNorm, and NDC. SCRIPT is a standard developed by National Council for Prescription Drug Programs (NCPDP) for the electronic transmission of medical prescriptions in the United States. Transmissions can occur between prescribers, pharmacies, payers, and other entities. Transmitted information includes new prescriptions, changes of prescriptions, prescription refills, status notifications, prior authorizations, and

other transactions. RxNorm is produced by the National Library of Medicine (NLM). It provides normalized names and unique identifiers for generic and branded medications. The goal of RxNorm is to allow computer systems to communicate drug-related information efficiently and unambiguously. NDC is a 10-digit 3-segment number, a unique identifier for each drug in the United States. The code is present on all medication packages. The three segments of the NDC identify the labeler, the product, and the package size. The FDA assigns the labeler code while labeler assigns the product and package code.

Over 1000 standards are currently in use in health care, some comprise pharmacy components. For example, Systematized Nomenclature of Medicine—Clinical Terms (SNOMED CT), distributed by the NLM, is a standardized medical terminology used by physicians and other providers for the electronic exchange of health information. Utilizing SNOMED CT for documentation provides means to consistently capture and share clinical data across multiple sites of care and is fundamental to an interoperable electronic documentation system. Clinical data coded in SNOMED CT terms can be mapped to International Classification of Diseases 10th (ICD-10) codes for reimbursement and analytical purposes. Many aspects of pharmacy services are uniquely identified in SNOMED CT. This allows pharmacists to document the clinical activities they perform.

Pharmacy Informatics Education

Despite that pharmacy informatics has grown to be an integral component within the clinical informatics domain, many pharmacists and students know little more than the basic concepts. According to ASHP, the role of pharmacy informaticians encompasses five categories: data, information, and knowledge management; information and knowledge delivery; practice analytics; applied clinical informatics; and leadership and management of change.[56] To fulfill these responsibilities, pharmacy informatics education becomes a top priority.

Education in Doctor of Pharmacy Programs

The Accreditation Council for Pharmacy Education (ACPE) has identified informatics as a core competency required of pharmacy graduates in order to successfully transition to the practice environment. Pharmacy informatics was included as a requirement in the 2007 ACPE Guidelines.

The guideline identifies three levels of competencies: "basic terminology (data, information, knowledge, hardware, software, networks, information systems, information systems management); reasons for systematic processing of data, information, and knowledge in health care; and the benefits and current constraints in using information and communication technology in health care." In the ACPE 2016 Standards for the Didactic PharmD Curriculum, the outcome in health informatics is stated as "Effective and secure use of electronic and other technology-based systems, including EHR, to capture, store, retrieve, and analyze data for use in patient care, and confidentially/legally share health information in accordance with federal policies." Recognizing that informatics is now a requirement in pharmacy education, informatics courses have been developed and integrated into the PharmD curriculum to prepare pharmacists for the evolving role with HIT.[57-60]

Course format is either classroom or online, covering topics such as HIT, EHR, CPOE, CDS, and pharmacy IS. For example, faculty members at the University of California, San Francisco School of Pharmacy, have developed an online pharmacy informatics curriculum, known as Partners in E.[61] In addition to the fundamental informatics education for all students, advanced training can be offered to students who are interested in becoming informatics experts. Advanced

training covers design, development, implementation, and evaluation of new and potentially better systems to support pharmacy practice.[62]

Residency Programs

Pharmacy informaticians are dual specialists, who possess knowledge about both pharmacy practice and informatics. Some obtain formalized training while others have had extensive experience in utilizing health IS/IT. There are a growing number of residency programs available within the United States.[63] A total of 22 pharmacy informatics residencies have been identified with 20 deemed as second post-graduate year residencies. Ten residencies were accredited by the ASHP, while eight were candidates for accreditation. Most of the pharmacy informatics residencies are large hospital affiliated (>500 beds), such as Vanderbilt University, University of Utah, University of Michigan, and Oregon Health and Science University.

▶ IV. Future Trends

A future pharmacy practice model will heavily rely on pharmacy informatics, which focuses on the use and integration of data, information, knowledge, and technology involved with medication use processes to improve outcomes.[64] The growing use of HIT requires increased pharmacist knowledge of health informatics regardless of practice setting. Future pharmacists must utilize IT and automation to create a safer and more effective medication-use system.

There are plenty of research opportunities in the arena of pharmacy informatics. Pharmacogenomics studies how systems of many genes exert an impact on drug response phenotypes. It is an integral part of personalized medicine, tailoring treatments to individual genetic makeup to enable more precious ways to prevent and treat disease. The presentation of pharmacogenomics information in useful ways can improve prescribing decisions in the form of CDS alerts.[65] Pharmacogenomics has a widespread impact on the practice of medicine and will continue to grow together with the initiatives of precision medicine and personalized medicine.

Telehealth is another area where technology innovations can be used by allowing pharmacists to practice at locations far away from where they are. These kinds of systems can enhance practice in rural areas and allow specialists including pharmacists to project their expertise where they normally would not be able. For example, Avera eCARE Telemedicine has transformed healthcare delivery in South Dakota and beyond by partnering with Avera's proven virtual healthcare solution.[66] In total, up until 2018, 330 sites were served, $188,000,000 healthcare costs were saved, and 1,069,000 patients were touched. Avera eCARE Pharmacy provides pharmaceutical needs 24/7/365 to ensure that patients receive the safest and most effective medications. ePharmacists deliver pharmaceutical knowledge to rural and critical access areas when local pharmacists are unavailable. ePharmacists can verify providers' orders, perform clinical consults and medication dosing, and are able to collaborate with onsite nursing, providers, and patients to provide optimal pharmaceutical care to patients.

▶ V. Conclusion

In this chapter, we analyze the current state of technologies as applied in the medication use process. The medication use process has four sequential steps. The first step is the prescription of a medication from a provider. We discussed CPOE, CDS, and e-prescribing. The second step is dispensing from a pharmacy. We discussed procurement and packaging, automated dispensing cabinet, compounder and robotics. The third step is administration of the medication to a patient. Technologies utilized are electronic medication administration record, bar coded medication administration, and smart pump. The final step is monitoring for efficacy and potential adverse effects using pharmacy clinical surveillance systems. In addition, we elaborated the pharmacy interoperability, which is the ability to exchange information across systems and to make meaningful use of the information being exchanged. Pharmacy-specific terminologies were discussed. Finally, we reviewed the current status of pharmacy informatics education. Informatics courses have been integrated into the PharmD curriculum and over 20 pharmacy informatics residencies have been identified.

The expansion in technology use throughout health care provides substantial opportunities for pharmacists to improve the medication-related systems. As medication experts, pharmacists have a responsibility to ensure the best use of technology as it relates to drug therapy. As pharmacists' roles and involvement with HIT continue to evolve, the profession must be prepared to engage technology appropriately within their practice to ensure safe and quality care for patients. All pharmacists need to have some knowledge of informatics to be effective in providing care. Additionally, specially trained pharmacists are needed to maximize the utility of information systems.

Notes

1. *SAPHIRE: Intelligent healthcare monitoring based on semantic interoperability platform.* Retrieved from www.ehealthnews.eu/content/view/282/27/
2. ASHP statement on the pharmacist's role in clinical informatics. (2016). *American Journal of Health-System Pharmacy, 73*(6), 410–413. doi:10.2146/ajhp150540
3. ASHP guidelines on pharmacy planning for implementation of computerized provider-order-entry systems in hospitals and health systems. (2011).

American Journal of Health-System Pharmacy, 68(6), 537. doi:10.2146/sp100011

4. Section of Pharmacy Informatics and Technology, American Society of Health-System Pharmacists. (2009). ASHP statement on bar-code-enabled medication administration technology. *American Journal of Health-System Pharmacy, 66*(6), 588–590. doi:10.2146/ajhp080414

5. Troiano, D., Jones, M. A., Smith, A. H., Chan, R. C., Laegeler, A. P., Le, T., … Chaffee, B. W. (2015). ASHP guidelines on the design of database-driven clinical decision support: Strategic directions for drug database and electronic health records vendors. *American Journal of Health-System Pharmacy, 72*(17), 1499–1505. doi:10.2146/sp150014

6. Fox, B. I., Flynn, A. J., Fortier, C. R., & Clauson, K. A. (2011). Knowledge, skills, and resources for pharmacy informatics education. *American Journal of Health-System Pharmacy, 75*(5), 93. doi:10.5688/ajpe75593

7. Siska, M. H., & Tribble, D. A. (2011). Opportunities and challenges related to technology in supporting optimal pharmacy practice models in hospitals and health systems. *American Journal of Health-System Pharmacy, 68*(12), 1116–1126. doi:10.2146/ajhp110059

8. Troiano, D. (1999). A primer on pharmacy information systems. *Journal of Healthcare Information Management, 13*(3), 41–52.

9. Pedersen, C. A., & Gumpper, K. F. (2008). ASHP national survey on informatics: Assessment of the adoption and use of pharmacy informatics in U.S. hospitals—2007. *American Journal of Health-System Pharmacy, 65*(23), 2244–2264. doi:10.2146/ajhp080488

10. Retrieved from www.pharmacyhit.org/

11. Fox, B. I., Pedersen, C. A., & Gumpper, K. F. (2015). ASHP national survey on informatics: Assessment of the adoption and use of pharmacy informatics in U.S. hospitals-2013. *American Journal of Health-System Pharmacy, 72*(8), 636–655. doi:10.2146/ajhp140274

12. Pedersen & Gumpper (2008).

13. Fox et al. (2015).

14. Retrieved from www.cms.gov/Regulations-and-Guidance/Legislation/EHRIncentivePrograms/downloads/1_CPOE_for_Medication_Orders.pdf

15. Fox et al. (2015).

16. Bates, D. W., Cullen, D. J., Laird, N., Petersen, L. A., Small, S. D., Servi, D., … Edmondson, A. (1995). Incidence of adverse drug events and potential adverse drug events. Implications for prevention. ADE Prevention Study Group. *The Journal of the American Medical Association, 274*(1), 29–34.

17. Nuckols, T. K., Smith-Spangler, C., Morton, S. C., Asch, S. M., Patel, V. M., Anderson, L. J., & Shekelle, P. G. (2014). The effectiveness of computerized order entry at reducing preventable adverse drug events and medication errors in hospital settings: A systematic review and meta-analysis. *Systematic Reviews, 3,* 56. doi:10.1186/2046-4053-3-56

18. Radley, D. C., Wasserman, M. R., Olsho, L. E., Shoemaker, S. J., Spranca, M. D., & Bradshaw, B. (2013). Reduction in medication errors in hospitals due to adoption of computerized provider order entry systems. *Journal of the American Medical Informatics Association, 20*(3), 470–476. doi:10.1136/amiajnl-2012-001241

19. Harrison, M. I., Koppel, R., & Bar-Lev, S. (2007). Unintended consequences of information technologies in health care—An interactive sociotechnical analysis. *Journal of the American Medical Informatics Association, 14*(5), 542–549. doi:10.1197/jamia.M2384

20. Westbrook, J. I., Baysari, M. T., Li, L., Burke, R., Richardson, K. L., & Day, R. O. (2013). The safety of electronic prescribing: Manifestations, mechanisms, and rates of system-related errors associated with two commercial systems in hospitals. *Journal of the American Medical Informatics Association, 20*(6), 1159–1167. doi:10.1136/amiajnl-2013-001745

21. Carayon, P., Xie, A., & Kianfar, S. (2014). Human factors and ergonomics as a patient safety practice. *BMJ Quality & Safety, 23*(3), 196–205. doi:10.1136/bmjqs-2013-001812

22. Her, Q. L., Seger, D. L., Amato, M. G., Beeler, P. E., Dalleur, O., Slight, S. P., … Bates, D. W. (2016). Development of an algorithm to assess appropriateness of overriding alerts for nonformulary medications in a computerized prescriber-order-entry system. *American Journal of Health-System Pharmacy, 73*(1), e34–e45. doi:10.2146/ajhp150156

23. Retrieved from www.healthit.gov/

24. Hines, L. E., Saverno, K. R., Warholak, T. L., Taylor, A., Grizzle, A. J., Murphy, J. E., & Malone, D. C. (2011). Pharmacists' awareness of clinical decision support in pharmacy information systems: An exploratory evaluation. *Research in Social and Administrative Pharmacy, 7*(4), 359–368. doi:10.1016/j.sapharm.2010.10.007

25. Kawamoto, K., Houlihan, C. A., Balas, E. A., & Lobach, D. F. (2005). Improving clinical practice using clinical decision support systems: A systematic review of trials to identify features critical to success. *British Medical Journal, 330*(7494), 765. doi:10.1136/bmj.38398.500764.8F

26. Kawamoto et al. (2005).

27. Retrieved from www.himss.org/library/pharmacy-informatics/e-prescribing

28. Retrieved from www.gpo.gov/fdsys/pkg/CFR-2012-title21-vol9/pdf/CFR-2012-title21-vol9-part1311-subpartC.pdf

29. Kaushal, R., Kern, L. M., Barron, Y., Quaresimo, J., & Abramson, E. L. (2010). Electronic prescribing

improves medication safety in community-based office practices. *Journal of General Internal Medicine, 25*(6), 530–536. doi:10.1007/s11606-009-1238-8

30. Rupp, M. T., & Warholak, T. L. (2008). Evaluation of e-prescribing in chain community pharmacy: Best-practice recommendations. *Journal of the American Pharmacists Association (2003), 48*(3), 364–370. doi:10.1331/JAPhA.2008.07031

31. Grossman, J. M., Gerland, A., Reed, M. C., & Fahlman, C. (2007). Physicians' experiences using commercial e-prescribing systems. *Health Affairs (Millwood), 26*(3), w393–w404. doi:10.1377/hlthaff.26.3.w393

32. Grossman et al. (2007).

33. Fox et al. (2015).

34. Retrieved from www.fda.gov/media/106198/download

35. Fox et al. (2015).

36. Retrieved from www.bd.com

37. Fox et al. (2015).

38. Retrieved from www.bd.com

39. Retrieved from www.medkeeper.com

40. Retrieved from www.baxter.com

41. Retrieved from www.medicalletter.ashp.com/-/media/assets/policy-guidelines/docs/guidelines/handling-hazardous-drugs.ashx?la=en&hash=E0DF626948227B0F25CAED1048991E8E391F2007

42. Retrieved from www.mckesson.com

43. Retrieved from www.aethon.com

44. Poon, E. G., Keohane, C. A., Yoon, C. S., Ditmore, M., Bane, A., Levtzion-Korach, O., … Gandhi, T. K. (2010). Effect of bar-code technology on the safety of medication administration. *The New England Journal of Medicine, 362*(18), 1698–1707. doi:10.1056/NEJMsa0907115

45. Marini, S. D., & Hasman, A. (2009). Impact of BCMA on medication errors and patient safety: A summary. *Studies in Health Technology and Informatics, 146*, 439–444.

46. Fox et al. (2015).

47. Koppel, R., Wetterneck, T., Telles, J. L., & Karsh, B. T. (2008). Workarounds to barcode medication administration systems: Their occurrences, causes, and threats to patient safety. *Journal of the American Medical Informatics Association, 15*(4), 408–423. doi:10.1197/jamia.M2616

48. Williams, C. K., & Maddox, R. R. (2005). Implementation of an i.v. medication safety system. *American Journal of Health-System Pharmacy, 62*(5), 530–536.

49. Infusion pump integration. (2013). *Health Devices, 42*(7), 210–221.

50. Pettus, D. C., & Vanderveen, T. (2013). Worth the effort? Closed-loop infusion pump integration with the EMR. *Biomedical Instrumentation & Technology, 47*(6), 467–477.

51. Allen, M. (2017). Clinical surveillance systems reduce risks that thrive in information gaps. *Health Management Technology*. Retrieved from www.healthmgttech.com/clinical-surveillance-systems-reduce-risks-thrive-information-gaps

52. Echevarria, K., Smith, G., Tierney, C., Patterson, J., & Cadena-Zuluaga, J. (2011). Utility of an electronic clinical surveillance system to facilitate tracking of Multidrug-Resistant Organisms (MDRO) and antimicrobial stewardship in a VA medical centre. *ElectronicHealthcare*. Retrieved from www.longwoods.com/content/22571

53. Samore, M. H., Bateman, K., Alder, S. C., Hannah, E., Donnelly, S., Stoddard, G. J., … Stevenson, K. (2005). Clinical decision support and appropriateness of antimicrobial prescribing: A randomized trial. *The Journal of the American Medical Association, 294*(18), 2305–2314. doi:10.1001/jama.294.18.2305

54. Stokes, L. B., Rogers, J. W., Hertig, J. B., & Weber, R. J. (2016). Big data: Implications for health system pharmacy. *Hospital Pharmacy, 51*(7), 599–603. doi:10.1310/hpj5107-599

55. Stokes et al. (2016).

56. ASHP statement on the pharmacist's role in clinical informatics. (2016).

57. Fox, B. I., Karcher, R. B., Flynn, A., & Mitchell, S. (2008). Pharmacy informatics syllabi in doctor of pharmacy programs in the US. *American Journal of Pharmaceutical Education, 72*(4), 89.

58. Fuji, K. T., & Galt, K. A. (2015). An online health informatics elective course for doctor of pharmacy students. *American Journal of Pharmaceutical Education, 79*(3), 41. doi:10.5688/ajpe79341

59. Hincapie, A. L., Cutler, T. W., & Fingado, A. R. (2016). Incorporating health information technology and pharmacy informatics in a pharmacy professional didactic curriculum-with a team-based learning approach. *American Journal of Pharmaceutical Education, 80*(6), 107. doi:10.5688/ajpe806107

60. Siska & Tribble (2011).

61. Retrieved from http://www.himss.org/library/pharmacy-informatics/partners-in-e

62. Flynn, A., Fox, B. I., Clauson, K. A., Seaton, T. L., & Breeden, E. (2017). An approach for some in advanced pharmacy informatics education. *American Journal of Pharmaceutical Education, 81*(9), 6241. doi:10.5688/ajpe6241

63. Blash, A., Saltsman, C. L., & Steil, C. (2017). A national survey on the current status of informatics residency education in pharmacy. *Currents in Pharmacy Teaching and Learning, 9*(6), 1160–1163. doi:10.1016/j.cptl.2017.07.016

64. ASHP statement on the pharmacist's role in clinical informatics. (2016).

65. Devine, E. B., Lee, C. J., Overby, C. L., Abernethy, N., McCune, J., Smith, J. W., & Tarczy-Hornoch, P. (2014). Usability evaluation of pharmacogenomics

clinical decision support aids and clinical knowledge resources in a computerized provider order entry system: A mixed methods approach. *International*

Journal of Medical Informatics, 83(7), 473–483. doi:10.1016/j.ijmedinf.2014.04.008
66. Retrieved from www.averaecare.org/ecare/

Chapter Questions

7-1   What is the definition of the term "pharmacy informatics"?

7-2   What elements of informatics are included in the medication use process?

7-3   How do you think a pharmacy information system (PIS) impacts the efficiency of pharmacy workflow?

7-4   How do you think a PIS impacts the patient experience of care?

7-5   How do you think a PIS impacts the cost of health care?

Biographies

Dr. Misty Jensen is a clinical pharmacist at Avera McKennan Hospital & University Health Center. She received her PharmD from South Dakota State University and completed her post graduate residency training at Avera McKennan Hospital and University Health Center. Finally Dr. Jensen received her master's degree in patient safety leadership from University of Illinois, Chicago.

Dr. Ping Ye is a research scientist at Avera McKennan Hospital & University Health Center. She is an Associate Professor in the Department of Pediatrics and Department of Internal Medicine at University of South Dakota School of Medicine and an Adjunct Associate Professor in the Department of Pharmacy Practice at South Dakota State University College of Pharmacy. Dr. Ye received her PhD from University of Michigan. Her postdoctoral training was at Johns Hopkins University Department of Biomedical Engineering.

Dr. Ye has research experience in computational biology and informatics. Her research efforts focus on identifying the relationship between prenatal environmental exposures, epigenetic alternations, and long-term outcomes of child development and reproduction.

Dr. Ye has published ~40 articles in peer-reviewed journals, including Nature Communications, PNAS, Cell Reports, and Genome Research. She has received funding from National Institutes of Health (NIH) and March of Dimes as a principal investigator. Dr. Ye is a standing member of NIH NICHD Reproduction, Andrology and Gynecology Study Section. She also serves as the Secretary of Society for Mathematical Biology, an international society to promote research at the interface between the mathematical and biological sciences.

Dr. Ye has taught a Bioinformatics course to graduate and undergraduate students, covering topics on computational tools to analyze protein and nucleic acid sequences; functional genomics and expression data; and proteomics and systems biology. Currently, Dr. Ye teaches a Health Informatics course, which introduces health professions graduate students to a diverse range of topics including electronic health records, clinical decision support, telehealth, and regulatory issues.

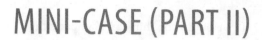

MINI-CASE (PART II)

The Case of Lose It!

Joseph Tan with Michael Dohan

▶ Introduction

Lose It! is one of a growing number of off-the-shelf calorie counting mobile applications, which can support any interested users trying to lose weight. It assists users in terms of self-care management for health and wellness with its core features that facilitate logging and monitoring of exercise, food intake, and weight, the first two being important to maintain and achieve an ideal body mass. Extended features include social networks, achievement badges, tools for specialized diets, integration with scales and other devices, and many others. According to Dohan & Tan[1], the official website of Lose It! (www.loseit.com) has boasted more than 17,000 "likes" on Facebook just only a few years after it was launched; moreover, it was further purported that Lose It! has helped many of its active users, on average, to shed 12.3 pounds per user, with 86% of these active users reporting losing weight positively, while over 90% of these same users confirming weight lost within a short period of product adoption, typically no more than a single month. Best of all, Lose It! had long been made available for free download on the iTunes App Store.

▶ Learning How to Use Lose It!

When launching the Lose It! app, beginning users typically do not need to learn its entire interface. Like many smartphone apps, Lose It! prominently features its core functions (i.e., "add food," "add exercise"), and these functions are very easy to use and learn. First, a user will enter a weight loss goal based on their current weight, their desired weight, and their desired rate of weight loss, and this will result in the setting of a daily net calorie goal for the user to adhere to. They will enter in their food intake (with the help of a food database) and exercise activity, with the intent to meet their daily calorie goal.

Users find that the steps needed to take to control each of these functions will be more or less intuitive, including having to simply scroll down a list, search, and select particular highlighted features. The user can monitor their progress throughout the day, and take action to meet their daily net calorie budget, whether this means to get more exercise or to make dietary choices. The daily net calories compared with the daily calorie budget over time is also easily understood. These are represented using color and graphs, with the implementation of a single-barred colored chart. The linear trend that appears on the resulting line graph across the bars makes tracking of one's wellness goals very convenient, and will also serve as a guiding visual tool to continually motivate the users in adhering to the Lose It! program.

More advanced functions can also be mastered as the user gains experience with the Lose It! app, for example, adding recipes and customizing food to be recorded. However, if there are too many ingredients in a particular dish to be recorded, or the food being consumed is unique (e.g., Durian), it may be convenient for most users to just record by looking up a close substitute in the existing food database, especially when the targeted dish is rarely eaten. For some users, it may be more efficient and convenient to forego the dish altogether; instead, estimated calories that are available on prepackaged (a prefixed sized-portion) food or from other familiar sources may be logged without having to record the specific food name, the portion size, and other less telling details. Notwithstanding, all these additional tasks can be mastered over time for the sole purpose of calculating and logging the relevant calorie data accurately, and adhering to calorie monitoring in the long run. Of course, users belonging to certain ethnic cultures may find that the specialty foods (such as Chinese herbal soup) frequently taken by them may in fact be nonexistent in the food database.

▶ Benefits Versus Downsides of Using Lose It!

There are many benefits that can be associated with use of smartphone apps such as Lose It! First, it is cheap, handy, and conveniently mobile. Second, when it comes to reaching one's fitness goals, actively taking steps to lose weight using a device like Lose It! is just the beginning. Importantly, Lose It! helps users track the different events throughout their daily routine—the activity, exercise, food, weight, and even sleep habits and water intake. It helps users to be continually motivated, to stay on track of achieving their self-set goals, and to be able to see how small successes can eventually lead to a significant impact on their life.

Even so, there are downsides to using any handheld devices, including Lose It! Like any handheld device, one downside of using Lose It! is that it may not always be accessible. For example, the battery could be running low and/or one may have accidently misplaced the device somewhere; perhaps it could be stolen and/or sustained some kind of damage (e.g., cracked screen). A complaint about earlier versions of these apps in particular are their interoperability with other systems and devices; that is, the data is stored independently on the device only, and cannot be accessible from any other. Many competing devices are now available in the digital fitness marketplace whose data may be offloaded to a cloud or synchronized wirelessly with another Internet of Things (IoT) device such as an Apple Watch or iPhone or be interconnected with a larger workplace computer that is located off-site (say, a laptop in one's own office or a physician's office or clinic). Here, there are many implications of risks when multiple devices are permitted to access the very same data being collected, for example, one's privacy, confidentiality, data security, and the ethical use of one's data.

▶ Conclusion

The question remains as to the potential of Lose It! or similar smartphone apps which are implemented in a socially relevant setting as well as in a relevant clinical setting. While we now know that weight loss is indeed a desired health outcome for those who are obese or have Type II diabetes, how can apps such as Lose It! and devices such as FitBit and others improve their effectiveness as tools for fitness and wellness monitoring? Also, could these devices be used as an augmented educational tool in a relevant clinical setting, for example, one in which good choices concerning diet and physical activity are taught in a clinical setting and/or memorized by the users for when the device is inaccessible?

Imagine that you have been asked to innovate the next-generation Lose It! and FitBit tools and devices. What would you do differently to significantly influence users to achieve their fitness and wellness goals while moving this innovation forward to achieve connected health not just for individuals but for targeted populations, for example, the aging population?

Note

1. Dohan, M., & Tan, J. (2011). Lose IT! *International Journal of Health Information Systems & Informatics, 6*(2), 60–65.

Biography

Michael S. Dohan, PhD (Business Administration), MSC (Management), HBComm (Information Systems), Dipl. B (Computer Programmer Analyst), is an Assistant Professor in the Faculty of Business Administration at Lakehead University in the Information Systems area, and the Director of Lakehead University's Center for Innovation and Entrepreneurship Research (CIER). He received his doctorate from McMaster University, with the dissertation titled, "*The Importance of Healthcare Informatics Competencies (HICs) for Service Innovation in Paramedicine: A Mixed-Methods Investigation.*" His research interests predominantly include digital health and digital transformation in health care, and he has published articles in journals, including *Communications of the Association for Information Systems, Health Policy and Technology, International Journal of Healthcare Information Systems and Informatics*, as well as in the proceedings of the *America's Conference on Information Systems, Hawaii International Conference on Systems Sciences*, and others. He enjoys teaching various topics in the information systems area, including Systems Analysis and Design, Design Thinking, Website Design and Administration, Business Intelligence, and Business Technology Management.

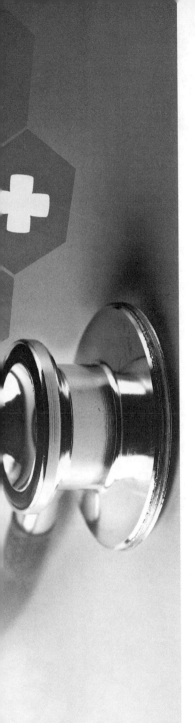

PART III

HMIS Planning and Management

CHAPTER 8

Digital Health Strategic Planning and Strategies for Health Systems

Joseph Tan and David Pellizzari

LEARNING OBJECTIVES

- Overview HMIS Strategic Planning and Strategy
- Rationalize Situation Analysis and Strategic Awareness
- Understand Strategy Conception and Formulation for Health Systems
- Actualize Strategy Implementation

CHAPTER OUTLINE

Scenario: *The Future Big Data, Big Health Gains Scenario*[1]

In this scenario, health and well-being becomes a central societal concern due to a major and profound cultural shift—the paradigm of adopting innovative programming for upbringing children and changing the lifestyle and behaviors of next-generation human race. One example cited is the Harlem Children's Zone for demonstrating the concept of health and well-being to encompass nutrition, housing, and education. Here, smart cities will promote access to locally grown, affordable healthy food via a community strategy by implementing open-source platforms, such as CreativeCommons.org, to allow the visualization of social problems and community-based solutions brought together by converging community resources to achieve the "healthy people, healthy places" vision. Accordingly, the communities, including the poorer neighborhoods, will begin to have access to healthier food sources and adopt healthier lifestyle changes.

Illustratively, it is purported that by 2032, new technologies will empower social connectivity among communities to draw on resources needed to transform investments at the local level. Changes will focus on healthier lifestyle behaviors, as well as a reorientation of entertainment and other services toward enhancing health—such projects are anticipated to experience major support from all participating citizens with the mandate to improve health from the cradle to the grave. Likewise, the new education system will be redesigned to produce an educated workforce focusing on working smart and living a healthier work-life balance.

A correlation between health and social equity will soon highlight the success of such health-oriented trending communities. It will be unveiled through the implementation of powerful analytics software resolving complex problems by feeding massive data on where best to deploy limited community resources and assets. New insights and knowledge will also be generated through sharing of innovative thinking, idle community resources, and more productive use of time toward galvanizing a broad-based commitment to achieving a more equitable and healthy society.

Initiatives such as *Healthy People 2020* and *2030* will increasingly shape the common dialogues among the millennials, academics, and trained healthcare professionals to highlight the central role of societal health and well-being. By drawing on big data applications, and with input from individual health records and environmental and national statistical data, such big data analytics will offer complex solutions for transforming ways to better deliver care for all people, especially the elderly and the disabled, providing a means toward achieving more responsible fiscal management, greater national security, privacy, and the human right to live healthier and stay healthy while maintaining economic vitality.

At the individual level, big data will drive the personal health agenda, facilitate self-care management, especially for those who may have to deal with chronic diseases, and offer the potential of personalized medicine and therapies in order to restore these individuals back to a healthy state. Similarly, the individual big data clouds could eventually be aggregated so as to feed into the generation of community health status reports for evaluating the differing health status across participating communities.

Imagine that you have been chosen to head and champion a community program with participants from various Detroit neighborhoods wanting to be part of the *Healthy People 2030* initiative with the vision of moving toward a healthier society as envisioned above. How would you go about attracting buy-ins from community members, leaders, academics, and businesses in the greater Detroit area to work together toward the aforementioned scenario? What types of big data analytics do you believe would be relevant and appropriate for implementation to empower you, as well as other participating individuals, toward achieving the vision of "healthy people, healthy places" throughout the greater Detroit area?

▶ **I. Introduction**

Senior managers of most organizations, including health systems organizations, are likely to use strategic planning and strategies as tools to convey effectively their vision and expectations on intermediate and longer-term performance, as well as future directions, to their direct reports. In health systems organizations, strategic planning teams often comprise top executives and other key advisory members of the organization who share unique perspectives and insights. These individuals meet once or twice a year to generate new perspectives, revise strategy, and update their insights on the organizational positioning in terms of fulfilling short- and long-term goals vis-à-vis established organizational policies and procedures. Generally, strategic plans are crafted with a 3- to 5-year planning horizon to guide complex decisions needed in directing, organizing, coordinating, and controlling the lower organizational echelon. Executives best coordinate stakeholders' efforts when strategic planning effectively communicates the organization's vision, mission or mandates, goals, and specific objectives.

Healthcare Strategy

In the healthcare industry, strategic planning is carried out not only by executives of regional and national healthcare systems but also by not-for-profit enterprises and government agencies. Key components of strategy often include an organization's vision, mission, and goals that shape high-level decision-making, and strategic and tactical objectives to influence operational, or lower level, activities. Cumulative efforts shared among healthcare executives to coordinate key stakeholders'

efforts to progress the area's health systems will eventually lead to a well-directed national and regional strategy; for example, the efforts of The Office of the National Coordinator for Health IT (ONC) in the United States have pursued a national and regional strategy that leads to pervasive electronic health record (EHR) adoption and meaningful use among U.S. care system organizations in recent years.

In the last several years, rapid technological developments have transformed the healthcare industry, with health information systems/technologies (health IS/IT) becoming an integral part of health systems organizations. Across the globe, regulatory bodies and national health institutes are developing top-down strategies that promote standards in health information sharing and health technology deployment, so that health systems organizations can independently provide continuous, collaborative care to patients via a wide range of clinical, administrative, and medical technology as well as health IT components and applications, including EHR, computerized order entries, virtual scheduling of examinations and imaging applications, big data and geospatial big data analytics, cloud hosting, and, increasingly, Internet of Things (IoT) connected devices. By optimizing health IT resources, health systems organizations can more effectively achieve their strategic objectives. Smart health IT strategies will eventually lead to desirable national health outcomes; aid in the prevention of debilitating and chronic disease among targeted population(s); ensure equitable, affordable, and accessible care for all citizens; improve patient-centered servicing; promote patient safety; and advance programs of care into a continuous improvement environment.[2]

ONC–CMS Strategy

In the United States, among the most influential agencies for Health IT development and adoption are the ONC and the CMS (Centers for Medicare and Medicaid Services).

The CMS provides care for a large proportion of the American public and procures services from many health systems organizations. CMS has also made health IT compliance a requirement for care providers. Likewise, the ONC, a department within Health and Human Services (HHS), was created in response to legislated mandates under the 2009 American Recovery and Reinvestment Act (ARRA), and more specifically, the Health IT for Economic and Clinical Health (HITECH) Act. To incentivize health IT adoption, HITECH allocated more than $20 billion to be distributed by the ONC and CMS to health systems organizations that implemented "meaningful use" certified health IT.[3] Meaningful use criteria are aligned with ONC and CMS strategy to create a nationally interoperable healthcare system to further progress the quality and capabilities of health IT infrastructure. HITECH catalyzes the adoption of health IT in health systems organizations by focusing on the triple aims of health care—increase patient safety and enhance the quality of care services while reducing wastes.[4] Health systems organizations that did not achieve meaningful use certification after a predetermined time would be penalized, while those that have successfully adopted health IT were rewarded. The ONC summarized the aim of its top-down strategy as, "Federal programs and policies aim to create an adaptive environment that stimulates market innovations that advance these transformational activities, while trying to prevent additional health and technical disparities."[5] By creating resources, including data samples, standards, and incentives, the ONC hopes to stimulate innovation and entrepreneurship in the strategic use of health IT.

U.S. healthcare leaders must be cognizant of the ONC and CMS strategy and vision throughout their health IT strategic planning, as these organizations' influence sets the futures of the U.S. health IS/IT ecosystem. In 2015, the ONC published the *Federal Health IT Strategic Plan (the Plan)* that outlined the strategic framework and directions envisioned for American health care. While *the Plan* is not legislation, it presents the ONC's intent for the transformation of the U.S. healthcare system and provides insight into future legislation. *The Plan* details the U.S. health system's transition to provide higher-value care motivated by alternative payment models. A survey of prominent individuals in the health IT industry found that reforming financing of health care to a risk-sharing model is a credible strategy to facilitate change. Researchers also report that respondents expect the ONC or CMS to be responsible for further U.S. healthcare reform.[6] Accordingly, the ONC has taken steps toward transforming U.S. health systems progressively; even so, many consultations and developments are underway. For example, the ONC has dedicated workshops to develop long-term strategies to reform U.S. healthcare funding, and researchers expect a transition to a payment model that incentivizes eliminating unnecessary and avoidable uses of health care.[7] Key factors facilitating this transition include increased attention to population health as well as teamwork and integration within organizations along the continuity of care as supported by advances in health IT.[8] The ONC, through such efforts, hopes to reduce the "digital divide" between organizations with mature health IT capabilities versus those that lack such capabilities, which is important not only for the provision of care but also for wider socioeconomic considerations.[9] *The Plan* highlights many of the ONC's key initiatives and outlines their strategy to progress American health IT infrastructure. Leaders in U.S. health systems organizations should therefore use *the Plan* to guide their corporate health IT strategy and decisions so that their organization remains competitive and in compliance.

ONC's Plan and Learning Health Systems

Today, U.S. health IT has generally progressed from isolated legacy systems into more integrated, interoperable networks—a fundamental change that has been aided via standardization as a result of meaningful-use certification. The next phase of the ONC's transition for the U.S. health systems is the Learning Health Systems (LHS). Here, greater abilities in information sharing and population health monitoring are key aspects of LHS. *The Plan* describes LHS with the Institute of Medicine's (IoM's) definition, "one in which science, informatics, incentives, and culture are aligned for continuous improvement and innovation, with best practices seamlessly embedded in the care process, patients and families active participants in all elements, and new knowledge captured as an integral by-product of the care experience.[10]" Essentially, in LHS, data are gathered by health IT throughout all care processes and are subsequently used to analyze care provision (analytics); in this way, meaningful metrics can be developed and tracked with positive versus negative evidence to motivate policy changes, embedding scientific innovations into the care process.[11]

The ONC's *Plan* has a vision and mission statement with four overarching goals. The vision is to achieve high-quality care at lower costs, resulting in a healthy and engaged population via healthcare transformation. ONC's mission to realize this vision is to improve the health and well-being of individuals and communities via technology and health information that is accessible when and where it matters most. Four goals support the ONC's mission: (a) advance person-centered and self-managed health; (b) transform healthcare delivery and community health; (c) foster research, scientific knowledge, and innovation; and (d) enhance the nation's health IT infrastructure.[12] ONC-led strategic leadership in health IT initiatives and guides to developing the national health IT infrastructure are underway as U.S. healthcare administrators, planners, managers, and key decision-makers adopt these strategies to improve ongoing care services delivery and optimize deployed resources.

Beyond progressing a national health IT strategy, LHS thinking will promote the strategic goals of health systems organizations. Driving LHS thinking with health IT can eventually aid U.S. care provider organizations to achieve the "triple aim of healthcare reform…(that is)…improving the quality, safety, and experience of care, enhancing population health, and reducing the per capita cost of healthcare."[13] At this juncture, U.S. health systems organizations must therefore progress their health IT capabilities to support LHS thinking and achieve the "triple aim." Strategic planning in health systems organizations must begin with an understanding of national plans that shape the organization and industry, to align their strategy with the progress of the industry. Moreover, health systems organizational strategies need to be robust and flexible to adapt to changing environments, and at the same time, contain enough detail to allow organizational policymakers and key stakeholders to carry out the organization's high-level goals. Parallel to implementing an organization's corporate strategy is the organization's health IT strategy or strategic plan, which should be aligned with the corporate goals and strategy. Health IT strategy is thus derived from the corporate vis-à-vis national health IT strategies. Vision and mission statements are translated into tactical strategies and specific programmatic aims that use health IT intelligently to achieve the care provider higher-level organizational objectives. A health systems organization's strategy could include health IT as a component to realize organizational objectives or include health IT components directly in its organizational strategy. Examples include being a low-cost provider of care or maintaining full compliance with health IT certification programs, respectively.

Put together, health IT investments yield the most benefit to stakeholders when planning is aligned with the organization's strategy. Senior managers within the organization should oversee the strategic planning of health IT portfolios and programs as plans are being

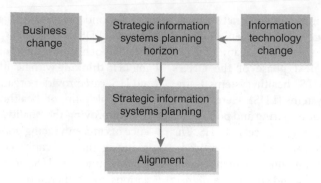

FIGURE 8-1 Strategic Alignment Concepts.

synthesized into health IT strategy. Aligning business-IT strategies have shown to enhance an organization's efficiency and increase customer value.[14] Such strategic alignment encompasses the process of creating IT targets and plans that achieve organizational objectives and goals, as shown in **FIGURE 8-1**.

In other words, one may assess an organization's strategic alignment by observing how closely the IT plan meets objectives of the business plan.[15] Ultimately, health IT planning must support the organization's strategy so as to provide quality patient care and to achieve strategic alignment.

▶ II. Strategic Information Systems Planning and Strategic Awareness

Strategic Information Systems Planning (SISP) is an important process driving the successful alignment between health IT and organizational strategy; that is, the degree to which health IT components facilitate organization's goals to be met. The task of aligning health IT with corporate strategy is the primary focus of planners through SISP and should be considered during each of its phases. The outcome of SISP is a portfolio of health IT components

that serve organizational strategy.[16] Development of health IT strategy and aligning its objectives with the organization is completed through SISP. Here, health systems organizations must use strategic thinking and planning to make decisions regarding health IT investments; standard methodologies of planning are used to ensure important planning aspects are not overlooked.[17] Core functions of strategic planning include the discovery of missing information, assessing future scenarios, examining resource flows, and pursuing goals systematically.[18] There are several published SISP models; each vary in exact detail but are generally created along the same basis. Major components of SISP include understanding of the desired state, what the organization would look like if the strategy was realized, current state analysis of health IT, and a gap analysis between the current and desired state,[19] as shown in **FIGURE 8-2**.

Understanding the desired state helps planners identify health IT capabilities most required to fulfill the organization's objectives and develop health IT plans that align with organizational strategy. The current state allows for the analysis of health IT systems, internal and external policies, and other components that aid or impede the organizations success. Gap analysis is then performed and differences between current and required health IT capabilities are highlighted. Strategically aligned plans then close the gap. It is through the SISP process that the

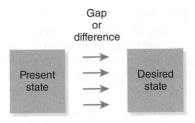

FIGURE 8-2 Gap Analysis Concepts.

organization's health IT benefits are optimized and the organization's strategy is carried out.

Effective management of healthcare information and processes require comprehensive SISP. Planning activities such as "gathering information, evaluating potential courses of action, limiting trial-and-error decision-making, delaying decisions until all alternatives have been evaluated, and determining a good course of action," contribute to successful planning outcomes.[20] A successful planning outcome of SISP is an effective health IT strategy that enables a health systems organization to provide quality care in an environment of rising costs, aging populations, and increased demand of patients living with long-term conditions.[21] Health IT can combat these constraints by managing care costs, increasing care quality, and making systems safer and more accessible.[22]

In this chapter, the SISP model chosen to outline the process was first published by Lederer and Sethi in 1988 and has been intensively studied.[23–25] This SISP method is conducted in five phases: (1) planning the health IT planning process, (2) analyzing the current environment or situational analysis, (3) conceiving strategy alternatives, (4) selecting strategy or formulating strategy, and (5) planning strategy implementation,[26] as shown in **FIGURE 8-3**.

These SISP phases are assessed within four dimensions, namely, alignment, analysis, cooperation, and capabilities. Alignment is how closely the health IT supports business strategy. Analysis examines the capability of the planning team to use and track impact measures of health IT components. Cooperation

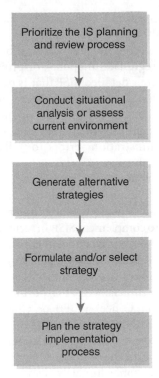

FIGURE 8-3 Five phases of strategic IS/IT planning (SISP).

measures how well team members can work together and with other parts of the organization. And capabilities investigate the processes used by planners to incorporate lessons learned into planning. Researchers have studied the correlation between the efforts spent during each of the above phases, vis-à-vis IS/IT implementation success in organizations. These researchers have also used well-defined criteria, which form the basis for guidelines within each phase to measure the degree to which they were completed. Lederer–Sethi's SISP model was traditionally applied to IS generally; more specifically, to tailor this model to health IT, we incorporate Sittig–Singh's socio-technical model[27] of health IT in complex adaptive systems (CAS) in the situational analysis phase as discussed next.

In the next few sections, we outline the five SISP phases with emphasis on key factors that pertain to health IT planning from an organizational perspective. Health IT plans, to be effective, should be crafted at the enterprise level; indeed, SISP can be carried out on a regional, functional, or project level as well. Finer detailed SISP that is performed for functional or project level may, however, only focus on one aspect of the organization's strategy, such as reducing medication order and administration errors or decreasing duplicate lab tests.

An organization's structure–culture will shape the SISP process and its outcome, which implies that structure–culture changes may be required to complement SISP. In terms of structural changes, for example, there may be the need to assemble an *ad hoc* planning team, to set up a project management office, and/or to re-assign a clinician's role to report to the Chief Information Officer (CIO) or Chief Digital Officer (CDO). Cultural changes may include the development of more collaborative relationships vertically or horizontally throughout the organization. Ultimately, changes that align organizational structure–culture to complement SISP lead to more effective planning.

Critical success factors (CSFs) of SISP can help planners plan-to-plan. Effective SISP is achieved by ensuring success factors are satisfied and required components are available prior to SISP. Examples of CSFs include SISP fit to an organization's structure-culture, planners are realistic and have access to needed resources, planners are capable of aligning health IT with organizational strategy, planners can perform situation analysis well, planners will be able to achieve an agreement and provide assessment-measurement to be integrated into the planning process, and so forth. Many of these CSFs are addressed directly in strategic awareness, the first phase of SISP.

Strategic Awareness

Four key components determine strategic awareness: (a) a planning team, (b) top management commitment, (c) key planning issues, and (d) planning objectives.

To begin SISP, a planning team is organized to carry out the analysis-planning activities. Effective selection of team members increases the probability of success. Representation from senior management will aid planners to be realistic with available resources based on their knowledge of strategies and/or increasing departmental budgets. Senior representation also makes experts in the organization's strategy available to health IT planners to align their plans. A key SISP success factor is the capability of the planning to analyze various aspects of health IS/IT. Other dimensions of expertise to include in the planning team are employees who are knowledgeable about external policy, internal workflow patterns-processes, clinical and medical information, and IT digitalization. The effectiveness of SISP teams are dependent on their ability to identify problem areas, anticipate crisis and surprises, adapt to change, and gain the support of health IT user groups.[28] Capable planning teams have the potential to implement changes in the organization that are required to optimize health IT use.

Planning Strategy Objectives

Once formed, the team members should lay out key planning issues and objectives. Planners should focus on high-level organizational strategy objectives to articulate key issues (and broad objectives) that will be addressed by SISP. With a high-level focus, health IT-organizational strategy can be better aligned. Additionally, planning activities that identify key issues will ensure team members not be carried away or be biased by assumed benefits of health IS/IT implementation while shifting the focus toward tangible and achievable goals.[29] Planners that assume any health IT improvement will benefit the organization are less likely to think critically or strategically of health IT plans. After studying key issues–objectives, the team should be well orientated with the organization's strategy and potential areas for achieving competitive organizational transformation via health IT. The team then summarizes these key issues and broad objectives into a planning proposal or scope statement. Included in the document is a table of contents with components planners can elaborate in the final planning document. The planning proposal document describes the strategic objectives that SISP is targeting—this important document will guide the efforts of the planning team toward achieving the desired and envisioned outcomes.

The final move in strategic awareness would be top-level management support. Communication between the planning team and senior management must occur in both directions; on the one hand, the team must ensure top management understands the need for corporate digitalization to achieve strategic IT-corporate alignment, while, on the other hand, the team must be informed of top management's perspective of evolving corporate strategic priorities.[30] It is in the best interest of executive-level managers, including the CEO, CIO, or CDO and medical officers in health systems organizations, to be included in the SISP process, as advisory or being represented within the planning team. Well-aligned and executed health IT investments provide the organization opportunity to realize substantial benefits, while failed investments present tremendous risk. Thus, the presence of executive managers in planning teams increases access to required resources and reduces risk of harmful events occurring.[31] Additionally, strategic awareness forms the foundation for maintaining managerial commitment.[32] Strong SISP planning team and top-level managerial coordination will more closely align health IT with corporate strategy, ensuring that targeted organizational objectives are rolled out.

▶ III. Situational Analysis (SA)

In SISP, situational analysis (SA) follows strategic awareness. SA allows for planners to get an understanding of the organization's current state. The general SISP methodology analyzes IS/IT in five dimensions, all of which will have to be modified to adapt to the uniqueness of health systems and the increasing complex health IT environment: (a) current business (or health services delivery) systems; (b) organizational or health systems; (c) IS or health IT; (d) external business or health services delivery environment; and (e) current external IS/IT or health IT environment. As noted, all five dimensions of analysis must be conducted within the unique context of the health systems so as to ensure efficient, precise, and meaningful analysis of the health organization's health IS/IT environment. In the extant literature, a similar issue appeared when studying implemented health IT; that is, further research is needed to generate a holistic methodology that better measure and characterize the complexity of health IT environments.

Qualitative and quantitative analysis of the current state will help planners to identify areas for improvement via health IS/IT, gain an understanding of health organizational processes and procedures, understand health information needs of subunits, understand the current technological landscape across the organization, and monitor the capabilities and needs of current health IS/IT.[33] Planners analyze the current state by modeling the health organization's data, information, and processes, with a focus on understanding requirements that lead to success.[34]

Sittig and Singh describe eight socio-technical dimensions, which are shown in **TABLE 8-1**, that can help the SISP team analyze the current state of an organization's health IT.[35] These dimensions are neither hierarchical nor independent, that is, issues may often arise in strategic planning that incorporate two or more socio-technical dimensions. For example, *the Plan* cites common criticism of health IT that include awkward layouts, disrupted workflows, decreased efficiency, and limited interoperability.[36] An example of a survey response of an end user of health IT that includes each criticism may be, "The computer system slowed

TABLE 8-1 Sittig–Singh Eight Socio-technical Dimensions

Hardware and software computing infrastructure	Clinical content
Human computer interface	People
Internal organizational policies, procedures, and culture	Workflow and communications
External rules, regulations, and pressures	System measurement and monitoring

me down, the text was too small, signing in and out interrupted my office time, I had to cancel appointments because I was late and for some patients, I did not have the lab results from a family doctor." The listed grievances could even be oversimplified and may be synthesized as, "I find use of computer systems to be disruptive to my practice" clinician found trouble using health IT components, but by analyzing health IT through each of the eight dimensional aspects, we can break down clinician perceived challenges. In the above example, awkward layouts are human–computer interface issues, disrupted workflow are workflow challenges, decreased efficiency is a measurement issue, and interoperability can probably be clinical content or incompatible hardware–software, a computing infrastructure problem.

Systems Measurement and Monitoring

Authors of the eight dimensions did not suggest a sequence in which to study them. However, system measurement and monitoring begins the team's analysis of the current state. By measuring aspects of health IT and the organization, planners can and will highlight areas for improvement, thereby setting a base benchmark against which progress can be measured. Health IT can be measured in four key aspects, specifically, systems' availability, systems' use in clinical settings, patient outcomes, and unintended consequences.[37]

Measurement of specific health IT components and interactions also occur throughout other dimensions, for instance, a survey of end users can be used by planners to qualitatively assess the human–computer interface dimension. For many stakeholders, having an understanding of the functionality and use of health IT components provide a tangible representation of the current state of health IT.

The importance of measurement is growing due to large volumes of data (Big Data) captured and stored by health IT, and the need for organizations to create value from Big Data. Health organizations following the ONC's plan will progress into an LHS that use measurement and analytics to create processes that can improve care continuously.[38] Metrics that measure and monitor such care processes as well as patient outcomes allow for clinicians and administrators to determine which solutions are most appropriate and effective in their organization's environment. The current state analysis should begin with pretested measurements—this will establish the need to understand current process performance and the outcomes desired after implementing health IT strategy.

The ONC annually publishes three measuring tools for data collection to assess health systems progression toward a health IT-enabled LHS. The ONC measures the percent of physicians that have patient information available from outside of their organization, percent of hospitals that have necessary patient clinical information from other organizations when providing care, and percent of individuals that experienced gaps in clinical information while receiving care.[39] Tracking these metrics inside organizations indicate to planners the effectiveness of health IT toward alignment with the ONC's national strategy.

External Rules, Regulations, and Pressures

Owing to rapid changes in the health IT environment, the impact of externalities such as external rules, regulations, and pressures have been alluded to earlier in the chapter. Indeed, health systems today are increasingly being subjected to changes in the external regulatory environment. In the United States, the ONC developed the national health IT strategy for guiding health systems organizations in handling external pressures imposed upon by regulators and other external influential stakeholders.[40] *The Plan*, which outlines the evolution of U.S. health IT infrastructure, notes: "federal action will supplement existing stakeholder work or encourage additional activities to begin."[41]

According to the ONC, "federal efforts will also focus on improving accessibility, technical standards, services, policies, federal data, and governance structures that support person-centered outcomes research."[42] Here, the ONC is signaling to organizations that health payment reform is likely to occur, and that health IT components may need to be changed as well. Health leaders, planners, decision-makers, and policymakers need to understand the progression of health systems into an LHS.

Hardware–Software Computing Infrastructure

This dimension includes technical components such as computers, keyboards, and other devices that process clinical applications and receive information from medical instruments. Health IT components to be analyzed include storage devices, network equipment, clinical–administrative applications, and operating system (OS) software, as well as the computing infrastructure that maintains the care facility's operation and medical devices.[43] To better understand each component of the computing infrastructure dimension, the technology under analysis may be classified into three categories: clinical tools and clinical and administration systems. Generating such a functional health IT capabilities taxonomy allows planners to assess if and how the computing infrastructure in place is fulfilling its intended requirements. Beyond the analysis of current systems, dividing components of this dimension allows planners to see what, where, and how available health IT resources can best be applied or redeployed to achieve specific clinical, administrative, and/or medical strategies.

Internal Organizational Policies, Procedures, and Culture

Internal policies are the structures and norms that drive the operations of other health IT dimensions on a routine basis. Senior managers are most influential in shaping the organization's procedures as they create the organizational policies, structure, and culture.[44] Managers and SISP planners, if given the responsibility to appropriately adapt the organization to health IT changes, must be mindful that health IT planning, implementation, and use occur within the defined organizational procedures. Planners need to align the process of creating strategic plans with organizational procedures to optimize health IT use.

Workflow and Communication

Workflow and communication are the procedures that members of the organization carry out to facilitate care provision. Process analysis techniques are used to measure workflow within organizations. While studying this dimension, planners should concentrate on processes that support the organization's objectives via qualitative–quantitative analysis.[45] Analysis of key processes prior to health IT strategy implementation is used as a baseline measurement to monitor improvements. For newly developed health IT strategies to be successful, care processes and procedures need to be adapted. New health IT capabilities are not used optimally if workflow processes do not change to complement health IT.

Clinical Content

This dimension describes elements of data, knowledge, and information that are created and stored during care. Information is essential for clinicians to provide quality care, but due to the lack of financial incentives and incomplete information, clinicians may not have access to needed information. The ONC included these concerns in their justification for healthcare payment reform into a system that is pay-for-outcome.[46] To achieve an environment of continuous improvement that aligns with the ONC's strategy, both the collection of health data and applications that manage such information need to be tailored to capture *process data* and *clinical outcomes*.

Data and applications should meet the needs of both primary caregivers and secondary users of information.[47] Primary caregivers need information to be complete and accessible, while researchers (an example of secondary users) use mostly de-identified data to preform studies. Knowledge is better extracted for continuous improvement from data that was created and stored in a structured format. Therefore, aggregating data on individuals across a region, state, or nation allows for the analysis of population health, an outcome of LHS and a component of the ONC's long-term vision. The aggregated finding then can be used in decision support, quality measurement, population health management, and research.[48] Standardization also facilitates information sharing and improved interoperability. The ONC health IT Certification

Program promotes the adoption of information standards for care provision that is seamless and secure.[49] In the clinical content of an LHS, quality improvement in care delivery is central. Accordingly, embedding information that supports care provision into health IT allows clinicians to offer patients preventative care options, monitor patients' conditions on an ongoing basis, and coordinate care between providers.[50]

Human–Computer Interface

Human–computer interfaces are the touch points between end users of a system and hardware-software components of health IT that allow end users to access and interact with clinical content. User interfaces impact caregivers' workflow and communication by enabling or restricting information access. It is important to reduce the complexity end users face when navigating through the health IT systems so that their workflow is not being inhibited; at the same time, health IT must include appropriate redundancies to ensure safe care. Ergonomic factors of health IT should also be considered, for example, the straining of eyesight during use of health IT systems.

People

Finally, health IT stakeholders must be considered. Key stakeholders, such as clinicians, computer scientists, administrators, researchers, and patients, are major users of health IT systems. Thus, an intelligent analysis of stakeholders' behaviors allows planners to tailor specific health IT components to different user groups. As human capital is measured, planners can assess if there is further need for knowledge, skillsets, and training capabilities that may be required to fulfill the health IT strategy.[51] Stakeholder analysis is also completed to identify resistors and champions of change. The planning team might then devise a communication plan to mitigate the risk of resistance and optimize the driving forces and influential attitude of champions.

Examining all eight dimensions of health IT components stresses the interdependence of many factors and that analysts should not be myopic. These eight dimensions holistically measure the impact, effectiveness, and unintended consequences of health IT use.[52]

▶ IV. Strategy Conception and Formulation

Analysis completed during the first two SISP phases is used in strategy conception by the planning team to create high-level health IT strategy that is aligned with the organization's strategy.[53] Studies that examine the amount of resources devoted to strategy conception by the planning team do not predict successful SISP outcomes.[54,55] Planners therefore do not need to develop elaborate health IT strategies to align with their organization's strategy.

Strategy Conception (SC)

The four components of the SC phase include: (a) identify major IT objectives, (b) identify opportunities for improvement, (c) evaluate opportunities, and (d) identify high-level strategy.[56,57] In completing the SISP strategy conception phase, planners should use simple tools to align the health IT strategy they create with the organization's strategy.

Results of situational analysis, the prior phase, can be organized into a matrix of strengths, weaknesses, opportunities, and threats (SWOT). For example, an organization's strengths may be its capability to store and manage clinical content on hardware–software components. Examples of organization's weaknesses are undertrained employees–clinicians or dated human–computer interfaces. As well,

the organization can benefit from government incentives or a more technologically engaged public, while faced with the threat of an aging and increasingly chronically ill population. Results of the SWOT analysis often assist planners on how to align health IT plans with the organization's strategy and environment. Components of an organization's health IT infrastructure that are considered strengths are used to seize opportunities, reduce the likelihood and impact of threats, and carry out the organization's objectives. Weaknesses in organizations are alerted to management and, where possible, corrected to reduce the risk of threats having a negative impact on the organization. Gaps, or weaknesses, between an organization's capability and those required to achieve organizational strategy are highlighted. SISP plans incorporating health IT components to close the gap and achieve strategic outcomes are creatively generated.

Examples of health IT strategies generated during the SC phase may include using health IT initiatives to: (a) enable caregivers to offer higher quality care; (b) achieve regulatory guideline compliance; (c) better inform decisions within and outside of the hospital, for example, increase safety, improve research, and promote population health; (d) create a broader representation for health IT governance structure and future investment decisions; and (e) improve clinician–patient communications.[58] Specific goals resulting from high-level health IT strategy may include the following: (a) providing follow-up care to more outpatients, (b) decreasing inpatient hospital length of stays, (c) improving collaboration among internal workers and with other organizations, (d) becoming more competitive and productive with improved health IT features, and (e) increasing profit.[59]

Strategy Formulation (SF)

Components of planning contained in the SF phase include: (a) identifying new ways to deliver care by changing care processes, (b) identifying new opportunities to upgrade existing health IT infrastructure, (c) identifying new health IS/IT projects, and (d) setting priorities for new projects. SF components cover such activities as to assess the degree health IT plans and opportunities support the organization's strategy, the degree planned health IT aligns with strategic change, and the degree to which the impact of emerging technology is understood by end users.[60] Also, during this phase planners must agree upon a method for deciding which projects to complete, given risks versus rewards, and in what order projects will be completed.[61]

During SF, the planning team often creates new care processes. Such activities are often required to align health IT components with the organization's strategy. Planners use the situation analysis of the workflow and internal structure dimension to assess the need to revise organizational components. If an organization's practices and structure remain unchanged, the organization may fail to realize the benefits to be leveraged from health IT investments.[62] SF is the phase in which planners decide on the specific health IT projects and components to be contained within the SISP scope. Projects and initiatives should be considered again through the eight dimensions of measuring health IT. The results of SC phase are used to determine what components within each of the eight socio-technical dimensions of health IT yield the most benefit when incorporated into health IT strategy.

The strategic planning team will then develop alternative projects suited to meet the organization's strategic health IT needs. When identifying projects and priorities that are to be implemented, it is helpful for planners to choose "low hanging fruit," as objectives to begin with. "Low hanging fruit," projects are potential health IT initiatives that do not require large investments but

will closely align health IT to an organization's strategy. Researchers have found that common opportunities for improvement are present in care quality and safety as wells as potential cost saving with many health IT initiatives.[63] Easier projects build goodwill between health IT implementers and end users, and set the momentum for future projects.

▶ V. Strategy Implementation (SI)

During the SI phase, health IT strategy is conveyed into policies, procedures, and structures to be carried out within the organization. SI components include: (a) defining the change management approach; (b) defining, then evaluating, an action plan; and (c) defining control procedures.[64] During SI, planners develop plans and guidelines for managerial responsibility throughout health IT implementation, communicate plans throughout the organization, and coordinate subunit efforts to carry out the plan.[65] Change management is required when implementing a new health IT strategy. An organization's investment in health IT will provide long-term benefits to an organization if new capabilities are embedded in organizational practice.[66] An aspect of change management that complements long-term health IT investment is the creation of structures and procedures that facilitate SISP.

Defining and evaluating alternative action plans to transform the organization's competitiveness via implementation of health IT strategy is often achieved by reaching a consensus among planning team members on key initiatives. Once consent decisions have evolved, action plans are then drafted that may include sourcing of available resources such as personnel and estimated budget and setting of predetermined project deadlines, milestones, and deliverables.[67]

▶ VI. Conclusion

At the end of all SISP phases, planners should have crafted a new health IT strategy that includes agreed upon projects and initiatives geared toward accomplishing the organization's broader strategy. Altogether, the five SISP phases represent a useful guide or map for health IT planners to align its health IT plan with (or to) the health systems organization's strategy. Incorporating health IT domain-specific knowledge into the five SISP phases allows planners to better understand the strategic planning processes as they pertain to unique settings of health systems.

Notes

1. *Health & Health Care in 2032: Report from the RWJF Futures Symposium.* (2012, June 20–21). Retrieved from www.altfutures.org/pubs/RWJF/IAF-Health andHealthCare2032.pdf
2. Federal Health IT Strategic Plan. (2015). p. 18. Retrieved from www.healthit.gov/sites/default/files/9-5-federalhealthitstratplanfinal_0.pdf
3. *A new socio-technical model for studying health information technology in complex adaptive healthcare systems.* (2010). Retrieved from www.ncbi.nlm.nih.gov/pmc/articles/PMC3120130/pdf/nihms297306.pdf 6
4. Sheikh, A., Sood, H.S., and Bates, D.W. (2015). "Leveraging health information technology to achieve the "triple aim" of healthcare reform." *JAMIA* 22(4), 849–56. doi: 10.1093/jamia/ocv022. Epub 2015 Apr 15. Retrieved from www.ncbi.nlm.nih.gov/pubmed/25882032
5. Federal Health IT Strategic Plan. (2015), *ibid.*, p. 19.
6. Triple aim. (2015), *ibid.*, p. 5.
7. *Ibid.*, p. 6.
8. Federal Health IT Strategic Plan. (2015), *ibid.*, p. 19.
9. *Ibid.*, p. 14.
10. National Research Council. (2011). *Institute of Medicine "The learning health system and its innovation collaboratives".* Retrieved from www.nationalacademies.org/hmd/~/media/Files/Activity%20Files/Quality/VSRT/Core%20Documents/ForEDistrib.pdf
11. Federal Health IT Strategic Plan. (2015), *ibid.*, p. 21.
12. *Ibid.*, p. 6.
13. Triple aim, (2015), *ibid.*, p. 2.
14. *Technology alignment in the presence of regulatory changes: The case of meaningful use of information technology in healthcare.* (2017), p. 42. Retrieved from www.ncbi.nlm.nih.gov/pubmed/29331254
15. *Aligning IT strategy with business strategy through the balanced scorecard in a multinational pharmaceutical company.* (2007), pp. 2–3. Retrieved from ieeexplore-ieee-org.libaccess.lib.mcmaster.ca/stamp/stamp.jsp?tp=&arnumber=4076857&tag=1
16. *The effectiveness of strategic information systems planning under environmental uncertainty.* (2006), p. 2. Retrieved from www.sciencedirect.com/science/article/abs/pii/S0378720606000024
17. *IT strategic planning in a pediatric hospital: Overview of the process and outcomes.* (2012), p. 2. Retrieved from https://ieeexplore-ieee-org.libaccess.lib.mcmaster.ca/stamp/stamp.jsp?arnumber=6149178
18. *"Less is More:" Information systems planning in an uncertain environment.* (2012), p. 20. Retrieved from https://ieeexplore-ieee-org.libaccess.lib.mcmaster.ca/stamp/stamp.jsp?arnumber=6149178
19. *A critical inquiry of strategic information systems planning (SISP) analysis approaches.* (2015), p. 3. Retrieved from www.researchgate.net/publication/255634369
20. *The effectiveness of strategic information systems planning under environmental uncertainty.* (2006), *ibid.*, p. 3.
21. Triple aim (2015), *ibid.*, p. 1.
22. *Strategic information systems planning in healthcare organizations.* (2015), p. 2. Retrieved from www.researchgate.net/publication/273338864_Strategic_Information_System_Planning_in_Healthcare_Organizations
23. *The implementation of strategic information systems planning methodologies.* (1988). Retrieved from https://dl.acm.org/citation.cfm?id=59195
24. The effectiveness of strategic information systems planning under environmental uncertainty. (2006), *ibid.*, p. 2.
25. "Less is More," (2012), *ibid.*, p. 14.
26. A critical inquiry of SISP analysis approaches. (2015), *ibid.*, p. 5.
27. Or, C., Dohan, M., & Tan, J. (2014). Understanding critical barriers to implementing a clinical information system in a nursing home through the lens of a socio-technical perspective. *Journal of Medical Systems,* 38(9), 1–10.
28. "Strategic information systems planning," *Encyclopedia of information science and technology.* (2018), p. 6.

Retrieved from www.igi-global.com/chapter/strategic-information-systems-planning/183802

29. *Ten key considerations for the successful implementation and adoption of large-scale health information technology.* (2015), p. 1. Retrieved from www.ncbi.nlm.nih.gov/pmc/articles/PMC3715363/d

30. "Strategic information systems planning," (2018), *ibid.*, p. 6.

31. "Less is More," (2012), *ibid.*, p. 14.

32. *"Ibid.*

33. "Strategic information systems planning," (2018), *ibid.*, p. 6.

34. A critical inquiry of SISP. (2015), *ibid.*, p. 3.

35. A new socio-technical model. (2010), *ibid.*, pp. 4–6.

36. Federal Health IT Strategic Plan. (2015), *ibid.*, p. 16.

37. A new socio-technical model. (2010), *ibid.*, p. 6.

38. Federal Health IT Strategic Plan. (2015), *ibid.*, p. 21.

39. *Ibid.*, p. 33.

40. A new socio-technical model. (2010), *ibid.*, p. 6.

41. Federal Health IT Strategic Plan. (2015), *ibid.*, p. 6.

42. *Ibid.*, p. 29.

43. A new socio-technical model. (2010), *ibid.*, p. 4.

44. *Ibid.*, p. 5.

45. A critical inquiry of SISP. (2015), *ibid.*, p. 7.

46. Federal Health IT Strategic Plan. (2015), *ibid.*, p. 11.

47. *Ibid.*, p. 12.

48. *Ibid.*, p. 26.

49. *Ibid.*

50. *Ibid.*, p. 19.

51. A new socio-technical model. (2010), *ibid.*, p. 5.

52. *Ibid.*, p. 8.

53. "Less is More," (2012), *ibid.*, p. 14.

54. *Ibid.*, p. 21.

55. The effectiveness of strategic information systems planning under environmental uncertainty. (2006), p. 4.

56. "Less is More," (2012), *ibid.*, p. 23.

57. "Strategic information systems planning," (2018), *ibid.*, p. 6.

58. IT strategic planning in a pediatric hospital. (2012), *ibid.*, p. 7.

59. *Strategic information management plans: The basis for systematic information management in hospitals.* (2001), p. 8. Retrieved from https://pdfs.semanticscholar.org/46e7/34ec46851ff5c7ffd6f8e6a2828c34a089a9.pdf

60. "Strategic information systems planning," (2018), *ibid.*, p. 6.

61. *Ibid.*

62. *Information systems use as strategy practice: A multi-dimensional view of strategic information system implementation and use.* (2014), p. 47. Retrieved from www.sciencedirect.com/science/article/pii/S0963868714000055

63. Triple aim, (2015), *ibid.*, p. 6.

64. "Strategic information systems planning," (2018), *ibid.*, p. 6.

65. *Ibid.*, p. 5.

66. Information systems use as strategy practice. (2014), *ibid.*, p. 45.

67. Strategic information management plans: The basis for systematic information management in hospitals, *ibid.*

Chapter Questions

8-1 Differentiate between "strategic planning" and "strategy." Why is understanding the different terminologies important for planners?

8-2 As mentioned in the chapter, planners in a health systems organization strategically plan and produce the health IT vision and define its strategic objectives. What are some of the inputs that the planning team would consider when developing the health IT strategic plans?

8-3 How do you think members of the planning team work to get the health IT strategy aligned with the organization's strategy? Illustrate your answer with a case scenario.

8-4 What makes strategic planning of health IT appear to be unique and more complex than most other business systems? Who are key stakeholders in health systems organizations?

8-5 How do advances in health IT impact the strategic planning process?

Biography

David Pellizzari has a Bachelor of Commerce degree from McMaster University, Hamilton, Ontario (Canada). Through his studies, David has focused on diversifying his understanding of Information Management and Information Technology. To maintain successful and effective Healthcare Management Information Systems, David believes strategic planning is essential and must permeate the culture and processes of the organization. David looks forward to continuing his studies.

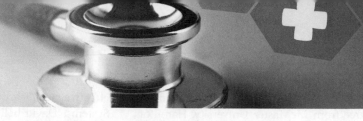

POLICY REVIEW II

Roles and Responsibilities of Health Systems Leaders and Managers

Joseph Tan with Phillip Olla and Joshia Tan

Abstract

With rapid growth and advances in technology and the need for a technological revolution in healthcare systems, leadership and proper management of health management information systems (HMIS) cannot be overly emphasized. This opens up a discussion of the critical roles played by the chief executive officer and others in health systems organizational c-suites. These executives are responsible for providing an appropriate vision for future HMIS directions. They are responsible for aligning IT departmental goals and strategies with corporate goals and strategies, and they are also responsible for strategizing appropriately, executing intelligently, and evaluating wisely on the system's performance of healthcare services delivery with the application of effective and efficient business processes and information technologies throughout the corporation.

POLICY REVIEW OUTLINE

▶ Vision

Health executives and managers over-seeing health information systems/technologies (health IS/IT) projects in any health learning systems require the mastery of a certain set of strategic, tactical, and operational competencies. Essentially, these leaders (and/or managers) are expected to think quickly and strategically, solve problems intelligently in many areas of health IS/IT specializations, and advocate influentially on the use of available and advancing technologies to close the gap between departmental IS/IT goals and strategies vis-à-vis the corporate goals and strategies.

Healthcare organizations are undergoing tremendous changes, including the need to integrate an increasing array of scientific and technological innovations into the day-to-day operations of the organization. Innovations, such as artificial intelligence, health personalization, and precision medicine, are transforming the current landscape. In addition, they are also altering the role of health IT leaders, who must not only adapt themselves but also influence the transformation within their staff.[1]

Among the most critical roles, then, is having a vision—this involves the creation of future scenarios and possibilities to drive health IS/IT development, future growth, and investments. Apparently, crafting such a "vision" is a long-drawn-out process whereby a set of shared and related notions in the form of a vetted "proposal" supported by top management should be generated via a planning team. Above all, there is the need to sell both the professional staff and other corporate employees the same vision; that is, a large majority of organizational members should be aware of, must be willing to support, and must be able to participate in some fashion to bring about the realization of this vision over time. Surveys of management, professional staff, and other employees are some of the ways to promote an understanding and keen awareness of such a visionary step.

To turn articulated vision into reality, however, top management will need to take a practical approach to understand and detail the "strategies" in the context of unfolding the health IS/IT envisioned plan.

▶ Strategy

Whereas vision relates primarily to mandates (or, mission with a sense of purpose), strategy relates to how one goes about achieving the vision. Among major classes of strategies health managers should be acquainted include corporate, competitive, and functional strategies, as depicted in **FIGURE PR2-1**.

Following a detailed scanning of the corporate environment at its highest level, corporate strategies may be further grouped into four types: growth, diversification, turnaround, and defensive strategies. *Growth strategies* are aggressively followed if and when market opportunities for a health system become apparent; for example, aging population growth, increased chronic ailments, and inflationary fuel (public transportation) costs signal a time of growth for tele-home healthcare services. *Diversification strategies* represent an approach to risk management; for example, delays in reading digitized images taken for ER patients may be a justification for outsourcing in-house radiological services via tele-radiology. *Turnaround strategies* serve to retrofit the organizational strengths and internal capabilities via methods such as outsourcing, organizational restructuring, business process reengineering, assets reallocation, or even service downsizing, for example, the use of expert-based courseware in integrative medicine to combat the strong growing market forces in the complementary-alternative medicine services. Finally, *defensive strategies* come into play with a steady decline in market demands due to growing competition, for example, eliminating traditional paper-based prescribing that is error-prone but still used by

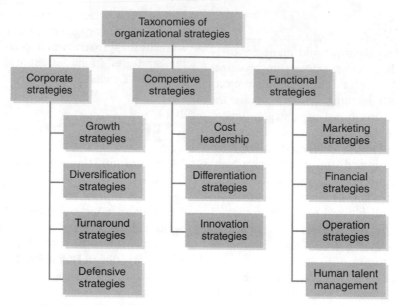

FIGURE PR2-1 Taxonomies of Strategies.

many physicians, the merger of clinical practices that can leverage on efficient and effective technological deployment, and so forth.

For a health organization to stay competitive, Porter's classical work alludes to a different class of strategies[2]: cost leadership, differentiation, and innovation strategies. In *cost leadership*, cost advantage is gained via economies of scale and cost-effectiveness, such as participating in a large-scale well-managed supply chain. *Differentiation* highlights the uniqueness of certain aspects of the business activities, such as implementing a *unique paperless corporate environment*. Lastly, *innovation strategy* requires an organization to be constantly thriving at the leading edge, such as launching a Health Innovation Center (HIC)[3] to capture health digitalization research and development efforts.

Functional strategies, another class of strategies typically employed at the more operational level of managing health systems organizations, include marketing strategy, financial strategy, operation strategy, and human talent management. *Marketing strategy* touches on how product-services are being propagated

and promoted in the marketplace. *Financial strategy* has to do with the intelligent use of financial information to make key decisions on resource allocation and financing of new programs while *operation strategy* focuses on quality improvement and greater efficiencies to achieve greater patient satisfaction in care services. Thus, well-implemented financial-operation strategies are key to achieving immediate, intermediate, and longer-term goals vis-à-vis the increased competition faced in today's healthcare marketplace. Above all, *human talent management* is critical to determine the success of any organization because it is the people who work for the organization who put a face to how the organization really is perceived by its customers, third parties, and external relations.

▶ Execution

The McKinsey 7-S organization framework[4] of strategy, structure, systems, style, staff, shared values, and skills, as illustrated in **FIGURE PR2-2**, is often used to guide the evaluation and

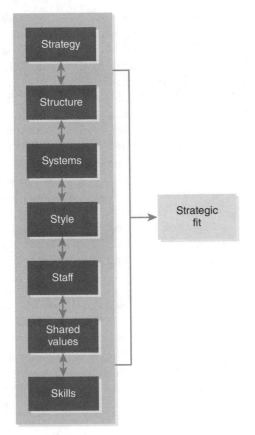

FIGURE PR2-2 McKinsey's 7-S Strategic Fit Framework.

implementation of organizational strategies, amounting to the seven areas and/or steps that must be completely changed via executive orders—essentially, the steps of leading and managing change in the operational execution of realizing the vision and strategies.

Strategy is the set of activities or actions targeted at achieving a competitive edge in the marketplace through organizational process improvements, intelligent capital management, and systemic resources allocation. *Structure* is the reporting hierarchy of the organization as determined by the placement of personnel within the organization and the accompanying division and/or integration of organizational tasks, roles, and responsibilities to be accomplished on a daily and longer-term basis. *Systems* are the task and informational processes

and workflow that together determine how the organization conducts its daily affairs, for example, the performance evaluation, quality control, and capital budgeting systems. *Style* refers to the way management behaves within the organization, not just what is being communicated—the tangible evidence of how the organization spends time, pays attention, and performs collectively. *Staff* refers to the human resources—the people hired by the organization to perform its daily functions—although it is important to think of this not in terms of individuals, but of corporate demographics. *Shared values* portray the common goals, objectives, and beliefs of most members of the organization and may be indicative of both the organizational identity and corporate destiny. Finally, *skills* may be conceived as the total competencies of the organization due not simply to individual expertise in isolation but, more appropriately, to the interactive coordination among the hired employees. In essence, it is a derivative of the other six organizational elements noted in the 7-S framework.

▶ Characteristics of Healthcare Leaders and Managers

At this point, we discuss key characteristics of health leaders and managers in order to successfully carry out (execute) their roles and responsibilities. Key traits include being: (1) trustworthy, (2) inspirational and a motivator of others, (3) an effective communicator, and (4) a collaborative leader with foresight.

Being Trustworthy

Regardless of the managerial position, trustworthiness is an essential trait of effective leadership. As "trust" is the essence of managerial effectiveness, extraordinary leaders must have the ability to exude trust from their direct reports and corresponding followers. To lead others, health managers should be able to command the highest respect from their subordinates; that is, mutual trust and respect between the superiors and their direct reports must exist to building a lasting and successful working relationship. Closely related to trustworthiness and respect is the concept that those who lead should not upset their followers with any unannounced surprises—which requires that they stick to their principles, keeping precisely to what they have articulated or promised, with a clear and open attitude about how and why certain things are or are not being executed. Effective leadership can then result naturally in having the highest trust and respect from others.

At times, some employees may become frustrated because there is more work to be completed than there are people assigned to the task—due, perhaps, to budgetary constraints, regulatory changes, and/or economic downturns. This frustration may result in employees having difficulty understanding where they should focus their time—it is the job of an effective leader (manager), then, to prioritize tasks for the employees: framing major issues, simplifying complex assignments, and spelling out what is the most to the least important. By eliminating the unnecessary distractions to employees and focusing on what should be the central issue, the employees will be less frustrated with their work. Not only will they become more satisfied, but they will also be more creative and productive in achieving the key goals set for them.

Being Inspirational and a Motivator of Others

Health leaders (and managers) want to ascertain that all health IT projects are delivered on time and within budget. It requires these individuals to provide in-depth inspiration and be self-motivated as well as able to motivate others. *Motivation* is the art of inspiring

others, giving them a sense of confidence and/or the desire to accomplish certain goals. As it is an "art" form, motivation requires that these leaders (and managers) have special skills and elevated expertise before they can effectively manage and inspire others. Among the first critical steps is effective communication, which will be discussed later. Additionally, it is the job of the leaders (and managers) to support their subordinates to become skilled and ever ready to complete the most challenging tasks at hand. Above all, instituting a collaborative spirit with a strong sense of team belonging and task information sharing among subordinates is critical to success when faced with executing any complex health IT-related project goals.

Another key step in motivating others is measurement; that is, for subordinates to remain motivated, not only must they have a clear grasp of their assignments, but they must also be clearly informed on how they are performing at any given time. Providing constructive feedback as opposed to micro-managing and unnecessary criticisms is therefore the key to successful goal attainment among employees. Conversely, employees often need to be encouraged and recognized for their achievements, which would give them a sense of being valued while they seek to improve further. Without individualized recognition, the employees are not motivated to do their best—to work past their potentials and to reach out for the top or to perform to the best of their abilities.

Being an Effective Communicator

Effective communication is essential for forming all kinds of work relationships, in particular, to build strong social networks among key stakeholders. Communication is the core of effective management; without it, chaos and dissatisfaction will emerge and evolve over time.

Clearly, one-sided communication is ineffective, which means that it is essential for a leader (manager) to learn to listen. Listening requires patience and having eye contact with others; spending time to acknowledge what others have articulated with appropriate gestures; and being able to provide feedback, whenever necessary, by rephrasing what others may have articulated to achieve clarity of thoughts. In turn, this will build a good rapport between the conversing parties. As well, effective communicators are media-sensitive; that is, they understand the media used in the communication is crucial as different types of information may be received under each setting. For example, certain means of communication, such as face-to-face versus a general meeting, may be appropriate for specific or more formal messages to be conveyed, whereas other means, such as e-mail and telephone communications, are useful for informal, humorous, and/or lighthearted exchanges. Moreover, having specific knowledge about your audience or those to whom you will be communicating is critical in effective communications as every audience is different with different needs to be satisfied.

Need for Foresight and Collaborative Leaders

Healthcare Systems leaders need to be collaborative in their management style. The need to disregard the ingrained behavior of just managing technology under their control to developing meaningful partnerships with other leaders both within the organization and at external entities. It is important that these leaders have foresight and are preemptive in outlining an effective partnership policy for their organizations with external partners that goes beyond the traditional technology procurement model. They need to position the organization as an innovative healthcare system inventing the future of health care. Health IT leaders will now need to be more attentive to business outcomes than their predecessors, and will need to be extremely collaborative to ensure the innovation being adopted by other

leaders in the organization provides the outcomes needed to sustain the operations and grow the organization. This requires foresight, not only to build and capitalize on technological innovations within the organization, but also to ensure that legacy systems are also stable and secure.

▶ Specific Health IT Roles and Responsibilities

Broadly speaking, to lead IT initiatives in a health systems organization so as to reduce human errors and improve the organizational service quality, efficiencies, and productivity, a health executive (or manager) is expected to work intelligently in a diversely cultured and growing socio-political environment.

Today, the job of health IT leaders (managers) has become increasingly stressful, more business oriented, and less hands-on; for example, this individual must direct the planning and implementation of enterprise-wide health IT initiatives in order to improve health information exchanges within and outside of the organization so as to enhance overall cost-effectiveness, operational efficiencies, and care services delivery quality. Additionally, most health IT managerial responsibilities now have expanded beyond the traditional role to include concerns about enhancing "customer satisfaction" and being "customer-centric."[5] The formal education and on-the-job training for such an individual can differ significantly, but having a university degree in a related field, such as industrial engineering, computer science, and/or business administration, is a very good start.

Geared with knowledge and experience in managing and directing increasingly sophisticated health IT operations, this health IT leader (manager) must possess acumen in routine business operations, periodic performance evaluation activities, and strategy and human resource management. Such a leader must be able to execute strategic as well as tactical IT planning effectively. He or she is expected to demonstrate the ability to apply health IT concepts in real-world business problem-solving situations and will also be largely responsible for negotiating, outsourcing, and/or managing vendor contracts on health IT products, services, and other related projects (such as ensuring the compliance of the health organizational IS with the Health Insurance Portability and Accountability Act [HIPAA] rules and standards). Overall, the key role of this individual is to develop and preserve tight integration between health IT decisions and corporate business goals. The health IT leader must have superior understanding of both the organization's and health IS/IT departmental goals and objectives so as to align these goals and objectives seamlessly. This single set of responsibilities calls upon every political, negotiation, and project management skills of the health IT leader (manager) in response to an increasingly hyper-competitive health IT marketplace.

Finally, aside from learning to focus on external relations, such as customer satisfaction concerns, health IS/IT security issues, technology acceptance and evaluation ratings, budgeting, staffing, outsourcing, hosting, and return on investment (ROI) analysis, the role of a health IT leader (manager) will continue to evolve over the next several years with advancing technology and a more computer-literate U.S. population; most likely, the future health IT leader (manager) will be expected to act as a change agent and as a business change leader. Ultimately, a combination of strong technological-business skills with leadership, persuasion, and communication skills will be needed of health IT leaders (managers) to ensure success at their jobs.

▶ Conclusion

Management students should pay particular attention to the roles–responsibilities of health

IT leaders (managers) if they want to follow in their footsteps. Importantly, real-world practices are not easily replicated and cannot be learned by merely reading published theories or cases in textbooks. Indeed, successful practices have to be learned on the job and must be orchestrated in a variety of social settings. Hence, the use of the word *inspiration* in this brief does a great justice to the idea; that is, it is vital for health IT leaders and managers to be "inspirational" and "on fire," doing what the employees are not able to "articulate" clearly for themselves; these leaders are, in fact, the "mouthpieces" of the organization in crafting the organization's future visions, strategic directions, and strategic thinking. They must meet and talk with everyone who is a part of the organization, both at the top and on the front line. It is the inspiration from these individuals that will ultimately make a difference in transforming the organization.

Moreover, an effective leader (manager) must also possess several specific traits, each of which significantly affects the performance of subordinates. The abilities to communicate effectively, to motivate others, and to lead followers are all essential for being a good leader. By earning the trust and respect of their employees, these individuals will help and allow their subordinates to work to the best of their abilities. This not only generates personal success for the employees but, ultimately, for the organization. Another essential point is the importance of continuing to "sharpen the saw" when it comes to effective management skills.[6] The leaders (managers) have to be willing to learn from their own mistakes and understand that learning is a part of the total process of becoming an effective manager. It is not always possible to get things right the first time; thus, good managers learn from their "first" mistakes, turning those mistakes to their advantage at the earliest point of opportunity.

Finally, a key differentiating point between effective versus non-effective leaders (managers) is that of seeking feedback from their direct reports. Using such feedback to turn the noted weaknesses of the leader (manager) into additional strengths makes him or her that much more effective; in other words, being an effective leader is a continuous process. By possessing and continuing to sharpen those effective management skills, he or she can positively affect the morale of the organization's employees. It also naturally enlarges the circle of influence as direct reports can then be inspired to follow through with the outstanding model exemplified by those above them. Effective management inspires everyone, from your employees (who will manage successfully in the future) to other managers (who will immediately manage more effectively). By effectively managing people, the success of subordinates can be ensured, which will ultimately translate into the organization's success.

In sum, senior leaders (managers) play critical roles in their organizational successes. They need to exploit and manage data from all over the enterprise that is being generated at an explosive rate and ensure that leaders within the healthcare system are using it wisely. With the adoption of the emerging technologies and business concepts, such as artificial intelligence, predictive technologies, patient centric care, and value-based care, health IT leaders are entering a new era in healthcare technology with plenty of challenges and opportunities.

The overall performance standard of a health systems organization depends not only on the quality and work productivity of its employees but also on the training, quality, and active participation of the administrative and professional staff in supporting the services of the organization. It also depends on the extent to which IT support has empowered and enabled these various individuals to perform as productively as possible. The sharing of a technology vision among top management team members, professional staff members, and employees within the organization is also critical in determining the success of the health IT leadership. The culture of a health systems organization can transform because of changes in health IT implementation, as well as the extent to which employees are accepting the health IT innovation and working collaboratively with each other, and with the organization's customers. Under the supervision of a proactive, productive, and politically astute health IT leader (manager), the health organizational IT support and services can grow and expand effectively and quickly, leading to a transformed organization that is the envy of all its competitors.

Notes

1. Ellis, L. D. *The changing role of health IT leaders: Positioning for success moving forward*. Retrieved from www.hsph.harvard.edu/ecpe/changing-role-health-cio-leaders/
2. Porter, M. E. (1985). *Competitive advantage*. (Ch. 1, pp 11–15). New York, NY: The Free Press.
3. Retrived from www.fiercehealthcare.com/special-report/5-healthcare-innovation-centers-to-watch
4. Waterman, R. H., Jr. (1982). The seven elements of strategic fit. *Journal of Business Strategy, 2*(3), 69–73.
5. Cindy, W. *The 2008 state of the CIO: The imperative to be customer-centric IT leaders*. Retrieved from www.cio.com
6. Covey, S. R. (1989). *The 7 habits of highly effective people*. New York, NY: Free Press.

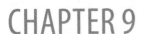

CHAPTER 9

Decision Aiding and Predictive Systems: A Framework for Data Mining and Machine Learning for Health Systems Management

Saumil Maheshwari, Anupam Shukla, and Joseph Tan

LEARNING OBJECTIVES

- Overview Data Mining–Machine Learning (DM–ML) techniques
- Differentiate between descriptive and predictive analytics
- Develop a framework for DM–ML applications for health systems management
- Recognize the use of social network analysis for health surveillance

CHAPTER OUTLINE

Scenario: Open Health Tools for Interoperable Health Care[1,2]

Open Health Tools (OHT), a collaborative health information technology (HIT) open-source site, continues to develop ways to create an ecosystem focused on producing reusable software tools for health systems organizations to promote the exchange of medical and health information across geographic, political, socio-cultural, and technological barriers. Previously, the OHT community has added code from the United Kingdom's National Health Service (NHS) and incorporated an academic outreach project to motivate developers across the world to embrace its programming tools. With support from major healthcare services organizations in the United States, Canada, the United Kingdom, and Australia; vendor giants, including IBM and Oracle; and health standards organizations such as HL7 and the International Health Terminology Standards Development Organization, OHT hopes that health systems organizations will use its open-source technology as the backbone for HIT infrastructure.

Specifically, OHT is focused on bringing value to its stakeholders by developing a free software platform that allows electronic health record (EHR) data to be exchanged among various commercial products. Essentially, OHT is the translator that permits various legacy databases to communicate with one another. This involves processes such as message and document interchanges, static model designers, simulators, adaptors, data transformers, and device access. The underlying frame is available under an open-source license so organizations can design and build applications without any payment required for the software.

OHT hopes to duplicate the success of the Eclipse, a popular non-profit, open-source community whose projects are focused on developing an open platform for building, deploying, and managing software across its lifecycle. Skip McGaughy, one of Eclipse's founders and OHT's executive director, envisions OHT to mimic a "satellite" of Eclipse.

"We're going to be using Eclipse technology," McGaughy claims, "but our governance is under the direction and control of the health and computer industry. We use the same development and intellectual property process, the same paradigms, and many of the same people. The Eclipse code has been downloaded and used by millions of programmers, so it's thoroughly tested and debugged. Programs using the Eclipse framework, through the use of plug-ins, are compatible."

As high-quality medical decisions are based on the reliability of health data, the need for reliable and accurate coding in healthcare services is essential. With increasing complexity of HIT, it is argued that OHT's dynamic, open-source software tools have a unique advantage over other competitive commercial products. McGaughy further clarifies, "It's componentized, it's modular, and it's done in the open, so everyone understands what the requirements are, and there's a dialogue about the requirements."

McGaughy also maintains a perspective of HIT as a means to achieving the goal of improving health. "At the end of the day, what's really important is reducing costs, but also saving lives and improving care. And what is unique is the number of really good software developers who are joining this effort. So instead of just moving little bits on the screen, they can now save lives."

How do you feel about saving lives as a result of the willingness of the human spirits to join forces, to share and to collaborate on HIT software development—isn't this, in and of itself, a noble cause? Yes, but it all begins with planning and strategizing, which are precisely the focus of the previous chapter. Then, what's next? Making the right choice at the right time, sharing and using the right tool sets for software products that would be compatible with one another—so, this is a chapter about the way software should be designed and the tools that HIT developers and users can rely on to make sense of the massive amounts of data being produced in our current health systems.

▶ I. Introduction

Quality of life is the right of every human being. As one's health status is often considered a key determinant of one's quality of life, health consumers all around the globe are expecting their caregivers (physicians) to work hard in updating their knowledge on ground-breaking findings and/or discoveries from the latest research.

Owing to the limits of the human brain, regardless of how well trained and experienced these caregivers may be in providing treatments to patients, they cannot be expected to memorize or follow all the best practices and guidelines for every situation; hence, their diagnosis probably cannot always be correct.[3] Moreover, the shortage of medical experts in many places challenges the efficient–effective delivery of care services due to healthcare resource-constrains (e.g., personnel, facilities, third-party funding, and more) as well as limited accessibility–availability of timely health data and health data analysis presently.

Indeed, the healthcare industry is being transformed by the increased availability of data, specifically EHR data that are cumulated through patient visits to the hospital and other care facilities in their life span. In essence, the EHR contains the patient's centric digital records, such as personal demographic profile, diagnosis, treatments referrals, and more.[4] With the generation of this massive amount of EHR data, these data have become a valuable resource not only for primary care services, but also for secondary medical data analysis and research in various academic fields,[5-7] similar to what the financial and retail services industries have experienced in the last decade.

While these records are real-time, patient-centered data available to authorized users for secured and immediate access, in many cases, the assembled information is too complicated and volumetric for the purpose of analysis by standard methods.[8] Further analytical processing needs to take place to reduce this voluminous data into key insights that may be hidden and/or embedded within or throughout the dataset. In this sense, data mining provides the means to transform data into useful information for aiding key clinical decision-making. Advances in automated data processing with the data mining and machine learning techniques now allow researchers to thoroughly sift through vast digital traces that we collectively leave behind each day.[9,10] This chapter aims to provide the framework for applying data mining and machine learning in various healthcare applications.

▶ II. Data Mining (DM) and Machine Learning (ML) for Health Care

We are at the dawn of a new data-driven age. Voluminous EHR data generated from various private–public healthcare settings, coupled with continuous flow of data from connected medical devices and other HIT tools imply the need for innovative methodologies to deal with the aforementioned data deluge problems. Accordingly, the development of advanced healthcare decision support systems via DM and ML has become more and more popular, if not increasingly necessary. The broad range of clinical decisions to be aided via data analytics includes disease diagnosis, the mortality prediction, the prognosis of a patient's future quality of life, or even the treatment selection of individual patients.

- DM, which is generally a well thought-out, recently developed methodology, aims to identify novel, meaningful, and useful patterns embedded in data— patterns that are complex and too difficult for humans to uncover.[11–13] A general framework for DM is that provided by CRoss-Industry Standard Process for Data Mining (CRISP-DM)[14] decribing the activities with six phases: business understanding, data understanding, data preparation, modeling, evaluation, and deployment. CRISP-DM is an iterative process[15] for the analysis of data as shown in **FIGURE 9-1**.

- The first phase (business understanding) helps in identifying the business objectives, such as data mining goals. The second and third phases are data understanding and data preparation, respectively; these are important as "no data means no mining." Also, data sampling and data transformation are all part of the data preparation phase. The fourth phase is significant as this is the actual analysis, the modeling phase. Most DM methodologies such as clustering, classification, regression analysis, association, and others are part of this phase. We will detail this phase for health care later. Next is the evaluation stage, which is the fifth phase. The evaluation stage allows the assessment of post-mining results in terms of charts, graphs, or other significant structures. Finally, the sixth and last phase,

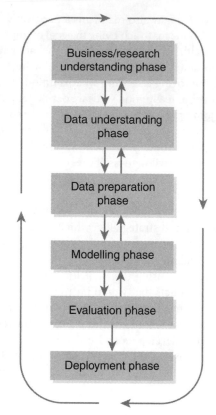

FIGURE 9-1 Iterative process of the CRISP-DM model.

Reproduced from Lobov, Andrei, & Martinez Lastra, Jose Luis. (2007). Data Mining of Systems State Spaces.

deployment, relates to actual implementation and operation of the DM model.[16,17]

Specific to healthcare DM, researchers have focused on various challenges and issues.[18,19] To date, various DM techniques had been discussed for analysis and prediction of different diseases.[20–29] Some modifications on the available DM applications on healthcare services have also been proposed with improved results.[30–32]

As early diagnosis of disease is critical for effective, precise, and timely treatment to be administered appropriately to patients, it is important to consider a classification of diseases. Although various types of disease taxonomies can be done, **FIGURE 9-2** describes the types of diseases based on the medium of disease transmission. Airborne diseases spread

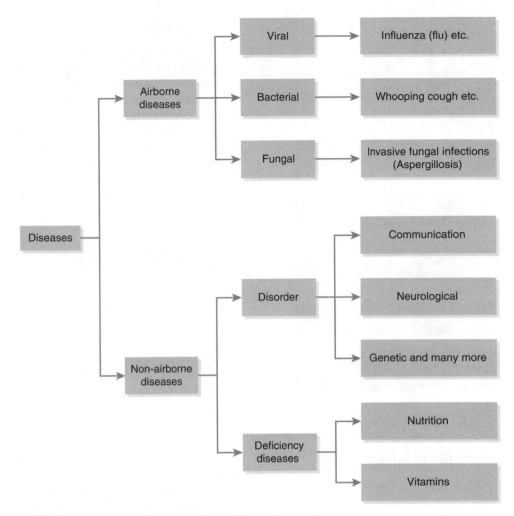

FIGURE 9-2 Arrangement of diseases based on medium of transmission.

through coughing, sneezing, laughing, and close personal contact with the infected person discharging pathogenic microbes throughout such disease-spreading activities.

DM can be used for diagnostic analysis of both airborne as well as non-airborne diseases with improved accuracy and efficiency.

▶ III. Framework

The design of predictive–decision aiding systems via DM–ML techniques is a non-trivial process and requires careful planning and preparation. The clinical decision support system (CDSS) yields insights on the causes and nature of the disease and thus plays a constructive role in the effective diagnosis of disease, predicting the rate of mortality, and more. Much of the extant literature available highlights new methodology and framework for the design and development of effective decision aiding systems.[33–38]

FIGURE 9-3 shows a five-step framework: (i) data preprocessing, (ii) feature engineering, (iii) DM, (iv) representation of results, and (v) development of the system, as discussed next.

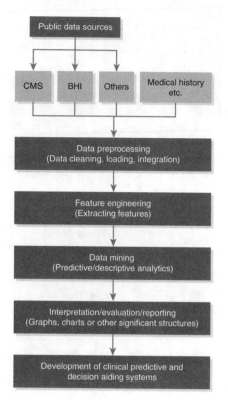

FIGURE 9-3 Framework for clinical predictive and decision aiding systems.

Data Preprocessing

- The data available and captured from public sources often contain noise, outliers, errors, and more. As poor quality data produces poor results, we need to improve the data quality by using data cleaning techniques. Also, as data are collected from multiple sources, we also need to integrate these data as well.

Feature Engineering

- Feature extraction plays a key role in the effective analysis of the data. Here, we transform the raw data in bulk and classify them into key features, which will allow for the simplification of the data processing and ease the interpretation of results.

Data Mining (DM)

- DM task, in general, can be categorized into predictive versus descriptive analytics. The predictive analytics always involves the response variable (i.e., it always performs some prediction that can be categorical or numerical based on the method used). In contrast, the descriptive analytics aims at finding patterns or associations between the datasets. Both predictive and descriptive analytics have been deployed in health care.

DM: Predictive Analytics

- Predictive modeling is probably the most common and important applications in DM. Predictive analytics involves the use of statistical methods and technology over voluminous data to predict the outcome of each patient, to predict fraud in health care, or to predict the requirement of resources, and so on.

Prediction in medical servicing extends from disease diagnosis to mortality prediction, from fraud detection to hospital readmission, and more, for example, determining the possibility of an infectious disease, predicting infections from methods of suturing, diagnosing a disease with real-time prediction, and/or predicting one's wellness for the shorter or longer-term time frame. **FIGURE 9-4** explains some basic uses of predictive analytics.

Popular methods of predictive DM methods may be classified as classification versus regression.

Classification. Among the most popular techniques for predictive analytics, this technique categorically partitions data points. It predicts the output variable that is categorical in form, for example, while classifying the medical database for the diagnosis of a disease for each patient; output can be a positive or negative report. The output variable can be partitioned

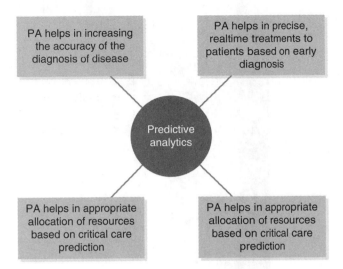

FIGURE 9-4 Uses of predictive Analytics.

into two classes known to be a binary classification or into more than two classes such as low, medium, and high.

Classification is a supervised learning approach. Consider a medical database of a heart disease patient with attributes defined in **TABLE 9-1**.[39] Here, the training set value of output variable is *known* (used for generation of the classification model) but the *prediction set output variable is unknown* and is predicted using the classification model. The derived classification model can be represented as IF-THEN rules, decision-tree, or neural networks, as shown in **FIGURE 9-5**. Because classification technique is the most popular for predictive modeling, we will discuss some of the classification algorithms used in health care.

- *k-NN classifier*: k-Nearest Neighbor classifier (k-NN classifier) is one of the simplest classifiers, also known as lazy learner.[40] Lazy learner implies that the classifier, when given with the training data, simply stores it and waits for the test tuple. When the test tuple is given, then it classifies the unknown test tuple based on the closeness of k-training tuple with the test tuple.[41] K-training tuples are the k "nearest neighbors" of test tuple. It uses a direct comparison of distance (i.e., euclidean distance) between tuples of training data with test tuple. Certain points to be consider for k-NN classifier include: (a) deciding the good value of k, (b) need for data normalization, (c) computing the distance for non-numeric attributes, and (d) dealing with the missing value, as no value can be missing in any dimension.

  k-NN classifier finds its application in various domains including health care, clustering, image or pattern recognition, and more. The algorithm is very time consuming and requires a large memory but can yield a better accuracy when data size is large. Hence, for the sake of classification accuracy, time can be managed as health care demands more accuracy.

- *Discriminant Analysis:* Linear discriminant analysis is a widely used discriminant-based classification method. It uses a discriminant function that takes an input vector x and classifies it to one of the classes C_k.[42] There can be two or more number of classes in which data can be classified. This method is suited for datasets that are easy to separate into classes.

TABLE 9-1 Sample of Attributes for Heart Disease Prediction

Patient ID	Input Attributes/Variables									Output Attribute/Variable
	Age	Gender	CPT*	FBS**	RECG***	Cholesterol	Slope#	Thalach##	...	Diagnosis classes: Heart disease; No heart disease
→										

* Chest Pain Type (value 1:angina; 2: non-angina; 3:asymptotic)
** Fasting Blood Sugar (value normal:1; else 0)
*** Resting Electrocardiographic
# Slope of peak exercise ST segment
maximum heart rate achieved

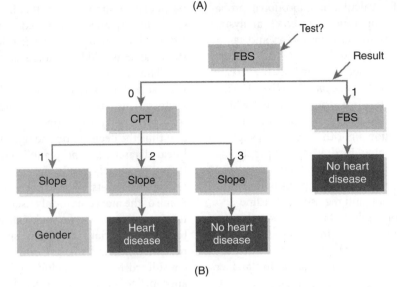

IF (Age = 50 AND Gender = MALE and FBS = 0) THEN Class = Heart disease
IF (Age = 30 AND Gender = FEMALE and FBS = 1) THEN Class = No heart disease
IF (Age = 50 AND Cholesterol = HIGH) THEN Class = Heart disease

(A)

(B)

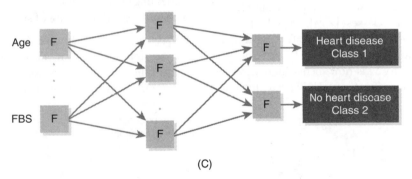

(C)

FIGURE 9-5 (a) IF-THEN rules; (b) Decision tree; and (c) Neural network model for classification.

- *Decision Tree (DT)*: DT is a tree-like structure where each non-leaf node represents a test on attribute; each branch represents the outcome of the test and leaf node represents the class prediction.[43] Figure 9-5b explains the classification using DT where non-leaf node like fasting blood sugar (FBC), chest pain type (CPT), etc. are attributes on which test is performed. The branch represents the outcome of the test (attribute value), and

the leaf node represents the class to which the tuple may belong. Certain points to be considered for DT classifier include: (a) generally good with categorical data (gives simple structure of the tree) and (b) deciding the attribute sequence on which test is to be performed.

Selection of the attribute on which the test is to be performed can be decided based on the maximum information gain,[44] and hence, the best available alternative attribute can be used. DT is the most popular and interpretable classifier representation. The most common use of DT is for calculating conditional probabilities in operational research analysis.[45] DT results are self-explanatory and can be transformed into IF-THEN rules effortlessly. DT is used extensively in health care.

■ *Support Vector Machine (SVM)*: In 1995, Vapnik introduced the concept of SVM,[46] which is now one of the most popular ML classification algorithms based on supervised learning. By drawing a hyperplane, which would act a separator between the classes,[47-50] SVM supports both data classification and regression. The line separator is selected in such a way that it would give maximum distance from the support vector of both classes and thus is also known as maximum margin classifier.

Initially used for binary classification (i.e., could separate a set of training examples in two different classes $[x_1,y_1]$, $[x_2,y_2]...[x_m,y_m]$, where $x_i \in R^2$ denoting feature vector in d-dimensions and $y_i - \in -1, +1$ is a respective class label), SVM is now increasingly used for multiclass classification.[51] **FIGURE 9-6** illustrates

the functioning of linear kernel-based SVM in which there is a mapping of nonlinear input space into newly linear separable state space. In particular, all input vectors that lie on one side of the hyperplane are assigned value different from the ones lying on another side. Typically, these values would be denoted as −1 and +1.

The training instances that are present nearest to the hyperplane are called support vectors. These support vectors are then used to determine the margin of the hyperplane and thus the decision boundary. In the case of linear datasets, a hyperplane itself can divide them into two classes. In the case of nonlinear separable datasets, SVM uses kernel functions. Some of the most commonly used kernel functions are linear, polynomial, Gaussian, radial basis, exponential radial basis, sigmoidal kernel functions, and so on. Certain points to be considered for SVM include: (a) selection of appropriate kernel functions, (b) estimation of values of gaussian parameters, and (c) number of feature selection in case of smaller datasets.

■ *Artificial Neural Networks (ANNs)*: ANNs are implemented to model the human brain for the purpose of processing the information. The main objective of developing a

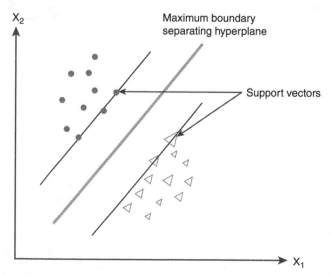

FIGURE 9-6 Support Vector Machine (SVM).

neural network (NN) system is to perform various computational tasks at a faster rate. Thus, for implementing the NN system, high-speed digital computers are used. NNs possess a large number of interconnected elements called neurons or nodes. These neurons usually operate in parallel.[52] NNs are used for performing tasks such as classification, pattern matching, approximation, and more. Before the introduction of DT and SVM, NN was considered the best classification algorithm.[53]

NN-based models are revived due to the success of deep learning methods. Deep NNs or DNNs, which are synonymous with deep learning, are ANNs that model complex nonlinear relationships using multiple hidden layers of units between the input and output layers.[54,55] Some points to be considered for ANNs include: (a) deciding number of hidden layers, (b) number of units per layer, and (c) number of connections per unit. These attributes define the deep learning based systems' behavior and structure. Researchers have recently solved various clinical problems using deep learning methods.

- *Bayesian Methods (BM)*: BM uses Bayes theory for the purpose of classification.[56] There are two kinds of Bayesian classification methods based on Bayes theory namely, Naïve Bayesian classification and Bayesian Belief Networks. Naïve Bayesian classification works on the concept of attribute independence (i.e., it considers that attributes are not related to each other). But this is not the case with the medical dataset as the attributes are related to each other. Despite this attribute independence concept, Naïve Bayesian classification has provided decent results in the field of health care.

Regression. Classification techniques discussed till now are used for the classification or prediction of the categorical data. Regression is one of the critical tools for predicting a response from a wide variety of data types.[57] Thus, both classification and regression are used for the purpose of prediction of output variable, but classification deals with categorical data whereas regression deals with continuous data. Regression involves generation of a mathematical model using a training dataset. Once the model is constructed, it is used for the prediction of a test dataset.

Regression involves two kinds of variables: one is the predictor variable and the other is the response variable, represented as X and Y, respectively. Regression can be classified as linear versus non-linear regression; that is, when the relationship between predictor variable is linear, a linear regression (LR) would fit well. Otherwise, a non-linear regression strategy should be followed. LR is further classified as simple versus multiple LR. Simple LR involves only one predictor variable, X, for predicting the response variable, Y. Conversely, multiple LR involves more than one predictor variable, say X_1, X_2, ..., X_n, for predicting the response variable Y. The non-linear relationship between predictor and output variable can be achieved through polynomial regression, step functions, and more. Typically, multiple LR and non-linear regression is used in the field of health care, for example, when predicting the disease based on the symptoms. Some key points to consider for using regression include: (a) finding the outliers as response variable is greatly affected by outliers, (b) deciding on the high leverage points, and (c) non-constant variance of error terms.

DM: Descriptive Analytics

Descriptive analytics focuses on finding the patterns, association, or relationship between the attributes or objects of the dataset by considering the whole database. Descriptive analytics does not require any response variable; thus, it is also known as unsupervised learning. Popular methods of descriptive DM can be classified as clustering, association, etc.

Clustering. This approach groups data objects into different clusters such that objects within a group are similar to each other, but are dissimilar to the objects in another group.[58] The primary objective here is to maximize the intraclass similarity while minimizing the interclass similarity. Clustering differs from "classification" as it is unsupervised technique with no predefined class labels. This essentially partitions data objects based on similarity index. In health care, disease symptoms can be used to predict the risk of disease; for example, if we have the data recordings (blood pressure and cholesterol level) of various patients, we can partition them into two groups: high-risk versus low-risk patients for heart disease based on their recorded data. The following are the various clustering methods used in health care:

- *Partitioning Methods*: For a set of n objects, a partitioning method is to divide these data objects into k clusters, where $k \leq n$. Each partition represents a cluster. The partition of data objects into different clusters can be exclusive or fuzzy; in exclusive partition, each data object belongs exclusively to one cluster only while in fuzzy partitioning this requirement is relaxed (i.e., a data object can belong to different clusters). There are various algorithms for partitioning methods such as K-means, K-medoids, CLARA, CLARANS, and more. The partitioning method requires defining the number of clusters as input to the algorithm. K-means, a centroid-based algorithm that partitions the data object into k clusters based on minimum distance criteria,[59] is the most popular algorithm. A proper initialization of K-means is important for obtaining good final results. Therefore, Modified K-mean algorithm known as K-mean ++ is also available in the literature.[60] K-mean ++ allows getting the initial clusters center that will probably prove to be the best optimal solution.

- *Hierarchical Method*: The hierarchical method facilitates by moving ahead without specifying the number of clusters in advance. The method works by grouping data objects into a hierarchy or tree of clusters. The tree of clusters is important for data summary.[61] There are two approaches for hierarchical clustering method: one is Agglomerative Hierarchical clustering and the second is Divisive Hierarchical clustering. The former uses a bottom-up strategy, starting by considering each data object as its own cluster and then merges the objects iteratively based on certain features to form larger and larger clusters. The process continues until all the objects are in one single cluster or some termination criteria are satisfied. Conversely, the latter uses a top-down strategy, starting by placing all objects in one group or cluster and then dividing the clusters into smaller and smaller clusters until the lowest level is reached. Various algorithms for hierarchical clustering are Balanced iterative reducing and clustering using hierarchies (BIRCH), Chameleon, and others.[62]

- *Density-based Method*: Methods discussed so far have used distance as criteria for partitioning the data objects into clusters. It is difficult to get clusters of arbitrary shape as the shape of the clusters is spherical when only distance is used for constructing the cluster.[63] So, density-based clustering allows the cluster to grow, provided that the density (number of data objects in neighborhood) crosses some predefined threshold. This allows the arbitrary shape of clusters and finds an important role in the field of health care. There are various approaches for density-based clustering, for example, density-based spatial clustering of applications with noise (DBSCAN), density-based clustering algorithms (DENCLUE), and more. The approaches require the $\in$ (density threshold) to be defined in advance.

Frequent Patterns Mining (FPM). Frequent patterns are the patterns that occur frequently in datasets. FPM allows the discovery of associations between itemsets. Interesting association discovery can impact the healthcare industry significantly, for example, the disease-symptoms association lends a hand for the detection of diseases based on the symptoms. In 1994, R. Agrawal & R. Shrikant[64] introduce the *a priori* algorithm or frequent itemset mining algorithm, which has two main steps: join step and prune step. The working of the algorithm requires the input of two values, support and confidence. Support signifies the frequency of occurrence of itemsets while confidence specifies the accuracy of association of itemsets. Support and confidence conveys the interestingness of the association rule.

Social Network Analysis (SNA). SNA is a special branch of DM that focuses on applying analytic techniques to make out the relationships between individuals and groups.[65] The social network can be represented as a graph $G = (V, E)$, where V is a set of nodes and E is edges connecting the nodes. A node can represent individual, city, country, or organization, while edges represent the communication, friendship, or ties between them. These ties can have some form of weight that defines the differences (bonding) between the ties.[66] SNA can be performed using centrality measures, which allow the central node or key node in a network to be discovered. There are various methods for finding the centrality measures such as degree, betweenness, closeness, eigenvector centrality, and more.[67]

Predictive analysis helps in the accurate diagnosis of airborne diseases and non-airborne diseases. Apart from an effective diagnosis of the disease, controlling the further propagation of disease is also important. Hence, SNA can be used in health care to prevent the outbreak of airborne diseases. A framework, which will aim at preventing the further spread of airtborne disease and also for early diagnosis for those who were in direct contact with the infected person, can be designed based on a social network of an infected person. The social network can be formed based on the location traversing and call logs of the infected person.

Interpretation–Evaluation

Once the task of DM is complete, we have the extracted data patterns that can be represented in the form of graphs, charts, values, or other significant structures. How interesting these patterns would be can or has to be evaluated using interestingness measures. The interpetation of output is important to identify the knowledge from the extracted data. Also, deciding on the visualization tool for showing the DM results is considered during this phase.

Development of Clinical Predictive and Decision Aiding Systems

Finally, with the extracted knowledge, visualization and knowledge representation techniques can be used to develop the clinical predictive and decision aiding system. The novel information gained with the use of clinical predictive–decision aiding system is beneficial to administrative as well as medical decision-making. Examples include preventing disease outbreak, estimating medical staffing, assessing health insurance policy and options, detecting health insurance fraud, suggesting treatments, predicting disease, and many more possibilities.[68-72]

▶ IV. Contributions of DM–ML in Health Care

DM provides significant advantages to the healthcare industry in the fields of diagnosis of disease, mortality prediction, fraud detection, and many more. Both predictive and descriptive analytics have played key roles in the field of health care. Examples of application areas are discussed next.

Diagnosis of Disease

Researchers had worked on the diagnosis of diseases such as heart disease, breast cancer, Parkinson's, hypertension, kidney failure, diabetes, asthma, chest pain, and more using DM–ML techniques. Research on the diagnosis of disease started as early as 1970s. In 1973, Willcox et al.[73] attempted to use a computer and applied Bayesian theory to identify a bacterial disease. In 2010, Abeel et al.[74] proposed to identify biochemical features in the diagnosis of cancer. The authors studied a feature selection algorithm and used a Support Vector Machine (SVM) classification algorithm to apply the integrated feature selection technique to disease diagnosis. Concerning the efficient diagnosis of heart diseases and neural diseases, Ahmed[75] merged an artificial bee colony algorithm and a modified full Bayesian network classifier for effective prediction of disease, therein achieving a nearly 100% accuracy. Patil[76] used the Jelinek-Mercer smoothing method and the Bayesian model to predict and diagnose heart diseases. Milan Kumari et al.[77] performed a comparative study of classification method for the prediction of cardiovascular disease. These authors compared four classification techniques in DM to predict cardiovascular disease in patients: rule-based RIPPER techniques, DT, ANNs, and SVM. The results showed that the SVM model turned out to be best classifier for cardiovascular disease prediction.[78] Various other bodies of literature for heart disease prediction establish the important role of different DM and ML algorithms.[79–85]

Breast cancer is one of the most critical and perilous diseases in women. The Weka tool has been used by Potter et al.[86] for performing an experiment on the breast cancer dataset and then comparing the performance of different classification methods. Huang et al.[87] used hybrid SVM-based strategy for developing a predictive model for breast cancer diagnosis. Many diagnosis algorithms for breast cancer have since emerged.[88–90]

Various other diseases are also effectively diagnosed using the DM–ML techniques. Osofisan et al.[91] used the ANN for kidney failure detection. DT algorithms such as Iterative Dichotomiser 3 (ID3), Classification and Regression Trees (CART), and C4.5 have been used for medical diagnosis of diabetes, hepatitis, and heart disease in Kumar et al.[92] Results convey the superior performance of CART algorithm versus C4.5 and ID3. Barakat et al.[93] used SVM for the diagnosis of diabetes mellitus. Results on a real-life diabetes dataset show that intelligible SVMs provide a promising tool for the prediction of diabetes, where a comprehensible rule-set has been generated, with a prediction accuracy of 94%. Patil et al.[94] used an *a priori* algorithm for generating association rule to classify the patients suffering from type-2 diabetes.

TABLE 9-2 gives insight into different healthcare research methodologies for disease diagnosis. The table highlights the database used, method, and accuracy of the developed method.

The aim of using DM–ML techniques is to provide human-like, informative automated diagnosis system. This will not only reduce waiting times for patients but also minimize the substantial time, effort, and manpower required of their caregivers.

Mortality Prediction in ICU

The ICU is a special care area where severely ill patients are treated using medical devices by doctors and nurses. The main focus of researchers is to improve the safety, quality, and cost-effectiveness of the treatment for these patients. Mortality prediction helps in effective allocation of additional ICU resources to those with higher chances of survival due to resource constraints.

TABLE 9-2 Summary of Studies on Disease Diagnosis

Ref.	Database	Method	Accuracy (%)	Disease
Sadiq[75]	Iraqi hospitals	Modified Full Bayesian Classifier	93	Heart Disease Prediction
Patil[76]	Cleveland Heart Disease database	Naïve-based Classifier	78	
Kumari[20]	Cleveland cardiovascular disease dataset	Decision Tree	79.05	
		SVM	84.12	
		ANN	80.06	
Kumar[92]	UC-Irvine archive of machine learning datasets	Decision Tree: CART ID3 C4.5	72 70 61	
Cheng[79]	Cleveland Heart Disease database	C4.5 Naïve based	81.11 81.48	
Dangare[82]	Cleveland Heart Disease database and Statlog Heart Disease database	Naïve Bayes	90.74	
Resul[83]	Cleveland Heart Disease database	Neural Network Ensembles	89.01	
Avci[84]	Acuson Sequoia 512 Model Doppler Ultrasound system in the Cardiology Department of the First Medical Center	Genetic-SVM classifier	95	
Shouman[85]	Cleveland Heart Disease database	KNN	97.4	
Huang[87]	Chung-Shan Medical University Hospital	SVM	86	Breast Cancer Diagnosis
Qi[89]	SEER Public-Use Data 2005	Decision Tree	71.17	
Resul[83]	Wisconsin Breast Cancer Dataset (WBCD)	Decision Trees	95	

(continues)

TABLE 9-2 Summary of Studies on Disease Diagnosis				*(continued)*
Barakat[93]	Data from 4682 subjects of age 20 years and above were collected using a questionnaire	SVM	94	Diabetes Mellitus Diagnosis
Patil[94]	Pima Indian Diabetes dataset, UCI repository	Association rule (AR)	AR generation— 100% accuracy	

In aiding ICU effectiveness, many severity scores, such as Simplified Acute Physiology Score (SAPS)[95] and Acute Physiology and Chronic Health Evolution (APACHE),[96] have been proposed since the early 1980s. These metrics have been used for predicting the mortality of patients via patient characteristics recorded during their ICU visits. The predictions using these scores were limited to a few biological–clinical variables selected by domain experts. Since the 1980s, these scores have been modified repeatedly to improve their performance.[97–99] However, SAPS-II[100] and APACHE-II[101] scores remain the most widely accepted for predicting critical illness in intensive care. Katsaragakis et al.[102] had compared these two measures in a single ICU study.

Notwithstanding, the development of an acceptable prediction tool in the field of critical care is a non-trivial task due to the complexity and inconsistency associated with the data collection. Most of the prediction tools adopt a logistic regression model and have been rated by critical care professionals.[103–105] Presently, new approaches using ML algorithms such as DTs, ANNs, SVM, and an ensemble of ML techniques have resulted in various mortality prediction models.[106–110] These approaches have been adopted in different critical care or locally customized settings in the context of specific disease or specific age of the population and other factors. These efforts affirm the importance of ML approaches for modeling mortality prediction.

Beyond these, researchers have implemented alternate DT algorithms and deep NNs for predicting the mortality of patients in ICU.[111–114] Using deep learning algorithms, the performance of such mortality prediction systems for ICU can be improved. Orr,[115] for example, presented an ANN to estimate the risk of death in cardiac surgical patients and used only seven variables from patient's database. The area of receiver operating characteristics (ROC) curve is only 0.74, but the model has a good calibration. To estimate mortality risk after cardiac operation, the implemented NN proved to be very useful.

Fraud Detection

With the dawn of a new era, healthcare insurance rates continue to escalate. As more people and/or organizations are forced to invest a huge sum of money within the healthcare industry for themselves and their employees, it increases the risk of fraud activities in the healthcare insurance domain. With advances in DM and ML techniques, HIT applications toward fraud detection will significantly reduce healthcare costs via a more robust detection of fraud.

While DM is a useful tool to detect fraud,[116] one may also use electronic fraud detection as a safeguard during claims preprocessing by identifying any irregularities or searching for fraud indicators when analyzing processed claims.[117–119] Richard Bauder et al.[120]

discuss an analysis on up-coding fraud, which can be done by obtaining high reimbursement for certain services by coding it as more expensive service than the case actually is worth. Guido van Capelleveen et al.[121] use fraud detection via outlier analysis in medical dental domain. These authors also provide a case study of future applications via outlier analysis for fraud detection within health care.

Preventing Outbreak of Airborne Disease Control

By forming the social network via the call logs and location tracking of the infected person, SNA can be used for the control of airborne diseases. On further analysis of the social network of the infected person, we can prune the persons who have a major chance of disease infection, which can be done by calculating the outbreak role index for every user.[122] Rajinder Sandhu et al.[123,124] discussed the framework for preventing the outbreak of any airborne disease. These authors proposed a framework for effective analysis of the social network of infected persons so that further propagation of the disease can be prevented. Gambhir et al.[125] used ML methods such as ANN, DT, and Naïve Base for the diagnosis of Dengue disease. The authors established that the ANN approach outperforms other approaches of ML.

Readmissions Prediction

The accelerating cost of hospitalization demands the use of DM–ML algorithms to unveil the cause of readmission of patients, thereby avoiding high chances of readmission. Researchers are working on preventing patients being readmitted to hospitals. Various models have been generated to predict early hospital readmission. Joseph et al.[126] compared five models including logistic regression, random forest, SVM, penalized logistic regression, and deep NNs to predict the probability of patients being readmitted. Their result shows

that random forest, penalized logistic regression, and deep NNs perform better than other previously tested algorithms. Beata et al.[127] discussed the role of HbA1c measurement for readmission. These researchers establish a significant role of HbA1c as a useful predictor for predicting the readmission probability of diabetes patient, which will help in reducing the chances of readmission after the first hospitalization with proper actions and/or decisions.[128–131]

Other Contributions

Aside from the aforementioned contributions, DM–ML algorithms have been utilized in areas such as analyzing the hospital details for determining the hospital ranking, hospital resource management, providing consistent patient safety and quality, health policy planning, and customer relationship management (CRM).

Also, the recording from the biosensors may now be analyzed with the use of ML-DM techniques. Biosensors are embedded in the device that senses the biological component of an individual such as sweat, saliva, and more. The analysis of these components offers insight for disease prediction. Lee et al.[132] proposed a sweat-based glucose monitoring wearable device. The developed system provides closed-loop solution for sweat-based management of diabetes mellitus.

▶ V. Conclusion

In summary, DM–ML techniques for health systems have been reviewed in this chapter. More specifically, the chapter discussion shows that the accuracy of these approaches varies due to the different characteristics of health dataset available for analysis, and the accuracy also varies depending on the appropriateness of the chosen DM–ML methodologies for the data.

Many healthcare datasets are complex due to their inextricable nature. Size of the dataset is also unpredictable, a cause of concern for the development of advisable prediction and decision aiding systems. Nonetheless, the development of real-time health decision aiding systems can benefit both patients and their caregivers in obtaining more precise guidance on ways to restore one's health and well-being. For example, sometimes, the advising system would not recommend anything more than continuing to track the symptoms actively; conversely, the recommendation may be a minor intervention such as prescribing a suitable form of medication. Finally, if the patient has lived with the chronic illness for a long while, the recommendation may be able to predict how best to conduct one's future care services in order to maintain an affordable, safe, and high quality of life.

In the end, having the DM–ML embedded in the decision aiding and predictive systems would be especially helpful for patients in the early stages of problem diagnosis; otherwise, its applications may be useful to alert the caregivers toward providing personalized medicine when certain known patterns of disease are automatically matched via clever mining of the patient data characteristics and ML of patient behavioral lifestyles.

Notes

1. McGaughey, S., & Rubin, K. (2008). *Open health tools: Tooling for interoperable healthcare.* Retrieved from https://timreview.ca/article/206
2. Atoji, C. Open health tools hopes to repeat eclipse's success. *Digital HealthCare and Productivity.* Retrieved from www.eclipse.org
3. Winters-Miner, Linda A. (2014). Seven ways predictive analytics can improve healthcare.
4. Lee, H., Song, C., Hong, Y. S., Kim, M. S., Cho, H. R., Kang, T., … Kim, D. H. (2017). Wearable/disposable sweat-based glucose monitoring device with multistage transdermal drug delivery module. *Science Advances, 3*(3), e1601314.
5. Liu, C., Wang, F., Hu, J., & Xiong, H. (2015). Temporal phenotyping from longitudinal electronic health records: A graph based framework. *Proceedings of the 21th ACM SIGKDD International Conference on Knowledge Discovery and Data Mining* (pp. 705–714). Sydney, NSW, Australia: ACM. doi:10.1145/2783258.2783352
6. Sideris, C., Shahbazi, B., Pourhomayoun, M., Alshurafa, N., & Sarrafzadeh, M. (2014). Using electronic health records to predict severity of condition for congestive heart failure patients. *Proceedings of the 2014 ACM International Joint Conference on Pervasive and Ubiquitous Computing: Adjunct Publication* (pp. 1187–1192). Seattle, WA: ACM.
7. Li, H., Li, X., Jia, X., Ramanathan, M., & Zhang, A. (2015, September). Bone disease prediction and phenotype discovery using feature representation over electronic health records. *Proceedings of the 6th ACM Conference on Bioinformatics, Computational Biology and Health Informatics* (pp. 212–221). Atlanta, GA: ACM.
8. Koh, H. C., & Tan, G. (2011). Data mining applications in healthcare. *Journal of Healthcare Information Management, 19*(2), 65.
9. Bates, M. (2017). Tracking disease: Digital epidemiology offers new promise in predicting outbreaks. *IEEE Pulse, 8*(1), 18–22.
10. Internet: Retrieved from www.crisp-dm.org/
11. McGregor, C., Catley, C., & James, A. (2011, July). A process mining driven framework for clinical guideline improvement in critical care. *Proceedings of the Learning from Medical Data Streams Workshop.* Bled, Slovenia.
12. Han, J., Pei, J., & Kamber, M. (2011). *Data mining: Concepts and techniques.* Atlanta, GA: Elsevier.
13. Larose, D. T., & Larose, C. D. (2015). *Data mining and predictive analytics.* Hoboken, NJ: John Wiley & Sons (Published simultaneously in Canada).
14. Internet: Retrieved from www.crisp-dm.org/
15. Larose, C. D., & Larose D. T. (2015). *Data mining and predictive analytics* (Wiley Series on Methods and Applications in Data Mining). Hoboken, NJ: John Wiley & Sons.
16. Koh, H. C., & Tan, G. (2011). Data mining applications in healthcare. *Journal of Healthcare Information Management, 19*(2), 65.
17. McGregor, C., Christina, C., & Andrew, J. (2012). A process mining driven framework for clinical guideline improvement in critical care. *Learning from Medical Data Streams 13th Conference on Artificial Intelligence in Medicine (LEMEDS),* 765. Retrieved from http://ceur-ws. org
18. Canlas, R. D. (2009). Data mining in healthcare: Current applications and issues. *School of Information Systems & Management.* Carnegie Mellon University, Australia. https://pdfs.semanticscholar.

org/0acb/878637612377ed547627dfdeeb266204dd97.
pdf?_ga=2.56418603.1600134081.1561554282-
535543275.1561554282

19. Hosseinkhah, F., Ashktorab, H., & Veen, R. (2009). Challenges in data mining on medical databases. *Database Technologies: Concepts, Methodologies, Tools, and Applications* (pp. 1393–1404). Hershey, PA: IGI Global.

20. Kumari, M., & Godara, S. (2011). Comparative study of data mining classification methods in cardiovascular disease prediction 1. *International Journal of Computer Science and Technology, 2*(2), 304–308.

21. Soni, J., Ansari, U., Sharma, D., & Soni, S. (2011). Predictive data mining for medical diagnosis: An overview of heart disease prediction. *International Journal of Computer Applications, 17*(8), 43–48.

22. Dangare, C. S., & Apte, S. S. (2012). Improved study of heart disease prediction system using data mining classification techniques. *International Journal of Computer Applications, 47*(10), 44–48.

23. Srinivas, K., Rani, B. K., & Govrdhan, A. (2010). Applications of data mining techniques in healthcare and prediction of heart attacks. *International Journal on Computer Science and Engineering (IJCSE), 2*(02), 250–255.

24. Aljumah, A. A., Ahamad, M. G., & Siddiqui, M. K. (2011). Predictive analysis on hypertension treatment using data mining approach in Saudi Arabia. *Intelligent Information Management, 3*(6), 252.

25. Delen, D. (2009). Analysis of cancer data: A data mining approach. *Expert Systems, 26*(1), 100–112.

26. Osofisan, A. O., Adeyemo, O. O., Sawyerr, B. A., & Eweje, O. (2011). Prediction of kidney failure using artificial neural networks. *European Journal of Scientific Research, 61*(4), 487.

27. Bodkhe, A. (2017). Predicting Pancreatic Cancer Using Support Vector Machine. Masters Project, San Jose State University.

28. Huang, M. J., Chen, M. Y., & Lee, S. C. (2007). Integrating data mining with case-based reasoning for chronic diseases prognosis and diagnosis. *Expert Systems with Applications, 32*(3), 856–867.

29. Gupta, S., Kumar, D., & Sharma, A. (2011). Data mining classification techniques applied for breast cancer diagnosis and prognosis. *Indian Journal of Computer Science and Engineering (IJCSE), 2*(2), 188–195.

30. Parvathi, R., & Palaniammal, S. (2011). An improved medical diagnosing technique using spatial association rules. *European Journal of Scientific Research ISSN*, 49–59.

31. Ha, S. H., & Joo, S. H. (2010). A hybrid data mining method for the medical classification of chest pain. *International Journal of Computer and Information Engineering, 4*(1), 33–38.

32. Kavitha, K. S., Ramakrishnan, K. V., & Singh, M. K. (2010). Modeling and design of evolutionary neural network for heart disease detection. *International Journal of Computer Science Issues (IJCSI), 7*(5), 272.

33. Nalavade, J., Gavali, M., Gohil, N., & Jamale, S. (2014). Impelling heart attack prediction system using data mining and artificial neural network. *International Journal of Current Engineering and Technology, 4*(3), 1–5.

34. Shukla, A., Tiwari, R., & Kaur, P. (2009, March). Knowledge based approach for diagnosis of breast cancer. *Advance Computing Conference, 2009. IACC 2009. IEEE International* (pp. 6–12). IEEE. Patiala, India.

35. Duan, L., Street, W. N., & Xu, E. (2011). Healthcare information systems: Data mining methods in the creation of a clinical recommender system. *Enterprise Information Systems, 5*(2), 169–181.

36. Kumar, B. S. (2018). Adaptive personalized clinical decision support system using effective data mining algorithms. *Journal of Network Communications and Emerging Technologies (JNCET), 8*(1). Retrieved from www.jncet.org

37. Palaniappan, S., & Awang, R. (2008, March). Intelligent heart disease prediction system using data mining techniques. *IEEE/ACS International Conference on Computer Systems and Applications. AICCSA 2008.* (pp. 108–115), IEEE, Doha Qatar.

38. Rao, A. R., Chhabra, A., Das, R., & Ruhil, V. (2015, October). A framework for analyzing publicly available healthcare data. *17th International Conference on E-health Networking, Application & Services (HealthCom), 2015* (pp. 653–656), IEEE, Boston, MA.

39. Kalaiselvi, C. (2016). Diagnosis of heart disease using K-nearest neighbor algorithm of data mining. *International Conference on Computing for Sustainable Global Development (INDIACom)* (pp. 3099–3103), IEEE.

40. Han et al., (2010), *ibid.*

41. *Ibid.*

42. James, G., Witten, D., Hastie T., & Tibshirani, R. (2013). An introduction to statistical learning. New York, Heidelberg, and London: Springer.

43. Han et al., (2010), *ibid.*

44. Apté, C., & Weiss, S. (1997). Data mining with decision trees and decision rules. *Future Generation Computer Systems, 13*(2–3), 197–210.

45. Goharian & Grossman, Data Mining Classification, Illinois Institute of Technology. (2003). Retrieved from http://ir.iit.edu/~nazli/cs422/CS422-Slides/DM-Classification.pdf

46. Andrew, A. M. (2000). *An introduction to support vector machines and other kernel-based learning methods* by Nello Christianini and John Shawetaylor

(2000, xiii+ 189 pp.). Cambridge: Cambridge University Press.

47. Vapnik, V. (1998). The support vector method of function estimation. *Nonlinear Modeling: Advanced Black-Box Techniques, 55*, 86.

48. Chistianini, N., & Shawe-Taylor, J. (2000). *An introduction to support vector machines, and other kernel-based learning methods*. Cambridge: Cambridge University Press.

49. *Ibid.*

50. Andrew, (2000), *ibid.*

51. Hsu, C. W., & Lin, C. J. (2002) A comparison of methods for multiclass support vector machines. *IEEE Transactions on Neural Networks, 13*(2), 415–425.

52. Sivanadam, S. N., & Deepa, S. N. *Principles of soft computing* (2nd ed.). India: Wiley India Publications.

53. Obenshain, M. K. (2004). Application of data mining techniques to healthcare data. *Infection Control & Hospital Epidemiology, 25*(8), 690–695.

54. Scott, J. (2000). *Social network analysis, A handbook* (2nd ed.). London: Sage Publications.

55. Opsahl, T., Agneessens, F., & Skvoretz, J. (2010). Node centrality in weighted networks: Generalizing degree and shortest paths. *Social Networks, 32*(3), 245–251.

56. Silver, M., Sakata, T., Su, H. C., Herman, C., Dolins, S. B., & O'Shea, M. J. (2001). Case study: How to apply data mining techniques in a healthcare data warehouse. *Journal of Healthcare Information Management, 15*(2), 155–164.

57. James, G., et al., (2013), *ibid.*

58. Han et al., (2010), *ibid.*

59. *Ibid.*

60. Bahmani, B., Moseley, B., Vattani, A., Kumar, R., & Vassilvitskii, S. (2012). Scalable k-means++. *Proceedings of the VLDB Endowment, 5*(7), 622–633.

61. Han et al., (2010), *ibid.*

62. *Ibid.*

63. *Ibid.*

64. Agrawal, R., & Srikant, R. (1994). Fast algorithms for mining association rules. *Proceedings of the 20th International Conference on Very Large Data Bases*, VLDB. Vol. 1215. Santiago de Chille, Chille.

65. Scott, (2000), *ibid.*

66. Opsahl et al., (2010), *ibid.*

67. *Ibid.*

68. Silver et al., (2001), *ibid.*

69. Harper, P. R. (2005). A review and comparison of classification algorithms for medical decision making. *Health Policy, 71*, 315–331.

70. Stel, V. S., Pluijm, S. M., Deeg, D. J., Smit, J. H., Bouter L. M., & Lips, P. (2003). A classification tree for predicting recurrent falling in community-dwelling older persons. *Journal of the American Geriatrics Society, 51*, 1356–1364.

71. Bellazzi, R., & Zupan, B. (2008). Predictive data mining in clinical medicine: current issues and guidelines. *International Journal of Medical Informatics, 77*, 81–97.

72. Neesha, J., & Husain, W. (2015). Data mining in healthcare – A review. *Procedia Computer Science, 72*, 306–313.

73. Willcox, W. R., Lapage, S. P., Bascomb, S., & Curtis, M. A. (1973). Identification of bacteria by computer: Theory and programming. *Microbiology, 77*(2), 317–330.

74. Abeel, T., Helleputte, T., Van de Peer, Y., Dupont, P., & Saeys, Y. (2009). Robust biomarker identification for cancer diagnosis with ensemble feature selection methods. *Bioinformatics, 26*(3), 392–398.

75. Sadiq, A. T., & Mahmood, N. T. (2014). A hybrid estimation system for medical diagnosis using modified full Bayesian classifier and artificial bee colony. *Iraqi Journal of Science, 55*(3A), 1095–1107.

76. Patil, R. R. (2014). Heart disease prediction system using Naive Bayes and Jelinek-mercer smoothing. *International Journal of Advanced Research in Computer and Communication Engineering, 3*(5), 2278–1021.

77. Kumari & Godara, (2011), *ibid.*

78. *Ibid.*

79. Kononenko, I. (2001). Machine learning for medical diagnosis: History, state of the art and perspective. *Artificial Intelligence in Medicine, 23*(1), 89–109.

80. Karaolis, M. A., Moutiris, J. A., Hadjipanayi, D., & Pattichis, C. S. (2010). Assessment of the risk factors of coronary heart events based on data mining with decision trees. *IEEE Transactions on Information Technology in Biomedicine, 14*(3), 559–566.

81. Lakshmi, K. R., & Kumar, S. P. (2013). Utilization of data mining techniques for prediction and diagnosis of major life threatening diseases survivability-review. *International Journal of Scientific & Engineering Research, 4*(6), 923–932.

82. Dangare, C. S., & Apte, S. S. (2012). Improved study of heart disease prediction system using data mining classification techniques. *International Journal of Computer Applications, 47*(10), 44–48.

83. Das, R., Turkoglu, I., & Sengur, A. (2009). Effective diagnosis of heart disease through neural networks ensembles. *Expert Systems with Applications, 36*(4), 7675–7680.

84. Avci, E. (2009). A new intelligent diagnosis system for the heart valve diseases by using genetic-SVM classifier. *Expert Systems with Applications, 36*, 10618–10626.

85. Shouman, M., Turner T., & Stocker, R. (2012). Applying K-nearest neighbour in diagnosing heart disease patients. *International Conference on Knowledge Discovery (ICKD-2012)*. Bali, Indonesia.

86. Potter, R. (2007, July). Comparison of classification algorithms applied to breast cancer diagnosis and prognosis. *Advances in Data Mining, 7th Industrial Conference, ICDM 2007* (pp. 40–49), Leipzig, Germany.

87. Huang, C. L., Liao, H. C., & Chen, M. C. (2008). Prediction model building and feature selection with support vector machines in breast cancer diagnosis, *Expert Systems with Applications, 34*, 578–587.

88. Osareh A., & Shadgar, B. (2010). Machine learning techniques to diagnose breast cancer. *Health Informatics and Bioinformatics (HIBIT)*, IEEE. Antalya, Turkey.

89. Fan, Q., Zhu, C. J., & Yin, L. (2010). Predicting breast cancer recurrence using data mining techniques. *Bioinformatics and Biomedical Technology (ICBBT), 2010 International Conference on* IEEE, Chengdu, China.

90. Resul et al. (2009), *ibid*.

91. Osofisan, A. O., Adeyemo, O. O., Sawyerr, B. A., & Eweje, O. (2011). Prediction of kidney failure using artificial neural networks. *European Journal of Scientific Research, 61*(4), 487.

92. Kumar, D. S., Sathyadevi, G., & Sivanesh, S. (2011). Decision support system for medical diagnosis using data mining. *International Journal of Computer Science Issues, 8*(3), 147–153.

93. Barakat, N., Bradley, A. P., & Barakat, M. N. H. (2010). Intelligible support vector machines for diagnosis of diabetes mellitus. *IEEE Transactions on Information Technology in Biomedicine, 14*(4), 1114–1120.

94. Patil, B. M., Joshi R. C., & Toshniwal, D. (2010). Association rule for classification of type-2 diabetic patients. *Second International Conference on Machine Learning and Computing* (pp. 330–334). IEEE Computer Society, Washington, DC, USA.

95. Le, J. G., Loirat, P., Alperovitch, A., Glaser, P., Granthil, C., Mathieu, D., … Villers, D. (1984). A simplified acute physiology score for ICU patients. *Critical Care Medicine, 12*(11), 975–977.

96. Knaus, W. A., Zimmerman, J. E., Wagner, D. P., Draper, E. A., & Lawrence, D. E. (1981). APACHE-acute physiology and chronic health evaluation: A physiologically based classification system. *Critical Care Medicine, 9*(8), 591–597.

97. Le Gall, J. R., Lemeshow, S., & Saulnier, F. (1993). A new simplified acute physiology score (SAPS II) based on a European/North American multicenter study. *JAMA, 270*(24), 2957–2963.

98. Knaus, W. A., Draper, E. A., Wagner, D. P., & Zimmerman, J. E. (1985). APACHE II: A severity of disease classification system. *Critical Care Medicine, 13*(10), 818–829.

99. *Ibid*.

100. Le Gall et al., (1993), *ibid*.

101. Knaus et al., (1985), *ibid*.

102. Katsaragakis, S., Papadimitropoulos, K., Antonakis, P., Strergiopoulos, S., Konstadoulakis, M. M., & Androulakis, G. (2000). Comparison of Acute Physiology and Chronic Health Evaluation II (APACHE II) and Simplified Acute Physiology Score II (SAPS II) scoring systems in a single Greek intensive care unit. *Critical Care Medicine, 28*(2), 426–432.

103. Clermont, G., Angus, D. C., DiRusso, S. M., Griffin, M., & Linde-Zwirble, W. T. (2001). Predicting hospital mortality for patients in the intensive care unit: A comparison of artificial neural networks with logistic regression models. *Critical Care Medicine, 29*(2), 291–296.

104. Nguile-Makao, M., Zahar, J. R., Français, A., Tabah, A., Garrouste-Orgeas, M., Allaouchiche, B., … Clec'h, C. (2010). Attributable mortality of ventilator-associated pneumonia: Respective impact of main characteristics at ICU admission and VAP onset using conditional logistic regression and multi-state models. *Intensive Care Medicine, 36*(5), 781–789.

105. Rosenberg, A. L. (2002). Recent innovations in intensive care unit risk-prediction models. *Current Opinion in Critical Care, 8*(4), 321–330.

106. Dybowski, R., Gant, V., Weller, P., & Chang, R. (1996). Prediction of outcome in critically ill patients using artificial neural network synthesised by genetic algorithm. *The Lancet, 347*(9009), 1146–1150.

107. Dursun, D., Walker, G., & Kadam A. (2005). Predicting breast cancer survivability: A comparison of three data mining methods. *Artificial Intelligence in Medicine, 34*(2), 113–127.

108. Sierra, B., Serrano, N., LarrañAga, P., Plasencia, E. J., Inza, I., JiméNez, J. J., … Mora, M. L. (2001). Using Bayesian networks in the construction of a bi-level multi-classifier. A case study using intensive care unit patients data. *Artificial Intelligence in Medicine, 22*(3), 233–248.

109. Vieira, S. M., Mendonça, L. F., Farinha, G. J., & Sousa, J. M. (2013). Modified binary PSO for feature selection using SVM applied to mortality prediction of septic patients. *Applied Soft Computing, 13*(8), 3494–3504.

110. Pirracchio, R., Petersen, M. L., Carone, M., Rigon, M. R., Chevret, S., & van der Laan, M. J. (2015). Mortality prediction in intensive care units with the Super ICU Learner Algorithm (SICULA): A population-based study. *The Lancet Respiratory Medicine, 3*(1), 42–52.

111. Mathias, J. S., Agrawal, A., Feinglass, J., Cooper, A. J., Baker, D. W., & Choudhary, A. (2013). Development of a 5 year life expectancy index in older adults using predictive mining of electronic health record

data. *Journal of the American Medical Informatics Association, 20*(e1), e118–e124.

112. Rodriguez, J. J., Kuncheva, L. I., & Alonso, C. J. (2006). Rotation forest: A new classifier ensemble method. *IEEE Transactions on Pattern Analysis and Machine Intelligence, 28*(10), 1619–1630.

113. Freund, Y., & Mason, L. (1999). The alternating decision tree learning algorithm. *Proceedings of the Sixteenth International Conference on Machine Learning (ICML)*. San Francisco, USA.

114. Choi, E., Schuetz, A., Stewart, W. F., & Sun, J. (2016). Using recurrent neural network models for early detection of heart failure onset. *Journal of the American Medical Informatics Association, 24*(2), 361–370.

115. Orr, R. K. (1997). Use of a probabilistic neural network to estimate the risk of mortality after cardiac surgery. *Medical Decision Making, 17*(2), 178–185.

116. Aral, K. D., Güvenir, H. A., Sabuncuoğlu, İ., & Akar, A. R. (2012). A prescription fraud detection model. *Computer Methods and Programs in Biomedicine, 106*(1), 37–46.

117. Forgionne, G. A., Gangopadhyay, A., & Adya, M. (2000). An intelligent data mining system to detect healthcare fraud. *Healthcare Information Systems: Challenges of the New Millennium,* (pp. 149–168). Hershey, PA, USA: IGI Global.

118. Bolton, R. J., & Hand, D. J. (2002). Statistical fraud detection: A review. *Statistical Science, 17*(3), 235–255. Retrieved from https://projecteuclid.org/download/pdf_1/euclid.ss/1042727940

119. Ortega, P. A., Figueroa, C. J., & Ruz, G. A. (2006). A medical claim fraud/abuse detection system based on data mining: A case study in Chile. *DMIN, 6,* 26–29.

120. Bauder, R., Khoshgoftaar, T. M., & Seliya, N. (2016). A survey on the state of healthcare upcoding fraud analysis and detection. *Health Services and Outcomes Research Methodology, 17*(1), 31–55.

121. van Capelleveen, G., Poel, M., Mueller, R. M., Thornton, D., & van Hillegersberg, J. (2016). Outlier detection in healthcare fraud: A case study in the Medicaid dental domain. *International Journal of Accounting Information Systems, 21,* 18–31.

122. Sandhu, R., Gill, H. K., & Sood, S. K. (2016). Smart monitoring and controlling of pandemic influenza a (H1N1) using social network analysis and cloud computing. *Journal of Computational Science, 12,* 11–22.

123. *Ibid.*

124. *Ibid.*

125. Gambhir, S., Malik, S. K., & Kumar, Y. (2018). The diagnosis of dengue disease: An evaluation of three machine learning approaches. *International Journal of Healthcare Information Systems and Informatics (IJHISI), 13*(3), 1–19.

126. Futoma, J., Morris, J., & Lucas, J. (2015). A comparison of models for predicting early hospital readmissions. *Journal of Biomedical Informatics, 56,* 229–238.

127. Strack, B., DeShazo, J. P., Gennings, C., Olmo, J. L., Ventura, S., Cios, K. J., & Clore, J. N. (2014). Impact of HbA1c measurement on hospital readmission rates: Analysis of 70,000 clinical database patient records. *BioMed Research International,* 2014.

128. Choudhry, S. A., Li, J., Davis, D., Erdmann, C., Sikka, R., & Sutariya, B. (2013). A public-private partnership develops and externally validates a 30-day hospital readmission risk prediction model. *Online Journal of Public Health Informatics, 5*(2), 219.

129. He, D., Mathews, S. C., Kalloo, A. N., & Hutfless, S. (2014). Mining high-dimensional administrative claims data to predict early hospital readmissions. *Journal of the American Medical Informatics Association, 21*(2), 272–279.

130. Kansagara, D., Englander, H., Salanitro, A., Kagen, D., Theobald, C., Freeman, M., & Kripalani, S. (2011). Risk prediction models for hospital readmission: A systematic review. *JAMA, 306*(15), 1688–1698.

131. Yu, S., Farooq, F., Van Esbroeck, A., Fung, G., Anand, V., & Krishnapuram, B. (2015). Predicting readmission risk with institution-specific prediction models. *Artificial Intelligence in Medicine, 65*(2), 89–96.

132. Lee, H., Song, C., Hong, Y. S., Kim, M. S., Cho, H. R., Kang, T., … Kim, D. H. (2017). Wearable/disposable sweat-based glucose monitoring device with multistage transdermal drug delivery module. *Science Advances, 3*(3), e1601314.

Chapter Questions

9-1   How is predictive analysis different from descriptive analysis? Illustrate your answers with examples from healthcare scenarios.

9-2   Why and how do you think ML techniques can be used intelligently to deal with airborne diseases?

9-3   Provide examples of applications where ICU recordings of patients may be utilized to provide safer, higher quality, and cost-effective care to patients.

9-4   Early diagnosis of disease is important. State ways in which ML can be utilized for this purpose.

Biographies

Saumil Maheshwari is a research scholar at ABV-Indian Institute of Information Technology and Management (ABV-IIITM), Gwalior, India, under the supervision of Professor Anupam Shukla. He has Bachelor of Engineering and Masters of Technology degree in Computer Science and Engineering. He has published six research papers in International Journals and conferences. His primary area of research interests are data mining, social network analysis, and machine learning. He has worked as an Assistant Professor at Madhav Institute of Technology and Science from 2014 to 2016.

Anupam Shukla is a Director at the Indian Institute of Information Technology (IIIT), Pune, India. Before joining IIIT, Pune, as director, he was a Professor in the Department of Information and Communication Technology (ICT) at ABV-Indian Institute of Information Technology and Management (ABV-IIITM), Gwalior, and a visiting faculty at Indian Institute of Management (IIM), Rohtak. He has 28 years of administrative, research, and teaching experience. He is globally renowned for his research on artificial intelligence, which has won him several academic accolades and resulted in collaborations with academics across the world. He is the author of three patents; four books, published by international publishers such as CRC Press USA, and Springer-Verlag, Berlin; 166 peer-reviewed publications; editor of three books published by IGI Global Press, Hershey, PA, USA; and mentor of 107 doctorate and post-graduate theses. He has successfully completed 13 government-sponsored projects worth Rs. 10 crores.

CHAPTER 10

The Role of Informatics in Public Health

April Moreno Arellano

LEARNING OBJECTIVES

- Understand the role of informatics in the promotion of public health
- Describe key applications of public health information
- Identify the common data frameworks for the use of electronic health information
- Recognize the use of relevant data for chronic disease surveillance

CHAPTER OUTLINE

Scenario: Aligning Clinical and Public Health Data Standards Through Partnership with the Public Health Data Standards Consortium[1]

In October 2014, the American Health Information Management Association (AHIMA) announced their interest in combining efforts with public health agencies for establishing data standards, and has partnered with the Public Health Data Standards Consortium (PHDSC), a U.S.-based organization of public health government agencies, professional associations, universities, public and private organizations, and individuals. This collaboration offers the opportunity to advance health IT (HIT) data standards while strengthening the infrastructure of health information, to align data standards for clinical and public health. Both organizations have a commitment to the advancement of their professions through HIT and standards. They both work toward the standardization of HIT data use for population health.

> "We are thrilled to welcome PHDSC and its former Executive Director, Dr. Anna Orlova, into the AHIMA family, and look forward to furthering our join expertise and impact in the public health/data standards field,"[2] Angela Kennedy, EdD, Med, MBA, RHIA, CPHA, AHIMA Board President and Chair announced. She further stated that "This partnership directly ties to AHIMA's strategic initiatives in informatics and public good and will increase our collective influence within the industry."[3]

Imagine that you have been asked to lead the coordination of the partnership of AHIMA and PHDSC. You have been commissioned to provide a vision and a plan for the development of the strategy to establish the commonality of data standards among the clinical and public health sectors. What would be important to focus on first, and how would you structure the management of this endeavor?

Describe your vision, plan, and any future-oriented functionalities that you would envision for supporting clinical and public health providers and consumers. Be sure to address workforce, workflow, and population health considerations, as well as commonalities and differences between clinical and public health data use and exchange processes.

▶ I. Introduction

Public health is the promotion of health at the community, national, and global levels, involving environments where people *live, learn, work, and play.*[4,5] Public health concerns many aspects of our daily lives—from the air we breathe to the smoking policy of neighborhood restaurants; from the safety of highway travel to the control and immunization of diseases affecting animals as well as children and adults; and, even from the quality of our drinking water to the quality of water found in public beaches and swimming pools.

As a discipline, public health is focused on promoting healthy lifestyles and research for the *prevention, detection, and control* of diseases.[6] Three core functions of public health are generally highlighted as: (i) Assessment, (ii) Policy Development, and (iii) Assurance. As part of these three core functions, the Centers for Disease Control and Prevention (CDC) has identified 10 categories of activities expected of public health[7] (**FIGURE 10-1**).

These 10 essential activities may be described as:

    i. Assessment:
        1. Monitoring the status of community health to address community health issues
        2. Diagnosing and investigating community health risks and problems

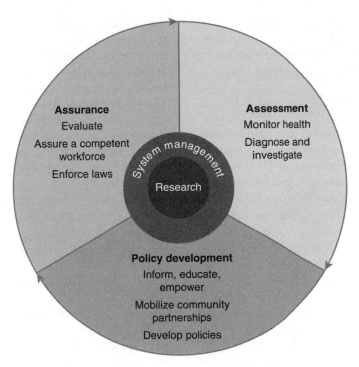

FIGURE 10-1 The 10 essential public health services (CDC, 2014).

Data from the Public Health System & the 10 Essential Public Health Services. From https://www.cdc.gov/publichealthgateway/publichealthservices/essentialhealthservices.html

ii. Policy Development:
3. Providing education and information to empower individuals to improve health
4. Catalyzing community partnerships to discuss and solve health issues
5. Developing policy and planning to support efforts in improving the health of individuals and communities

iii. Assurance:
6. Enforcing regulations and laws, which serve to protect or ensure health and safety
7. Providing linkages to personal health care and providing healthcare services when availability is a challenge
8. Assuring a competent workforce of public and personal health care

9. Evaluating the quality, effectiveness, and accessibility of individual and population health services
10. Researching insights and innovations to address health issues.[8]

Recent discussions of public health have included the realm of translational methods for public health research, which provides a broader, more *non-linear* and *intersectoral* scope to the factors influencing health, known also as the *determinants of health*.[9] As an example of the intersectoral nature of public health, a wide range of professions are involved, such as researchers, scientists, health educators, epidemiologists, biostatisticians, social workers, urban and community planners, policymakers, and occupational health and safety professionals.[10] A broad range of professionals is needed to work with the challenges and complexities of public health. Additionally, emerging developments in technology and the increasing emphasis of electronic medical and health records have prompted the need for public health informatics professionals.

Public Health Informatics

Public health informatics is a field involving a variety of skills and competencies related to the strategic management of IT knowledge, information, and data to support public health programs.[11] In the relatively new environment of public health informatics, the combined use of electronic health records (EHR) analytics on the prevalence of chronic diseases and effective data communication with public health agencies can contribute to our understanding of chronic disease trends so as to improve targeted population health outcomes. This can take place through the collaboration of public health, clinical, laboratory, and other providers for a particular region, ideally sharing de-identified EHR data in an interoperable manner. The future of health informatics places critical demands on public health to become more increasingly focused on data. Similarly, future health informatics research depends upon meaningfully transforming clinical data into information and, with aggregated data from clinics, transforming information into knowledge.[12] Much of this information comes from clinical providers sharing patient data with public health agencies in order to expand knowledge from the individual patient level to improve population health.[13]

Beyond Data, Information, and Knowledge

Although several researchers have differentiated the concepts of data, information, and knowledge,[14,15] Chaim Zins[16] has also outlined the difference between these three concepts as an order of sequence, in which data is the smallest of the units, consisting of the raw material that is used to build information,

and information serves as the raw material for knowledge. In the context of public health informatics, these three concepts have been expanded to include wisdom, practice, and healthier communities to develop a discipline in the design of information systems to improve the practice of public health.[17] Rather than being the main collector of information, the field of public health will become focused on the interpretation and distribution of data through EHR.[18] In the case of accessing the data for public health systems, three functions can be identified: raw data acquisition, cleaning and managing data, and analyzing the data in ways that these data will become meaningful and available to the user.[19] Additionally, the spatial component of these data will provide insights into community and population health through the EHR. Public health agencies will soon become increasingly responsible for the review and aggregation of data from a variety of sources, while providing accessibility of information in ways that can be interpreted.[20]

▶ II. Global Public Health

Public health can require participation and collaboration across national borders, for example, emerging infectious and communicable diseases taking place in other countries may require immediate response and control. Through processes such as international travels or cross-border logistics, disease can spread quickly across borders. The effort of disease prevention and control requires a range of stakeholders and a range of professionals across the health systems, more specifically, epidemiologists, nurses, and physicians, in addition to community organizations, government officials, and patients.[21]

Although it has been acknowledged that global health does not have a determined definition and also has an unclear understanding of its achievements, approaches, skills, and

TABLE 10-1 Comparing Global and Public Health (Koplan et al., 2009)

	Global Health	Public Health
Geographic Focus	Directly or indirectly affecting health across national borders	Affecting the population health in a community or a country
Cooperation Level	Global cooperation is often required for developing and implementing solutions	Developing and implementing solutions generally does not need global cooperation
Individual or Population	Includes disease prevention in populations and through individual clinical care	Focuses on disease prevention programming for populations
Health Equity	Health equity is a major focus for nations and all people	Health equity is a major focus within nations or communities
Disciplines	Very interdisciplinary and multidisciplinary, and can include fields outside of health	Encourages a multidisciplinary approach in health and social sciences

required resources,[22] a general consensus on its definition can include the promotion of health at a global scale. As seen in **TABLE 10-1**, global health involves the need for interdisciplinary and multidisciplinary cross-borders cooperation, with a focus on health equity, and the work of global health can be population or individual based.

The work of global health includes the improvement of health systems, the promotion of health at all stages of life, preparation or prevention, control, and surveillance of diseases internationally.[23] This can also include the work of humanitarian assistance and response services, to reduce or eradicate the spread of diseases such as malaria, polio, and measles.[24]

Global Health Informatics

Global health informatics has the capability for programs to have access to critical health information for decision makers, and can be in the creation of improving health systems efficiency. This can be conducted through the standardization of data collection, as well as the analysis and storage of these systems, for the improvement of disease surveillance and response.[25] The work of global health informatics can provide health improvements to "resource-constrained" countries, through the application of emerging technology research and through the evaluation of interventions, which have been conducted through the use of informatics.[26]

Informatics is an important aspect of the response to global public health problems and can also be utilized for monitoring incidence, tracking to identify disease trends, and predictive modeling of diseases for prevention. Global health informatics can be utilized at the emergency response level for disease epidemics, as well as for more gradual chronic disease conditions such as hypertension, diabetes, and obesity. Recent developments in technology have allowed for health information technology to provide real-time surveillance data, available without geographic limits. Surveillance networks at a global scale are now available, and current systems developed by the World Health Organization (WHO) include surveillance for flu, dengue, and other global outbreak data.[27,28] International standards for data are useful in working with global health informatics. As discussed later, standards and systems such as Health Level Seven (HL7), LOINC, SNOMED-CT, and even ICD codes allow for a level of consistency internationally.

Applications of Public Health Information

With advances in health technology, various types of public health reporting and electronic innovations are taking place. According to the Office of the National Coordinator (ONC) for HIT, the trend in public health is moving from traditional paper health reports (such as lab reporting and manual data recording and abstraction) to unidirectional health data from patient EHR to registries and systems for reportable conditions surveillance. From there, technological advancement is allowing for bidirectional health data exchanges to take place. With this capability, data will utilize transport standards (such as HL7, SNOMED-CT, and LOINC) to communicate between EHR and more specific registries and systems almost instantly.[29] The following are several examples of electronic public health data and reporting applications in existence.

Reporting Systems

These systems often are electronic recordings of reporting health data for purposes such as performance measurement and evaluation generally taking place within public health agencies. For instance, at the county level, Los Angeles County Public Health utilizes the Los Angeles County Participant Reporting System (LACPRS) for Substance Abuse Prevention

and Control data, now known as Sage. This system is available only to the county as well as to the individual substance abuse service provider facilities to report required data on patient/client admissions and discharge dates, modalities of service, allowing for comparisons of outcomes across modalities, programs, and provider locations.[30]

Hospitals use these reporting systems for statistical reporting such as the Healthcare Effectiveness Data and Information Set (HEDIS) measures as required. Reported by over 90% of health plans, HEDIS measures aid in performance tracking for 81 measures and 5 care domains. As the measures are very specific, it is possible for health plan performance to be compared and audited using a National Committee for Quality Assurance (NCQA) designed process. Some of the data include measures for childhood and adult weight and BMI, child/adolescent immunizations, and comprehensive diabetes care. The information is available to the public through the Quality Compass tool where data can be provided in graphs to compare health plans, measures, and data for up to 3 years.

Registries

Public health registries traditionally contain data on disease cases (both required and not required data) such as syndromic surveillance and reportable hospital lab results. Registries can be seen as systems designed to monitor diseases, their duration and treatment outcome as well as incidence. They are usually known as having been established to respond to specific legislation requiring them. They are also known for being able to keep reports on individual cases for a long period of time.[31] Registries can be used for non-infectious diseases as well. A traditional example is the National Cancer Registry of all cases that are reportable to health agencies. Registries also exist where disease is still a focus, but the tracking of actions and effectiveness for preventing disease can be the focus. For example, the San Diego

Immunization Registry is used to report vaccinations to share patient immunization information and to identify what immunizations are required in the future, as well as determining the effectiveness of immunization interventions. Chronic disease surveillance systems are another example; it is different from infectious or communicable disease surveillance because it allows more time to report and analyze the data and to intervene, particularly as many of these conditions are generally not required reportable conditions.[32] Also, public health agencies are seeking data from undiagnosed patients (non-cases), which makes it different from a traditional registry. Working with community clinics, laboratories, and hospitals in the region, the key is to collect data from patients across the county in order to identify prediabetes and undiagnosed hypertension. In Colorado, the Colorado Health Observation Regional Data Service (CHORDS) shares the data from various health providers in the region to form registries by topic area such as tobacco use, chronic disease, and mental health (see section on *Electronic Knowledge Resources*).

Surveys

Public health surveys are sets of questions designed to gather data on many diseases, including chronic diseases and behavioral risk factors influencing the development of disease. These surveys are generally collected on a regular basis for a particular geographic region, by age group and in several languages. All of the data tend to be self-reported which can be a limitation for accuracy of information. Survey information is often collected by telephone through random digit dialing (or face-to-face for some surveys).

One of the best examples of a survey is the Behavioral Risk Factor Surveillance System (BRFSS), which collects data on health behaviors, chronic health conditions, and prevention. It is administered throughout the year on a continuous basis. The National Health and Nutrition Examination Survey (NHANES) is another classic survey example assessing the health and nutrition of individuals in the nation. In addition to the interview and survey questions, it combines interviews (either by telephone or face-to-face) and physical exams. A third interesting example is the CDC Health-Related Quality of Life Survey (HRQOL), which provides a set of questions, including "healthy days" measures about individual physical and mental health status. The instrument is available for public use; HRQOL measures also include asking questions about pain, depression, and anxiety as well as how these conditions may cause limitations to normal activities.

Electronic Knowledge Resources

These resources can include a variety of information such as linking health data and patient information. Data sharing through a Health Information Exchange (HIE) takes place regionally, where health data from a variety of sources is available through one source may be cited as an example. San Diego Health Connect, for instance, is a county-level HIE where data from a variety of sources are made available through a federated model in which data files are stored with their own respective organizations but are shared securely through the HIE. Data from a variety of sources such as from hospitals, healthcare providers, patients, and other stakeholders can also be connected through HIE to share important patient information across organizations. In Colorado, CHORDS sounds more like a public health network but shares the data to form registries by topic area via working with EHR data for monitoring health in the region. It also is used to measure efficacy in public health interventions.

Networks for Linking Public Health Professionals

These networks are professional groups designed to connect public health professionals.

They exist for a variety of purposes, including sharing of data and information about national, regional, and local HIT vis-à-vis the role of public health in this process. A strong example of this is the CDC Public Health Information Network (PHIN), which provides tools, resources, and a network for public health agencies to develop capacity for electronic health data and information exchange. This includes a directory of people, organizations, and regional jurisdictions, resources, standard vocabularies, and standards for interoperability.

Launched in 2012, the Massachusetts eHealth Institute launched the Massachusetts Department of Public Health Network (MDPHnet), which is designed to enable public health professionals to query patient data from health centers and hospitals or clinics for the identification of illnesses and chronic conditions without accessing personal information. This allows for public health professionals to collaborate as a network to share aggregated patient data to identify conditions such as diabetes and influenza across the state.

Another type of network for public health professionals in HIT is the Academy Health Electronic Data Methods (EDM) group, Population Health Community of Practice. Here, a group of public health agency officials meet monthly by phone to discuss various issues in public health electronic data research and reporting for quality improvement.

▶ III. EHR as a Comprehensive Tool for Health Care

Across multiple healthcare settings, EHR is the electronic location of where patient data exist with the potential for comprehensive and interoperable data sharing. EHR provides a way for improved data quality and for timely information to be made available.[33]

EHR are differentiated from electronic medical records (EMR) in the following ways: EMR are simply electronic data from traditional clinical paper charts originally designed simply for diagnosis and treatment, while EHR contain the data and information found in EMR, but also involve the interoperability of more comprehensive "total health," including general patient allergies, laboratory results, family medical history, and demographic information, as well as administrative information such as billing and insurance details.[34] EMR are strictly medical patient records data while EHR are more comprehensive in scope. Additionally, in EHR, data must be collected, communicated, and shared first at the individual patient scale, then analyzed at the population level through the transmission of information in an interoperable format. The EHR contains a full spectrum of information from the individual prescription and procedure, onward to the demographic and geographic factors of community-level characteristics, to the greater population level of health plan and state and federal health program eligibility. Unlike EMR, EHR data are stored and shared through the use of EHR software via the many vendors such as Epic, Cerner, AllScripts, and eClinicalWorks. At the vendor level, many of the EHR providers currently do not distinguish between EMR and EHR and still regard the products as EMR, even in cases where the platform involves more comprehensive data beyond the traditional patient health record. The Practical Playbook has defined the EHR as *EMR with the information exchange of other systems for longitudinal patient data access from across various* providers.[35]

Likewise, in the case of chronic disease, information provided from EHR data can be utilized to develop knowledge in the form of a community level snapshot of health trends within populations. At this level, a greater systems awareness and approach to geo-graphically specific chronic disease care is the objective, fully keeping in mind the ultimate goal of improved patient-centered outcomes.

Data Standards for EHR

With the advancement of health technol-ogy, various types of public health reporting and electronic innovations are taking place. According to the ONC for HIT, the trend in public health is moving from traditional paper health reports (such as lab reporting and man-ual data recording and abstraction) to uni-directional health data from patient EHR to registries and systems, generally for reportable conditions surveillance. From there, techno-logical advancement is allowing for bidirec-tional health data exchanges to take place. With this capability, data will utilize transport standards (such as HL7, SNOMED-CT, and LOINC) to communicate between EHR and more specific registries and systems almost instantly.[36]

Originally designed for health insurance and patient billing, the most commonly used standard for storing, sharing, and commu-nicating clinical patient data within EHR is through HL7 standards. Other commonly used standards for patient data for communi-cating information such as diagnoses, clinical and laboratory data include ICD-10, LOINC, and SNOMED-CT (**TABLE 10-2**).

EHR Data for Chronic Disease

EHR data for chronic disease can involve a variety of data components form a patient's medical record, as well as additional demo-graphic and environmental data to develop a community and neighborhood-level snap-shot for data visualization and analysis. For the purpose of chronic diseases such as type 2 diabetes, clinical data such as BMI and HbA1c are collected from the patient's record. Addi-tionally, for the purposes of surveillance for chronic disease prevention, data from *all* clin-ical patients (including the undiagnosed) are

TABLE 10-2 Common Standards for Storage, Sharing, and Communication of Patient Data

Data Standard	Description/Purpose
HL7	Health Level Seven. Managed by Health Level Seven International. Originally designed for health insurance billing purposes, now the common standard for sharing clinical patient data.
ICD-10	International Classification of Diseases. Managed by the National Center for Health Statistics (NCHS) in the United States. The 10th is the most recent update. Comprehensive index of clinical diagnosis codes.
LOINC	Logical Observation Identifiers Names and Codes. Managed by the Regenstrief Institute. Used to standardize laboratory data, provides the request for laboratory testing ("the question") transmitted through HL7 messages.
SNOMED-CT	Systematized Nomenclature of Medicine—Clinical Terms. Managed by IHTSDO. Used to standardize laboratory data, provides the result of laboratory testing ("the answer").

TABLE 10-3 HL7 Messages Relevant to Chronic Disease Surveillance

HL7 Message Name	Description of Message	HL7 Segment Name	Description of Segment
ADT	Admissions Discharge Transfer	PID	Patient Identification (and demographic information)
		PV1	Patient Visit
		PV2	Patient Visit: Additional Information
		OBX	Observation (and results)
ORU	Order Result Message	OBX	Observation (and results)
		OBR	Observation Request
PPR	Patient Problem Message	PRB	Problem Details
		DG1	Diagnosis

Data from Corepoint Health, (n.d.-a); Health Level Seven (2007).

required in order to identify patients at risk of these diseases (**TABLE 10-3**).

HL7 data are developed in a highly structured format composed of approximately 200 different messages and a similar number of segments. In working with HL7 for chronic disease surveillance, useful data in the HL7 data are located in the Admission, Discharge, and Transfer (ADT), unsolicited transmission of an observation (ORU), and patient problem message (PPR) messages. Most relevant data is likely to exist in the ADT message of clinical data which document details of the patient's counter and reason for visiting in addition to basic vital details such as blood pressure, height, weight, date of birth, and address.

The Patient ID (PID) segment of the HL7 message contains patient identification and demographic information, such as medical record number, name, sex, date of birth, marital status, citizenship, and home address.[37]

▶ IV. HL7 Message Examples

The following are examples of HL7 messages relevant to chronic disease and diabetes.

HL7 Message Example of a Patient with Heart Disease[38,39]

MSH|^~\&||NEFACIL^1234567890^NPI||SSEDON|201102091114||ADT^A01^ADT_A01|201102091114-0078|P|2.5 EVN||201102181114|||||NEFACIL^1234567890^NPI
PID|1||20060012168^^^^MR||~^^^^^S

```
||19500923|F||U^^CDCREC|^^^^65101
|||||||||U^^CDCREC|||||||N PV1||I||||||||||||||||
20110217_0064^^^^VN|||||||||||||||||||||||||20110
217144208PV2|||^SOB,TIGHTNESSINCHEST
OBX|1|TX|18684-1^BLOOD PRESSURE^LN
||165/127|mmHG^F^UCUM|||||
F|||20110217145658
DG1|1||58258-5^MYOCARDIAL
INFARCTION^LN||20110217163455|F
PR1|1||36.91^Repair of aneurysm of coronary
vessel^I9CP|201102171600
```

In the heart disease example above, the patient's first visit (PV1) included very little information about the initial visit, which took place on 2/17/2011. During the second visit (PV2) on 2/17/2011, a hypertensive-level blood pressure measurement of 165/127 was recorded, and a diagnosis (DG1) of myocardial infarction was reported, with the repair of the coronary vessel taking place.

HL7 Message Example of a Patient with a Prediabetic Glucose Reading[40]

```
MSH|^~\&|GHH LAB|ELAB-3|GHH OE|
BLDG4|200202150930||ORU^R01|
CNTRL-3456|P|2.4<cr>
    PID|||555-44-4444||EVERYWOM-
AN^EVE^E^^^^L|JONES|19620320|F|||153
FERNWOOD DR.^
    ^STATESVILLE
^OH^35292||(206)3345232|(206)752-
121||||AC555444444||67-
A4335^OH^20030520<cr>
    OBR|1|845439^GHH OE|1045813^GHH
LAB|15545^GLUCOSE|||200202150730|||||||||
    555-55-5555^PRIMARY^PATRICIA
P^^^^MD^^|||||||||F||||||444-44-4444^HIP-
POCRATES^HOWARD H^^^^MD<cr>
    OBX|1|SN|1554-5^GLU-
COSE^POST 12H CFST:MCNC:PT:SER/
PLAS:QN||^182|mg/dl|70_105|H|||F<cr>
```

In the above example, a request (OBR) for a glucose reading was made on 2/15/2002. The pre-glucose reading (OBX) was conducted after the patient fasted for 12 hours before the reading was taken. The glucose level was read at 182 mg/dl, in the prediabetic range.

▶ V. Relevant Data Elements for Chronic Disease Surveillance of Prediabetes and Hypertension

In the selection of required data elements for the design of chronic disease surveillance of prediabetes and hypertension, the following data elements were identified.

Demographic Information

Patient demographic information in the form of patient ID (patient clinical or insurance member number in this case), date of birth, sex, race, ethnicity, and address were of relevance. Public health is able to request this information from clinics (which does not face the same academic or clinical restrictions), particularly when protected health information (PHI) is necessary to conduct public health work.[41,42] In the case of chronic disease surveillance, the relevance of a patient identifier/member number is necessary in order to de-duplicate patient data, for example, if the patient has sought treatment at several clinics or hospitals. Additionally, patient address data is relevant in mapping as well as analyzing data on the prevalence of chronic disease at the neighborhood level in the design of public health prevention and intervention programs. Also, it is relevant to note that comorbid chronic and heart disease risk factors such as hypertension and diagnoses may exist with patient conditions, and data elements for several conditions may be required[43,44] (**FIGURE 10-2**).

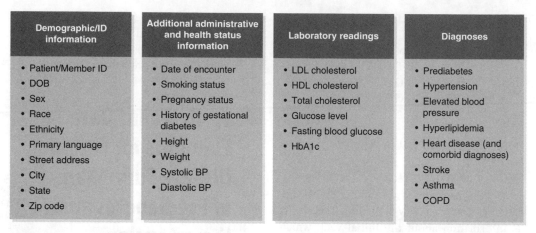

Demographic/ID information	Additional administrative and health status information	Laboratory readings	Diagnoses
• Patient/Member ID • DOB • Sex • Race • Ethnicity • Primary language • Street address • City • State • Zip code	• Date of encounter • Smoking status • Pregnancy status • History of gestational diabetes • Height • Weight • Systolic BP • Diastolic BP	• LDL cholesterol • HDL cholesterol • Total cholesterol • Glucose level • Fasting blood glucose • HbA1c	• Prediabetes • Hypertension • Elevated blood pressure • Hyperlipidemia • Heart disease (and comorbid diagnoses) • Stroke • Asthma • COPD

FIGURE 10-2 Example list of relevant data elements from HL7 queries for chronic disease surveillance.

Health Informatics in the Context of Chronic Disease Surveillance

Currently, very few public health agencies have been involved in chronic disease surveillance activities due in large part to funding priorities for health agencies, where surveillance of reportable communicable diseases such as Zika and infectious diseases such as antibiotic-resistant bacterial infections are understandably of importance. Nonetheless, understanding the need to curb the current obesity epidemic requires strategies in support of chronic disease prevention for diseases often associated with obesity such as heart disease, stroke, and type 2 diabetes.

Chronic disease surveillance of risk factors such as prediabetes is different from infectious or communicable disease surveillance for a few reasons. Surveillance for chronic diseases such as diabetes is not of urgent importance when compared to emerging infectious and communicable diseases, and allows time to query patient data on a periodic basis as well as data analysis and the design of intervention programs.[45] Additionally, surveillance for chronic disease prevention requires data from undiagnosed patients (non-cases). Although the concept of surveillance of non-cases is currently uncommon, the CDC has defined public health surveillance as referring to collecting, analyzing, and using data for the goal of public health prevention, which does meet this process.[46]

▶ VI. Conclusion

While population health focuses on more targeted approaches to individual care within specific populations, public health is focused on the *promoting healthy lifestyles* and research to prevent, detect, and control diseases in a geographic region. The core functions of public health can be identified as assessment, policy development, and assurance. The emergent developments of technology in health care, combined with the established need for EHR have called for public health informatics professionals to conduct this work. But this cannot be done without the collaboration of clinical and other sectors. Much public health electronic information comes from clinicians sharing patient data with agencies for the improvement of population and public health. Public health surveillance is both responsive, in tracking reportable conditions from clinics, and is also proactive, where much of the work of prevention and control of diseases takes place through community health education programs and outreach, working with community members who may either be diagnosed with disease, but working also with those who are healthy.

Notes

1. *AHIMA, PHDSC Unite to Strengthen Public Health Data Standards.* (2018, October). Retrieved from www.phdsc.org/about/pdfs/AHIMA-PHDSC_%20 Press_Release_10022014.pdf

2. *Ibid.*

3. *Ibid.*

4. APHA. (2017). *What is public health?* Retrieved from https://www.apha.org/what-is-public-health

5. CDC Foundation. (2017). *What is public health?* Retrieved from www.cdcfoundation.org/content/what -public-health

6. *Ibid.*

7. CDC. (2014, May 29). *The public health system and the 10 essential public health services.* Retrieved from www.cdc.gov/nphpsp/essentialservices.html

8. *Ibid.*

9. Ogilvie, D., Craig, P., MacIntyre, S., & Wareeham, N. (n.d.). A translational framework for public health research. *BMC Public Health, 2009*(9), 116.

10. APHA. (2017).

11. Centers for Disease Control and Prevention. (2017, March 16). *Global public health informatics program.* Retrieved from www.cdc.gov/globalhealth /healthprotection/gphi/index.html

12. Hoyt, R. E., Yoshihashi, A., & Bailey, N. (Eds). (2012). *Health informatics: Practical guide for healthcare and information technology professionals* (5th ed.). Retrieved from www.lulu.com/us/en/shop/robert -e-hoyt-and-ann-k-yoshihashi/health-informatics -practical-guide-for-healthcare-and-information -technology-professionals-sixth-edition/paperback /product-21723648.html

13. Savel, T. G., & Foldy, S. (2012). The role of public health informatics in enhancing public health surveillance. *Morbidity and Mortality Weekly Report, 61*(03), 20–24.

14. Aamodt, A., & Nygard, M. (1995). Different roles and mutual dependencies of data, information, and knowledge—An AI perspective on their integration. *Data & Knoweldge Engineering, 163*(2), 191–222.

15. Chen, M., Ebert, D., Hagen, H., Laramee, R. S., Van Liere, R., Ma, K. L., & Silver, D. (2009). Data, information, and knowledge in visualization. *Computer Graphics and Applications, IEEE, 29*(1), 12–19.

16. Zins, C. (2007). Conceptual approaches for defining data, information, and knowledge. *Journal of the American Society for Information Science and Technology, 58*(4), 479–493.

17. LaVenture, M., Brand, B., & Zeleznak, K. (2005). *Diagram of an informatics-savvy organization (Adapted).* Bloomington, IN: Bloomington Division of Public Health.

18. RESOLVE. (2014, May). The high achieving governmental health department in 2020 as the community chief health strategist—The-High -Achieving-Governmental-Health-Department -as-the-Chief-Health-Strategist-by-2020 -Final1.pdf. Retrieved from www.resolv.org/site -healthleadershipforum/files/2014/05/The-High -Achieving-Governmental-Health-Department-as -the-Chief-Health-Strategist-by-2020-Final1.pdf

19. Magnuson, J. A., & Fu, P. C. (2014). *Public health informatics and information systems—Springer.* Retrieved from http://link.springer.com.ccl.idm.oclc .org/book/10.1007%2F978-1-4471-4237-9

20. RESOLVE. (2014). The High Achieving Governmental Health Department in 2020 as the Community Chief Health Strategist. Retrieved from www.resolv .org/site-healthleadershipforum/files/2014/05/The -High-Achieving-Governmental-Health -Department-as-the-Chief-Health-Strategist-by -2020-Final1.pdff Health Strategist

21. World Health Organization. (2017). *Engaging stakeholders.* Retrieved from www.who.int/national policies/processes/stakeholders/en/

22. Koplan, J., Bond, T., Merson, M., Reddy, K., Rodriguez, M., Sewankambo, N., & Wasserheit, J. (2009). Towards a common definition of global health. *The Lancet, 373*, 1993–1995.

23. World Health Organization. (2017). *About WHO.* Retrieved from http://www.who.int/about/en/

24. United Nations Foundation. (2013). *What we do: Global health.* Retrieved from www.unfoundation .org/what-we-do/issues/global-health/

25. Centers for Disease Control and Prevention. (2017). *Global public health informatics program.* Retrieved from www.cdc.gov/globalhealth/healthprotection /gphi/index.html

26. American Medical Informatics Association. (2017). *Global health informatics working group.* Retrieved from www.amia.org/programs/working-groups/global -health-informatics

27. Castillo-Salgado, C. (2010). Trends and directions of global public health surveillance. *Epidemiologic Reviews, 32*, 93–109.

28. World Health Organization. (n.d.). *Global surveillance of Epidemic-prone infectious disease.* Retrieved from www .who.int/csr/resources/publications/introduction /en/index4.html

29. The Office of the National Coordinator for Health IT. (2014). *Health IT for public health reporting and information systems.* Retrieved from www.healthit.gov /sites/default/files/phissuebrief04-24-14.pdf

30. County of Los Angeles, Department of Public Health. Los Angeles County Participant Reporting System (LACPRS) and SAGE. Retrieved from publichealth.lacounty.gov/sapc/NetworkProviders /pm/100517/ProviderMeeting100517LACPRS.pdf

31. Hopkins, R. S., & Magnuson, J. A. (2014). *Informatics in disease prevention and epidemiology* (in Magnusson, JA and Fu, PC Public Health Informatics and Information Systems). London: Springer-Verlag.
32. Thacker, S. B., Qualters, J. R., & Lee, L. M. (2012). Public health surveillance in the United States: Evolution and challenges. *MMWR, 61*(3), 3–9.
33. Gliklich, R., Dreyer, N., & Leavy, M. (2014). *Registries for evaluating patient outcomes: A user's guide [Internet]* (3rd ed.). Retrieved from www.ncbi.nlm.nih.gov/books/NBK208625/
34. Office of the National Coordinator for Health Information Technology. (2011, January 4). *EMR vs EHR—What is the Difference?* Retrieved from https://www.healthit.gov/buzz-blog/electronic-health-and-medical-records/emr-vs-ehr-difference/
35. The Practical Playbook. (2016, January 18). *Using electronic health records for population health.* de Beaumont Foundation. Retrieved from www.debeaumont.org/programs/practical-playbook/
36. Office of the National Coordinator for Health IT. (2014). *Health IT for public health reporting and information systems.* Retrieved from www.healthit.gov/sites/default/files/phissuebrief04-24-14.pdf
37. Corepoint Health. (n.d.). *HL7 PID (Patient Identification) segment.* Retrieved from http://corepointhealth.com/resource-center/hl7-resources/hl7-pid-segment
38. Corepoint Health. (n.d.). *HL7 ORU - HL7 result message (Observation Result).* Retrieved from http://corepointhealth.com/resource-center/hl7-resources/hl7-oru-message
39. Syndromic Surveillance Event Detection of Nebraska (SSEDON). (2011). *HL7 Implementation guide—Inpatient syndromic surveillance.* Retrieved from http://dhhs.ne.gov/publichealth/EPI/Documents/SSEDON%20HL7%20Inpatient%20Surveillance%20Implementation%20Guide.pdf
40. Ringholm, B. V. (2007). *HL7 message examples: Version 2 and Version 3.* Retrieved from www.ringholm.com/docs/04300_en.htm
41. Thacker, S. B. (2003, April 11). *HIPAA privacy rule and public health : Guidance from CDC and the U.S. Department of Health and Human Services.* Retrieved from www.cdc.gov/mmwr/preview/mmwrhtml/m2e411a1.htm
42. U.S. Department of Health and Human Services. (2003, April 3). *Health information privacy: Public health.* Retrieved from www.hhs.gov/hipaa/for-professionals/special-topics/public-health/index.html
43. Robbins, J. M., Webb, D. A., & Sciamanna, C. N. (2005). Cardiovascular comorbidities among public health clinic patients with diabetes: The urban diabetics study. *BMC Public Health, 5*(15), 9.
44. Sowers, J. R., Epstein, M., & Frohlich, E. D. (2001). Diabetes, hypertension, and cardiovasuclar disease—An update. *Hypertension, 37*, 1053–1059.
45. Thacker, S. B., Qualters, J. R., Lee, L. M., & Centers for Disease Control and Prevention. (2012). Public health surveillance in the United States: Evolution and challenges. *MMWR, 61*(3), 3–9.
46. Centers for Disease Control. (2015, October 21). *Surveillance resource center.* Retrieved from www.cdc.gov/surveillancepractice

Chapter Questions

10-1 Briefly describe the difference between data, information, and knowledge and provide examples of each.

10-2 What is the distinct role of informatics in public health? For example, how and why is it distinguishable from clinical informatics?

10-3 How would you describe the difference between public and population health?

10-4 What are some of the common data frameworks for electronic health data and what are their purposes?

Biography

April Moreno Arellano is a postdoctoral researcher at UC San Diego Department of Biomedical Informatics. Dr. Moreno Arellano received her PhD in Health Promotion Science/Information Systems and Technology from the Claremont Colleges—Claremont Graduate University in Los Angeles, CA. She earned a master's degree in Public Administration from California State University Northridge in Public Sector Leadership and Management. Her research interests include health technology, public and population health, health equity, and user-centered design.

CHAPTER 11

Health IS/IT Project Implementation, Innovation Procurement, and Services Management

Joseph Tan with Phillip Olla and Joshia Tan

LEARNING OBJECTIVES

- Define critical success factors (CSFs) for health IS/IT implementation
- Understand the strategic planning and management issues
- Explore and illustrate systems implementation phases concepts
- Review IT services management concepts
- Understand the innovation procurement concept
- Review different innovation procurement models and their benefits

CHAPTER OUTLINE

Scenario: Wellcentive— Philips Population Health Management Solution[1]

In July 2016, Royal Philips, Amsterdam, the Netherlands, announced the acquisition of Wellcentive to expand its existing population health management services. Philips' existing portfolio in population health services include tele-medical services, personal emergency response systems (PERS), home monitoring, and general prevention and personal health programs for various groups within a targeted population to intensive ambulatory care for high-risk patients within the said population. Appointing Tom Zajac, then CEO of Wellcentive, to lead this business group, Philips' CEO Jeroen Tas notes:

> With this strategic acquisition, we will strengthen our Population Health Management business and its leadership, as health systems gradually shift from volume to value-based care, and provide more preventive and chronic care services outside of the hospital….Our sweet spot is at the point of care as we give consumers, patients, care teams and clinicians the tools, such as remote monitoring solutions and therapy devices, to optimize care. Wellcentive's solutions will provide our customers with the ability to collect data from large populations, detect patterns, assess risks and then

deploy care programs tailored to the needs of specific groups.[2]

Philips Wellcentive population health management software application aims to aid providers in changing the way health care is delivered, improving the use of data, and enhancing patient outcomes, especially for organizations having to shift to value-based care. In noting that Wellcentive has, over the past 11 years, successfully offered care management for over 30 million patients by focusing on "data-driven clinical, financial, and human outcomes" for their customers, Tom Zajac further asserts: "Combining forces with Philips and its broad portfolio of health technologies and global reach will create a great foundation to accelerate growth in connected care—from healthy living and prevention, to diagnosis, treatment and home care—enabling consumers, providers and health organizations to benefit from our combined, stronger offering in population health management."[3]

Imagine you are asked to go into competition with the Philips Wellcentive initiative and have been commissioned to provide a vision and a plan on the development of an innovative suite of next-generation software that would support key population health management needs, community health promotional and health preventive programs, as well as information sharing and shared patient–caregiver decision-making. Describe your vision, plan, and any future-oriented software functionalities that you would envision for aiding future healthcare providers and consumers on a global basis. Discuss and describe the different data analytics that you would like to see incorporated, how you would go about rolling out your vision, and the type of innovations that you would like to see harvested in your new software offering.

▶ I. Introduction

Health information systems/information technology (IS/IT) project implementation in health systems organizations entails a process whose success is dependent on the fulfillment of a number of key activities. These may include project planning, a thorough preliminary conception and initiation, broad and detailed project definition and planning, project launch or execution, project performance and control, and project closure. Health IS/IT project managers and analysts are among the best people overseeing such projects due to the project management skills that are needed to ensure a well-managed project that is completed on time and within budget. Another concept that is being explored among some healthcare organizations and governments is

innovation procurement. This approach allows healthcare organizations to explore partnering with vendors to procure innovation that does not currently exist on the market.

In practice, certain critical factors can influence the success of health IT implementation. For example, two broad areas have played key roles: (1) the application of well-tested guidelines and standard protocols and (2) the enforcement of ethical and legal concerns. Our focus here is on the health IT implementation process; some of these factors and challenges are addressed in Chapter 12 and the accompanying policy review (Policy Review III) on standards, both of which are provided in Part IV of this text. **FIGURE 11-1** shows that once health IT planning is fine-tuned to address success factors for health IT implementation, on the one hand, and organizational planning and management considerations, on the other, the actual steps including specific activities for health IT implementation can be specified, directed, monitored, and controlled by project planning and management directives.

This chapter highlights the steps necessary to achieve health IT implementation success within a health systems organizational

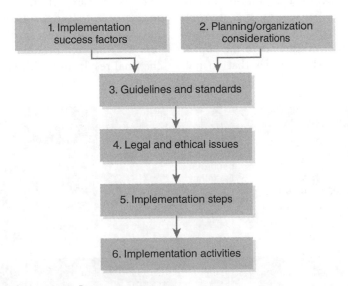

FIGURE 11-1 The implementation Process.

setting. It draws from previous parts of the book, in particular Chapters 8–10, to show how health IT implementation is no more than an outgrowth of strategic planning, decision aiding, and predictive systems development and public health informatics. Even so, with the growing complexity of health IT applications and the increased investments placed on health IT projects, all (or most) health systems organizations today require that success be a prime criterion in any health IT implementation effort. We begin with a look at the CSFs underscoring health IT implementation.

▶ II. Critical Success Factors for Health IT Implementation

Many critical factors have been found to affect the success of health IT implementation in health systems organizations. Top management should focus undue attention on these CSFs before any major health IT implementation exercise is undertaken. Generally, management should position the organization for health IT adoption. More particularly, management must pay special attention to those factors that are likely barriers or constraints to the implementation process. Minor issues that do not warrant top management consideration can be delegated to middle managers, who can oversee these issues or control them with inputs from top management on an ad hoc basis during the actual implementation. However, there may be times when minor issues are truly major issues in disguise, and if so, these should then be flagged for top management intervention.

In general, the CSFs for health IT implementation fall into one of three broad categories: user characteristics, systems design characteristics, and organizational characteristics. **FIGURE 11-2** shows specific examples of factors from each of the three categories that contribute to successful or unsuccessful health IT implementation.

User Characteristics

Among the factors believed to influence health IT success, user characteristics (i.e., the "people problem") are by far the most extensively studied.[4,5] Examples include individual differences, such as learning style, cognitive behavior, user attitudes, and user expectations of what the health IT can do for them.

Health IT implementation often carries with its great expectations. It is not unusual, for instance, to find that many end-users who have little or no direct involvement with system development become disappointed with the final results of health IT implementation

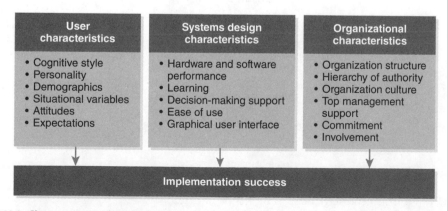

FIGURE 11-2 Characteristics of implementation Success Factors.

because the end-product does not match their expectations. Indeed, the argument that health IT applications are a "mirage" is familiar.[6] Clearly, the health IT solutions are not a panacea, in and of themselves, but the health IT, if developed properly, will certainly help managers make better choices as well as speed up processes that were previously handled manually. Adopting an attitude that health IT applications are the ends and not the means sets up impossible goals and expectations that can only result in unfulfilled expectations. Consequently, this is another reason to involve personnel from across all organizational units in health IT planning and implementation right from the beginning. In so doing, we can generate positive attitudes and feelings among end-users, with realistic expectations that can only enhance successful health IT implementation. Further, the adoption of a comprehensive user education program can serve to increase the likelihood of meeting operational objectives sought in initial health IT planning.

Among various personal reactions to health IT, resistance is the most destructive behavior related to health IT implementation. Dickson and Simmons noted five factors relating to resistance.[7] First, the greater operating efficiency of health IT often implies a change in departmental or divisional boundaries and a high potential to eliminate duplicating functions. This can create a sense of fear of job loss among operational and clerical workers. Second, health IT can affect the informal organizational structure as much as the formal one by creating behavioral disturbances, such as doing away with informal interactions. Third, whether individuals will react favorably to health IT implementation depends on their overall personalities (e.g., younger, inexperienced workers are less likely to resist than older, more experienced ones) and cultural background (e.g., the replacement of interpersonal contacts with human–computer interface). Fourth, the presence of peer pressure and previous experiences with health IT

implementation can also influence the organizational climate for success. Finally, the management techniques used to implement health IT (e.g., the use of project planning and scheduling methodologies) directly affect user perception of the system.

The recognition of potential dysfunctional user behaviors is a first step toward successful health IT implementation. User orientation, training, education, and participation are ways to minimize the behavioral problems that may follow the introduction of health IT in health systems organizations.

Systems Design Characteristics

Aside from user characteristics, systems design characteristics also play an important role in determining the eventual health IT acceptability. Examples here include hardware–software performance, the characteristics of information and decision-making support provided to the user, and systems interface characteristics, such as the availability or incorporation of easy-to-use and easy-to-learn features into the health IT.

The essential ingredients of any computer-based health IT are the hardware, software, firmware, and middleware. Common sense dictates that configuration of wares be applicable to the organizational performance and strategies. For an organization's information needs to be satisfied from a systems design perspective, they need to be articulated and documented during the early planning stages and acted upon using tailored implementation techniques. Further, the reliability of hardware, software, and middleware is critical to health IT performance. It is important to acknowledge, for example, that most information needs demand a certain amount of flexibility, notwithstanding the needs for completeness, accuracy, validity, reliability, frequency, and currency (timeliness) of information to be supplied to the user.[8] Flexibility necessitates an ability to cope with growth and variability in an ever-changing healthcare services environment.

Systems interface is a subject that could fill an entire chapter of its own and has been briefly discussed in previous editions of this text. To relate this topic to health IT implementation, examples are provided. First, health IT should be designed in the way end-users such as nurses organize themselves. For example, many nurses organize their thoughts about patients by using patient room numbers as a constant frame of reference.[9] Inevitably, when a dietetics system in a hospital uses the alphabet as an organizing scheme, the systems interface becomes inadequate to support the nurses in performing their routines. This has happened in real life, where a group of nurses and clerks who were exposed to the system complained about the time it took to enter diet orders and changes into the health IT. They became less efficient and increasingly anxious, frustrated, and dissatisfied with the system. The result was to abandon the system unless software would be redesigned to follow through with the patient room number organizing scheme.

Second, health IT interface design should incorporate favorable factors, such as the proper use of graphics and color.[10] One patient registration system used bright primary colors that were "hard on the eyes" and thus distracting during prolonged use. The system also produced graphics that were difficult to read and interpret. The system was almost abandoned until it was discovered that both the graphics and colors were changeable.

Third, the design of health IT should consider the users' previous knowledge. For instance, in a long-term care facility, nurses who, for years, had used large desktop screens to register new patient information have found the smaller screen-size bedside monitoring and tracking system extremely cumbersome for entering this information. In that case, the incorporation of a coded identification bracelet placed around the wrists of the patients along with an automated remote scanning device resolved the problem. Nurses quickly embraced the new bedside tracking system in place of the old desktop system.

These cases illustrate the significance of human–computer interface in health IT implementation success.

Organizational Characteristics

Organizational characteristics can also influence health IT implementation success. Examples of variables include organizational structure and power, organizational culture, and other managerial factors, such as top management support, commitment, and involvement.

One of the key areas affecting implementation success is the influence of top management. Exercising sound project control, resolving issues in a timely manner, allocating resources accurately, and avoiding short-lived changes or features additions in critical areas at the last minutes (sometimes known as *scope creeps*) are all serious management considerations.[11] The strategic alignment of corporate health IT planning and the application of proper project planning and scheduling can together serve to prevent costly delays in health IT implementation. Such an alignment also ensures that the organization is not forced into a reactive as opposed to a proactive role.[12] Here, a proactive strategy anticipates industry trends and instills innovative processes for competitive advantages and operational efficiencies, whereas a reactive strategy takes into account current industry trends and chooses to adopt a known process developed elsewhere.

Key strategies to achieve successful health IT implementation include a realistic situational assessment (or environmental scanning), accurate identification of necessary resources, and development of an action plan.[13] It is therefore critical to encourage top management involvement in many areas, and there should be a chief information officer or chief technology officer (CIO or CTO) or another knowledgeable senior member such as a chief knowledge officer or chief digital officer (CKO or CDO) of the management team taking charge of health IT implementation.

Health IT implementation in health systems organizations is no different than in business organizations. The degree of commitment and involvement of all end-users and especially the support, commitment, and involvement of top management affect long-term success. All users need to invest their energy in health IT planning and implementation in order to create a system that is going to be accepted and adopted. Top managers in particular must provide support and act as role models to their subordinates. Potential heavy users, such as middle managers, physicians, nurses, and support staff, also need to be committed and involved in the health IT implementation process in order to improve the likelihood of its long-term success.[14,15] In short, health IT success requires inputs that come directly from all users, not just systems professionals.

▶ III. Strategic Planning and Management Issues

Our analysis of CSFs for health IT implementation reveals a number of critical considerations involved in health IT planning and management. Often, careful attention to these details in the early planning stages can facilitate the creation of strategies that will enhance health IT success.

FIGURE 11-3 shows the various types of planning and management issues that will influence the process and the strategy chosen to optimize health IT implementation for health systems organizations. The key issues to be addressed are staffing issues, organizational project management, reengineering considerations, end-user involvement, and vendor involvement, as well as other additional considerations.

Staffing Issues

Health IT staffing issues can be addressed by first simply asking the question: "Do we have the adequate human resources and health IT expertise to carry out a successful implementation project?" The answer to this question was articulated in previous discussions, which essentially advocate the use of an internal audit of the current health IT staffing situation.

For new organizations, health IT development is relatively straightforward; that is, all individuals with the needed skills are simply to be recruited externally. However, once beyond that, it is a more complicated process. It becomes necessary to identify potential knowledge gaps in health IT staff that need to be filled. The following are more specific questions that need to be answered.

■   Are the current staff members already working at capacity?

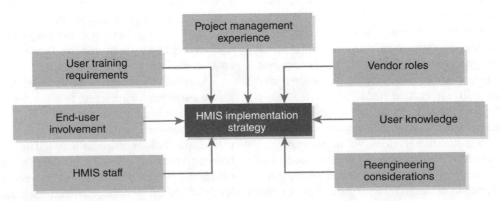

FIGURE 11-3 Planning and Management Issues.

- What level of knowledge and skills does the current staff have, and how does this affect recruitment and training?
- How many new staff members will be needed, and when will they be needed?

The answers to these questions enable the planning of staffing strategies to be layered into a health IT implementation plan. It is critical that these considerations be addressed so that arrangements can be made well in advance to hire the necessary staff or to plan for the needed training. For instance, carrying through with an implementation schedule requires data on the availability of staff members with health IT expertise for certain periods. Conversely, the training of staff members and the scheduling of recruitment depend on the overall implementation schedule. Clearly, a lack of needed expertise among existing personnel can slow the process of health IT implementation, often leading to increased pressure and frustration among the existing staff members and possibly resulting in missed opportunities associated with on-time and "seamless" project completion. A projection of future staffing needs is also warranted if the project has a long-term focus.

Although the staffing issues can be resolved at the health IT implementation stage, management of health systems organizations must establish clear reward policies to encourage the retention of experienced staff members. Gray documented that the demand for new systems personnel of all types grows at a rate of 15% per year, whereas the turnover of information systems personnel averages about 20% per year.[16] Reducing this high turnover rate can immediately improve productivity and reduce operation costs.

To reward good technical health IT personnel, health organizations can use a *dual career path* or a *professional stage model*.[17-20] In the former, a pathway of promotions in the technical level is created to parallel the managerial path in rank and salary. For example, a technical staff member would be promoted from programmer to systems analyst, then to systems specialist, and finally to senior analyst and technical expert/mentor. In the latter, the path for promotions can be from apprentice to colleague to mentor to project sponsor.[21] Both models provide significant incentives for the return of experienced staff members past the initial stage of health IT implementation, thereby sowing the seed for long-term success.

After examining various staffing issues at the system level, an important issue at the individual level—user knowledge—must be briefly examined. Health IT implementation in health systems organizations requires an assessment of in-house systems and expert knowledge. This assessment should take into account future user needs. Together with staffing needs assessments, management can ascertain the educational requirements of the organization. By doing so, the organization also avoids heavily diverting its resources to educating and training users during and after the online implementation. Thus, educational planning—including general training for managers, technical training for health IT professionals, and specific end-user training to satisfy the needs of various user groups—helps ensure a smooth and timely health IT implementation.[22]

Numerous difficulties, both expected and unexpected, associated with the initial 3 months of online operations can be prevented through proper orientation and health IT staffing and training. In certain cases, this responsibility can even be off-loaded to software vendors. This approach may be particularly desirable for "turnkey" systems prepackaged and serviced by a single vendor. However, the costs in the long run can be significant.

Alternatively, if the organizational structure is capable of supporting this role with an internal training department and knowledgeable personnel, it may be more cost-effective to provide the staff education in-house. If in-house training is to be conducted, the training personnel should be able to distinguish between two levels of training—holistic training and technical training. *Holistic* (or *ideological*) *training* here refers to training modules focused on the systems, and not the operational, perspective. Systems goals and benefits, systems constraints and limitations, organizational effects, and functional implications are sample topics for this level of training. In short, holistic training intends to bring the entire system into view and to analyze its relationship with its surrounding elements (the macro view). This kind of training should be directed primarily to managerial staff, who need to view health IT in its entirety, and secondarily to operational staff, who are more concerned with the day-to-day operations (the micro view).

Technical (or *operational*) *training* is aimed at familiarizing the appropriate personnel with the operational aspects of health IT that pertain to their tasks. This level of training may encapsulate such topics as completing forms, report abstracting, data-coding standards, data validation, standard data input or update procedures, and introduction of routine tasks. This kind of training is directed primarily to technical or operational staff, who are concerned with daily use of health IT, and secondarily to managerial staff, who also need to know the procedures of their subordinates.

In any event, it should be recognized that the use of a team approach in-house has the added benefit of increasing user acceptance and reducing resistance in the long run. Regardless of how a health systems organization is planning to conduct the needed staff training, the quality of the training should be emphasized, because well-managed training for health IT operations has the potential to reduce anxiety and potential user resistance and to promote an organizational climate toward health IT implementation success.

Organizational Project Management

The style of project management is extremely dependent on the organizational culture and on the depth of experienced personnel who are available to manage such a process. In many instances, experienced project managers with both technical and application knowledge are difficult to find. Consequently, outside consultants are often used. However, time is needed to educate these consultants on specific situational and historical characteristics, both internally and externally, that can at times be significant enough to make outside consultation counterproductive. As within the health systems organization, there is often a trade-off. Although team or committee management of the implementation process provides the benefits of internal knowledge, user acceptance, and overall effectiveness of implementation,[23] the need for a fresh look from an external, unbiased perspective should not be overlooked.

Although it is difficult to make specific recommendations with respect to health IT implementation, certain techniques are useful in project management. Here, a brief examination is given to some of the commonly used techniques for project scheduling and program coding. To ensure that the system implementation is completed by a certain date, a detailed and realistic schedule needs to be prepared and followed at the initial and subsequent planning stages. At the same time, the schedule should be flexible enough to accommodate some unexpected delays. Moreover, a detailed timetable for implementation is often essential to inspire management confidence in the installation plan. Here, two techniques to assist project scheduling are discussed—the critical path method (CPM) and Gantt charts.

When using the CPM, the duration of all the tasks involved and the sequence (indicated by arrows) of all tasks need to be compiled in a network representation, as shown in **FIGURE 11-4**. In the figure, the numbers in circles represent different stages of implementation, the letters represent different tasks involved, and the numbers beside the letters represent the number of days needed to complete the task.

After translating the implementation schedule into a network representation, the

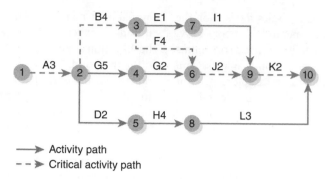

— Activity path
- - - Critical activity path

FIGURE 11-4 A Health IT Implementation Schedule in a Network Representation for the Critical Path Determination.

Note: Letter–numbered pairs represent the name of the path and the amount of time (in days) it takes to travel it. For example, "A3" indicates that path A takes 3 days.

Path	Days required
A → B → E → I → K	11
A → B → F → J → K	15
A → C → G → J → K	14
A → D → H → L	12

FIGURE 11-5 Possible Paths through the Critical Path Network in Figure 11-4.

critical path of the network can then be determined. The critical path is the sequence of activities that will take the longest period to complete. The time needed to complete all the activities on this critical path is the minimum period required to complete the entire project. **FIGURE 11-5** lists all the possible paths (activities in sequence) and the time needed to complete each. In this example, the path through activities A-B-F-J-K is the longest, requiring 15 days for completion. This is therefore the critical path of the project. Briefly, the project cannot be completed in less than 15 days unless certain tasks are started early or shortened.

Another way of representing the details in Figures 11-4 and 11-5 is to use Gantt charts, which represent project tasks with bar charts. They are often easier to construct and understand than CPM but may capture and generate less information. **FIGURE 11-6** shows a Gantt

chart for the same project described. It is worth mentioning that the exact start and end dates of certain noncritical tasks can be moved without causing delay to the overall schedule. For instance, if every other task in Figure 11-5 commences and finishes on time, task L can be postponed for a day without delaying the final completion date.

Program coding, or simply *programming*, refers to the process of writing instructions that the computer system can execute directly. This is usually a very labor-intensive task, and as a result, coordination among programmers needs to be emphasized. Here, two useful coordination techniques—data dictionaries and walkthroughs—are introduced.

Data dictionaries, containing definitions and proper uses of entities that are in alphabetical order, can be computerized or manually compiled. Data dictionaries should also have the identities of database programs used; the names of all the data fields found in the database, along with the names of the programmers that use them; and descriptions of the data and the personnel responsible for the data. Just like regular dictionaries, data dictionaries are useful in program coding coordination, because they allow the names of data elements to be cross-referenced, help programmers rapidly locate blocks of codes that are reusable in new applications, and ensure that all codes are consistent with the overall application.

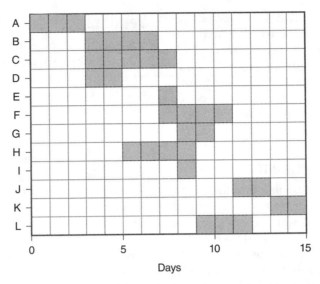

FIGURE 11-6 A Gantt Chart Representation of the Health IT Implementation Schedule in Figure 11-4.

Another very useful tool in program coding is conducting a *walkthrough* (or *review*). A walkthrough can take place at various stages of program design and development. It is essentially peer evaluation and testing of a programmer's work, with the primary objective of soliciting constructive feedback. In other words, walkthroughs act as control points in programming, making sure that what is programmed is in line with specific goals and objectives and other operational constraints. It is not in any way directed personally at the programmer.

Reengineering Considerations

Often when new health IT applications are implemented, work flows and processes may also change drastically because of the inherent differences of daily operations with the computerization. Even without the changes as a result of computerization, users may still find changes to daily operations as their tasks at work gradually change from time to time. Whereas adequate training initially helps better prepare end-users for some of these changes, end-user involvement in the reengineering process can greatly enhance satisfaction with computerization. This again relates to the importance of the "people aspect" in health IT.

To gain maximum benefit from health IT implementation, all operations must be redesigned periodically to accommodate environmental changes and maximize operational benefits, while still maintaining the necessary controls in the process. If the delivery systems are not reengineered to meet new organizational needs, the increase in efficiency brought about by the health IT implementation may be offset by the unmet demands in the environment.

Often, it is inefficient simply to automate old systems processes, because computerization lends itself to a new workflow, thus demanding extra personnel and resources. A good example of this is the attempt to automate patient charts to mimic paper-based systems currently in place. This document is primarily a legal document on paper, but once captured in health IT, it can become a much more versatile tool. Very often, health systems organizations are reluctant to rely totally on health IT and therefore opt to keep the paper copy for backup. Therefore, health professionals are required to continue filling out these forms manually, which essentially is a duplication of effort, thus creating an unnecessary workload.

To decide how health IT operations (or parts thereof) are to be reengineered, it is useful to solicit inputs from the staff already acquainted with existing procedures. Team or committee forums on system-supported group decision settings are excellent means to decide what should or should not be modified. This leads us to the topic of end-user involvement.

End-User Involvement

In health systems organizations, health IT planning and development are recognized to be slow compared with the rapid pace of change in the business world. However, lessons learned in the business sector have been found especially useful; one such lesson is the empowerment of end-users through their involvement in IT project planning and design.

Health IT planning and development require active (not passive) end-user involvement throughout the entire process in order for implementation to be truly successful. It has been recognized that unless health IT staff, physicians, and nurses are involved in systems planning and ongoing evaluation, health IT success will be short-lived.[24] In fact, in the health systems, which comprise a much broader group of individuals representing many technical and professional groups, it seems wise to extend this to users of all the different modules or areas of health IT. For this to materialize, adequate time and resources need to be allotted, and critical committees and internal and external liaisons have to be established such that all aspects of health IT can be optimized while generating organization-wide user acceptance.

Specific considerations with respect to acceptance of end-users include the effect of the change on the need satisfaction of the affected personnel, the position of those affected, and the leadership style of those managing the change. Further, direct involvement of application program vendors, which is the next topic of discussion, is often of critical importance.

Vendor Involvement

The traditional view that vendors specialize only in sales of equipment or computer software is fast giving way to the realities of the vendors of today. Although the primary function of computer systems vendors is and will continue to be the actual equipment sale, there is rapidly increasing emphasis on the sale of "services" beyond the realm of equipment maintenance. In the digital era, vendors can be—and in fact very often are—involved in some degree of technical support and servicing, including "Platform as a service" (PaaS); "infrastructure as a service" (IaaS); and "software as a service" (SaaS); and implementation, more specifically, health IT implementation. Cigna-Express Scripts, Amazon Cloud Services, and IBM Watson are prime examples of such vendors.

The options with respect to the roles of vendors vary between two extremes. Here, the term *vendor* usually refers only to software vendors because they dictate much of the implementation. However, the platform-network vendors are also important when considering outsourcing health IT services. On the one hand, there can be complete turnkey implementation by the software vendor (turnkey systems are prepackaged, ready-to-go application programs that are often products supplied by a single vendor). On the other hand, there is the option of exercising complete in-house organizational control. Between these extremes lies the most used option, a blend of vendor and organizational responsibilities, with each performing in areas of specialty to tailor the process to the needs of the health IT implementation.

Depending on the strengths of the organization and the vendor, areas of responsibility that can be shared include analyst support, project management, user training, hardware and facilities planning, software modification, interface development, conversion assistance, procedure development, and implementation audits. The means through which vendors can be involved vary from one organization to another. In some cases, a single vendor acts as the sole handling agent for all technical problems and even some user training; in others, several vendors may have to cooperate to deal with complex problems of the health systems organization.

Nevertheless, there are generally six steps through which a health systems organization can solicit and apply useful inputs from vendors.

1. Initial conceptualization.
2. Strategic planning.
3. Feasibility study.
4. Request for proposals.
5. Proposal evaluation and selection.
6. Physical implementation.

These, as well as post-implementation upkeep issues, are outlined later in the chapter.

Additional Considerations

A few other considerations that are not often described in the literature can help ensure smooth health IT implementation. The first of these is related to the concept of quality. Several methodologies can be adapted to address quality in the health services delivery industry. The methodology continuum consists of quality control, quality assurance, continuous quality improvement, total quality management, Six Sigma, and reengineering. Depending on the organization's information status, implementation may be facilitated by the inclusion of any one of these principles.

Another consideration that needs to be taken into account pertains to the manner in which health systems organizations have been changing the way they measure performance. Many organizations are progressing from an efficiency and throughput approach to an effectiveness and outcome measurement approach. Experiencing the economic pressure perceived by many businesses, health systems organizations are also increasingly being pressured to link the utilization of various

healthcare resources to their level of outcome and demand and, in many cases, to justify the utilization with the outcome produced.

Although almost all organizations are run differently with respect to performance measurements, management styles can directly affect health IT implementation. For example, the structure of management within organizations—such as departmental organization, program management, matrix design, hierarchical design, and circular design—can influence health IT implementation. In keeping with the changing priorities in the health services delivery system, there has been a demonstrated need for more highly integrated and interoperable health IT.[25] Thus, it is critical to keep these considerations in mind when making decisions regarding any health IT implementation project.

It is also crucial to keep in mind that leadership roles exhibited by the CEO and the CIO can affect the success of health IT implementation. Information technology, therefore, needs to be integrated from the cultural perspective of an organization. For this to occur, both the CEO and CIO must leverage health IT in achieving the goals and objectives of the organization and communicate this effectively within the organization.

In particular, Austin has called attention to several areas that should be addressed when monitoring and evaluating health IT implementation: productivity, user utility, value chain, competitive performance, business alignment, investment targeting, and management vision.[26] Although it is recognized that these criteria suit profit-oriented organizations, several seem equally applicable to nonprofit health systems organizations.

▶ IV. Health IT Implementation Stages

Regardless of the strategies utilized in health IT implementation, there are several steps most health systems organizations should take in order to optimize internal and external processes in a manner that ensures an efficient and effective outcome. In general, these steps fall into two broad stages: pre-implementation preparation and post-implementation upkeep, each of which is now discussed in greater detail.

Pre-implementation Preparation

The stage of pre-implementation preparation begins with the initial health IT conceptualization and ends with the initial online operation of the system. The major steps included are initial conceptualization, strategic planning, feasibility study, request for proposal, proposal evaluation and selection, and physical implementation.

Initial conceptualization can take place in a variety of ways. For instance, the CEO of a long-term care facility may be impressed by another health systems organization's health IT in the same community or regional area; the board of directors of a health facility may have discussed health IT in their 10-year plan; or staff members of a network of accountable care organizations (ACOs) may complain about their non-interoperable and aging islands of technological applications preventing them from sharing critical information for coordinated care. In short, the initial conceptualization represents a genuine wish to consolidate and improve the information flows, data storage, and information exchange capabilities in a health systems organization.

As stated previously, incorporating organizational *strategic planning* into health IT strategic plans is a desirable milestone in any health IT implementation. Health IT development must be based on a strategic information plan that is aligned with the organization's mission, vision, goals, and objectives. Adopting a strategic approach helps focus measurable goals and objectives for IS/IT implementation that best suit internal and external information

needs. Only in this way can the necessary factors and considerations (such as outcome measurement, future technological change, networking, and process reengineering) be included.

Once strategic information planning is completed, a *feasibility study* can be carried out. In general, this study aims to determine the extent to which the implementation and the health IT upkeeps are feasible. It includes results from various meetings with the board, middle management, and even staff members who are likely to be affected (user involvement) to solicit their input. It also incorporates financial (how much money is available) and physical (whether the facility is too crowded for extra equipment) feasibility research. Moreover, the feasibility study can also make recommendations on the schedule of implementation, its speed, and other issues of concern. In many health systems organizations, the reports for the feasibility study need to be approved or endorsed by the board of trustees. In these cases, the feasibility study report also acts as project proposals subject to extensive inquiries. The study reports should always be produced professionally and should be subjected to peer review.

Following the feasibility study, the detailed goals and objectives for the health IT project can be outlined on the basis of an internal and external needs assessment. Needs assessment makes it possible to formulate a *request for proposal* (RFP) for the various hardware, software, and servicing vendors to submit bids. The RFP can include details on the organization, its information needs, and the specifics of the organization's goals and objectives that the system is expected to fulfill. When vendor replies are received, it is then possible to correlate proposals on the basis of such internal objectives as budget and infrastructure compatibility issues in terms of existing hardware, software, and services. This leads to the next stage of proposal evaluation and selection, which is followed by physical implementation.

Separate discussion sections are dedicated to each of these important steps.

Proposal Evaluation and Selection

As soon as all the proposals have been submitted, it is time to evaluate them to make a selection. In the *proposal evaluation and selection* process, two methods commonly used are benchmark tests and the vendor rating system. In a benchmark test, the health systems organization provides the vendors with a set of mock data. This set of data then acts as inputs in a prototype of the proposed system. The prototype system then simulates the performance of the real system using this list of computations. The actual performance of the prototypes is then compared with the prespecified standards for evaluation.

Benchmark testing attempts to create an environment that is as close to the real clinical setting as possible. As the prototypes are being tested, it is not uncommon to find that the real, constructed system may, in fact, perform at a lower level due to the heavy load of information to be processed in real life. To some extent, benchmark testing gives the organization a "concrete" feel for what the implemented system would look like and how it would function in the clinical setting. In comparison, the *vendor rating system* is simply one in which the vendors are quantitatively scored as to how well their proposed systems perform against a list of weighted criteria. Commonly used criteria include user friendliness, data management, graphical and reporting capabilities, forecasting and statistical analysis capabilities, modeling, hardware and operating system considerations, vendor support, and cost factors.

The importance of the "people" aspect to the success of health IT implementation cannot be over emphasized. As a direct consequence, user friendliness should be a prime concern when evaluating system proposals from vendors. User friendliness can be manifested in a variety of ways. The consistency of language command, the use of natural language and touch screens, voice activation, automatic grammar checker and spelling correction, and the availability of the "Help" and "Undo" commands are examples of user-friendly hardware–software features. Moreover, menus and prompts, novice and expert modes, spreadsheet display of data and results, as well as what-you-see-is-what-you-get features also contribute to the user friendliness of the system.

Designed as advanced "data-processing" facilities, health IT should have adequate data management tools to handle the massive volumes of data to be processed in the day-to-day operation of a health systems organization. Such features as a common database manager, data security measures (log-in password, etc.), simultaneous access (without significant trade-off in performance), data selection, data dictionaries, data analytical capabilities, and data validation should be supported and included. The primary health IT function is to produce timely and accurate information for making intelligent healthcare decisions. Accordingly, health IT should have the capability to generate standard and custom reports; to generate basic graphical plots and three-dimensional charts; to allow multicolor support and the integration of graphical and text files; and to allow compatibility and interoperability with existing graphics devices, legacy systems, the Internet, new organizational IS/IT applications, or other IoT devices.

An important theme emphasized throughout this latest edition of our health IT text is data analytical capabilities and systems interoperability. The selection of health IT should take this matter into consideration. In practice, this can be viewed in terms of software and digital platform-network system considerations. Compatibility with various digital systems and iPads, IoT support, virtual workstation requirements, and printer and plotter support, as well as server and network compatibility, should all be considered when selecting health IT. Even so, the interoperability most likely is a matter of integrative software or middleware platform-network capabilities. As noted in other parts of this text, Web services and open-source systems provide interoperable solutions to many islands of health IT and legacy systems.

Finally, vendor involvement can positively influence health IT implementation. In selecting health IT, the amount of vendor support can definitely be a valid selection criterion. Vendor support can be provided in a variety of ways: consultation, training, active research and development, maintenance of local branch offices, technical support personnel, and continuing enhancements. Also, the financial stability and credibility of the vendor should be confirmed before reaching a final decision.

Probably the most important factor for all health systems organizations is the cost. In evaluating health IT proposals, it would be very helpful to bear in mind how the costs are calculated and which items are or are not included. A modular pricing approach combined with some form of "packaged offer" is one of the more common approaches. In this case, the management should pay particular attention to the initial license fees, license renewal fees, maintenance arrangements, documentation, and resource utilization, as well as to hidden conversion costs. Certainly, the cost of training and staffing has to be estimated by the management itself.

FIGURE 11-7 presents a sample evaluation sheet used in a vendor rating system. Note that although these criteria are generally applicable to all health systems organizations, specific criteria are more important to each organization by virtue of its unique environment. These should be specified separately and weighted accordingly.

VENDOR RATING							
Vendor:				Proposed system:			
Criteria	**Weight**	**Score**	**Weighted score**	**Criteria**	**Weight**	**Score**	**Weighted score**
User friendliness • Language command • Help command • Undo function • Others: _____				**Data management** • Common database manager • Security • Simultaneous access • Others: _____			
Reports and graphs • Report format • Basic graphs • Graph previews • Others: _____				**Forecasts and statistics** • Linear regression • Multiple regression • Curve fitting • Others: _____			
Modeling • Mathematical functions • User-defined functions • Procedural logic • Others: _____				**Hardware and operating system** • Hardware compatibility • Operating system compatibility • Workstation compatibility • Others: _____			
Vendor support • Consultation • Training • Technical support • Others: _____				**Cost factors** • Total budget • Leveraged payment • Maintenance cost • Others: _____			
Total score:							
Additional comments:							
Evaluated by: _____		Signed: _____			Date: _____		

FIGURE 11.7 Sample Evaluation Sheet for Health IT Proposal.

Physical Implementation

Once vendors are chosen, a contract is signed, thereby beginning the *physical implementation* stage—the stage when the most "action" takes place. This stage actually consists of several steps, including recruitment of personnel, training of staff, acquisition of equipment, installation of equipment, uploading of initial data, system testing, documentation, and online implementation.

All these steps are performed in a logical progression (some carried out simultaneously),

depending on the needs of the organization and how these needs are reflected in decisions based on the described factors and considerations. The keys to a smooth implementation process are effective planning and project management. Some variations may be necessary, depending on the differences in each organization, but some common steps (including some earlier steps) in initial health IT implementation are shown in **FIGURE 11-8**.

Among these steps, the recruitment of health IT personnel and training of existing staff members have already been discussed.

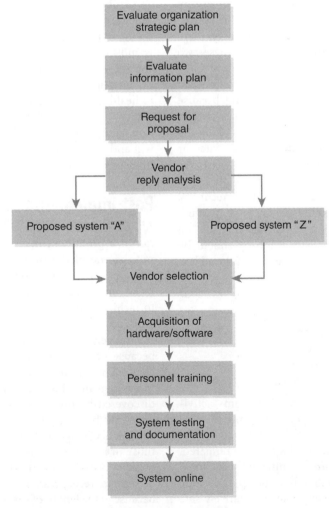

FIGURE 11-8 Common Steps of Initial Implementation of a Health IT.

The modes of acquisition and installation of the equipment are highly dependent on the characteristics of each health organization, as well as on the contract between the vendor and the management. In addition, whether the equipment is acquired over some period or at the same time ultimately depends on the payment scheme agreed upon by the vendors and the management.

The uploading of initial data and systems testing are sometimes conducted simultaneously. The initial sets of data are used to test whether the system is functioning at the desired level. If there are any significant discrepancies between the predesignated level of performance and the actual level, the system may have to be modified. Accordingly, there should be ample time allotted to these two steps.

Very often, documentation can proceed simultaneously with systems testing because the structural layout of the system is already fixed. Any additional modifications along the way can then be documented as updates or memos. Ideally, there should be at least one copy of the master documentation with details on how to operate the system at the technical level and on how to manage the system at the tactical and strategic levels. The distributing copies as well as the master copy should be updated periodically, incorporating the ad hoc updates or memos.

Online implementation involves four common approaches:

1. Parallel approach.
2. Phased approach.
3. Pilot approach.
4. Cutover approach.

In the *parallel approach*, systems activities are duplicated; the old system and the new system are both operated simultaneously for a time so that their results can be compared. In the *phased approach*, different functional parts of the new system become operative one after another. This approach is relatively safe and less expensive than the parallel approach

because the systems are not duplicated. The *pilot approach* requires the installation of the new system in sites that are representative of the complete system (e.g., in a small geographical area). This means that certain locations or departments are to serve as "alpha" pilot test sites first, followed by other "beta" pilot sites or departments until all sites operate under the new system. The *cutover approach* is also called the "cold turkey" or "burned bridges" approach. Essentially, this approach requires the organization to "flip the switch" to the new system all at once. If results are unsatisfactory, the system can be revised and activated again.

FIGURE 11-9 gives a diagrammatic representation of the four common approaches to online implementation. As to which approach is most suitable, it depends directly on the specific environment of each health systems organization. For instance, the general level of health IT knowledge in the staff, the availability of resources for systems implementation, and the amount of data handled per day will and should all affect the choice of online implementation approach.

Post-implementation Upkeep

Although full, online health IT implementation is a prominent milestone, it is definitely not the end of the story. Once the health IT becomes operational, ongoing maintenance kicks in—good maintenance is essential to achieve implementation success in the long run.

In general, ongoing upkeep is required because of problems within the system and changes in the environment. Problems within the system may be errors that have not been discovered by previous tests or may develop primarily because of an unexpectedly heavy workload. Changes in the environment include those in related systems, such as in inventory order systems, and those in the organization of human resources. In many cases, simply because of the length of time it takes to develop health IT, there are some deviations between

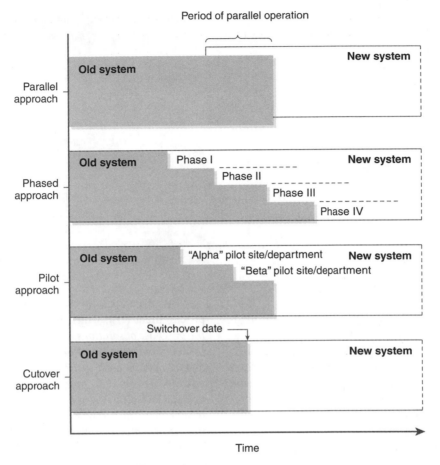

FIGURE 11-9 Common Approaches to Online Implementation.

the initial planning and final production; these deviations also contribute to the need for close post-implementation monitoring.

Regardless of why the system needs to be maintained and modified, the maintenance cycle depicted in **FIGURE 11-10** captures the major steps involved.

Problems are usually discovered in either unexpected events or periodic systems evaluations. Post-audits (or post-evaluations) are intended to evaluate the operational characteristics of the system, thereby acting as control points throughout the operation of the system. Once the problem is defined, a maintenance project can be initiated. Very often, because of creativity and the uncertainty involved,

this type of project is relatively unstructured, characterized by numerous attempts to search for the ultimate "ideal" solution. Here, the concepts of *IT services management*, which are highlighted in the next section, are very useful. After a feasible solution is found, it is then implemented and tested. If the problem is still not completely solved, it may need to be redefined. Attempts to search for an acceptable solution are then resumed. If the problem is solved, the project can be completed by making notations on maintenance logs and by producing the appropriate documentation for circulation.

It is also worth noting that documentation does not just take place at the end of the

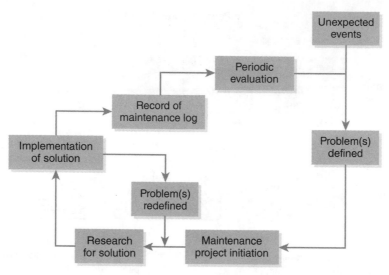

FIGURE 11-10 A Sample Maintenance Cycle for Health IT.

maintenance cycle. Rather, it occurs throughout the entire cycle in the form of documentation of problems, written requests for change, and memos on possible sources of problems and solutions. The documentation at the end of the cycle therefore emphasizes the incorporation of all these forms and memos into a mini-report that can be used for future reference or for incorporation into the system manual.

FIGURE 11-11 recaptures the main steps of the overall schema of health IT implementation. Throughout the entire implementation process (both pre-implementation preparation and post-implementation upkeep), active involvement of both the users and the managers cannot be overemphasized, for reasons described earlier.

▶ V. Innovation Procurement (IP)

Healthcare organizations are increasingly faced with requiring technological solutions that do not exist. One approach that has shown promise in addressing this challenge is innovation procurement (IP), which has been viewed *as the purchase of solutions not currently available in the marketplace, and/or need to be adapted or improved to meet specified needs and create value for users and the procuring organization.*[27] Canada, as well as Europe, has implemented IP models with research in Canada demonstrating the potential benefit of IP in health care.[28]

CSFs for IP

The key benefits of IP for healthcare organizations is that it allows the health IT leadership to identify and adapt innovative solutions that could potentially resolve existing system challenges that would lead to patient satisfaction and improved quality service delivery.[29]

Some CSFs that determine IP success within the different country contexts include:

Health IT Leadership Champion IP could fail due to a shift into a risk-adverse and/or other sensitive cultural issues as well as a lack of procedural knowledge. To avoid failure, it is important to include healthcare executive leaders in the process that act as champions to lead and steer the IP project intelligently within the organization.

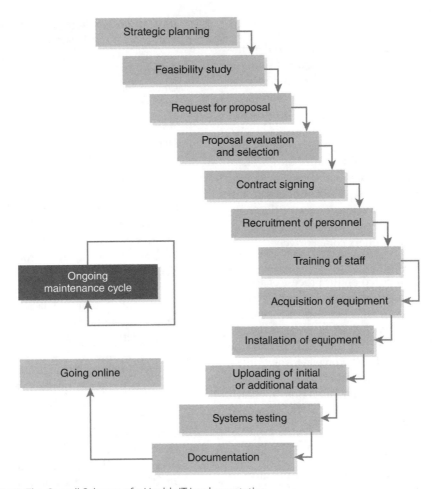

FIGURE 11-11 The Overall Schema of a Health IT Implementation.

Clear Understanding of Organizational Needs It is important for the organization to have a well-formed need statement that has been approved by all internal stakeholders. All stakeholders should have a clear understanding of the impact of the documented needs. The needs should be clear and well articulated and have easily understood potential outcomes.

Planning the Innovation Process Adequate time should be given to the planning process to ensure all the relevant considerations can be addressed. Some of the deliberations that should be addressed during the planning process include type of vendors eligible to participate, intellectual property ownership, evaluation criteria to be used, and the drafting of outcome-based specifications. It is critical to involve legal professionals, as well as business and health IT stakeholders and the user community in the planning process.

Risk Management To be successful with an IP project, it is important that organizations can identify and evaluate the potential risks involved at every phase of the procurement process and cultivate appropriate strategies to mitigate the risks.

IP Models

IP can be structured in different ways depending on the complexity of the required solution, solutions available in the market, and how the solution will be scaled up to address problems identified within the institution. The Canadian government has developed guidelines created by the Ontario Ministry of Government and Consumer Services' BPS Primer on IP. These guidelines outline six procurement models as shown in **FIGURE 11-12**. These models are differentiated by the various stages of the innovative product lifecycle while selecting among the qualifying suppliers competitively.

R&D Procurement Model (Stage 1): This model is focused on the process of acquiring research and development (R&D) stage products. They typically include prototypes or alpha/beta stage products; however, they do not incorporate the acquisition of the complete solution or finished product. An example of a model that aims to implement this approach for large-scale projects is the European Union's IP in health program titled "Horizon 2020: Health, demographic change and wellbeing." This project collects high-level challenges and develops initiative to support the R&D among member states.[30]

Model 1:	R&D procurement
Model 2:	Innovation partnership
Model 3:	Design contest
Model 4:	Competitive dialogue
Model 5:	Competitive procedure
Model 6:	Innovation-friendly competitive

FIGURE 11-12 Innovation procurement models.

Innovation Partnership Model (Stage 2): This process involves matching the healthcare provider with the selected vendor for a partnership to jointly conduct the R&D. Once a solution has been created, there is an agreement that the innovative solution is purchased to meet an identified need.

Design Contest Model (Stage 3): This model is a process by which potential vendors propose a design proposal or submit an invention to participate in a competition for an award. If successful, the vendor is typically contracted by the healthcare organization to develop the product further, and the completed product is purchased by the healthcare organization. The CreateIT Now initiative is an example of an organization that facilitates design contests to connect technology developers with healthcare organizations. CreateIT Now is a Canadian healthcare-focused innovation center for high-impact initiatives. They support product, service, and technology initiatives that solve healthcare problems. CreateIT Now creates design contest and challenges to fast-track ideas. They identify the key healthcare problems, vet viable solutions, and encourage input from patients, clinicians, and organizations in the evaluations of products.[31]

Competitive Dialogue Model (Stage 4): This process allows the healthcare organization to comprehensively explore the various components of the needs with potential suppliers before specifying the full requirements. Once the dialogue is complete, vendors are invited to submit full proposals to address the needs. Southlake Regional Health Centre in Newmarket, Ontario, Canada implemented a competitive dialogue approach for such an IP project. Specifically, the cardiac care unit worked with Medtronics, a global medical device company, to implement new technology that would transform the cardia care program. The following quote by the Regional Cardiac Care Program at Southlake Regional Health Centre highlights the problem "Traditional procurement strategies were trying to achieve the lowest price for the products....Whereas we were looking for a strategy that would not only achieve value for money but would also achieve our goal of adopting new innovation into our heart program."[32]

Using this IP approach, Southlake could consider the value of the innovation delivered by the new technology, as opposed to just considering the price. They could determine if the technology would improve health outcomes for their cardiac patients. They discovered that the medical devices helped the patients to recover faster, go home sooner, and potentially reduce their risk of returning to the hospital. During the dialogue process, they could also assess the longevity of the device and evaluate if it was more appropriate for a patient's specific condition. This would not have been possible if a traditional procurement model was adopted.

Competitive Procedure with Negotiation Model (Stage 5): This process can be used to address more complex needs in situations where innovative solutions currently exist in potentially different sectors. This process allows for some flexibility in requirements that will allow the health organization and vendor to discuss options to address the identified need(s). Research by the World Health Innovation Network (WHIN) provides a key summary of the Opportunities and Impact of Innovation Procurement in Ontario. After reviewing over 20 cases, they discovered that the approach was typically a positive experience for healthcare organizations and technology vendors participating in the process. Another key insight was that it provided important mechanisms for health organizations to work with industry partners.[33]

Innovation-Friendly Competitive Model (Stage 6): The main purpose of this approach is to allow for innovative solutions to be considered in the competitive process when they are assessed against rigid product specifications. Healthcare organizations would have the option to review alternative proposals, ensuring the competitive process is innovation-friendly.

▶ VI. IT Services Management Concepts

After examining the various steps of health IT implementation and innovation procurement in the previous sections, we now turn to discuss on the upkeep of health IT products after they have been implemented: IT services management concepts.

At present, a growing number of governmental bodies in the United Kingdom and nonprofit organizations around the world have been formed to assist in the establishment of best practices in IT services management based on core principles of IT Infrastructure Library (ITIL) standards and guidelines. ITIL, a registered community trademark of the Office of Government Commerce (OGC), is essentially a set of publications that together offers a framework of "best practices" management guidance for all aspects of IT services. Major categories include guidance for planning to implement service management, the business perspective, IT infrastructure management, application management, service delivery, service support, and security management.

In this text, concepts of health IT strategic *planning and implementation* have been covered primarily from a general organizational and management perspective, but not specifically along the IT service management perspective, which emphasizes a continuous service quality improvement process. Nonetheless, key processes underpinning IT services planning, implementation, and management are akin to those of health IT planning, implementation, and review—beginning with a vision; assessing the external marketplace and scouting the environments to surmise the best and most appropriate strategies that should be considered to improve expected outcomes; providing strong leadership support and directions to subordinates whenever possible and practical to do so; striking a balance among the different roles played by human resources, technology, and culture within the boundaries of an organization; setting goals; deciding on measurable targets; conducting process improvement cycles; and achieving goals based on specific predetermined measures and metrics.

The *business perspective* essentially conveys the message of the need for aligning IT goals and objectives with the broader corporate goals and objectives. To achieve a well-knitted alignment, the processes emphasized by ITIL include: (1) building long-term business relationships and recognizing the value chain as part of the business partnership management; (2) enhancing supplier relationships, including supply chain management (SCM); (3) reviewing, planning, and developing IT applications as these applications relate to the business goals and objectives; and (4) providing liaison, education, and communication on IT services so as to influence, gain support, and achieve changes through IT services for greater business competitive advantage. Many of these concepts have also been covered throughout parts of this new edition of the text.

In the domain of *IT infrastructure management*, IT managers are challenged to managing appropriately the people, products, processes, and partners (4 *P*s) associated with IT services throughout the different health IT life cycle stages. The key steps include, but are not limited to, feasibility analysis, systems requirements, design specifications, software development, testing, implementation,

operation, review, and retirement. All aspects of infrastructure management and administration, design and planning, technical support, and operational deployment are covered. The IT infrastructure manager coordinates among the different players to ensure that all necessary support processes are in place to aid service efficiencies and the effective use of IT services throughout daily operations, during periods of change management, and when in crisis management situations. Various aspects of these concepts relating to health IT planning and management have been discussed and illustrated in earlier sections of this and other chapters of this text.

In the domain of *application management*, it is important to relate service management concepts to application development and management in that all deployed applications should be designed for services. In this sense, all applications have to be more flexible, scalable, interoperable, available, reliable, maintainable, manageable, usable, and in compliance with design specifications and organizational requirements. Service management is concerned with the activities relating to the release, delivery, support, and optimization of the application. Again, a critical theme emphasized throughout this text has been the interoperability of health IT applications and the management of systems that do not support interoperability.

In the domain of *service delivery*, various forward-looking delivery aspects of IT servicing are covered, including availability management, capacity management, financial management for IT services, IT service continuity management, and service-level management. Availability ensures that IT services are reliable, available, secure, serviceable, and able to be maintained. It is the key to quality servicing in IT service management. Capacity management ensures that employee requests for capacity to meet business needs and goals are given priority consideration at all times. Financial management sees IT servicing run as a business within the larger corporate business operation. Essentially, employees and technicians are both cost-conscious about IT services and will minimize future expenditures by trying to take care of problems in the best way possible to the extent that these problems can be eliminated once and for all. IT service continuity management entails setting in place a recovery plan for crisis situations management and ensuring that a certain level of servicing be made available within an agreed-upon work schedule to minimize any unnecessary work disruption. Finally, service-level management (SLM) refers to the satisfactory delivery of services on a daily operational level based on the service-level agreement (SLA) acceptable to the organization.

In the domain of *service support*, daily maintenance and support services are covered, including: (1) incident management, where incident reports are filed with the support personnel manning the computer help line or help desk; (2) problem management, where a proactive approach is taken to reduce the adverse impacts from the same problem or persistent incidents; (3) change management, where a more centralized approach is taken at a higher level to control persistent problems; (4) release management, in which new releases are being considered due to major changes so as to reduce work discontinuity and improve business processes; and (5) configuration management, where IT assets, such as the centralized or enterprise-wide databases, are being managed for the successful running of the enterprise.

In the domain of *security management*, the IT services management must institute a security policy to ensure all personnel are aware of the significance of protecting IT assets and information resources and conduct risk analyses from time to time throughout the life cycle of the IT servicing, including planning and implementation, operation, evaluation, and auditing. Topics on regulatory policies related to the release and protection of health information and health IT resources have also been covered separately in other parts of this text.

▶ VII. Conclusion

In summary, successful health IT implementation and the continual evolution of health IT as the information backbone of health systems organizations are the ultimate objectives of the healthcare services delivery field. Among the various steps along the path from initial conceptualization to physical implementation to operation, the stage wherein health IT acceptance resides in the spotlight of organization-wide attention seems to be the post-implementation stage. This is when the employees of the organization are truly using health IT to perform key task activities and achieving the goals of the corporation. But it is also here that IP and IT services management concepts play a most critical role to determine whether health IT will be of value to assist the health systems organization in attaining the goals of high-quality healthcare services delivery at the optimal efficiencies and cost-effective levels.

This chapter has discussed various concerns to be addressed in health IT implementation and some general steps involved. It is, however, not expected that managers of all health systems organizations follow the same steps and address the same concerns in an identical fashion. Rather, it is hoped that the chapter has provided the "essentials" for healthcare managers and planners as well as health administration students interested in health IT implementation or expansion to oversee new projects in health IT, such as the digitalization of legacy systems in health systems organizations. With the lessons learned, the students will then be able to adapt this global knowledge to schemes suitable to the special environment of each health systems organization.

Notes

1. *Philips to expand its population health management business with the acquisition of Wellcentive.* Retrieved from www.philips.com/aw/about/news/archive /standard/news/press/2016/20160720-philips -to-expand-its-population-health-management -business-with-the-acquisition-of-wellcentive.html
2. *Ibid.*
3. *Ibid.*
4. Toole, J. E., & Caine, M. E. (1988). Laying a foundation for the future information systems. *Topics in Health Care Financing, 14*(2), 17–27.
5. Zmud, R. W. (1979). Individual differences and MIS success: A review of the empirical literature. *Management Science, 25*(10), 966–979.
6. Dearden, J. (1972). MIS is a mirage. *Harvard Business Review, 50*(1), 90–99.
7. Dickson, G., & Simmons, J. (1970). The behavioral side of MIS: Five factors relating to resistance. *Business Horizons, 13*(4), 59–71.
8. Kropf, K. (1990). *San bernadino county medical center implementation of a hospital information system* (pp. 7–8). New York, NY: New York University.
9. Staggers, M. (1991). Human factors: The missing element in computer technology. *Computers in Nursing, 9*(2), 47–49.
10. Tan, J. K. H. (1998). Graphics-based health decision support systems: Conjugating theoretical perspectives to guide the design of graphics and redundant codes in HDSS interfaces. In J. K. H. Tan with S. Sheps (Eds.), *Health decision support systems.* Gaithersburg, MD: Aspen Publishers.
11. Lemon, R., & Crudele, J. (1987). System integration: Tying it all together. *Healthcare Financial Management, 41*(6), 46–54.
12. Austin, H. (1988). Assessing the performance of information technology. *Computers in Health Care, 9*(11), 56–58.
13. *Ibid.*
14. Feldman, R. J. (1990). System evaluation and implementation strategies. In T. A. Matson & M. D. McDougall (Eds.), *Information systems for ambulatory care* (pp. 67–78). Chicago: American Hospital Publishing.
15. Ryan, H. W. (Summer 1993). User-driven systems development: Defining a new role for IS. *Information Systems Management, 10,* 66–68.
16. Gray, S. (1982). DP salary survey. *Datamation, 28*(11), 114–128.
17. Couger, J., & Zawacki, R. (1978). What motivates DP professionals. *Datamation, 24*(9), 116–123.
18. Bartol, K., & Martin, D. (1982). Managing information systems personnel: A review of the literature and managerial implications. *MIS Quarterly, 6*(Special Issue), 49–70.
19. Couger, J., & Colter, M. A. (1983). *Motivation of the maintenance programmer.* Colorado Springs, CO: CYSCS.
20. Baroudi, J. (1985). The impact of role variables on information systems personnel work attitudes and intentions. *MIS Quarterly, 9*(4), 341–356.
21. Laudon, K. C., & Laudon, J. P. (1988). *Management information systems: A contemporary perspective* (p. 698). New York, NY: Macmillan Publishing.
22. Austin, C. J., & Boxerman, S. B. (1998). *Information systems for health service administration* (5th ed.). Ann Arbor, MI: AUPHA Press/Health Administration Press.
23. Feldman (1990).
24. Ryan (1993).
25. Lemon and Crudele (1987).
26. Austin (1988).
27. BPS Primer Innovation Retrieved from www .doingbusiness.mgs.gov.on.ca/mbs/psb/psb.nsf/0 /df7388300f40aec68525814d004a00bf/$FILE/BPS _Primer_on_Innovation_Procurement_Interim.pdf
28. Retrieved from www.worldhealthinnovationnetwork .com/our-work/publications
29. Retrieved from www.conferenceboard.ca/docs/default -source/network-public/nov2017_cip_brochure_web .pdf?sfvrsn=2
30. Retrieved from ec.europa.eu/research/health/pdf /innovation_procurement_health_agenda.pdf
31. Retrieved from www.createitnow.ca/about/
32. Retrieved from www.medtronic.com/ca-en/about /news/Innovative_procurement.html
33. Retrieved from www.oce-ontario.org/docs/default -source/Presentations/opportunities-and-impact-of -innovation-procurement-in-ontario—renata-axler -win-health.pdf?sfvrsn=0

Chapter Questions

11-1   What are some of the critical success factors in health IT implementation?

11-2   With respect to health IT staffing, what are some of the major concerns for health IT planners?

11-3   Describe some useful tools in health IT implementation project management.

11-4   Why is end-user involvement important in health IT implementation? How can end-users be more involved in the process?

11-5   What are some of the models being used to implement innovation procurement?

11-6   What are the key benefits of innovation procurement?

11-7   What are the key concepts underlying IT services management? Why are these various concepts important, and how do these relate to the health IT post-implementation stage?

MINI-CASE (PART III)

Physician Intervention in Reducing Readmissions and Tele-Health Solution

Jacqueline S. Jones, Sam Kazziha, and Mohan Tanniru

▶ Introduction

Since the introduction of the Affordable Care Act (ACA), hospital administrators are under pressure to implement strategies that will reduce readmissions. One of the mandates that received significant attention is the penalties a hospital receives for unplanned readmissions within 30 days after discharge under the Readmission Reduction Program.[1]

Since the Center for Medicare & Medicaid Services (CMS) view the readmission program as an indicator of quality of care and/or post-discharge care planning,[2] there has been growing interest in understanding factors that contribute to frequent readmissions. Using a qualitative study that included semi-structured interviews with 12 hospital administrators at 6 different hospitals, Koh et al.[3] have identified several strategies to address readmission. These include tracking readmissions using prediction tools, implementing disease-specific or generic readmission reduction programs,

adopting electronic health record (EHR)-based strategies to improve care transitions, recruiting frontline staff for program leadership, and coordinating patient care with primary care providers. These results highlight the need for varying approaches to address the complexity of patient readmission.

The most commonly endorsed readmission preventive strategy is to provide patients with enhanced post-discharge instructions and/or support including improved self-management plan at discharge, greater engagement of home and community support, and provision of resources to manage care and symptoms after discharge. Most interventions targeted for Medicaid patients with mental health conditions include both home-based care and improved patient management in community-based care settings. Early follow-up was found to be an effective strategy for reducing readmissions among certain population groups, such as newborns and patients with sickle-cell disease.[4]

Other examples include enlisting the help of a community of caregivers, including dietitians and social workers, in the education of patients at a dialysis center[5,6]; engagement of nurses within an academic institution in support of discharge planning[7]; and participation of specialists in nursing home consultation as a follow-up for patients who underwent cardiac surgery.[8]

While not comprehensive, **TABLE MC-2.1** identifies select approaches discussed in the literature to address unplanned readmissions.[9-13] Additional ideas proposed by Kripilani et al.,[14] as a part of future directions to address patient readmission, include:

■ External stakeholder engagement in providing home-based services (e.g., home visits);

TABLE MC-2.1 Methods Used to Support Patients in Discharge Planning		
Research Scope	**Research Focus**	**Research Outcome**
Identify predictors of repeated readmission in intensive care unit	Patient with cardiac surgery (older, higher BMI, non-elective surgery, >4 hours of operation, post-operative CNS disorders)	Understanding patient mix/history of complication can help develop customized post-discharge planning[8]
Post-discharge intervention to reduce readmissions	Telephone intervention of Medicare population	Use of post-discharge interventions such as telephone call closer to the discharge[9]
Discharge planning from hospital to home	Reduced unplanned readmissions of older people with medical conditions	Use of tailored discharge plans can have an impact on patient readmissions and increase patient satisfaction[10]
Re-engineering discharge (RED) reduces 30-day discharge rates	Project RED components include patient education, clinical follow-up, contingency plan review, written discharge, engage post-care providers on specific intervention	Besides hospital-based discharge planning, engage post-acute care providers (e.g., dialysis centers), specifically focusing on making participating providers take responsibility and be accountable for hospital readmissions—motivation is patient readmission is a community problem and the need to work together[11]
Project BOOST: Better outcome by Optimizing Safe Transitions	Redesign discharge processes and strengthen hospitalist program (education, motivation, and process improvement), and communications on Palliative care	A greater understanding of basic symptom management and patient psychological support needs regardless of physician specialty reduces fragmentation of care[12]

- Use of special care providers (e.g., mental health conditions managed by ambulatory care centers with those experienced in these areas);
- Community-based organizations and other healthcare partners (e.g., the CMS supported Community-based Care Transition Program network, which organizes partnerships between acute care hospitals and community-based organizations); and
- Caregiver engagement and support through education, medication counseling, and outpatient follow-up.

In summary, multi-faceted and broadly applied interventions are more successful than those that rely on individual providers offering specific services based on perceived risk factors.[15] Next, we discuss a specific case study on how a hospital addressed patient readmission using a mix of the aforementioned techniques.

▶ Readmission Strategy of Cardiac Patients at a Nursing Home

Balaban et al.[16] has examined general medicine inpatients over 60 with an admission diagnosis of heart failure and chronic obstructive pulmonary disease. Patient navigators (PNs) provided coaching and assistance in navigating the transition from hospital to home through hospital visits and weekly telephone outreach. Other interventions included discharge preparation, medication management, scheduling of follow-up appointments, communication with primary care, and symptom management.

While overall, 30-day readmission rates did not differ between intervention and control patients, a patient navigator intervention among high risk, safety-net patients decreased readmission among older patients. The case study described next uses a physician-led

and an advanced nurse practitioner coordinated effort to reduce readmissions of cardiac patients at a nursing home. The organizational setting is a private hospital in southeast Michigan and the patient population that is considered for this intervention comprises patients over 65 with a diagnosis of cardiovascular disease. The program started in March 2011 and continued to date at a nursing home in Boulevard in Rochester, Michigan, with Meta Lodge in Rochester, Michigan, added in Summer 2016.

The primary goals of the intervention are to improve transitions of care by decreasing medication errors, improve the quality of care post-discharge, reduce readmissions to the hospital and elderly care facility (ECF), such as a nursing home, as well as improve knowledge deficits in cardiovascular disease. The cardiology department, ECF, and other sources such as CMS pilot funded the program. The cardiology team supporting the intervention includes the cardiologist, cardiology nurse practitioner (NP), and the administrative director, director of nursing, and medical director of the ECF.

The intervention program used the following steps:

1. All patients with diagnosis of cardiovascular disease are identified. A licensed practical nurse (LPN) assigned to cardiology services generates patient list (10–15/week), follows up on cardiology orders and ensures their completion, and communicates with the cardiologist or NP on urgent issues as they arise. The LPN is located in the skill nursing facility.

2. Cardiology NP evaluates new patients using extensive medical chart review and documentation, orders diagnostic tests, makes medication adjustments, and collaborates closely with the cardiologist.

3. Cardiology services are available during the week for urgent care issues and managed by the same cardiac team at the hospital whenever possible to improve transition of care.

Based on experience over four (4) years, the following areas are identified for success: follow-up plan post-discharge; documentation of previous cardiovascular procedures; correct medication reconciliation; management of protocols regarding medical devices. These protocols include pacemaker/internal cardiac defibrillator (ICD) registry, venous thromboembolism (VTE) prophylaxis, atrial fibrillation, coronary stent, peripheral arterial disease/ischemic foot, etc.; and initiation of a cardiovascular preventive medicine program.

Results since 2013 show a noticeable reduction of unplanned patient readmissions,

both at the hospital and the ECF, as shown in **FIGURE MC-2.1**, thus enabling the program to be expanded to three ECFs, with a fourth one planned.

There are, however, challenges in implementing such a program, including nursing knowledge deficit, insufficient documentation, lack of referrals by attending physicians, incorrect medication reconciliations, and lack of protocols on how to manage pacemakers and deep vain thrombosis (DVT).

Skilled nursing facilities have to start recruiting people to act as enablers to support interaction with the advanced nurse practitioner. Telemedicine as a technology can address some of these challenges such as faster communication and consultation, better training of patients through knowledge exchanges, and improved sharing of documentation.

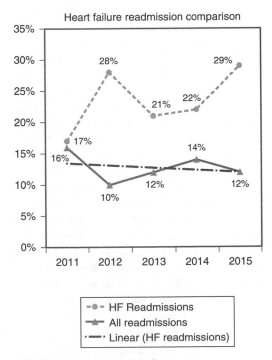

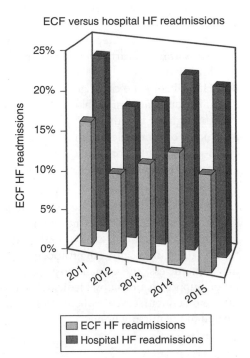

FIGURE MC-2.1 Readmission Comparisons.

Current Status

The nursing home at Boulevard hired a nurse practitioner in 2016 to provide greater coordination and higher care quality. Meta Lodge, which started its partnership in 2016, is slowly beginning to make improvements to care coordination as other nursing homes are being added. With more nursing care facilities, it becomes essential that scaling of the infrastructure to support collaboration has leveraged opportunities to increase the use of both medical and tele-health technologies.

Some of the medical and tele-health technologies include:

- Remote monitoring of cardiomems—wireless devices that measure the fluid level;
- Remote loop recorder—wireless devices—remote evaluation of heart rhythms;
- Pacemaker—today vendors have to check their functionality – newer devices have the ability to send reports remotely for evaluation of heart rhythm / battery longevity etc.
- Hand-held Echo cardiogram—faster ultrasound analysis of blood flow through the hearth
- Skype or other tele-health technologies—support virtual communication and monitoring of the patient condition.

Costs associated with this program are further budgeted with ongoing savings in various areas, for example, patient transport and logistics, physician office visits, better education of changing healthcare protocols, and so on. Nonetheless, the current cost of consultation support is borne by Medicare as a part of their reimbursement scheme for seniors treated in the nursing homes.

▶ Conclusion

In closing, in the context of initiatives to support the need for patient-centered medical care at an affordable cost, the onus of responsibility to meet these goals to reduce readmissions appears to be on the hospitals. Hospitals need to "recast readmission in a community context," such as providing community supported home care, use of special community-care providers; not simply because there is a readmission penalty, but because it is an effective way to deliver discharge services that are patient centric. Such an approach calls for the implementation of enterprise data and analytics systems in hospitals and extending such systems to post-discharge care when appropriate. Hospitals need to rethink each of the discharge services within their context and expand the talent pool available in the community to support professionals entering "transitional care" as well as to support vulnerable populations, including the use of health IT (e.g., tele-monitoring and social media based communication) to support coordination among care delivery professionals.

Imagine you are now asked to consult with a new hospital administrator in Detroit, Michigan that lacks the knowledge of the aforementioned approaches on how to go about preventing readmission of returning patients. What is of most concern is that this hospital has a growing number of returning patients who appeared to keep coming back due to lack of ability to self-manage their chronic illnesses, the difficulty of contacting them for post-discharge follow-up before they show up at the doorsteps of the hospital, and multiple other challenges (e.g., new to using remote monitoring devices). How would you use the lessons and knowledge drawn from the aforementioned case and the literature to handle this consultation?

Notes

1. Ahmad, F. S., Metlay, J. P., Barg, F. K., Henderson, R. R., & Werner, R. M. (2013). Identifying hospital organizational strategies to reduce readmissions. *American Journal of Medical Quality, 28*(4), 278–285.
2. Balaban, B. A., Galbraith, A., Burns, M. E., Vialle-Valentin, C. E., Larochelle, M. R., & Ross-Degnan, D. (2015). A patient navigator intervention to reduce hospital readmissions among high-risk safety-net patients: A randomized controlled Trial Richard. *Journal of General Internal Medicine, 30*(7), 907–915.
3. Koh, K. W., Wang, W., Richards, A. M., Chan, M. Y., & Cheng, K. F. (2016). Effectiveness of advanced practice nurse-led telehealth on readmissions and health-related outcomes among patients with post-acute myocardial infarction: ALTRA study protocol. *Journal of Advanced Nursing, 72*(6), 1357–1367.
4. Radley, E. H., Sipsma, H., Horwitz, L. I., Ndumele, C. D., Brewster, A. L., Curry, L. A., & Krumholz, H. M. (2014). Hospital strategy uptake and reductions in unplanned readmission rates for patients with heart failure: A prospective study. *Journal of General Internal Medicine, 30*(5), 605–611.
5. Burke, R. E., Kripalani, S., Vasilevskis, E. E., & Schnipper, J. L. (2013). Moving beyond readmission penalties: Creating an ideal process to improve transitional care. *Journal of Hospital Medicine, 8*, 102–109.
6. Costantino, M. E, Frey, B., Hall, B., & Painter, P. (2013). The influence of a post discharge intervention on reducing hospital readmissions in a medicare population. *Population Health Management, 18*(5), 310–316.
7. Haugaa, K. H., Martin, B., Tarrell, R. F., Mortan, B. W., Caraballo, P. J., & Ackerman, M. J. (2013, April). Institution-wide QT-alert system identifies patients with high risk of mortality. *Mayo Clinic Proceedings, 88*(4), 313–325.
8. Costantino et al., (2013), *ibid.*
9. *Health Care Forum.* (2013, May 9–10). *The physician practice: Emerging issues.* Rochester, MI: Oakland University.
10. Herzig, J. L., Schnipper, L., Doctoroff, C. S., Kim, S. A., Flanders, E. J., Robinson, G. W., … Auerbach, A. D. (2016). Physician perspectives on factors contributing to readmissions and potential prevention strategies: A multicenter survey shoshana. *Journal of General Internal Medicine, 31*(11), 1287–1293.
11. Jencks, S. F., & Brock, J. E. (2013). Hospital accountability and population health: Lessons from measuring readmission rates. *Annals of Internal Medicine, 159*(9), 629–630.
12. Kelly, M. D. (2011). Self-management of chronic disease and hospital readmission: A care transition strategy. *Journal of Nursing and Health Care Chronic Illness, 3*, 4–11.
13. Kelly, M. D., & Starr, T. (2013). Shaping service-academia partnerships to facilitate safe and quality transitions in care. *Nursing Economics, 31*(1), 6–11.
14. Kripalani, S., Theobald, C. N., Anctil, B., & Vasilekskis, E. E. (2013). Reducing hospital readmission rates: Current strategies and future directions. *Annual Reviews Medicine, 8*, 12–38.
15. Herzig et al., (2016), *ibid.*
16. Balaban, et al., (2015), *ibid.*

Biographies

Jacqueline S. Jones is a cardiology nurse practitioner currently consulting and evaluating cardiac residents in several extended care facilities in the northern Metro Detroit area. She was former Director of Cardiovascular Services at Crittenton Hospital Medical Center where she led both the Chest Pain and Heart Failure Centers ensuring high quality care and outcomes. She has been consulting in area nursing homes with the goal of ensuring residents receive the same quality of cardiac care as those in the acute care setting. She obtained her Bachelor of Science in Nursing in 2001 followed by a Master of Science in Nursing in 2003 through American Nurses Credentialing Center with certifications in both Emergency Nurse Certification (CEN) and Cardiac Medicine Certification (CMC).

She has presented to several groups on her heart failure work in extended care facilities including American College of Cardiology Michigan Chapter, Michigan Counsel of Nurse Practitioners, and IT National Conference. She has also coauthored a book chapter Advancing Professional Nursing Practice: Relationship-Based Care and the ANA Standards of Practice.

Samer Y. Kazziha, MD, FACC, is the Chief of the Heart and Vascular Institute at Henry Ford Macomb and prior to that, he worked at Crittenton/Ascension hospital system. He is a Clinical Associate Professor at Wayne State University School of Medicine. Besides his active teaching position, he is involved in outreach community service to advance patient participation and understanding of cardiac and vascular care. Currently, he is engaged in multiple research studies looking to improve clinical outcomes.

Dr. Kazziha completed his Internal Medicine Residency at Medical College of Virginia Hospital and completed the following Fellowships: Cardiology at Medical College of Virginia Hospital, Interventional Cardiology at Royal Oak Beaumont, Vascular Medicine/ Intervention at Cleveland Clinic Foundation, Cardiovascular Research Fellow at University Health Center of Pittsburgh.

Dr. Mohan Tanniru is a Senior Investigator at Henry Ford Health System in Detroit, Michigan, and Professor of Practice in the College of Public Health at the University of Arizona.

He is an Emeritus Professor of MIS in the Decision and Information Science Department, former Dean and Founding Director of Applied Technology of Business Program, all at Oakland University. He was the Department Head of MIS at the University of Arizona and taught at Syracuse University and the University of Wisconsin-Madison. He has a PhD from Northwestern University.

He published over 70 papers in journals, such as *ISR, MIS Quarterly, Decision Sciences, DSS, JMIS, IEEE Transactions in Eng. Management*, and *Communications of ACM*. His recent work in health care has been published in PAJAIS, *Healthcare Policy and Technology, Journal of Patient Satisfaction, Journal of Hospital Administration*, and *Journal of Healthcare Management*. He has coordinated numerous graduate and undergraduate projects with over 60 large companies, including GM, Chrysler, EDS/HP, Lear, Comerica, Carrier-UTC, MONY, Bristol Myers-Squibb, Honeywell, Intel, and Raytheon, and several healthcare organizations such as Kaiser Permanente, Beaumont Health Systems, St. Joseph Mercy-Oakland, and Henry Ford Health System.

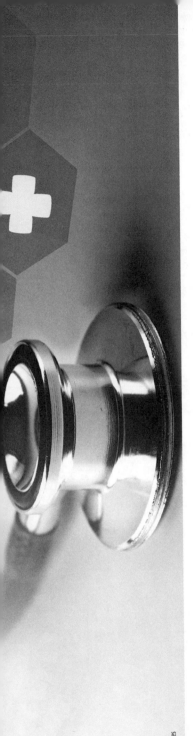

PART IV

HMIS Standards, Policy, Governance & Future

CHAPTER 12

Clinician Confidentiality, Privacy, and Ethical Issues in the Digital Age

Charie Faught

LEARNING OBJECTIVES

- Overview of health informatics competencies for clinicians and technologists
- Conceptualize the ethical and legal requirements regarding privacy and confidentiality with a focus on the HIPAA 1996 Privacy Rule and subsequent additions
- Recognize legal and ethical issues surrounding current types of health IT/IS used by patients and professionals
- Speculate future trends in HIPAA-related issues

CHAPTER OUTLINE

Scenario: Privacy and Security Policy and Subsequent Theft of Patient Information

A thriving multi-group practice has received numerous requests from patients to contact them using either e-mail or texts regarding lab and other results. Some of the newer physicians used messaging applications either personally or as part of their training.[1] Given the heightened awareness regarding privacy and security, many are worried about the risk of sending electronic messages to their patients.

The group has decided to formulate a single policy for all of the providers in the practice. What are the main risks that the policy should address? Should providers be allowed to use their own messaging or e-mail system, or should a specific technology be used? What are best practices regarding using technology to communicate directly to patients?

After implementing a new policy, including training, a provider laptop was stolen from a personal vehicle. The laptop contained notes from which the provider was intending to add to the medical record. The media was somehow alerted, and now the community is aware of the breach. If you were in charge of the situation, how would you go about repairing the damage? What changes would you like to see as a part of the practice?

▶ I. Introduction[2]

Since the time of the ancient Greeks, ethical challenges in the practice of medicine have existed. In fact, the concern of privacy is listed in the Hippocratic Oath. Along with privacy, certain ethical principles have stood the test of time. With sound legal understanding and practical tools and guidance, today's health systems providers have the ability to navigate the complex field of medicine and its interactions with technology.

In today's healthcare settings, clinicians face a changing landscape of health information technology (IT) and legal requirements. Both existing clinicians and future clinicians still in training are required to become increasingly proficient in the use of technology, while at the same time maintain high ethical and legal standards. This chapter provides an educational viewpoint for clinicians on the topics of confidentiality, privacy, and other relevant legal and ethical issues that surround the use of health IT. The purpose of the chapter is to highlight clinician competency requirements, potential issues that may arise, and ways to address these issues, including resources for future use.

▶ II. Current Perspective

Health IT Competencies

In order to frame the legal and ethical requirements relating to technology in the healthcare industry, an understanding of technology requirements is undertaken. The section reviews a select set of competencies applicable to health IT and clinical education as it pertains to the subjects of privacy, confidentiality, and legal and ethical responsibilities. Select competencies include the Certified Professional in Healthcare Information and Management Systems (CPHIMS) and the

Technology Informatics Guiding Education Reform (TIGER).

First, the Healthcare Information and Management Systems Society (HIMSS) "is a global, cause-based, not-for-profit organization focused on better health through information and technology. HIMSS leads efforts to optimize health engagements and care outcomes using information technology."[3] HIMSS currently has over 70,000 individual members, which represents the health IT industry as an association. HIMSS collaborates with other organizations, such as the Alliance for Nursing Informatics.[4]

HIMSS offers two professional certifications for its members, including the CPHIMS. The association publishes a CPHIMS Handbook, available on its website, which contains the competencies which a candidate must know in order to pass the exam.[5] The general areas of knowledge are the environment, systems, and administration. First, the environment competencies include the general healthcare environment and the technology environment. Second, systems include the categories of: analysis; design; selection, implementation, support, and maintenance; testing and evaluation; and privacy and security. Third, administration includes the categories of leadership and management.[6] In other words, the competencies encompass the technical components required to be a health IT professional, the prominent legal requirements including privacy and security, and also the knowledge of how health care works and how to be a leader in the field.

On a similar note, the HIMSS website also contains information regarding the TIGER Initiative.[7] The initiative started as a grassroots nursing effort to prepare "clinical workforce to use technology and informatics to improve the delivery of patient care."[8] The TIGER Initiative is now interdisciplinary in its approach. The TIGER Initiative developed a set of competencies, which includes the following categories: basic computer competencies, information literacy, and information management.[9] Within the information management competencies is the competency of due care, which includes:

> Confidentiality: assure confidentiality of protected patient health information when using Health Information Systems under his or her control. Access control: assure access control in the use of Health Information Systems under his or her control.
>
> Security: assure the Security of Health Information Systems under his or her control.[10(p. 12)]

In summary, the two sets of competencies list basic requirements that health information technologists and clinicians should obtain regarding the use of health IT. Levels of proficiency in clinical quality are not enough for clinicians to navigate the complex delivery of health care in today's setting.

In other words, clinicians are required to become adept at understanding how technology works in their practice, and use it to improve patient care while at the same time maintain privacy and confidentiality.

Privacy and Confidentiality

Privacy and confidentiality can be considered both ethical and legal terms, whose definitions are connected. Confidentiality is the "duty of an individual to refrain from sharing confidential information with others, except with the express consent of the other party."[11] Further, it can be stated that "Confidentiality is the keeping of another person or entity's information private."[12] In other words, the act of maintaining privacy is also the act of keeping information confidential. Another way of stating the terms is that privacy is a right, and confidentiality is the obligation to keep information private.[13] From an ethical standpoint, the act of keeping information private is one that is not concerned with the method of communication (verbal, written, or electronic) but rather that certain information is confidential and should be maintained as such unless consent is given.

From a legal perspective, the laws in the United States regarding privacy and confidentiality are varied. The broadest and perhaps most fundamental rights are found within the U.S. Constitution and the subsequent amendments. While the term privacy is not explicitly stated in the constitution, "the Supreme Court has concluded that the Fourth Amendment protects against government searches whenever a person has a 'reasonable expectation of privacy.'"[14] (p. 3) Further, many court cases and decisions regarding health have protected privacy against disclosures, and many states have included privacy in their constitutions.[15]

From a practical standpoint, however, health systems providers in the United States focus their attention on a more defined set of laws and regulations that form the requirements for privacy and confidentiality. The regulations are from a variety of agencies and departments, such as the U.S. Department of Health and Human Services (HHS—including the Office of Civil Rights), the Federal Trade Commission (FTC), and the Federal Communication Commission (FCC).[16]

The main agency relative to health care is the U.S. Department of HHS, which is charged with enhancing and protecting the health and well-being of all Americans.[17] Laws and regulations under the department include the Health Insurance Portability and Accountability Act of 1996 (HIPAA), which forms the most comprehensive and relevant requirements for healthcare professionals. Other laws include the Health Information Technology for Economic and Clinical Health (HITECH) Act, the 21st Century Cures Act, and the Alcohol And Drug Abuse Patient Records Privacy Law. Many of the relevant regulations may be found on the HHS website under the laws and regulations section. Another method that is relevant to providers can be found in the Regulations and Guidance section of the Centers for Medicare and Medicaid Services (CMS), which is an agency under HHS. While not exhaustive, the following section provides a basic overview of HIPAA and, more specifically, HIPAA privacy as it pertains to the topics in this chapter.

▶ III. 1996 HIPAA Rules

The original intent of HIPAA was to improve the efficiency and effectiveness of the healthcare system, using a set of "administrative simplifications" that includes standards for "electronic healthcare transactions and code sets, unique health identifiers, and security."[18] The act also provides guidance to keep information private given the advances in health IT. The relevant portions of HIPAA are the Privacy Rule, Security Rule, and new provisions under the HITECH Act (also called the final Omnibus Rule).[19]

HIPAA Privacy Rule

The Department of HHS provides the following overview of the HIPAA privacy rule:

> The HIPAA Privacy Rule establishes national standards to protect individuals' medical records and other personal health information and applies to health plans, health care clearinghouses, and those health care providers that conduct certain health care transactions electronically. The Rule requires appropriate safeguards to protect the privacy of personal health information, and sets limits and conditions on the uses and disclosures that may be made of such information without patient authorization. The Rule also gives patients rights over their health information, including rights to examine and obtain a copy of their health records, and to request corrections.[20]

The privacy rule is intended to keep information private while at the same time allowing necessary information for patient quality health care to be used.[21] The Office of Civil Rights has responsibilities for monitoring and enforcing the rule. Part of the enforcement includes civil monetary penalties and can include a criminal penalty as well.[22]

Perhaps two of the most important aspects of the HIPAA privacy rule are who must comply with the law and what information is protected. First, HHS clearly outlines each "covered entity" which is subject to HIPAA, which is easily accessible on the website under the heading of HIPAA for professionals. Among others, both healthcare professionals and providers (including both individuals and organizations) must comply with HIPAA.[23]

Second, the information that must be protected is called "Protected Health Information" (PHI).[24] PHI includes any information in any form (verbal, written, or electronic), that is information, including demographic data, that relates to the individual's past, present, or future physical or mental health or condition; the provision of health care to the individual; or the past, present, or future payment for the provision of health care to the individual, and that identifies the individual or for which there is a reasonable basis to believe it can be used to identify the individual. Individually identifiable health information includes many common identifiers (e.g., name, address, birth date, or Social Security Number).[25]

In general, a covered entity is required to keep PHI confidential, unless there is a permitted use or disclosure, or unless permission has been obtained.[26] Specific requirements for permitted use include using what is minimally necessary to perform certain tasks, such as clinical treatment. Each covered entity must also restrict access to PHI, develop policies and procedures, and perform training on the requirements.[27] In other words, healthcare providers working for a covered entity should be well versed in the HIPAA privacy requirements as it pertains to their position, and providers that own their own practice must also abide by the standards.

HIPAA Security Rule

Along with the HIPAA privacy rule, the HIPAA security rule also has specific requirements for the storage and transmission of protected health information in an electronic format, also called e-PHI. The same covered entities and what is considered protected are consistent with the privacy rule. Within the security rule is listed the definition of confidentiality: "The Security Rule defines 'confidentiality' to mean that e-PHI is not available or disclosed to unauthorized persons."[28] While this is a narrow definition, the HIPAA security rule covers in effect what many would consider to be private or confidential information with a focus on information that is electronically submitted, while the HIPAA privacy rule covers all private and confidential information, regardless of form.

Within the security rule lies the safeguards to protect e-PHI, such as having a security management process, information access, workstation and device security, and transmission security, among others.[29]

HITECH Act

The HITECH Act is "part of the American Recovery and Reinvestment Act of 2009, to strengthen the privacy and security protections for health information established under the Health Insurance Portability and Accountability Act of 1996 (HIPAA)."[30] The final rule of the HITECH Act does provide amendments to HIPAA, which are now in effect.[31] The final regulation has four final rules which include: modifications to HIPAA Privacy, Security, and Enforcement Rules; adopting a higher civil penalty structure; a higher standard of breach notifications; and a final rule for HIPAA as required by "the Genetic Information Nondiscrimination Act (GINA) to prohibit most health plans from using or disclosing genetic information for underwriting purposes."[32]

The HITECH Act does strengthen HIPAA in a variety of ways. First, it limits how healthcare organizations can use PHI for marketing and fundraising.[33] It also prohibits the sale of PHI, and increases the reporting of breaches. Lastly, the HITECH Act also increased penalties for noncompliance of the regulation and gives more auditing and enforcement capabilities.[34]

Other Agencies and Considerations

While HIPAA and its subsequent updates is perhaps the primary regulation pertaining to health information privacy and confidentiality, other considerations exist in the United States, in part based on the following:

> Health IT is defined by the federal government's Office of the National Coordinator for Health IT (ONC) as, "hardware, software, integrated technologies or related licenses, intellectual property, upgrades, or packaged solutions sold as services that are designed for or support the use by health care entities or patients for the electronic creation, maintenance, access, or exchange of health information."
>
> Health IT is the framework that enables the management of health information across multiple electronic systems and devices, such as wireless medical devices, hospital information systems, communications infrastructure, and electronic health record (EHR) systems. Three federal agencies, the Food and Drug Administration (FDA), ONC, and the FCC, each have unique responsibilities in the health IT arena.[35]

Having provided an overview of HIPAA, which includes responsibilities undertaken by the ONC, the next section focuses on the FTC, FDA and the FCC scope of control and guidance as well as intended regulations.

First, the FTC, in coordination with HHS, the ONC, and the Office of Civil rights, provides guidance for those who are developing mobile apps, which may be subject to the laws listed in this section. Second, in the case of patient information, the FTC guidance is relevant for both covered and non-covered entities.[36] "The FTC attempts to combat unfair or deceptive practices related to healthcare mobile device applications. This could include any false or misleading claims or omissions of material facts in relation to a mobile device or app."[37] "The FTC's Health Breach Notification Rule requires certain businesses to provide notifications following breaches of personal health record information."[38]

Next, the FDA regulates medical devices, including mobile devices that are intended to treat patients.[39] The FDA oversees a variety of technologies, including wireless medical devices, telemedicine, medical device data systems, and software as a medical device.[40] Lastly, the scope of the FCC can be said to complement those of the FDA in terms of mobile devices:

> The FCC's scope includes authorization of carriers whose networks are used by mobile devices to access, transmit, or store information—including health information. The FCC also authorizes a variety of radio frequency medical devices, such as implanted medical devices and patient monitoring devices. It also establishes the technical rules used by Wi-Fi or other similar networks for short transmissions.[41]

Notwithstanding, the FCC traditionally has not played a role in the enforcement of privacy standards.[42] In summary, the development and use of mobile device applications are subject to further scrutiny under FTC, FDA, and FCC regulations.

Canada and European Union Comparison

While this chapter focuses on U.S. regulations, a brief summary is provided on relevant laws in Canada and the European Union. First,

Canadian laws pertaining to privacy include the Privacy Act, which encompasses how the government handles personal information and the "Personal Information Protection and Electronic Documents Act (PIPEDA), which covers how businesses handle personal information."[43] Specific privacy laws also exist in each province and territory, which also include nonprofit organizations such as hospitals.[44]

In Europe, the Directive on the Protection of Individuals was created in 1995, designed to establish medical privacy laws in the member states.[45] The directive was later expanded to include further recommendations regarding the protection of medical data. Three articles in the recommendation are aligned with HIPAA: protecting patient identifiable information, the right to privacy in processing and collection of medical data, and establishing appropriate safeguards, such as communication of medical information only to those subject to the rules of confidentiality (similar to minimum necessary).[46] Further, a new regulation, the EU General Data Protection Regulation (GDPR) is in effect as of May 25, 2018.[47] The new law "applies to all companies processing the personal data of data subjects residing in the Union, regardless of the company's location."[48] The law includes stronger language regarding consent use of information, breach notification, right to access, right to be forgotten, data privacy and portability.[49]

In reviewing the U.S. laws in comparison to Canada and the EU, all three are "based on a layered approach."[50] First, the United States has a variety of federal laws, some of which have been illustrated in this chapter, there are also state laws, some of which preempt federal laws. Second, the Canadian approach also has national laws along with specific province and territory laws. Third, the EU has the aforementioned Directive and new GDPR, with individual member laws.[51]

On one end of the spectrum, the U.S. approach is more of a hands-off approach, with specific industry regulations, such as healthcare privacy.[52] At the other end, the European Union reviews privacy from a more global perspective; for example, instead of "protected health information" and "covered entities", the EU uses "protected information" for all member states. Interestingly, Canada is a mix of the two, with a closer alignment to the European Union with some provincial and territorial laws.[53]

In summary, while the chapter focuses on the United States, the principles of privacy and the establishment of safeguards are similar. As such, the proceeding sections will use the U.S. regulations as the main example. However, a practitioner should spend time familiarizing themselves with appropriate federal and local requirements, as they may differ.

▶ IV. Health Information Technology

According to the ONC, health IT may be defined as "a broad concept that encompasses an array of technologies to store, share, and analyze health information."[54] Further, the use of health IT has been highlighted as a method to improve patient care, including improving communications. The following section will highlight different types of health IT that providers or their patients may use for clinical care and communication. Types of health IT reviewed in this chapter are the EHR, mobile devices (m-health) and secure messaging, telemedicine and patient generated data, health information exchange (HIE), cloud computing, and social media.

EHRs and Mobile Devices

First, an EHR is an advanced electronic version of a medical record.[55] The difference between the EHR and the paper version is that it offers additional functionality, such as the use of evidence-based tools. It also has the opportunity to increase efficiencies and accuracy of patient information.[56] As such, from an ethical perspective, it may be considered a beneficial choice; however, the technology is not without potential legal and ethical problems.

Second, a mobile device includes a variety of devices that are not stationary, such as a desktop computer. Examples include a laptop computer, a tablet, or a smartphone.[57] Further, an "app" is a small, specialized program that is downloaded onto mobile devices, such as smartphones and tablets.[58(p. 222)] An estimated 1.7 billion users will have downloaded a healthcare, or "m-health" app. Of these, two categories may be defined: one for personal use outside of health care and one connected to other medical technologies within the healthcare sector.[59] For uses within health care, apps include checking medication interactions, diagnosing a condition, accessing EHRs, checking results, creating clinical results and notes, and prescribing electronically.[60] As mentioned previously, additional rules apply for those who are developing mobile health apps.[61]

Health Information Exchange (HIE)

Third, according to the ONC, an HIE "allows doctors, nurses, pharmacists, other healthcare providers and patients to appropriately access and securely share a patient's vital medical information electronically—improving the speed, quality, safety and cost of patient care."[62] Further, the types of HIE are as follows:

- Directed Exchange—the ability to send and receive secure information electronically between care providers to support coordinated care;
- Query-based Exchange—the ability for providers to find and request information on a patient from other providers, often used for unplanned care; and
- Consumer Mediated Exchange—the ability for patients to aggregate and control the use of their health information among providers.[63]

As illustrated, each HIE type has varying levels of information exchanged between providers or directly with patients, which is discussed next.

Telemedicine and Patient Generated Health Data

The World Health Organization (WHO) has defined telemedicine as:

> The delivery of health care services, where distance is a critical factor, by all health care professionals using information and communication technologies for the exchange of valid information for diagnosis, treatment and prevention of disease and injuries, research and evaluation, and for the continuing education of health care providers, all in the interests of advancing the health of individuals and their communities.[64(p. 9)]

Put simply, telemedicine is the delivery of health services via distance. One of the benefits of the technology is that it has the capability of bringing specialized care to rural areas.[65] Two basic types of telemedicine include store and forward, which allows sharing of information asynchronously, and real time, which is the synchronous transmission of information.[66] For both types, media such as video, audio, images, or text can be transmitted.[67]

Fourth, patient-generated health data (PGHD) are health-related data created, recorded, or gathered by or from patients (or family members or other caregivers) to help address a health concern. PGHD include, but are not limited to: health history, treatment history, biometric data, symptoms, [and] lifestyle choices.[68] A number of technologies can be used in PGHD, such as smart phones, mobile apps, remote monitoring devices, electronic health records, and patient portals.[69] The use of patient information in the form of patient reported outcomes in research has been in existence for years.[70]

Cloud Computing

According to the US National Institute of Standards and Technology (NIST), cloud computing is: a model for enabling convenient, on-demand network access to a shared pool of configurable computing resources (e.g., networks, servers, storage, applications, and services) that can be rapidly provisioned and released with minimal management effort or service provider interaction. This cloud model promotes availability and is composed of five essential characteristics, three delivery models, and four deployment models.[71]

Essentially, cloud computing relates not to the type of technology, but where data are stored. For instance, data captured in EHRs, mobile devices, HIE, or telemedicine can all become available and accessible via cloud computing as a way to retrieving those stored data.[72]

Social Media

According to Merriam-Webster, social media is defined as "forms of electronic communication (such as websites for social networking and microblogging) through which users create online communities to share information, ideas, personal messages, and other content (such as videos)."[73] Examples include Facebook, Twitter, and Instagram.[74] Other types of social media can include media sharing, content production, professional networking, or even online gaming.[75] From a provider's perspective, social media has a variety of professional uses, including accessing health news, communication with peers, marketing a practice, and communicating with patients.[76]

In summary, a variety of technologies are available for use both within a healthcare organization and for health consumers. Each one has benefits in terms of increasing efficiencies, communication, and access to information. However, each one also has potential legal-ethical risks, which are discussed next, starting with privacy and confidentiality.

▶ V. Potential Issues Arising from Technology Use

Privacy and Confidentiality

As noted, the U.S. HHS Office for Civil Rights (OCR) investigates and reports privacy breaches. Per the HITECH Act, the department posts "breaches of unsecured protected health information affecting 500 or more individuals" on the OCR Breach Portal.[77] The website lists all breaches reported in the last 24 months. For 2017, a total of 265 breaches were reported. The number of individuals affected in each breach ranges from 500 to 697,800. The types of breaches included 127 Hacking or IT incidents, 7 losses, 40 cases of theft, and 89 cases of unauthorized access or disclosure. The location of breached information included 25 cases of a desktop computer, 19 laptops, 20 electronic medical records, 60 e-mail, 59 network server, 29 others, 9 other portable electronic devices, and 39 paper or films.

A 2016 report indicated that almost 90% of covered entities surveyed have experienced a data breach in the last 2 years.[78] The average cost of a data breach is estimated to be more than 2.2 million dollars. While cyberattacks are a growing issue, many of the organizations studied are more concerned with negligent employees. The concern includes the use of mobile devices, including those owned by employees.[79]

Given the nature of privacy breaches, this section will review different types of health IT listed in the previous section, highlighting privacy and security issues. While the list will not contain every possible scenario, common issues are reviewed. Additionally, both secure messaging and social media will be addressed.

While the industry has moved toward "HIPAA compliant" software, the use of the software "comprises only a small fraction of safeguards required."[80] As previously noted in the discussion of types of breaches, EHRs are still at risk. One way in which they are at risk is inappropriate or unauthorized access to the EHR.[81] In one instance, a hospital employee downloaded patient names, addresses, and Medicare numbers in order to sell the information.[82] Another example was an employee sharing information seen in a record with someone outside of health care, or viewing a patient record when there is no need to do so, violating the minimum standard requirement.[83] A third example is the printing of information from an EHR, which also needs to be secured and protected in a similar manner to electronic information.[84] With paper-based PHI, unused or duplicate pages of a medical record must be disposed of using either a shredder or locked bins, with a business associate's agreement with the shredding company.

One type of breach which is of particular concern is that of mental health records, which are subject to two main rules: HIPAA and the Alcohol and Drug Abuse Patient Records Privacy Law.[85] Along with mental health records, the protected health information of individuals who receive drug and alcohol abuse treatment in federally funded programs is subject to additional privacy protections.[86] In one case, a patient psychiatrist's clinical notes were translated from paper record into EHR without appropriate data restrictions.[87] The patient later went in to see a medical doctor about an unrelated health issue, with the physician admitting that he read the notes and asked if the patient was seeing a psychiatrist. The patient then decided to see a therapist outside the clinical system, who agreed not to add the notes to an EHR.[88]

Due in part to their convenience and ease of use, a number of privacy and other risks also exist for mobile devices. The risks include the following: the use of a mobile device in a public setting; the interception of PHI while using an unsecure network; the loss of PHI if a device with data, such as pictures, is stolen; saving data in a cloud-based system that does not have a HIPAA business associate agreement; and the use of texting via an unsecure system.[89] For example, a contractor at a hospital downloaded the information for over 34,000 patients onto a laptop, which was later stolen.[90] The laptop was password protected, but the data was not encrypted.[91]

Another concern is the transfer of data from one device to another.[92] This concern exists across the types of health IT listed, including EHRs, mobile devices, HIE, and more. All types of technology, with mobile apps in particular, are threatened by the risk of cyber-attacks. Major threats include information that is sent via the Internet not using secure protocols, data stored on third-party servers (which can include cloud computing), and malicious software on a mobile device.[93]

Along the same lines, both HIE and telemedicine must comply with the same privacy and security standards as other aspects of health IT.[94] However, one potential risk area is the number of individuals across organizations that may have access to data. Other potential risk areas include administrative safeguards for keeping the data secure, and maintaining privacy and confidentiality using methods, such as keeping the area where the interaction takes place a private environment.[95]

Secure Messaging

The use of mobile devices, such as smartphones and text messaging, among physician residents has replaced the older technology of numeric paging.[96] However, one of the downsides of the newer technology is that it may be read or accessed by an unauthorized third party, thus leading to a HIPAA violation. Along the same lines, the Joint Commission in 2011 banned sending text messages containing patient information.[97]

One method to combat the risk is to use secure messaging, which can be downloaded as an app.[98] Notwithstanding, a 2016 study of programs in the Accreditation Council for Graduate Medical Education (ACGME) shows that violations have occurred. Among the results, the study found that over 58% of physician trainees and 40% of faculty "knowingly and admit to violating HIPAA with patient communication via text messaging."[99(p. 129)] The findings show that while the technology is available, further attention needs to be given to the area of secure use of mobile devices.

Alongside HIPAA requirements, it is important to note that CMS has issued a Memorandum regarding the use of texting for the purposes of order entry.[100] In a Memorandum dated December 28, 2017 and revised on January 1, 2018, CMS has clarified the requirements under Conditions of Participation for Hospitals standard §489.24(b) and for critical access hospitals (CAH's) under §485.638. The memo provides the following summary:

> Texting patient information among members of the Hospital and CAHs health care team is permissible if accomplished through a secure platform. Texting of patient orders is prohibited regardless of the platform utilized. Computerized Provider Order Entry (CPOE) is the preferred method of order entry by a provider.[101]

In other words, texting orders using a mobile device is not allowed, even if a secure messaging system is used.

Social Media

Given the use of social media in our society, special attention should be taken to maintain privacy and confidentiality. First, it should be noted that social media sites are not considered covered entities, and thus are not subject to HIPAA.[102] However, healthcare professionals are subject to HIPAA, and must become diligent in deciding what to post and what not to post.[103] Examples of privacy breaches include posting information, such as pictures of patient records, pictures of patients, or even comments about patients.[104] Further, one study indicated that "the utilization of social media is significantly correlated with nursing students' unethical behavior."[105] Another study found that "students and residents place protected health information on their publicly available social networking sites."[106]

Other Ethical and Legal Issues

For providers who may own their own practice, the purchasing and maintenance of an EHR may also pose liability risk.[107] The risks include: data accuracy; the ability to retrieve medical record data when needed, (not only for providing patient care but also for any malpractice claims); where the stored data is located and who maintains legal control of the data; who is responsible for maintaining security; physicians—not the vendor—being liable for the accuracy of clinical support tools; and system failure.[108] It is worth noting that as a covered entity, the provider is required to follow all of the HIPAA safeguards, and cannot rely on the vendor to have a "HIPAA compliant" product.[109]

Data Accuracy

Data accuracy is a concern for all medical record entries, even in the digital world. For instance, the diagnosis codes must be placed in the EHR in such a way that a provider can choose among the correct codes that correspond with the documentation narrative. In one instance, an EHR did not account for the four diagnosis possibilities under one code, thus creating the potential to document inaccurately.[110] Another issue of concern for data accuracy is the use of either cut and paste techniques or templates that automatically populate part of the documentation.[111] The bottom line is that the use of technology does not negate a clinician's responsibility to ensure that the information contained in a medical record is accurate and complete.

The legal issues in the realm of PGHD include data ownership, privacy, and the potential to make misleading claims.[112] Other concerns include determining that accuracy of the information provided (including authentication of the user), electronic security, and standardizing the data from multiple devices.[113] Patients are also concerned with privacy and security, and may lack health information literacy to fully participate.[114] Data accuracy is a concern in another way, in that the data from a variety of sources should also be contained in the medical record. In other words, how does the information from a mobile app make its way to the EHR, where it can be used for patient care purposes?

Medical Malpractice

Along with concerns about privacy, confidentiality, and data accuracy, another potential concern is medical malpractice.[115] For instance, under the circumstances of establishing the communication with a patient using mobile technology, a duty of care has been established, which is not dissimilar to the existing requirements. However, the change may be the "standard of care" in using a mobile device. Put simply, the expectations for failing to use an app, or not using it in a timely manner may be considered a breach of duty.[116] Like mobile devices, telemedicine may also be a risk for medical malpractice. For instance, one function of telemedicine is a patient using a medical device that can be monitored remotely. In this situation, there is the potential that patient misuse may result in injury, for which the physician may be held partially liable.[117]

Another potential concern similar to medical malpractice is licensure requirements. Given that technology transmission can cross boundaries such as state lines, healthcare providers must be wary of practicing medicine where they do not have a license.[118] Some states have made exceptions in areas of consultation and endorsement if they are working with a licensed professional in the state. However, the current licensing standards are such that each state and state board has its own set of regulations, for which, the technology currently being used have yet to be addressed.[119]

Social Media

While consent is part of the privacy and confidentiality requirements under HIPAA, the notion of informed consent is still at issue with the use of health IT. For instance, even if a patient's information may not be identifiable in a social media post, the patient may still not have given consent.[120] Another concern using social media in posting personal health information is data ownership.[121] Depending on the terms of service, the creator of the data may have some rights, but the social media site may be the owner of the content. As such, transferring data to other tools, such as an EHR for medical use, may cause legal challenges. Social media sites may or may not address privacy rights,[122] as they are not subject to the same requirements in the United States (because they are not considered covered entities). Further, social media sites may also change their "privacy settings at any time, without consent."[123]

From another viewpoint, communicating with a patient via social media, even when requested, may violate a patient's personal boundaries.[124] From the standpoint of health literacy as indicated in the competencies, information found in many social media sites may not be reliable or valid. An ethical concern is the potential to damage one's reputation. Others, including potential employers, patients, or professional associations, may view information on social media sites. Equally as serious, unprofessional behavior on social media is subject to disciplinary actions, including licensure and credentialing. Cases in which students were expelled have also occurred.[125]

▶ VI. Solutions and Recommendations

The risks of a privacy breach, loss of licensure, or a malpractice case are serious considerations for all healthcare professionals. Fortunately, resources that are fairly easy to find exist to help professionals. The solutions and recommendations can be attained using three methods: (a) the use of official sources, including licensure requirements and professional competencies; (b) the use of expert advice, including privacy and security experts and legal advice; and (c) the use of educational material by professional associations. A fourth recommendation is to receive education on specific ethical and legal risk areas, either formally in an academic setting or as a continuing education credit. The following section will provide recommendations using the first three of these methods.

First, government websites such as those provided by the HHS, especially the ONC, provide tools for healthcare professionals and practices. For instance, the ONC provides the following recommendations to help ensure privacy for EHRs[126]:

■ Access controls to make sure only those who are authorized can access health information
■ Audit functions that track who has accessed what pieces of health information
■ Internet-based portals that allow patients to access their own health records, see who else has viewed their records, and check the accuracy of the records.

For mobile devices, the ONC recommends the following[127]:

1. Install and enable encryption to protect health information stored or sent by mobile devices.
2. Use a password or other user authentication.
3. Install and activate wiping and remote disabling to erase the data on your mobile device if it is lost or stolen.
4. Disable and do not install or use filesharing applications.
5. Install and enable a firewall to block unauthorized access.
6. Install and enable security software to protect against malicious applications, viruses, spyware, and malware-based attacks.
7. Keep your security software up to date.
8. Research mobile applications (apps) before downloading.
9. Maintain physical control of your mobile device. Know where it is at all times to limit the risk of unauthorized use.
10. Use adequate security to send or receive health information over public Wi-Fi networks.
11. Delete all stored health information on your mobile device before discarding it.

Here are some questions to consider when using a mobile device to access an organization's network or system, such as an EHR[128]:

1. Does your organization have a mobile device use policy?
2. Does your organization allow you to use your personally owned mobile device for work?
3. Do you know who your organization's Privacy Officer and Security Officer are?
4. Does your organization require you to register your mobile device with the organization?
5. Does your organization have a Virtual Private Network (VPN) that allows you to access, receive, or transmit health information securely with your mobile device?

6. Does your organization have a policy about storing health information on your mobile device?

7. Does your organization require you to backup health information from your mobile device to a secure server?

8. Does your organization require you to enable remote wiping or remote disabling on your mobile device?

9. Does your organization offer mobile device privacy and security awareness and training?

Further advice for mobile devices includes reporting a stolen device, addressing policies and training in the organization, and working in a team-based approach to minimize any risks.[129]

For private practices, advice includes[130] (pp. 34–36):

- conducting and documenting a risk analysis, which HHS defines as "an accurate and thorough assessment of the potential risks and vulnerabilities to the confidentiality, integrity, and availability" of electronic PHI in your practice;

- reviewing the practice's policies and procedures for when PHI is lost or stolen or otherwise improperly disclosed, and making sure your staff members are trained in them;

- ensuring that the electronic PHI your practice holds is encrypted so that it cannot be accessed if it is lost or stolen;

- modifying the practice's EHR system so that you can flag information a patient does not want shared with an insurance company;

- having the ability to send patients their health information in an electronic format;

- reviewing your contracts with any vendors that have access to your practice's PHI; and

- updating your practice's notice of privacy practices.

One of the major threats to existing laws, such as HIPAA security, is that "It is not a framework, nor an industry standard, and not sufficient to base an organization's cybersecurity readiness on."[131(p.4)] A prominent firm specializing in healthcare security recommends the use of an enterprise risk management approach, which can be defined as "the culture, capabilities, and practices, integrated with strategy and execution, that organizations rely on to manage risk in creating, preserving, and realizing value."[132(p.14)] In short, the risk of each type of health IT, location, and use, should not be isolated, but rather considered in its entirety in a systemized approach.

From the viewpoint of professional associations, one article provides a summary of recommendations compiled from healthcare professional guidelines as provided and detailed in **TABLE 12-1**.

Applying the Four-Principles Approach

While this chapter focuses mainly on legal concerns and the use of health IT, taking a step back and reviewing the concerns from an ethical perspective may offer clinicians a more balanced and holistic approach. While the main ethical concern stated is one of privacy, the four-principle approach of autonomy, beneficence, non-maleficence, and justice may be applied.

First, autonomy can be considered the right for patients to make their own decisions in deciding what is best for themselves.[133] Second, beneficence is the principle of promoting the good, while non-maleficence is avoiding harm. Lastly, justice can be described as the benefits, risks, and costs which should be distributed fairly; patients in similar positions should be treated in a similar manner.[134] For issues described in the chapter, one can use the varying technologies in ways that promote the

TABLE 12-1 Social Media Guidelines for Healthcare Professionals	
Content credibility	■ Share only information from credible sources. ■ Refute any inaccurate information you encounter.
Legal concerns	■ Remember that the content you author may be discoverable. ■ Comply with federal and state privacy laws. Respect copyright laws.
Licensing concerns	■ Know professional licensure requirements for your state.
Networking practices	■ Do not contact patients with requests to join your network. ■ Direct patients who want to join your personal network to a more secure means of communication or to your professional site.
Patient care	■ Avoid providing specific medical advice to nonpatients. ■ Make appropriate disclosures and disclaimers regarding the accuracy, timeliness, and privacy of electronic communications.
Patient privacy	■ Avoid writing about specific patients. ■ Make sure you are in compliance with state and federal privacy laws. ■ Obtain patient consent when required. ■ Protect patient information through "de-identification." ■ Use a respectful tone when discussing patients.
Personal privacy	■ Use the most secure privacy settings available. ■ Keep personal and professional profiles separate.
Professional ethics	■ Disclose any in-kind or financial compensation received. ■ Do not make false or misleading claims.
Self-identification	■ Specify whether or not you are representing an employer

Reproduced from Ventola, CL. (2014). Social media and health care professionals: Benefits, risks, and best practices. P&T Community, 39(7), 491–499, 520. Retrieved from https://www.ptcommunity.com/journal/article/full/2014/7/491/social-media-and-health-care-professionals-benefits-risks-and-best

four principles, or in ways that detract from them. As an example, a privacy breach may take away a person's autonomy and cause harm.

▶ VII. Future Trends and Conclusion

Given the advantageous nature of health IT, its use will only continue to expand. Further, the ways in which different technologies will be used will cross industries, such as health care and social media. As such, the ethical and legal issues discussed here are likely to be as challenging in the future as they are today. As technology changes, the need to review both ethical principles and update relevant laws regarding their use are important aspects of education and continuing education as professionals.

Further, given the amount of privacy breaches and the varying ways in which a breach may occur, perhaps the biggest underlying question is further guidance or regulation on the subject. Given the scope of the laws in the United States based on industry, perhaps looking to other countries such as Canada or the European Union may provide better practices. Along with staying current in the field in terms of maintaining competencies and licensure, healthcare professionals also have the opportunity to voice their concerns, especially as it relates to patient care.

Notes

1. McKnight, R., & Franko, O. (2016). HIPAA compliance with mobile devices among ACGME programs. *Journal of Medical Systems, 40*(5), 1–8. doi:10.1007/s10916-016-0489-2

2. *Caveat*: The author of this chapter is not a lawyer, and therefore cannot offer legal advice. The chapter is designed to provide information on current perspectives, and is generalized. It is not intended to offer legal opinions, and may not be applicable to all healthcare providers or circumstances.

3. Healthcare Information and Management Systems Society. (2018a, March 10). *About HIMSS*. Retrieved from www.himss.org/himss-faqs

4. *Ibid.*

5. Healthcare Information and Management Systems Society. (2017). CPHIMS Candidate Handbook. *HIMSS.org*. Retrieved from www.himss.org/health-it-certification/cphims/handbook

6. *Ibid.*, (2018a).

7. Healthcare Information and Management Systems Society. (2018b). The TIGER Initiative. *HIMSS.org*. Retrieved from www.himss.org/professional development/tiger-initiative

8. *Ibid.*

9. Healthcare Information and Management Systems Society. (2010, October 21). Informatics Competencies. *HIMSS.org*. Retrieved from www.himss.org /informatics-competencies

10. *Ibid.*, p. 12.

11. Confidentiality. (2018, February 28). *Legal dictionary*. Retrieved from legaldictionary.net /confidentiality/

12. *Ibid.*

13. Kerr, P. (2009). Protecting patient information in an electronic age: A sacred trust. *Urologic Nursing, 29*(5), 315–319.

14. Solove, D. J. (2008). Understanding Privacy. Harvard University Press; GWU Legal Studies (Research Paper No. 420, p. 3); GWU Law School Public Law (Research Paper No. 420). Retrieved from SSRN ssrn .com/abstract=1127888

15. *Ibid.*

16. Washington, V., DeSalvo, K., Mostashari, F., & Blumenthal, D. (2017). The HITECH era and the path forward. *New England Journal of Medicine, 377*(10), 904–906. doi:10.1056/NEJMp1703370

17. United States Department of Health and Human Services. (2018a, March 7). About HHS. *HHS.gov*. Retrieved from www.hhs.gov/about/index.html

18. United States Department of Health and Human Services. (2018b, March 7). HIPAA for Professionals. *HHS.gov*. Retrieved from www.hhs.gov/hipaa/for -professionals/index.html

19. *Ibid.*

20. United States Department of Health and Human Services. (2015a, April 16). HIPAA Privacy Rule. *HHS.gov*. Retrieved from www.hhs.gov/hipaa/for -professionals/privacy

21. *Ibid.*

22. *Ibid.*

23. United States Department of Health and Human Services. (2013, July 26). Summary of the HIPAA Security Rule. *HHS.gov*. Retrieved from www .hhs.gov/hipaa/for-professionals/security/laws -regulations/index.html

24. *Ibid.*, (2015a).

25. *Ibid.*

26. *Ibid.*

27. *Ibid.*

28. *Ibid.*, (2013).

29. *Ibid.*

30. United States Department of Health and Human Services. (2015b, October 30). Omnibus HIPAA Rulemaking. *HHS.gov*. Retrieved from www .hhs.gov/hipaa/for-professionals/privacy/laws -regulations/combined-regulation-text/omnibus -hipaa-rulemaking/index.html

31. Rothstein, M. A. (2013). HIPAA Privacy Rule 2.0. *Journal of Law, Medicine & Ethics, 41*(2), 525–528. doi:10.1111/jlme.12060

32. United States Department of Health and Human Services. (2013). Modifications to the HIPAA Privacy, Security, Enforcement, and Breach Notification Rules Under the Health Information Technology for Economic and Clinical Health Act and the Genetic Information Nondiscrimination Act; Other Modifications to the HIPAA Rules (Vol. 78(17), pp. 5566–5700): Federal Register 45 CFR Parts 160 and 164.

33. Terry, N. (2017). Existential challenges for healthcare data protection in the United States. *Ethics, Medicine and Public Health, 3*(1), 19–27. doi:10.1016/j.jemep .2017.02.007

34. *Ibid.*

35. United States Food and Drug Administration. (2015, September 22). Digital Health: Health IT Risk-Based Framework. *fda.gov*. Retrieved from www.fda .gov/MedicalDevices/DigitalHealth/ucm338920 .htm

36. Office of the National Coordinator for Health Information Technology. (2017). *Conceptualizing a data infrastructure for the capture, use, and sharing of patient-generated health data in care delivery and research through 2024*. Washington, DC: Office of the National Coordinator for Health Information Technology.
37. Washington et al., (2012), *ibid.*
38. Federal Trade Commission (Producer). (2016, April). Mobile Health Apps Interactive Tool. *Federal Trade Commission*. Retrieved from www.ftc.gov/tips-advice/business-center/guidance/mobile-health-apps-interactive-tool
39. Washington et al., (2012), *ibid.*
40. United States Food and Drug Administration. (2018, February 15). Medical Devices: Digital Health. *fda.gov*. Retrieved from www.fda.gov/medicaldevices/digitalhealth/
41. Washington et al., (2012), *ibid.*
42. Yang, Y. T., & Silverman, R. D. (2014). Mobile health applications: The patchwork of legal and liability issues suggests strategies to improve oversight. *Health Affairs (Millwood), 33*(2), 222–227. doi:10.1377/hlthaff.2013.0958
43. Office of the Privacy Commissioner of Canada (2018, January 31). Summary of Privacy Laws in Canada. *Office of the Privacy Commissioner of Canada*. Retrieved from www.priv.gc.ca/en/privacy-topics/privacy-laws-in-canada/02_05_d_15/
44. *Ibid.*
45. Institute of Medicine (US). (2000). Committee on the Role of Institutional Review Boards in Health Services Research Data Privacy Protection. Protecting Data Privacy in Health Services Research. Washington, DC: National Academies Press (US). APPENDIX D, Confidentiality of Health Information: International Comparative Approaches. Retrieved from www.ncbi.nlm.nih.gov/books/NBK222816/
46. *Ibid.*
47. European Union General Data Protection Regulation. (2018, March 24). GDPR Portal: Site Overview. *edgdpr.org*. Retrieved from www.eugdpr.org/eugdpr.org.html
48. *Ibid.*
49. *Ibid.*
50. Quebec Lawyers Abroad (Producer). (2015, June 8). Privacy at the Crossroads: A Comparative Analysis of Regulation in the US, the EU and Canada. *Advocats Hors Quebec*. Retrieved from www.avocatshorsquebec.org/site/fr/les-nouvelles/articles/302-privacy-at-the-crossroads-a-comparative-analysis-of-regulation-in-the-us-the-eu-and-canada.html
51. *Ibid.*
52. *Ibid.*
53. *Ibid.*
54. Office of the National Coordinator for Health Information Technology. (2014). Learn EHR Basics. *HealthIT.gov*. Retrieved from www.healthit.gov/providers-professionals/learn-ehr-basics
55. *Ibid.*
56. Office of the National Coordinator for Health Information Technology. (2018, January 26). Patient-Generated Health Data. *HealthIT.gov*. Retrieved from www.healthit.gov/policy-researchers-implementers/patient-generated-health-data
57. Terry, M. (2015). HIPAA and your mobile devices. *Podiatry Management*, 99–104.
58. Yang & Silverman, (2014), *ibid.*, p. 222.
59. *Ibid.*
60. Petersen, C., & DeMuro, P. (2015). Legal and regulatory considerations associated with use of patient-generated health data from social media and mobile health (mHealth) devices. *Applied Clinical Informatics, 6*(1), 16–26. doi:10.4338/ACI-2014-09-R-0082
61. Federal Trade Commission, (2016), *ibid.*
62. Office of the National Coordinator for Health Information Technology. (2014a, May 12). What Is HIE? *HealthIT.gov*. Retrieved from www.healthit.gov/providers-professionals/health-information-exchange/what-hie
63. *Ibid.*
64. World Health Organization. (2010). Telemedicine: Opportunities and developments in Member States: Report on the second global survey on eHealth. *Healthcare Informatics Research, 18*(2), 153–155. Retrieved from www.who.int/goe/publications/goe_telemedicine_2010.pdf
65. Cloud Standards Customer Council. (2017). Impact of Cloud Computing on Healthcare (v. 2.0). *cloud-council.org*. Retrieved from www.cloud-council.org/deliverables/CSCC-Impact-of-Cloud-Computing-on-Healthcare.pdf
66. World Health Organization, (2010), *ibid.*
67. *Ibid.*
68. Office of the Privacy Commissioner of Canada, (2018, January 31), *ibid.*
69. *Ibid.*
70. Petersen & DeMuro, (2015), *ibid.*
71. Takabi, H., Joshi, J. B., & Ahn, G.-J. (2010). Security and privacy challenges in cloud computing environments. *IEEE Security & Privacy, 8*(6), 24–31.
72. Cloud Standards Customer Council, (2017), *ibid.*
73. Merriam-Webster Online Dictionary. (2018). Retrieved from www.merriam-webster.com
74. *Ibid.*
75. Ventola, C. L. (2014). Social media and health care professionals: Benefits, risks, and best practices. *Pharmacy and Therapeutics, 39*(7), 491–520.
76. Petersen & DeMuro, (2015), *ibid.*

77. United States Deparment of Health and Human Services Office of Civil Rights. (2018, March 23). Breach Portal: Notice to the Secretary of HHS Breach of Unsecured Protected Health Information. *ocrportal.hhs.gov.* Retrieved from ocrportal .hhs.gov/ocr/breach/breach_report.jsf

78. Ponemon Institute. (2016). Sixth Annual Benchmark Study on Privacy & Security of Healthcare Data. Retrieved from www.ponemon.org/local /upload/file/Sixth Annual Patient Privacy%26 Data Security Report FINAL 6.pdf

79. *Ibid.*

80. Nelson, G. (Producer). (2017, June 20). HIPAA Misconceptions Still Plague Healthcare Providers. *AHC Media.* Retrieved from www.ahcmedia.com /articles/140984-hipaa-misconceptions-still-plague -healthcare-providers

81. Neal, D. (2011). Choosing an electronic health records system: Professional liability considerations. *Innovations in Clinical Neuroscience, 8*(6), 43–46.

82. Ozair, F. F., Jamshed, N., Sharma, A., & Aggarwal, P. (2015). Ethical issues in electronic health records: A general overview. *Perspectives in Clinical Research, 6*(2), 73–76. doi:10.4103/2229-3485.153997

83. Kerr, (2009), *ibid.*

84. Cynergistek. (2018). Improving Readiness: Meeting Cyber Threats.

85. Substance Abuse and Mental Health Services Administration. (2016, March 14). Medical Records Privacy and Confidentiality. *samhsa.gov.* Retrieved from www.samhsa.gov/laws-regulations-guidelines /medical-records-privacy-confidentiality

86. United States Department of Health and Human Services. (2018c). Memorandum to State Survey Agency Directors Regarding Texting of Patient Information among Healthcare Providers. *CMS. gov.* Retrieved from www.cms.gov/Medicare /Provider-Enrollment-and-Certification /SurveyCertificationGenInfo/Downloads/QSO-18 -10-ALL.pdf

87. Kaplan, A. (2012). Electronic Health Records and Patient Privacy–An Oxymoron? *Psychiatric Times, 29*(8), 1–7.

88. *Ibid.*

89. Terry, (2015), *Ibid.*

90. Ozair et al., (2015), *Ibid.*

91. *Ibid.*

92. Bhuyan, S., Kim, H., Isehunwa, O., Kumar, N., Bhatt, J., Wyant, D. K., ... Dasgupta, D. (2017). Privacy and security issues in mobile health: Current research and future directions. *Health Policy and Technology, 6*(2), 188–191. doi:10.1016/j.hlpt.2017.01.004

93. *Ibid.*

94. Telehealth Resource Centers (Producer). (2018, March 24). *Privacy, confidentiality, and security.* Retrieved from www.telehealthresourcecenter.org /toolbox-module/privacy-confidentiality-and-security

95. *Ibid.*

96. McKnight & Franko, (2016), *ibid.*

97. Flaherty, J. L. (2014). Digital diagnosis: Privacy and the regulation of mobile phone health applications. *American Journal of Law & Medicine, 40*(4), 416–441.

98. McKnight & Franko, (2016), *ibid.*

99. *Ibid.*, p. 129.

100. United States Department of Health and Human Services, (2018c), *ibid.*

101. *Ibid.*

102. Terry, (2017), *ibid.*

103. *Ibid.*

104. Smith, G. C., & Knudson, T. K. (2016). Student nurses' unethical behavior, social media, and year of birth. *Nursing Ethics, 23*(8), 910–918. doi:10.1177/0969733015590009

105. *Ibid.*, p. 917.

106. Thompson, L. A., Black, E., Duff, W. P., Paradise Black, N., Saliba, H., & Dawson, K. (2011). Protected health information on social networking sites: ethical and legal considerations. *Journal of Medical Internet Research, 13*(1), p. 8. doi:10.2196/jmir .1590

107. Neal, (2011), *ibid.*

108. *Ibid.*

109. HIPAA Misconceptions Still Plague Healthcare Providers. (2017). *Healthcare Risk Management, 39*(7), 10–10.

110. Kaplan, (2012), *ibid.*

111. Neal, (2011), *ibid.*

112. Petersen & DeMuro, (2015), *ibid.*

113. Office of the National Coordinator for Health Information Technology, (2017), *ibid.*

114. *Ibid.*

115. Yang & Silverman, (2014), *ibid.*

116. *Ibid.*

117. *Ibid.*

118. *Ibid.*

119. *Ibid.*

120. Ventola, (2014), *ibid.*

121. Petersen & DeMuro, (2015), *ibid.*

122. *Ibid.*

123. Polito, J. M. (2012). Ethical considerations in internet use of electronic protected health information. *Neurodiagnostic Journal, 52*(1), 34–41.

124. Ventola, (2014), *ibid.*

125. *Ibid.*

126. Office of the National Coordinator for Health Information Technology, (2014), *ibid.*

127. Office of the National Coordinator for Health Information Technology, (2018, January 26), *ibid.*

128. *Ibid.*

129. HCPro. (2015). Use mobile devices without increasing risk. *Strategies for Health Care Compliance, 19*(1), 1–5.
130. Bendix, J. (2013). What the HIPAA omnibus rule means for your practice. *Contemporary OB/GYN, 58*(6), 34–42.
131. Cynergistek, (2018), *ibid.*, p. 4.
132. *Ibid.*
133. Gordon, J.-S., Rauprich, O., & Vollmann, J. (2011). Applying the four-principle approach. *Bioethics, 25*(6), 293–300. Retrieved from doi:10.1111/j.1467-8519.2009.01757.x
134. Polito, (2012), *ibid.*, p. 39.

Chapter Questions

12-1 How are the HIMSS and the corresponding TIGER Initiative competencies relevant to clinical professionals?

12-2 Since most, if not all, EHR vendors supply security software, why should providers be concerned with security issues?

12-3 While some entities are covered under HIPAA privacy and security, others are not. What risk does a non-covered entity pose to a healthcare provider?

12-4 What should providers consider in the use and storage of mental health records?

12-5 Does the requirement for accurate medical documentation change with new technology? If so, how?

12-6 List and define the different types of health IT introduced in the chapter. Based on use and functionality, do some types inherently have more legal and ethical risks? If so, how are the risks greater?

12-7 Other than privacy and security, what are other legal and ethical risks that are involved with the use of health IT?

12-8 The end of the chapter describes the "four principles approach" to healthcare ethics. In contemplating the scenario at the beginning of the chapter, how are each of the four principles either promoted or detracted?

Biography

Charie Faught is an Associate Professor of Business IT, Health Information Technology at Montana Tech. She received her Bachelor of Arts in Chemistry from the University of Montana in Missoula, Montana, and Master of Health Administration from Tulane University, School of Public Health and Tropical Medicine in New Orleans, Louisiana. She also completed her PhD in Human Services specializing in Health Care Administration from Capella University, Minneapolis, Minnesota. Her dissertation is on the use of clinical decision support on adult type 2 diabetes process and outcomes measures.

Dr. Faught's teaching and professional experience cover a variety of positions. She was a Director of Corporate Integrity for Health Partners, Inc. in Bloomington, Minnesota, and was an Integrity Liaison for Providence Health Systems in Seattle, Washington. Her teaching experience includes work as a Teaching Assistant for the Department of Health Systems Management at Tulane University. She also served as a United States Peace Corps Volunteer. She has taught high school math, chemistry, and biology in Lautoka, Fiji, at Jasper Williams High School.

Her recent work has focused on ethical and legal concerns regarding the use of health information technology, including regulatory requirements for mobile devices.

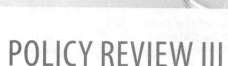

POLICY REVIEW III

Health IT Standards Adoption in Health Systems

Sanjay Sood and Joseph Tan

Abstract

Health IT standards, a topic of increasing significance for HMIS students, practitioners, and researchers, relate to data-coding standards (vocabulary), data-schema standards (structure and content), data-exchange standards (messaging), and Web standards. Adoption of these standards can bring about a common language for sharing health information digitally among care providers. This review discussed the different major standards in health IT with specific application examples highlighted. More specifically, it focuses on the adoption of standards required for increasing efficiencies in health data exchange among multiple care providers so as to ensure the transition of higher quality and safer care for patients among these providers. The topic is central to understanding HMIS as it links earlier parts of the text on new health IT perspectives pertaining to the innovative use of health data (and analytics) for clinical decision making and guidelines development, commercial ventures and for online data seeking (Part I); health IT technology and applications across the various patient-centric care domains (Part II); health IT strategic planning and management, data stewardship, and health learning systems implementation and maintenance; and finally to health IT governance, privacy and confidentiality as well as cyber security issues and health data misuse prevention.

▶ Introduction

Today, major standards have been applied across many hospital-based information systems, such as electronic health records (EHR), clinical decision support (CDS), computerized physician order entry (CPOE), radiological information systems (RIS), laboratory information systems (LIS), and pharmacy information systems (PIS). Without these standards in health IT, the medical field would have been at a standstill in terms of rapid IT adoption and diffusion. This explains why, in the past decades, nurses and physicians were particularly resistant to new technologies and why it took years for many routine hospital activities, such as nurse scheduling, prescription orders, and physician workflow, to be computerized.

Indeed, the laudable effort on the part of concerned standards development organizations (SDOs) in their quest of bridging the gap between the medical field and IT cannot be ignored. Well-established and influential SDOs, like HL7, the Institute of Electrical and Electronics Engineers (IEEE), the American National Standards Institute (ANSI), and the World Wide Web Consortium (W3C), among many others, are engaged in developing and promoting the adoption and diffusion of pertinent gold standards to ease the exchange of complex medical and other forms of information. Although these burgeoning standards exist in niche areas, significant effort still needs to be made so that nations and government agencies around the world are willing to trust and adopt a good number of the more established standards and embrace new ones, such as Logical Observation Identifiers Names and Codes (LOINC), Systematized Nomenclature of Medicine (SNOMED), Medical Information Bus (MIB), American Society for Testing and Materials (ASTM), Healthcare Informatics Standards Board (HISB), and Comité Européen de Normalisation (European Committee for Standardisation; CEN).

Next, we highlight some of the more established and widely accepted standards, including International Classification of Disease (IDC) standards, Health Level 7 (HL7), Digital Imaging and Communication in Medicine (DICOM), and web standards.

▶ ICD and Other Standards

ICD, developed under the auspices of the World Health Organization (WHO), refers to an internationally recognized standard classification of diseases in the form of standardized diagnostic codes with ICD 10th Revision, Clinical Modification, June 2003 (ICD-10-CM) representing a progression of ICD 9th Revision, Clinical Modification (ICD-9-CM) coding standards' capability to cover an expanded vocabulary and new requirements

generated by the Health Insurance Portability and Accountability Act of 1996 (HIPAA). MS-DRG, which is based on Medicare Severity DRG derived from ICD-9-CM, is a classification system primarily used by health systems organizations, such as the Centers for Medicare and Medicaid Services (CMS), for inpatient prospective payment services and billing. Additionally, MS-DRG coding can be used for utilization review, such as aiding in the planning of hospital inpatient discharge services by providing the hospital wards with critical information pertaining to the most prevalent groupings of inpatient services and average length of stays.

CPT, published by the American Medical Association (AMA), provides standard procedure codes for professional reimbursement and billing. The CPT codebook, maintained by the CPT Editorial Panel, is structured according to specialty, body system, or service provided. LOINC is a classification system used for identifying laboratory results and clinical observations. Therefore, two major sections of LOINC are Lab LOINC and Clinical LOINC. SNOMED, developed and maintained by the College of American Pathologists (CAP), is a coding scheme meant to integrate the data accumulated from multi-provider care processes by mapping with ICD, LOINC, and various other data classification standards. CCC, previously known as Home Health Care Classification (HHCC), offers a taxonomic framework for documenting holistically hospital-based patient care process along two interrelated dimensions: (1) CCC of Nursing Diagnoses and Outcomes and (2) CCC of Nursing Interventions and Actions. ICPC-2, developed by the International Classification Committee of the World Organization of National Colleges (WONCA), Academies, and Academic Association of General Practitioners/Family Physicians is a coding taxonomy that maps to ICD-10 for primary care services. A severity of illness checklists and functional status assessment charts are included in ICPC-2. Not surprisingly, new versions of codes have continued to evolve, including ABC codes and numerous others (e.g., CRM or Galen Common Reference Model, LOINC, UMLS, NDC, and NANDA).[1,2] **TABLE PR3-1** summarizes a sampling of the more popular codes.

Data-exchange standards (messaging) use a standardized interconnecting system protocol to predictably transmit electronic data; that is, it standardizes the order and sequence of data during transmission between two points across a network or sub-network. Open-systems interconnection (OSI) is an open architecture having seven layers, each demanding a different level of functionality for data exchange to materialize among different systems. These OSI levels include physical, data link, network, transport, session, presentation, and application. As discussed in the previous edition of this work, other standards for system networking include IBM's system network architecture (SNA), DEC's DNA (DEC network architecture), Transmission control protocol/Internet protocol (TCP/IP), and MUMPS (Bourke, 1994).[3]

Data schema standards (structure and content) involve defining essential data elements in the database, such as a minimum data set (MDS), and specifying the structure, domains, rules, and relationships among these data elements to be maintained within the records to facilitate data retrieval. In the manual system, the data entry was serial and not random at the functional level. Computerization allows the data representation to become functionally complex. Here, the data comes with different type, categorization, and transaction identities assigned at each functional level. This led to the development of widely used data schema, such as hierarchical, network, and relational data models, which were detailed in one of the *Technology Briefs* earlier in this text. Complex data object models have also evolved, which allow users to view data at a high conceptual level.

Coupled with HIPAA, all of these data standards will serve to minimize potential misuse of patient information and limit access to medical records by so-called covered entities, including physicians, clearinghouses, healthcare providers, hospital administrators, clinical researchers, and other employees. Because of the potential for serious harm through discrimination, loss of insurance, unemployability, or stigmatization, HIPAA regulations, which are detailed in other parts of the current edition, provide federal protection for this health information.[4]

▶ HL7

HL7, as accredited by ANSI, is a system development organization whose aim is to promote interoperability for the interchange of health data. "Level Seven" refers to the highest level of the International Organization for Standardization (ISO) communications model for OSI—the application level.[5] HL7 was built on existing production protocols, predominantly those of ASTM Standard 1238. It operates as a nonprofit volunteer-, vendor-, and provider-supported organization to encourage information scientists and various experts in the healthcare field to endeavor toward the development of standards for the management, processing, integration, and exchange of electronic healthcare information.

■ The Vocabulary Problem

The chief aim of HL7 is to address the *vocabulary problem*, which has paralyzed health IT developers, implementers, and users of computer-based applications in medicine. The vocabulary problem is best characterized by the failure among communities of health information end users to find a common denominator for representing health knowledge and discoveries. Despite countless efforts invested by medical terminology developers and informatics specialists, the vocabulary

TABLE PR3-1 A Summary of Coding Systems Representing Healthcare Concepts

Standard	Description
Read codes	Detailed set of codes used to explain patient care and treatment information.
LOINC	Standard codes and classifications for identifying laboratory and clinical terms.
ICD-10 codes	New diagnostic codes developed by the WHO, not yet used in North America.
IFC	International Classification on Functioning, Disability, and Health; a taxonomy to describe bodily functions and structure, domains of activity and participation, and environmental factors interacting with these components.
CPT4 codes	Procedure codes developed by the American Medical Association for professional billing and reimbursement for outpatient and ambulatory care.
HCPCS	Healthcare Common Procedure Coding System; provides codes used for reporting physician services for Medicare patients.
APC	Ambulatory Payment Classification system; refers to outpatient reimbursement based on groupings of CPT/HCPCS–coded procedures.
CDT-2005	Code on Dental Terminology; a dental procedural and nomenclature standard.
NANDA	North American Nursing Diagnosis Association code; set of nursing diagnoses.
National Library of Medicine (NLM) Unified Medical Language System (UMLS)	A cross-referenced collection of codes and related information sources.
APA DSM-IV	Diagnostic codes organized by the American Psychiatric Association (APA).
ECRI	Codes used to identify medical equipment.
Others	Diagnosis-related group (DRG) databases, SNOMED, IUPAC Codes, Arden Syntax, etc.

problem remained until the emergence of HL7. HL7 provided a common interface among the various user communities in terms of the nomenclature of health-related knowledge— its growing popularity hinges on its promise to realize the semantic interoperability of the HL7 Message Development Framework (MDF), which aims at easing the exchange and use of clinical information among disparate systems as well as enhancing clinical research and promoting population health management.

HL7 is responsible for driving the development of specifications for messaging standards that will enable disparate healthcare applications to exchange key sets of clinical and administrative data. Current core clinical standards available through HL7 include order entry, scheduling, medical records management, imaging, patient administration, observation (laboratory results, radiographic reports, examination findings, and so on), and patient financial messages.[6] Being a message standard protocol, HL7 handles clinical information communication, such as diagnostic results, scheduling information, clinical trials data, and master file records. HL7 serves the purpose of data sharing among disparate vendors or sources of electronic data interchange within the healthcare organizational environment. HL7 acts as a means to reduce, if not eliminate, the level of interface programming and program maintenance. It, therefore, ensures timely data exchange with minimal deficit of clinical knowledge.

■ *HL7 Development*

In 1999, a complete revision of HL7, which was based on the common Reference Information Model (RIM), was undertaken and appeared as HL7 version 3. All the data content for HL7 messages would now originate from the HL7 RIM, serving as a coherent and mutual information model. More recently, Health Level 7 has also been developing standards for the representation of clinical documents, such as discharge summaries and progress notes.[7] Bakken et al.[8] discussed the development of two sets of principles to provide guidance to terminology stakeholders: (1) principles for HL7-compliant terminologies and (2) principles for HL7-sanctioned terminology integration efforts. To help health systems organizations achieve HL7 compliance, the key activities undertaken by HL7 organizations today include the completion of a survey of terminology developers, the development of a process for HL7 registration of terminologies, and the maintenance of vocabulary domain specification tables.

■ *HL7 Adoption*

The relentless efforts put forward by HL7 have paid off in that countries such as Argentina, Australia, Canada, China, the Czech Republic, Finland, Germany, India, Japan, Korea, Lithuania, The Netherlands, New Zealand, the Republic of South Africa, Switzerland, Taiwan, Turkey, and the United Kingdom have now become part of HL7 initiatives. Presently, HL7 is also being used by about 2000 leading hospitals in countries like Japan, Germany, Sweden, and Holland. In the United States alone, HL7 standards have been influential— more than 150 U.S. healthcare institutions, the U.S. Centers for Disease Control and Prevention (CDC), large referral laboratories, and eminent universities have adopted these standards. Moreover, countries like New Zealand and Australia have already adopted HL7 as their national standards. Today, HL7 is known to be the most widely implemented healthcare data-messaging standard.

▶ DICOM

DICOM, which has emerged to fulfill the need for transferring digital images of various formats as well as related information between devices (irrespective of the device manufacturer), is a nonproprietary data interchange protocol.[9] Originally, the joint committee of the American College of Radiology (ACR) and the National Electronic Manufacturers

Association (NEMA) oversaw the development of DICOM standards. The comprehensive specification of DICOM includes the detailed engineering information used as a blueprint for information structures and procedures. These engineering details will enhance the network connectivity among the community of vendors' products, thereby enabling exchange of various formats of medical information within and outside the health systems organizations through the far-fetched abilities of telemedicine and other technologies. In 1985, DICOM version 1.0 was developed by ACR/NEMA; since then, it had undergone two consecutive revisions. Today, DICOM version 3.0 is recognized as the improved and most recent version.

■ *Purpose of DICOM*

The DICOM message standard, in collaboration with other standard groups, vies for the compatibility of digital information between medical imaging systems across the different health services delivery environments globally. With its growing success, DICOM brings together the medical societies, universities, governmental and nongovernmental agencies, and nonprofit as well as for-profit organizations to participate in the DICOM Standards Committee. Awareness and knowledge of the DICOM standards will create ample room for its adoption and diffusion, as well as its further extension.

Adopted by virtually every medical profession that utilizes images within the healthcare industry, such as cardiology, dentistry, endoscopy, mammography, ophthalmology, orthopedics, pathology, pediatrics, radiation therapy, radiology, and surgery, the DICOM standards are even used in veterinary medical imaging applications. There is an escalating interest regarding the efficient management of digitizing medical images for easy transfer between electronic devices. These standards are structured to support the formatting and exchanging of complex medical imaging applications in all the major medical disciplines noted earlier. Tele-radiology has emerged as the bridge to

close the gap between the general physicians and the referral specialists, including radiologists, cardiologists, orthodontists, ophthalmologists, pathologists, radiation therapists, pediatricians, surgeons, and other medical specialists who are used to reading radiological images to support the continuing care of their patients. Today, these encoding and communications protocols have largely moved into electronic storage, exchange, pre-fetching, real-time retrieval, and return of diagnostic and therapeutic images and image- and non-image-related information in emergencies and other high-stress medical environments.

The DICOM standards aim to bridge the gap through interoperability while enhancing the workflow efficiency between medical imaging equipment and other medical image–intensive departments on a global scale. By so doing, DICOM standards will enhance communication among image acquisition, waveform, picture archiving, and information system components. During the 1990s, laudable effort was made to achieve filmless radiology. The strides of DICOM standards were recognized in achieving this goal. The flexible nature of DICOM standards enables users to create an image management system. Designing a system around DICOM can prevent a department from being "trapped" by a single vendor and limited to a proprietary family of products; still, naive implementation of DICOM standards does not guarantee this flexibility.[10]

The DICOM standards allow proper organization of information objects by aggregating images having similar attributes. It further provides free-text and coded-data entry as well as fields for structured encoding. This increases the direct benefits of information retrieval through precise encoding. With the compatibility provided by DICOM standards, it is anticipated that use of image management systems will soon become a "plug-and-play" channel suitable for handling by any non-technically oriented physician. The DICOM standards also minimize duplicate data entry at the modality console due to the work lists received by the imaging modality. Additional facilities like query, storage, retrieval, print, and other functionalities are also supported by the DICOM standards. These cooperative standards promote network connectivity through interoperability of multi-vendor devices by specifying levels of conformance. DICOM standards maintain nomenclature of a multipart document to support the evolving standards by the addition of new features. DICOM standards will accommodate explicit hierarchy of information objects ranging from images, graphics, texts, reports, waveforms, and printings. Service classes are used to uniquely identify information objects from the hierarchy as part of the DICOM standards. A lexicon having the nomenclature in groups defines the hierarchy of information objects, while each data element defining the individual object consists of a data tag, a data-length specification, and the data value.

▶ Adoption of DICOM Standards

One of the reasons DICOM standards have been popularly accepted and adopted across a wide variety of clinical imaging contexts is that these standards specify a conformance statement that improves the communication of software specifications for imaging equipment.[11] Being a part of cooperative standards, DICOM connects every major diagnostic medical imaging vendor for cooperating individual testing. The participation of the vendor's professional societies around the world will also support and further enhance these standards.

With such a long list of well-tested benefits provided by DICOM, concerned organizations, such as imaging vendors, physician users, SDOs, and those of general interest, would not need to hesitate to embrace DICOM standards. In an effort to improve healthcare imaging, these standards have long been used and adopted by highly reputed academic

institutions, such as Harvard Medical School and other major medical establishments. The radiology department at Massachusetts General Hospital (MGH), for example, adopted DICOM standards years ahead of others for all of its tele-radiological programs.

▶ Web Standards

In 1994, Tim Berners-Lee founded the World Wide Web Consortium (W3C)—a consortium formed to ensure compatibility and agreement among industry members in the adoption of new web standards. W3C's mission is "To lead the World Wide Web to its full potential by developing protocols and guidelines that ensure long-term growth for the Web."[12]

Among the more popular conceptualization of web standards is that these standards are linked to the trend of endorsing a set of established best practices for building websites and a philosophy of web design and development that includes those methods. Many interdependent standards and specifications exist, which can directly or indirectly affect the development and administration of websites and web services. Web standards, when translated, can be separated generally into two different categories, namely, a table-free site or a site using valid code. Even so, web standards themselves involve broader aspects. A website built to comply with web standards should adhere to commonly accepted standards, such as Hypertext Markup Language (HTML), XHTML and Modularization, Extensible Markup Language (XML), Cascading Style Sheets (CSS), Document Object Model (DOM), and others (e.g., MathML), while utilizing valid code practices, accessible code, semantically correct code, and user-friendly universal resource locators (URLs). Generally, web standards comprise the following accepted specifications:

- *HTML*: HTML 4.0 is widely used on the web for adding structure to text documents. Web browsers interpret these documents, representing the structure in media-specific ways to the user.

- *XHTML and Modularization*: XHTML 1.0 is a reformulation of HTML as an XML application; XHTML 1.1 is an upgrade.
- *XML*: XML 1.0 is a markup language that allows you to define your own elements.
- *CSS*: CSS is a mechanism for changing the appearance of HTML or XML elements by assigning styles to element types, self-defined classes of elements, or individual instances.
- *DOM 1*: DOM allows the full power and interactivity of a scripting language, such as ECMA Script, the standardized version of JavaScript, to be exerted on a web page.
- *MathML: Document Markup for Mathematics*. MathML is an XML enabling application for sharing mathematical documentation through standardized notations adoption for conveying both the structure and content of web-based mathematical information.

Complying with web standards can give web pages greater visibility in web search engines, such as Google. The structural information present in standards-compliant documents makes it easy for search engines to access and evaluate the information in those documents. Websites get indexed more accurately due to the use of web standards, making it easier for server-side as well as client-side software to understand the structure and content of the document. Web standards are adopted so that old browsers will still understand the basic structure of a document. Writing web pages in accordance with the standards shortens site development time and makes pages easier to maintain. Debugging and troubleshooting become easier as the code follows a standard of web page development. This all ties in with the W3C mission statement to help ensure positive long-term growth for the web.

▶ Conclusion

During the past century, the medical field has experienced thrilling changes, such as new drugs, new devices, and new techniques. These mega-changes are being constantly adopted, but the real metamorphosis will be seen when the concepts of health IT and informatics help build real-world solutions for the administrative, clinical, and relevant systems that would enhance seamless interoperability and multilateral communication between the business units of the enterprise, whereby a cohesive information model can be maintained to promote the strategic goals of the enterprise. If we want to enjoy the benefits of information management technologies, we must embrace and even streamline many of these standards for the welfare of the planet. Heterogeneity of clinical knowledge and the continuing diversity that preclude effectiveness have plagued users, developers, and implementers of computer-based applications in medicine. International standards in health IT for health systems have provided the pivotal backbone to integrating clinical knowledge discovery. Standards such as ICD-9, HL7, and DICOM have been so overwhelmingly accepted that when strengthened by an enforceable law like HIPAA, these standards promise to satisfy the demanding capabilities of the electronic and digital needs in medicine.

Notes

1. Physicians' Current Procedural Terminology (CPT) is a coding system established in 1966 by the American Medical Association to provide a uniform language to accurately describe medical, surgical, and diagnostic services. Each procedure or service is identified with a five-digit code.

2. Detailed descriptions of ICD-10 codes and many other coding schemes can be found in various websites or from links to the Duke University Medical Center site (www.mcis.duke.edu).

3. Bourke, M. K. (1994). *Strategy and architecture of health care information systems.* New York, NY: Springer-Verlag.
4. O'Herrin, J. K., Fost, N., & Kudsk, K. A. (2004). Health Insurance Portability Accountability Act (HIPAA) regulations effect on medical record research. *Annals of Surgery, 239,* 772–778.
5. About HL7. Retrieved from http://www.hl7.org/about/
6. *Ibid.*
7. Dolin, R. H., Alschuler, L., Beebe, C., Biron, P. V., Boyer, S. L., Essin, D., … Mattison, M. D. (2001). The HL7 clinical document architecture. *Journal of the American Medical Information Association, 8,* 552–569.
8. Bakken, S., Campbell, K. E., Cimino, J. J., Huff, S. M., & Hammond, W. (2000). Toward vocabulary domain specifications for health level 7-coded data elements. *Journal of the American Medical Information Association, 7*(4), 333–342.
9. Ramos, A. T. (2002). Information object definition-based unified modeling language representation of DICOM structured reporting. A case study of transcoding DICOM to XML. *Journal of the American Medical Information Association, 9,* 63–71.
10. Bidgood, W. D., Hori, S. C., Prior, F. W., & Syckle, D. E. V. (1997). Understanding and using DICOM, the data interchange standard for biomedical imaging. *Journal of the American Medical Information Association, 4,* 199–212.
11. *Ibid.*
12. W3C. Retrieved from www.w3.org/consortium

Biography

State Awardee (Chandigarh Administration, 2014) *Dr. Sanjay P. Sood's* rich experience (24 years) spans various geographies. Dr. Sood holds a PhD. in Information Technology (telemedicine) and has a global outlook. He has been associated with the domain of telemedicine for two decades. He is actively into cutting edge research and development and implementations pertaining to Telemedicine and eHealth systems. He led the team that developed Indian Government's first indigenous Telemedicine Technology at Centre for Development of Advanced Computing (C-DAC), Mohali, Punjab (India) and has implemented telemedicine systems in around 150 hospitals in India and overseas. He has been a telemedicine consultant with World Health Organization in Africa and has also been an eHealth expert on the panel of the United Nations and is advising the Government of Andhra Pradesh (India) on Teleradiology Services. He is the Founder Director and Head of School of C-DAC School of Advanced Computing in Mauritius (University of Mauritius) and was also a Senate Member at the University of Mauritius (2004–2008). He is a Senate Member at Punjab Engineering College, Chandigarh (India).

Dr. Sood has authored numerous world-class publications and book chapters on Telemedicine and eHealth. He is serving on editorial boards of six international journals on Telemedicine, eHealth, and Healthcare IT. One of his telemedicine publications is amongst the world's most cited telemedicine research. He is a recipient of prestigious international fellowships (such as the Young Investigator Scholarship by University of Michigan and the SIDA Scholarship by the Swedish Government) and has traveled to over 25 countries. He is presently working as the Associate Director and Head (Health Informatics) at Centre for Development of Advanced Computing (C-DAC) Mohali, Punjab (India). One of his most recent developments include MyHealthRecord—Personal Health Records Management System for the citizens of India. It is slated to be rolled out in near future by Ministry of Health and Family Welfare, Govt. of India. At present, he is working towards roll-out of telemedicine (using eSanjeevani—an indigenous integrated telemedicine solution developed by Health Informatics Department of C-DAC Mohali, India) across India, at over 155,000 Health and Wellness Center for the Government of India.

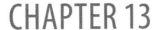

CHAPTER 13

AI and Social Media Analytics for Health Systems: Understanding Consumers' Preferences in Healthcare Services

Adela S. M. Lau, Kristine Baker, Katherine Kempf, Katie Grzyb, Sijuade Oke, Eric Tsui, Liege Cheung, Marie-Claire Slama, and Min Su

LEARNING OBJECTIVES

- Provide an overview of consumer shopping, behavioral changes, and e-health services
- Conceptualize social media analytics and artificial intelligence (AI)
- Illustrate Zocdoc use of social media analytics for health systems
- Speculate the future of social media analytics

CHAPTER OUTLINE

Scenario: Use AI and Social Media Analytics for Healthcare Consumer Preference Analysis

I. Introduction
II. Consumer Shopping, Behavioral Changes, and E-Health Services

III. Social Media Analytics (SMA) and AI
- *SMA*
- *Natural Language Processing (NLP)*
- *Knowledge Base and AI for Named Entity Extraction, Sentiment Analysis, and Relation Extraction*

Scenario: Use AI and Social Media Analytics for Healthcare Consumer Preference Analysis

Between a growing elderly population and a shrinking number of healthcare professionals, the United States faces a serious healthcare problem. To address this problem, health institutions and professionals are looking to innovative technologies, such as tele-health and artificial intelligence (AI). Madonna University's Master of Science in Health Services Administration is one of the leading programs in Michigan for preparing students to face today's healthcare challenges, participating in the development of health-focused technologies. One of the courses of the program worked with institutions and associations for exploring innovative solutions for our fast-paced, everchanging healthcare environment. A leading global digital health team with a passion for pioneering new health technologies worked with the authors to explore how AI can be used to identify the consumers' preferences in healthcare services. Using these AI-based models, leaders in health care can more confidently build their future roadmaps for and investments in e-health services. Such services are largely believed to be key in solving the current and future supply and demand problem in the healthcare industry.

Social media, rather than traditional questionnaires, is a readily available and affordable means of collecting data concerning consumers' healthcare preferences. Social media allows researchers to tap directly into a consumer's publicly-shared thoughts and opinions. However, social media as a data source has its downsides. Firstly, the volume of data is extreme, so identifying starting and ending points for research can present a challenge. Secondly, social media data can be complicated to efficiently summarize, classify, and group for the purposes of analysis, evaluation, and presentation. By combining AI's symbolic and mathematical methods for classifying and grouping data with the use of dashboards to display the analyzed results, healthcare institutions and professionals can visualize customer preferences and identify needs on a market-by-market basis.

▶ I. Introduction

AI simulates human perception and thinking processes and uses mathematical symbols, logic, rules, semantic networks, and knowledge representations to model the human cognitive thinking model.[1,2] The types of AI models may be classified into statistics, computational intelligence (neural networks or NNs, fuzzy logic, and evolutionary algorithms), and symbolic methods.[3-5] Importantly, the analysis of the social media posts will require the extraction of the entities from text, the classification of the entities into different categories, and the definition of the relationship of the entities to draw conclusions.

In the AI family, natural language processing (NLP) decomposes the social media text into entities (words, punctuation, and other elements). The AI models, such as regression model, support vector machine (SVM), decision tree (DT), NN, k-nearest neighbor (k-NN), Gaussian mixture model, Bayesian network, and Naïve Bayes, use statistical or probabilistic methods to classify the entities into different categories.[6,7] Other AI models, such as Bayesian network,[8] hidden Markov model,[9] neuro-fuzzy system,[10] and SVM,[11] use probabilistic or statistical methods to reason the relationships in and between the entities and extract the similar entities for sentiment analysis. The symbolic AI models, such as propositional logic, expert system, fuzzy logic,[12] and more, use a network of production rules to connect symbols (related entities) and to make deductions for drawing the conclusions from the social media posts.[13,14] The analyzed results and trends are then presented visually in a dashboard for health providers to review.

In recent years, consumers have used social media as a popular means for sharing product opinions and providing instant feedback of services.[15] In order for health providers to understand consumers' satisfaction levels and demands, mining physician reviews from social media is an important undertaking. This chapter presents the study of several social media websites on e-health services offered in the United States, Hong Kong, Malaysia, Indonesia, Taiwan, and Singapore. Zocdoc is one of the popular physician-reviewing websites in the United States and was selected in this study for further analysis. The social media analytics (SMA) methods and techniques are reviewed and some are applied, in the case of Zocdoc, to analyze consumers' comments regarding physicians' services. The study results demonstrate that the use of AI and vocabulary databases could extract and summarize consumers' comments and opinions on topics such as physician's review, appointment scheduling, and new services. The dashboard and key performance indicators (KPIs) are used to summarize the trends and provide feedback needed to allow physicians to improve their services as well as determine which new services to offer. Concerns regarding the use of SMA for health services are discussed at the end of the chapter.

In summary, this chapter demonstrates the use of AI in analyzing consumer opinions and preferences regarding e-health services. The steps and procedures for analyzing social media posts are first discussed. Following this, the case of Zocdoc is presented to demonstrate how AI is applied in SMA to find out consumers' opinions and expectations on e-health services. Finally, issues regarding SMA are highlighted.

▶ II. Consumer Shopping, Behavioral Changes, and E-Health Services

As the population ages and tele-health use becomes more prevalent, understanding e-health services' capacity and consumer behaviors are essential to the success of e-health development. With increasing healthcare services delivered online, and the integration of social media into consumers' daily lives, consumers frequently seek comments and opinions from other consumers via social media platforms before making decisions. To this end, SMA has recently been used to determine consumers' emotions, sentiments, and preferences of health services related to consumer relationship management (CRM), marketing, and new product research.[16]

An intelligent agent with the capability of monitoring and analyzing the social media discussion enables health providers to improve and develop new health services to consumers. It provides the autonomy, self-direction, self-organization, and self-learning capabilities to search,[17] classify, and group the social media discussions. Further, the agent can analyze and conclude consumers' satisfaction levels and preferences on the health services. Since consumers' intentions and actual behaviors surrounding e-health services change with their experiences regarding its usability (i.e., observed consumer satisfaction) and sociability (i.e., recommendation from the community),[18,19] AI (i.e., machine learning built into the agents) provides a mechanism for analyzing, learning, and adjusting the changes of these observations for consumers' preferences analysis. The SMA results can be visualized and presented in a dashboard to prompt health providers on how they might improve their services.

▶ III. Social Media Analytics (SMA) and AI

SMA

SMA analyze the content of social media websites. The techniques used in SMA include NLP, named entity extraction, text analysis, sentiment analysis, and relation extraction.[20] SMA use a knowledge base (text corpus), such as stop-word corpus,[21] vocabulary databases,[22] ontology databases,[23] and rule-based engines[24] for parsing and extracting key concepts from the social media posts. AI provides models, such as SVM, NN, and Bayesian network, to conceptualize and determine the pragmatic meanings of the opinions, emotions, and sentiments of the consumers, as well as summarize the conclusion of their discussion.[25-27] With the analyzed sentiments, AI is able to learn and predict the patterns of the consumer behavioral changes and find out the new services for the consumers. Health systems providers can also visualize these changes in a dashboard for new-services research. Hence, SMA is a new method to find out consumers' satisfaction, shopping behaviors, and preferences beyond the traditional marketing survey analysis as the consumers' shopping behavior has been changed from web searching into social opinions searching and referencing.

NLP

To perform the sentiment analysis of the social media content, NLP is used to preprocess the social media posts.[28] NLP decomposes the social media text into meaningful entities. The NLP processes include sentence segmentation, tokenization (word segmentation), part-of-speech tagging, stemming, lemmatization, name entity extraction, chunking (noun phrase extraction), parsing, and coreference resolution. After a paragraph of text is segmented into sentences, tokenization segments the sentence into units (tokens) of words, punctuation, numbers, alphanumeric, and more. Part of speech tagging assigns parts of speech (i.e., noun, verb, adjective, and other parts) to each word. To standardize the text presentation format, stemming chops off the end of the words and removes the inflectional suffixes and derivational affixes. Lemmatization returns the base or dictionary form of the text (i.e., lemma) of the stemmed word so that named entity extraction can then locate and classify the named entities of the tokens into predefined categories, such as person, occupation, locations, descriptor, and services for sentiment analysis.

To determine a sentence's syntactic structure for relation extraction analysis, the chunking (noun phrase extraction) segments and labels multi-token sequences to represent a phase or a meaning. A parsing tree then parses the tagged tokens into a syntactic structure and displays the tagged tokens in a tree-structure sentence. Within or between sentences, coreference resolution finds all tokens that refer to the same entity and cross-references them for relation extraction analysis. An example on how a social media post is preprocessed using NLP for sentiment and relation extraction analysis is shown in **TABLE 13-1**.[29]

Knowledge Base and AI for Named Entity Extraction, Sentiment Analysis, and Relation Extraction

To find out the named entity of the tokens, a knowledge base and AI models are used together. The knowledge base, which is constructed from a stop-word corpus, vocabulary

TABLE 13-1 An Example of Social Media Posts Decomposition

NLP tasks and its open sources	Social Post Example: I visited Dr. Bob two times. He is a nice and responsible physician.
Step 1: Sentence segmentation: *OpenNLP, CoreNLP*	Sentence 1: I visited Dr. Bob two times. Sentence 2: He is a nice and responsible physician.

Tokenization: *Natural Language Toolkit (NLTK), OpenNLP*

Sentence 1:

I	visited	Dr.	Bob	two	times

Sentence 2:

He	is	a	nice	and	responsible	physician

Step 2: Part of speech tagging: *NLTK, OpenNLP, CoreNLP*

Sentence 1:

I	visited	Dr.	Bob	two	times
Pronoun (PN)	*Verb (VB)*	*Noun (NN)*	*Noun (NN)*	*Determiner (DET)*	*Noun (NN)*

Sentence 2:

He	is	a	nice	and
Pronoun (PN)	*Verb (VB)*	*Determiner (DET)*	*Adjective (AJ)*	*Conjunction (CJ)*

responsible	physician
Adjective (AJ)	*Noun (NN)*

Step 3: Lemmatization: *WordNet*

Sentence 1:

I	visit	Dr.	Bob	two	time
Pronoun (PN)	*Verb (VB)*	*Noun (NN)*	*Noun (NN)*	*Determiner (DET)*	*Noun (NN)*

Sentence 2:

He	is	a	nice	and
Pronoun (PN)	*Verb (VB)*	*Determiner (DET)*	*Adjective (AJ)*	*Conjunction (CJ)*

responsible	physician
Adjective (AJ)	*Noun (NN)*

(continues)

TABLE 13-1 An Example of Social Media Posts Decomposition   *(continued)*

| Step 4: Named Entity Extraction: *CoreNLP, NLTK* | Sentence 1: |

I	visited	Dr.	Bob	two	times
		Title	*Person*		
Pronoun (PN)	*Verb (VB)*	*Noun (NN)*	*Noun (NN)*	*Determiner (DET)*	*Noun (NN).*

Sentence 2:

He	is	a	nice	and
			Descriptor	
Pronoun (PN)	*Verb (VB)*	*Determiner (DET)*	*Adjective (AJ)*	*Conjunction (CJ)*

responsible	physician
Descriptor	*Health Professional*
Adjective (AJ)	*Noun (NN)*

| Step 5: Chunking: *NLTK, OpenNLP* | Sentence 1: |

I	visit	Dr.	Bob	two	time
		Title	*Person*		
Pronoun (PN)	*Verb (VB)*	*Noun (NN)*	*Noun (NN)*	*Determiner (DET)*	*Noun (NN)*
Pronoun (PN)	*Verb (VB)*	*Noun Phase (NP)*		*Noun Phase (NP)*	

Sentence 2:

He	is	a	nice	and
			Descriptor	
Pronoun (PN)	*Verb (VB)*	*Determiner (DET)*	*Adjective (AJ)*	*Conjunction (CJ)*

responsible	physician
Descriptor	*Health Professional*
Adjective (AJ)	*Noun (NN)*
Noun Phase (NP)	

Step 6: Parsing tree: *NLTK, OpenNLP, CoreNLP*	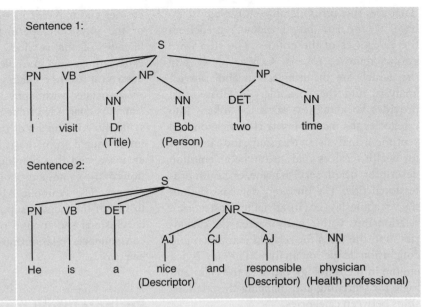

Step 7: Coreference resolution: *OpenNLP, CoreNLP*

Sentence 1:

I	Visit	Dr.	Bob	two	time
		Title	*Person*		
Pronoun (PN)	*Verb (VB)*	*Noun (NN)*	*Noun (NN)*	*Determiner (DET)*	*Noun (NN)*
Pronoun (PN)	*Verb (VB)*	*Noun Phase (NP)*		*Noun Phase (NP)*	

Sentence 2:

He	is	a	nice	and
			Descriptor	
Pronoun (PN)	*Verb (VB)*	*Determiner (DET)*	*Adjective (AJ)*	*Conjunction (CJ)*

responsible	physician
Descriptor	*Health Professional*
Adjective (AJ)	*Noun (NN)*
Noun Phase (NP)	

database, thesaurus database, ontology database,[30,31] and rule-based engine,[32] predefines the categories of the entities. The stop-word corpus removes tokens, such as *a, an,* and *the,* which are meaningless vocabularies for analysis, and the vocabulary database, that provides vocabularies, maps the tokens into categories for named entity classification and sentiment analysis. In this study, the categories for health services analysis can be an emotion descriptor, health service name, or health professional title. The ontology database defines the vocabularies (i.e., its attributes), categories, relationships within and between the categories, and the rules for relation extraction and conclusion deduction analysis. The rule-based engine in the ontology provides the rules and logic for searching and mapping the relationships between categories.

Commonly used AI models for named entity extraction[33] include SVM, conditional random field (CRF), hidden markov model (HMM), maximum entropy, and DTs. The AI models map the tokens to the vocabularies of the vocabulary and ontology databases to find out the token's named entity. After the named entities of the tokens are determined, another AI model, such as Term Frequency–Inverse Document Frequency (TF-IDF), *n*-grams, Naive Bayes, or linear SVM, is used for sentiment analysis. These AI models classify and calculate the total scores of the similar tokens (e.g., descriptor cluster 1: happy, nice, helpful...; descriptor cluster 2: rude, slow, late...) to identify which groups of consumers are sharing the same opinions and find out the total score of the consumers' opinions.

Even so, relation extraction uses other AI models,[34,35] such as logistic regression, CRF, Bayesian networks, HMM, maximum entropy models (MEM), or SVM to find out the relationship of the identified named entities (e.g., descriptor and physician appear together to describe the physician's service performance). Symbolic AI models, such as propositional logic, fuzzy logic, and similar others, use a set of production rules to connect the related

entities and make deductions for conclusions of the physician's performance, consumers' likeness of the services, and new services expectation. For example, if the identified descriptor tokens contain good comments that are associated with a physician A, then Physician A is concluded to be a good physician in symbolic AI. The set of production rules are implemented from the rules in the ontology database, and that ontology models the relations of the names entities in a specific domain context. The symbolic AI methods are used to search the facts to support the satisfaction conclusions and to find out the causes-and-consequences relationship of the consumers' behavior.

Business Intelligence (BI) Visualization Tools for Knowledge Visualization and Trend Analysis

To visualize the results of the sentiment analysis and the patterns of the behavioral changes on consumers' preferences and opinions in different consumer groups, business intelligence (BI) visualization tools are used. The KPIs and reporting tools, such as a "balanced scorecard" or "dashboard report" in BI[36] gives management a fast and comprehensive glimpse of performance in relation to meeting service quality and operational goals. Therefore, the use of a visual, real-time dashboard allows health systems professionals to monitor patients' satisfaction and visualize the consumers' behavioral changes on service selections, their service consumption patterns, and their new health services preferences. From the physician perspective, they can understand and receive feedback on their services (via social media users) and make real time performance improvement. From a business perspective, organizations can use the dashboard for forecasting the needs of their population based on the demographic stratification. Organizations could, potentially, assess what services are in high demand in their location and partner that information with what physicians are correlating with high satisfaction scores.

▶ IV. Zocdoc Case: SMA Use and Consumer's Preference on E-Health Services

The Zocdoc[37] physician reviewing website was selected for analysis here. It demonstrates how AI can be used in SMA on health services. The vocabulary database was built. NLP and AI were applied to analyze the social media posts, and a dashboard was used to demonstrate the analyzed results and its trends on behavioral changes of consumers' opinions and services preference.

Background and Objectives

With the advent of social media as a research medium, patients are turning to the Internet for help during their physician search. In order for providers to understand what people are looking for in a physician (general practitioner or specialist), gaining feedback on physician's services via social media analysis become essential. Hence, this case study is aimed at mining the data from social media sites that provide physician services' review. Social media websites from the United States, Hong Kong, Malaysia, Indonesia, Taiwan, and Singapore were studied. The study included a correlation analysis among the ratings issued by patients, a vocabulary used for describing the satisfaction of services, and calculation of the likelihood of a patient scheduling an appointment. By knowing the correlation of patient input to future patient engagement, health systems providers can determine if changes are needed in their practice in order to maintain their current patients or attract new patients.

Additionally, the SMA results help the health systems providers understand what services patients are seeking in which demographic areas.

A Review on the E-health Services Websites

Four physician reviewing websites were selected. The Singapore Medical Council (SMC) provides a physician reviewing website that allows patients to search for physicians either by provider name or by region and search for specialists, family physicians, or any physician in that region as shown in **FIGURE 13-1**.

After viewing the list returned, users can then view more information about the physician selected, as depicted in **FIGURE 13-2**. Users are able to view the doctor's credentials, but not see how other patients have evaluated him or her. FindDoc[38] is a website that services areas in and around Hong Kong, Taiwan, and Singapore. This site allows patients to apply filters related to the specialty, location, and other details, as shown in **FIGURE 13-3**, and review the comments of the returned list of physicians' meetings (see **FIGURE 13-4**). Also, on the "Doctor Details" page, patients can find contact information, service details, qualifications, and regular business hours of the clinics. In order to schedule an appointment on FindDoc, however, patients must use the smart phone app.

Mydoc.asia is another sophisticated website in Malaysia and Indonesia that offers all the features of FindDoc and allows new patients to attach information about their clinical history, complete new patient documentation online, and schedule appointments, as shown in **FIGURE 13-5**. Mydoc.asia also includes ratings from other patients, allows new patients to add information for their doctor, and allows for searches on the feedback from other patients (see **FIGURE 13-6**). ZocDoc in the United States marries all of these services into one page and allows physician search filtering, displays the details about each

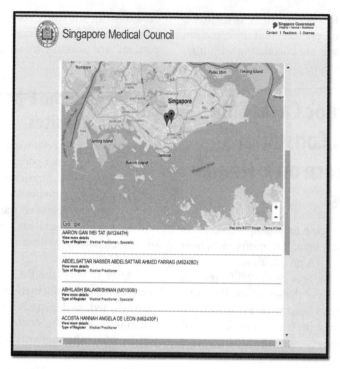

FIGURE 13-1 Singapore Medical Council (SMC).
http://www.healthprofessionals.gov.sg/smc

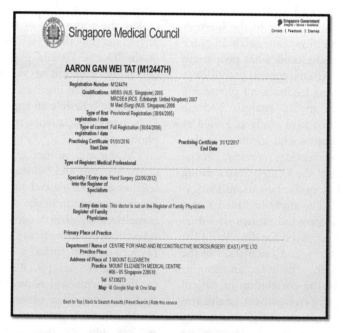

FIGURE 13-2 Singapore Medical Council (SMC) Sample Physician Profile.

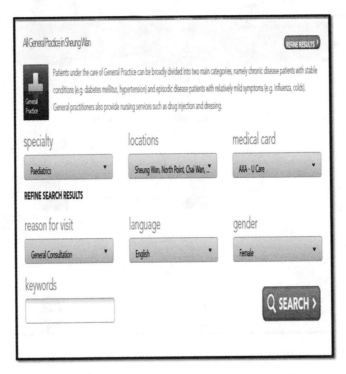

FIGURE 13-3 Search Window on FindDoc.com.

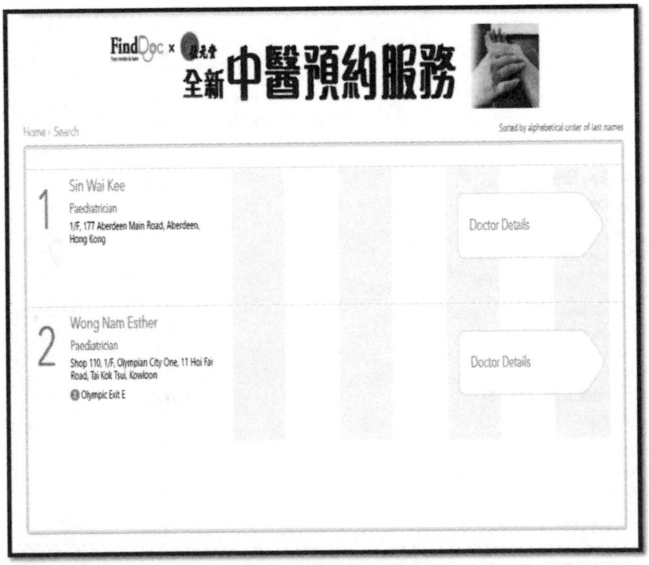

FIGURE 13-4 Returned Results on FindDoc.com.

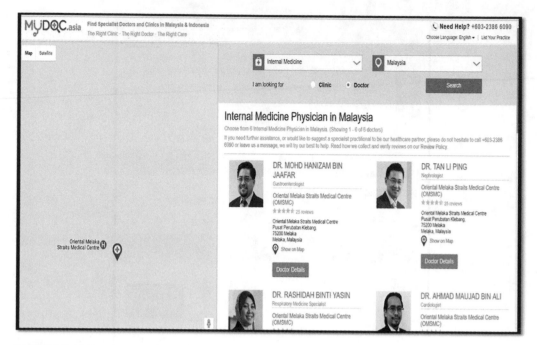

FIGURE 13-5 MyDoc.Asia search results, including star ratings.

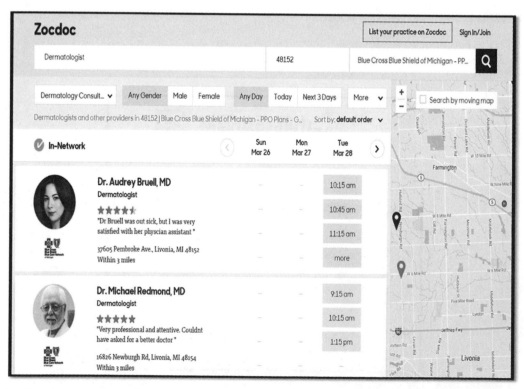

FIGURE 13-6 MyDoc.Asia Doctors' Next-Available Appointments.

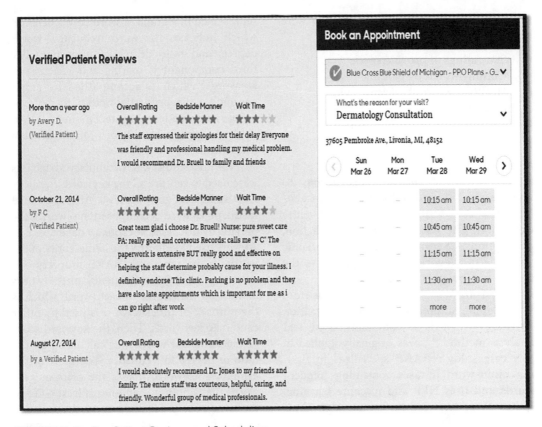

FIGURE 13-7 ZocDoc Patient Reviews and Scheduling.

returned physician and their patient ratings, and allows patients to schedule an appointment online, as depicted in **FIGURE 13-7**.

All in all, the most sophisticated online physician websites not only allow patients to rate physicians or find a physician by qualifications, specialty, practice locations, and insurance coverage, but also allow patients to review ratings and schedule appointments. As previously noted, examples of these websites include ZocDoc (zocdoc.com), FindDoc (finddoc.com), and MyDoc[39] (mydoc.asia). These sites are a means of cutting the time between needing a physician and scheduling an appointment. Additionally, consumers' opinions and expectations can be learned by examining the comments from patients on these sites, the patients' rating of the doctors, and, when applicable, how these comments and ratings correlate to

the likelihood of new patients seeing a specific clinician. Also, researchers or clinicians can review which particular healthcare services patients are most interested in and how all that social media information correlates to specific demographics. Even simpler, the data do not just provide insight into the type of information that the consumers are seeking, their perceived state of health, and their choices in healthcare services and providers, but also allow conclusions to be drawn about the consumer's preferences, lifestyle, and preference.

Application of AI (Machine Learning) and KPI for SMA

Data Sources and Target Information: To analyze the consumers' opinions on the health services, 2 years of the following data were extracted from the ZocDoc website:

- Star ratings of providers
- Comments left by patients
- Healthcare and physician service information
- Appointment scheduling statistics
- Demographic information of the social media users

Vocabulary Databases Construction: To analyze the chosen websites, four vocabulary databases were built for named entity extraction. The databases encompass action, descriptions, services, and demographic vocabulary categories. **TABLE 13-2** shows the sample vocabularies in the databases.

SMA Methods: To extract keywords from text, Rapid Automatic Keyword Extraction (RAKE), which is a commonly used text analysis method,[40,41] was originally applied in this case study.[42] RAKE specializes in finding multi-word phrases containing frequent words and uses NLP and machine learning. It has three keyword extraction algorithms to do sentiment analysis.[43] Candidate selection captures all possible keywords, including words, phrases, terms, or concepts. A property calculation then calculates the scores for each candidate keywords and defines the sum of its member word scores.[44] The metrics for calculating word scores are then evaluated, based on the degree and frequency of each word. This is represented in a graph of word co-occurrence, which indicates the word frequency, words degree, and ratio degree of frequency. The third component is scoring and selecting of keywords, which is accomplished by either combining the properties into a formula or using machine-learning technique (AI) to determine the probability of a candidate being a keyword.

In this study, the vocabulary databases were used to capture all the keywords to calculate the KPIs of good reviews. After the social media posts were decomposed into words, the previously discussed vocabulary databases and AI were used to identify the name-entity of the words in the sentences. RAKE property calculation counted the frequency of the words and found the degree of each word, which is the number of times a word is used by other candidate keywords. Then, the keyword score of the extracted words was calculated by the ratio of degree to frequency. The score of the candidate keyword, that is the pairs of keywords that adjoin one another at least twice in the same post and in the same order, was calculated by the sum of these adjoint keywords score. Finally, the top one third of the scoring candidate keywords were selected to represent the keywords for concluding the opinions of health services.

However, the drawback of RAKE is its inability to determine the semantic meaning of the post that may result in the inaccuracy of

TABLE 13-2 Action Vocabulary Database				
Expect	Document	Refer	Upset	Yell
Buy	Guide	Diagnose	Drain	Comfort
Compare	Help	Administer	Suture	Sooth
Schedule	Prescribe	Console	Charge	Correct
Admit	Heal	Treat	Influence	Evaluate

opinion analysis. It uses the "exact word" mapping method to extract keywords from text to calculate the keyword score and candidate keywords score of the adjoint keywords.[45,46] There are two primary problems: (a) The adjoint keywords may not be related to each other but are adjoined together to calculate the candidate keywords score; for example, the post has a comment of "the fee for service is low". The keywords of "fee + low" and "service + low" are determined as adjoint keywords but the "service + low" should not be adjoined together to calculate the candidate keywords score. Instead, it should only adjoin "fee + low" in the candidate keywords score calculation as the post is to give a comment of the service charge but not a service quality; and, (b) consumers may use different wordings (i.e., different keywords) to express the same opinion that may result in the errors of frequency counting and degree counting for keyword score calculation; for example, one post has a comment of "the physician's fee is reasonable" and another post has a comment of "the charge for the consultation is inexpensive." They both provide a positive sentiment on the clinical fee but use different wordings ("fee + reasonable" and "charge + inexpensive"). RAKE will classify these two posts as two different comments to calculate the keyword score and candidate keywords scores for conclusions may cause the opinion conclusion error in the final step, as only one third of the highest candidate keywords scores will be selected for the opinion conclusion.

In the end, this study used a novel approach of clustered ontology-based machine learning, which incorporated integrating ontology,[47,48] NLP,[49] support vector space,[50] TF-IDF,[51] Bayesian network,[52,53] and Neuro-fuzzy.[54] In this novel method, ontology databases, which were designed in a clustered-structure, as shown in **FIGURE 13-8**, were built on the top of the vocabulary databases. After the keywords were extracted from the social media posts, the NLP part of speech (POS) *n*-grams, Bayesian network,

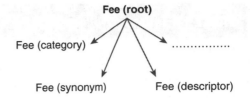

FIGURE 13-8 "Fee" ontology in a Clustered-Structure.

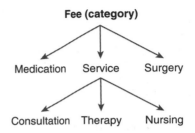

FIGURE 13-9 "Fee {Category}" ontology Sub-Tree.

and the ontology databases were then used to find out the keyword phrases for adjoint keywords pairing. For example, the post has a comment of "the fee for a service is low." The keywords of "fee," "service," and "low" are extracted from the vocabulary databases. The NLP tags {Noun, Noun, Adjective} of the keywords are found using wordnet.[55] By using POS *n*-grams, ontology databases, and Bayesian network, the keywords of "fee" and "service" are mapped in the "fee" ontology,[56] which the keyword "service" is a branch node of the "Fee category" ontology tree (see **FIGURE 13-9**). The "service fee" is then tagged as a keyword phrase in NLP tagging and the keyword "fee" is used as the dominator of the keyword phrase for keyword or candidate keywords score calculation.

The candidate keywords score of the adjoined keywords (i.e., fee + low) were finally calculated using the support vector space, TF-IDF method, and Bayesian network method (see **TABLE 13-3**). The significant candidate keywords were selected using the neuro-fuzzy method to conclude the opinions.

Similarly, consumers may use different keywords to express the same opinion. In the previous example of "fee + reasonable" and "charge + inexpensive," if the keywords "fee" and "charge"

TABLE 13-3 Descriptive Vocabulary Database

Professional	Welcoming	Condescending	Exceptional	Inattentive
Good	Genuine	Pleasant	Best	Rude
Understanding	Comforting	Helpful	Informative	Great
Great	Caring	Disengaged	Satisfied	Dumb
Nice	Dismissive	Positive	Polite	Angry

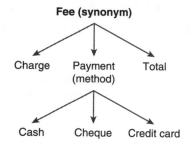

FIGURE 13-10 "Fee {Synonym}" ontology Sub-Tree.

can firstly map in the "Fee {Synonym}" ontology databases (see **FIGURE 13-10**), the two posts can then be classified as the same post (i.e., clinical fee) for keyword score calculation.

KPIs in the Dashboard: To understand which healthcare services patients are the most interested in and which physicians have higher and lower service satisfaction rates, KPIs were used in developing the dashboard. A physician's "scoring" KPI was established by combining the average star rating and the positive versus negative word count association and frequency for each physician in this study. Healthcare service KPI was established by a combination of the frequency count on services discussed on the site and the volumes of appointments scheduled via the social media site based on service and specialty. All of these KPIs were associated or able to be drilled-down based on the patient's location and demographic information for health systems providers to analyze

the satisfaction of the services and the trends of health service to be expected.

Dashboard Prototype and Screenshots

A prototype was developed using the Tableau visualization tool. The purposes of the dashboard are to provide a determination of:

- the healthcare services patients are most interested in (determined by patient comments on preference);
- what services physicians are receiving high and low satisfaction ratings (determined by average stars and word count of vocabulary database selection);
- how the comments and ratings correlate to the likelihood of new patients seeing a specific clinician; and
- how the provider selection, ratings, comments, and discussion on services relate to the demographics of the social media users.

The screenshots in **FIGURES 13-11**, **13-12**, and **13-13** highlight the dashboard pages and subsequent options for analysis. The initial page provides the selection of state, county, and city for analysis (see Figure 13-11). After the selection of one particular hospital or health system (see Figure 13-12) in that location, the

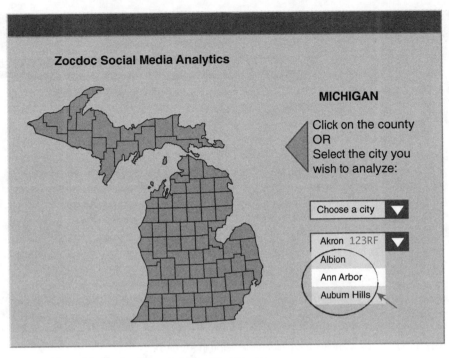

FIGURE 13-11 Dashboard Example of County Verse City Selection.

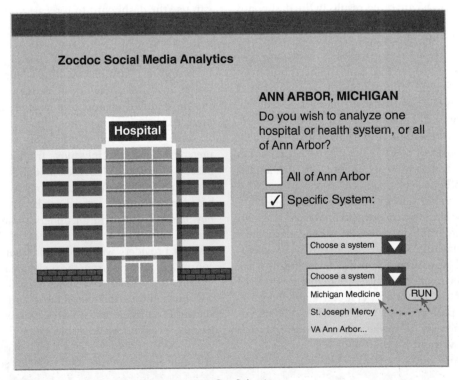

FIGURE 13-12 Dashboard Example of County Verse City Selection.

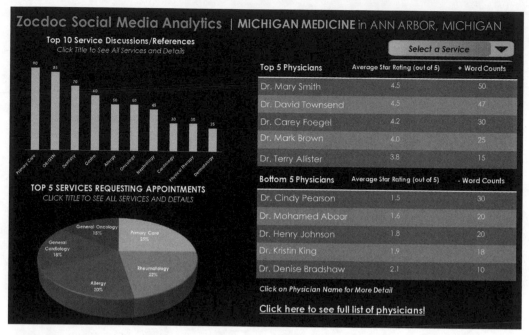

FIGURE 13-13 Dashboard Example for Michigan Medicine in Ann Arbor.

social media analyzed results in the dashboard were returned (see Figure 13-13).

The dashboard provided a real-time distribution of the top ten services being discussed or referenced by patients and the top five services appointments were requested for. On the right side, the dashboard lists the top five and bottom five most popular physicians, as calculated by their star ratings, and the counts of positive or negative word counts in the timeframe considered. The dashboard also allows one to look at a specific service (such as cardiology) by narrowing the scope of the dashboard outputs in service corner. All the graphs and lists of the feedback were summarized in the dashboard. The dashboard also allowed users to drill down for extracting the analysis-related information. From the physician perspective, feedback on their performance (via social media users) may be used to make real-time performance improvement on their services. From a business perspective, health systems providers can use the dashboard to forecast population needs based on captured demographics. They could also find out which services are in high demand in a particular location and partner with physicians who have high satisfaction scores to make appropriate business collaborations and decisions about offering new services.

The future trend of analyzing consumer preferences will certainly move from a survey-based to a social media-based model. Since survey data may not truly reflect the opinions of the broader consumers,[57] social media provides a new analytics platform for understanding consumers' opinions and preferences.[58,59] Health systems providers will collect and analyze the consumers' opinions from the social media websites. As the social media data is huge, SMA use AI to decompose the text, filter it, and extract keywords to mine the opinions. However, the trustfulness of the social media data is the problem in SMA.[60] Breaches in patient privacy are of major concern, especially in health services discussions. The degree to which consumers have confidence that their personal information remains private will impact how they interact with these websites and how much information they are willing to disclose. Hence, it is imperative that privacy-security issues be addressed for SMA to provide valuable insight.

Benson et al.[61] explored the use of social media and consumers' perceptions of privacy. The findings indicated that three facets of concern impacted consumers' self-disclosure of information. First is consumers' perception of online trust; that is, a greater sense of trust will result in an increase in self-disclosure, while a perceived risk to privacy will drive a decrease in self-disclosure. Second is the degree to which consumers feel they could remain anonymous; that is, consumers are more likely to divulge information if they feel less vulnerable through perceived anonymity. The final facet is the degree of control over personal information; that is, the availability for consumers control of their information on websites via opt-out. In other words, if consumers do not wish their information to be shared, they do not have to participate or disclose information. While this seems to be a reasonably effective way to protect information, it also drastically limits the consumers' ability to access healthcare information and care.

Even so, voluntarily providing safeguards to secure patient information develops an environment of trust. Consumers will feel less vulnerable and will be more likely to utilize the website, offering their personal health information more freely. Besides, Benson et al.[62] also suggest that companies can adopt a policy of transparency by self-regulation. Companies may post a notice to consumers in the form of a privacy policy statement or notice. Such statements outline for consumers in advance how data will be protected and may potentially be used. As well, privacy seals serve to establish a higher standard of security. Examples cited in Benson et al.[63] include TRUSTe™ and VeriSign™.

▶ V. Conclusion

The application of NLP, AI, and dashboard creation is key to delivering actionable data for health systems providers. This chapter focuses on studying the websites providing e-health services information and physician reviews. The methodology used can be applied in analyzing many other social media websites or other business areas. The issues that need to be considered before deploying the methods in other social media analytics studies are highlighted next.

- *Culture and Term Definitions*: The vocabulary and taxonomy terms presented in this chapter are specific to the use case identified and reflect a westernized culture. Future applications could include a review of the vocabulary used to create the knowledge base. It is important that the terms defined are appropriate for the demographic area selected; for example, if the demographic selected is known to be sarcastic or employ an idiom specific to the use case being studied, the vocabulary defined should include consideration for the population's speech and writing nuances.
- *Context Settings of the Analysis*: The settings under consideration here leaned largely toward ambulatory, or outpatient, experiences. To this end, the terms included in the sample databases included a variety of services. If this methodology is applied in a specific care setting, such as a hospital or even a particular unit of a hospital, or some other business setting, the database terms will again need to be updated to reflect the granularity of the data needed. A dashboard presented exclusively in a particular setting could also be further refined.
- *Information Sources*: In the future, it is important to consider the nature and typical use cases of the sources themselves when using the discussed methodology.

This source consideration will allow developer to again refine the NLP vocabulary terms, based on a careful evaluation of the source's audience. For example, if the source of the data being mined is from a more casual media outlet, such as Facebook, it will be critical to consider slang words, local idiom, and use of non-alphanumeric indicators (e.g., emojis) as elements for the NLP engine to identify.

▶ **Acknowledgments**

We would like to acknowledge Madonna University for providing an MSc course opportunity for the first five authors and the last two authors working on this project. This project was initiated by Marie-Claire Slama and Min Su, and Professor Adela Lau of A&A Research, Training, and Consultancy Ltd. (A&A). Marie-Claire Slama, Min Su and Professor Lau at Madonna University provided their guidance and input on the scope of the case study throughout the project. Some of the materials in the case study were extracted and used in this chapter. The other materials of this chapter were completed after the MSc course by Professor Lau of A&A and the sixth and seventh authors. In the chapter, Professor Lau discussed e-health services, consumers' shopping behavioral change, social media analytics, and artificial intelligence in the first two sections of chapter. Kristine Baker did the websites review and vocabulary databases. Sijuade Oke used RAKE for social media analysis. Professor Lau, Professor Tsui, and Liege Cheung researched and designed a novel social media analytics method for the case study. Katie Grzyb designed and implemented the dashboard prototype. Katherine Kempf researched the security and privacy issues of social media to conclude the future trend section of the chapter.

Notes

1. Flasinsk, M. (2016). Symbolic artificial intelligence. *Introduction to Artificial Intelligence* (pp. 15–22). Cham, Switzerland: Springer International Publishing.
2. Hartley, R. T., & Barnden, J. A. (1997). Semantic networks: Visualizations of knowledge. *Trends in Cognitive Sciences, 1*(5), 169–175.
3. Hatzilygeroudis, I., & Prentzas, J. (2004). Neuro-symbolic approaches for knowledge representation in expert systems. *International Journal of Hybrid Intelligent Systems, 1*(3–4), 111–126.
4. Duch, W. (2007). *What is computational intelligence and what could it become?* Retrieved from www.cogprints.org/5358/1/06-CIdef.pdf
5. Sordo, S., Vaidya, M., & Jain, L. C. (2008). An introduction to computational intelligence in healthcare: New directions. *Advanced Computational Intelligence Paradigms in Healthcare, 3*, 1–26.
6. Aliwy, A. H., & Abdul Ameer, E. H. (2017). Comparative study of five text classification algorithms with their improvements. *International Journal of Applied Engineering Research, 12*(14), 4309–4319.
7. Xhemali, D., Hinde, C. J., & Stone, R. G. (2009). Naïve Bayes vs. Decision Trees vs. Neural Networks in the classification of training web pages. *International Journal of Computer Science Issues, 4*(1), 1694–1784.
8. Ghahramani, Z. (2015). Probabilistic machine learning and artificial intelligence. *Nature, 521*, 452–459.
9. Jagtap, B., & Dhotre, V. (2014). SVM and HMM based hybrid approach of sentiment analysis for teacher feedback assessment. *International Journal of Emerging Trends & Technology in Computer Science, 3*(3), 229–232.
10. Rustamov, S., & Clements, M. A. (2013). *Sentence-level subjectivity detection using Neuro-Fuzzy models.* Proceedings of the 4th Workshop on Computational Approaches to Subjectivity, Sentiment and Social Media Analysis, Atlanta, GA (pp. 108–114).
11. Wang, Z., Bai, G., Chowdhury, S., Xu, Q., & Seow Z. L. (2017). *TwiInsight: Discovering topics and sentiments from social media datasets.* Retrieved from https://arxiv.org/ftp/arxiv/papers/1705/1705.08094.pdf
12. Howellsa, K., & Ertugana, A. (2017). *Applying fuzzy logic for sentiment analysis of social media network data in marketing.* 9th International Conference on Theory and Application of Soft Computing, Budapest, Hungary (Vol. 120, pp. 664–670).
13. Kashyap, S. (2017). Predicting human behaviour on social media using expert system tool CLIPS. *International Journal of Engineering Development and Research, 5*(2), 1522–1538.
14. Hatzilygeroudis & Prentzas, (2004), *ibid.*
15. Hajli, M. N. (2013). A study of the impact of social media on consumers. *International Journal of Market Research, 56*(3), 387–404.
16. Cordoş, A. A., Bolboacă, S. D., & Drugan, C. (2017). Social media usage for patients and healthcare

consumers: A literature review. *A Trust Framework for Online Research Data Services, 5*(2), 1–10.

17. Rudowsky, I. (2004). *Intelligent agents*. Proceedings of the Americas Conference on Information Systems, New York, NY (pp. 1–8).

18. Vaiciukynaite, E., Massara, F., & Gatautis, R. (2017). An investigation on consumer sociability behaviour on Facebook. *Inzinerine Ekonomika-Engineering Economics, 28*(4), 467–474.

19. Ozer, S. (2012). *The effect of social media on consumer buying decision process* (A dissertation of MSc in Management at National College of Ireland).

20. Fragkow, P. (2016). *Text segmentation using named entity recognition and co-reference resolution in English and Greek texts*. Retrieved from https://arxiv.org/pdf/1610.09226.pdf

21. Blanchard, A. (2007). *Understanding and customizing stopword lists for enhanced patent mapping?* (pp. 1–15). Retrieved from https://hal.archives-ouvertes.fr/hal-01247971/document

22. Chakraborty, R. (2013). Domain keyword extraction techniques: A new weighting method based on frequency analysis. *ACER, 109*–118. Retrieved from http://airccj.org/CSCP/vol3/csit3211.pdf

23. Chau, Q. N., & Tuoi, T. P. (2009). *An ontology-based approach for key phrase extraction*. Proceedings of the ACL-IJCNLP 2009 Conference Short Papers (pp. 181–184).

24. Christen, D. (2013). *Rule-based semantic tagging. An application undergoing dictionary*. Retrieved from https://arxiv.org/abs/1305.3882

25. Aliwy et al., (2017), *ibid*.

26. Xhemali et al., (2009), *ibid*.

27. Jagtap & Dhotre, (2014), *ibid*.

28. Farzindar, A., & Inkpen, D. (2015). *Natural language processing for social media*. In Graeme Hirst (Eds.), Morgan & Claypool Publishers.

29. Singapore Medical Council. Retrieved from https://prs.moh.gov.sg/prs/internet/profSearch/main.action?hpe=SMC

30. Chau & Tuoi, (2009), *ibid*.

31. Lau, A., Tsui, E., & Lee, W. B. (2009). An ontology-based similarity measurement for problem-based case reasoning. *Expert systems and Application, 43*(3), 6547–6579.

32. Recski, G. (2014). Hungarian noun phrase extraction using rule-based and hybrid methods. *Acta Cybernetica, 21*, 461–479.

33. Kaur, D., & Verma, A. (2014). Survey on named entity recognition used machine learning algorithm. *International Journal of Computer Science and Information Technologies, 5*(4), 5875–5879.

34. Wang, T., Li, Y., Bontcheva, K., Cunningham. H., & Wang, J. (2006). *Automatic extraction of hierarchical relations from text*. European Semantic Web Conference (Vol. 3, pp. 215–229), Springer-Verlag, Berlin/Heidelberg, Germany.

35. Konstantinova, N. (2014). *Review of relation extraction methods: What is new out there?* International Conference of Analysis of Images, Social Networks and Texts (Vol. 3, pp. 15–18). Springer International Publishing, Cham, Switzerland.

36. Curtright, J. W., Stolp-Smith, S., & Edell, E. S. (2000). Strategic performance management: Development of a performance measurement system at the mayo clinic. *Journal of Healthcare Management, 45*(1), 58–68.

37. ZocDoc.com. Retrieved from www.zocDoc.com

38. FindDoc.com. Retrieved from www.finddoc.com/en/

39. MyDoc.Asia. Retrieved from www.mydoc.asia/doctors/internal-medicine/malaysia

40. Dutt, A. (2016). A novel extension for automatic keyword extraction. *International Journal of Advanced Research in Computer Science and Software Engineering, 6*(5), 160–163.

41. Subramanian, L., & Karthik, R. S. (2017). Keyword extraction: A comparative study using graph based model and RAKE. *International Journal of Advanced Research, 5*(3), 1133–1137.

42. Baker, K., Kempf, K., Schwalm, K., & Oke, S. (2017). *An application of social media in health care analytics*. MIS 5230 Coursework Report, Madonna University, Livonia, Michigan, USA.

43. Wang et al., (2017), *ibid*.

44. Rose, S., Engel, D., Cramer, N., & Cowley, W. (2010, March 4). Automatic keyword extraction from individual documents. In M. Berry & J. Kogan (Eds.), *Text mining: Applications and theory* (pp. 1–20). Chichester, West Sussex, UK: John Wiley & Sons, Ltd.

45. Dutt, (2016), *ibid*.

46. Subramanian & Karthik, (2017), *ibid*.

47. Lau et al., (2009), *ibid*.

48. Yasavur, U., Amini, R., Lisetti, C., & Rishe, N. (2013). *Ontology-based named entity recognizer for behavioral health*. Proceedings of the Twenty-Sixth International Florida Artificial Intelligence Research Society Conference (pp. 249–254).

49. Kathait, S. S., Tiwari, S., Varshney, A., & Sharma, A. (2017). Unsupervised key-phrase extraction using noun phrases. *International Journal of Computer Applications, 162*(1), 1–5.

50. Jadav, B. M., & Vaghela, V. B. (2016). Sentiment analysis using support vector machine based on feature selection and semantic analysis. *International Journal of Computer Applications, 146*(13), 26–30.

51. Ghag, K., & Shah, K. (2014). SentiTFIDF—Sentiment classification using relative term frequency inverse document frequency. *International Journal of Advanced Computer Science and Applications, 5*(2), 36–43.

52. Tang, J., Li, J., Liang, B., Huang, X., Li, Y., & Wang, K. (2006). Using Bayesian decision for ontology mapping. *Web Semantics: Science, Services and Agents on the World Wide Web, 4*(4), 243–262.

53. Jadav & Vaghela, (2016), *ibid*.

54. Rustamov & Clements, (2013), *ibid.*

55. Miller, G. A., Beckwith, A., & Fellbaum, C. (1993). *Introduction to WordNet: An on-line Lexical database.* Princeton, NJ: Princeton University. Retrieved from http://wordnetcode.princeton.edu/5papers.pdf

56. Lau et al., (2009), *ibid.*

57. Haji, A. E. (2015). *All the reasons your surveys cannot be trusted.* Retrieved from https://greenbookblog .org/2015/12/01/why-surveys-cannot-be-trusted/

58. Schein, B., Wilson, K., & Keelan, J. (2010). *Literature review on effectiveness of the use of social media: A report for peel public health* (pp. 1–63). Retrieved from www .peelregion.ca/health/resources/pdf/socialmedia.pdf

59. WIPRO Ltd. (2010). *Why is social media important in Healthcare?* Retrieved from www.wipro.com /documents/resource-center/library/impact_of _social_media_in_healthcare.pdf

60. Pee, L. G., & Lee, J. (2016). Trust in user-generated information on social media during crises: An elaboration likelihood perspective. *Asia Pacific Journal of Information Systems, 26*(1), 1–21.

61. Benson, V., Saridakis, G., & Tennakoon, H. (2015). Information disclosure of social media users. *Information Technology & People, 28*(3), 426–441.

62. *Ibid.*

63. *Ibid.*

Chapter Questions

13-1 Why is social media analytics (SMA) an appropriate means of understanding consumers' preferences on e-health services? Compare and contrast SMA with the survey method.

13-2 Discuss how artificial intelligence can improve SMA. Discuss and illustrate some of the major challenges in AI-enhanced SMA.

13-3 How and why are visualization tools useful in identifying consumer preferences?

13-4 Give one example on the use of SMA in digital health. What are the challenges and difficulties of using SMA in digital health?

13-5 What are key performance indicators (KPIs)? Why may their use be important for information displayed on a dashboard?

13-6 What are the potential breakthroughs of digital health in the age of artificial intelligence?

Biographies

Adela Lau is currently an Assistant Professor and the Director of Center for Business Development at Madonna University and teaches healthcare informatics, social media and big data analytics, and management information system, and is also the Consultant at A&A Research, Training and Consultancy Ltd. in the United States. Her research specialties are in: (i) risk management and business intelligence/big data analytics in finance/enterprise/healthcare/marketing; (ii) e-learning and knowledge management; and (iii) e-business strategies, informatics, and applications. She was funded to research over 30 applied research and consultancy projects in the areas of machine learning, business intelligence, BPR, big data

analytics, taxonomy/ontology building, portal development, knowledge management, IS adoption, market research, healthcare studies and e-learning, etc. Her achievements include gaining the NANDA Foundation Research Grant Award, Inaugural Teaching and Learning Showcase Award, and Faculty Merit Award in Services at her prior institutions.

Katie Grzyb is a Continuous Improvement Specialist in the Department of Internal Medicine at Michigan Medicine. She has a bachelor's degree in Industrial Engineering and a master's degree in Health Services Administration. Her expertise is healthcare quality improvement, lean principles, and management system processes and operations. In her current role, she manages quality improvement projects through facilitation of improvement methodologies, tools, and data support. Her experience in developing innovative methodologies to achieve project objectives provides value through measurable outcomes.

Kristine Baker is the Director of Population Health IT Applications at Trinity Health in Livonia, Michigan. Kristine has a bachelor's degree in Technical Communications and a master's degree in Health Services Administration from Madonna University. She has experience and expertise in the areas of acute care EHR deployment and management, with a special interest in pharmacy informatics. In her current Population Health role, Kristine is focused on providing IT solutions to support alternate payment models in Trinity's Accountable Care Organizations and Clinically Integrated Networks. Her professional goal is to provide the IT tools and guidance necessary for enabling well-coordinated, safe patient care across the Trinity Health enterprise.

Kathy Kempf is currently pursuing a Master's Degree in Health Services Administration through Madonna University. She has been a Registered Nurse for over 30 years, with a Surgical Intensive Care and Trauma background. She has been in various leadership positions and is currently the Trauma Program Manager at St. Joseph Mercy Hospital Ann Arbor.

Sjiaude Oke, born in Nigeria, came to United States in 1999. He grew up in Michigan, received a Bachelor of Science during his undergraduate studies, and received his Master in Health Services Administration from Madonna University. Currently, Sjiaude works as a Process Specialist for an automotive company. His future aspiration is to work in the healthcare system as a hospital administrator.

Liege Cheung is a grade 12 student at International Academy of Macomb and is the voluntary helper at A&A Research, Training and Consultancy Ltd. He is working on his IB personal project of using social media, like Instagram, to motivate people. He analyzes the behavioral changes, such as navigation frequency and discussions, of followers on Instagram. His research interests are in the areas of medical science and emerging intelligent technologies. He adopted the Bayesian network method, that he researched in his previous project, to analyze the social media posts for this case study.

Eric Tsui is a Professor and the Director of the Knowledge Management and Innovation Research Centre (KMIRC) at The Hong Kong Polytechnic University. Previously, he was the Chief Research Officer, Asia Pacific of Computer Sciences Corporation (CSC). His research interests are on Knowledge Management technologies, Personal Knowledge Management, Cloud Services, and Learning pedagogies. His qualifications include BSc (Hons.), PhD, and MBA.

Marie-Claire Slama is leading Digital Health at AIA Group, Digital Platforms and Innovation. She joined AIA Edge – Group Innovation in 2016 and is based in Hong Kong. Prior to joining the Group, she spent 5 years with Leading Consumer Goods Supply Chain Group Li & Fung in Hong Kong, responsible for Digital and Tech initiatives, fostering innovation and technology servicing American and Pacific brands and retailers. She previously helped to found e-com department at Antalis in Europe and was in charge of Marketing for Asia Pacific region at Arjowiggins. She has lived and worked in Asia for 15 years. Marie-Claire holds an MSc in Management from ESSEC Graduate School of Management in France. She has also joined with success Fung Group Leadership Program (2013) at MIT, Sloan School of Management, Li & Fung Leadership Program by Stanford University in collaboration with The University of Hong Kong.

Dr. Min Su has had over 20 years of experience leading healthcare analytics initiatives and informatics transformation and consultation at Fortune 500 companies. She was an epidemiologist and a practicing pediatrician before working in insurance. At AIA, Min is responsible for leading healthcare analytics across the region and building analytical capabilities and developing data governance, structure, and quality control both centrally and locally. Min is a graduate of the University of Toronto and received her MD from Shanghai Jiao Tong University. Min published three peer-reviewed articles that lead to clinical guideline adjustments.

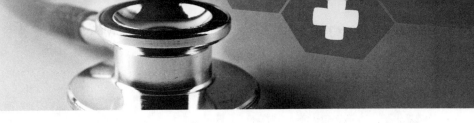

CHAPTER 14

Health Care Globalization Through Health Information Technology Enabled Initiatives

Anantachai Panjamapirom and Philip F. Musa

LEARNING OBJECTIVES

- Understand the globalization concepts in the contexts of the healthcare services industry
- Conceptualize the economic and societal values of health IT adoption
- Illustrate the applicability of tele-health in a global e-health initiative
- Speculate on the barriers to e-health adoption and the roles of different stakeholders

CHAPTER OUTLINE

Scenario: UPMC and KingMed Diagnostics Collaboration[1]

The World Health Organization (WHO) and many of its member countries have adopted health IT as an integrated component in the transformation of their healthcare services delivery models. While the use of health IT mainly begun with the goals of achieving a local agenda, it has accelerated the concept of globalized business partnership in the healthcare industry around the world. The partnership between UPMC and KingMed Diagnostics is a clear example of turning such concept into reality.

Since the turn of the decade, China has experienced unprecedented rates of cancer and associated mortality, accounting for up to half of the worldwide cases for some cancer types. Such demand in cancer diagnoses and treatments has created a high need for expertise in some pathology subspecialties, which China lacks, especially in small hospitals and some rural areas. The leadership and experts of KingMed Diagnostics, the largest independent clinical laboratory network in China, understood the importance of diagnostic pathology and its effects on better treatment selection for cancer patients.

In order to support and enhance the capabilities of local pathologists, KingMed formed a partnership with UPMC. In this relationship, UPMC has provided second-opinion pathology consultations. Both parties worked to design an image storage system that allows a UPMC pathologist to review and access digital microscopy files. During the implementation phase, Dr. Michalopoulos, chairman of the Department of Pathology at UPMC and professor of pathology at the University of Pittsburgh School of Medicine stated that "Information technology (IT) obviously was—and remains—a critical piece of the equation. Not surprisingly, one of the biggest hurdles we faced involved technology, including challenges with digital imaging, internet speed and firewalls. But those matters were relatively easy to overcome, particularly considering the size and expertise of the IT departments on both sides." (*ibid.*)

The service and collaborative efforts were quite simple and straightforward, but have realized significant values for patients' diagnoses and treatment. Basically, once the KingMed pathology images for a case were readily available, UPMC's pathology department was notified and an appropriate pathology specialist was identified to examine the imaging files. Additionally, the UPMC pathologists also "discussed the case with both the referring pathologists and the patients' physicians in China." (*ibid.*)

The number of referred cases for second-opinion services quadrupled in the second year. By 2014, UPMC served as the primary diagnosis entity for almost half of the referred cases. Approximately 54% of the remaining cases resulted in significant modifications to the primary diagnosis, which in turn led to a more appropriate and precise treatment option. "With the remote pathology consultation service, the pathologists at UPMC were able to provide more accurate and faster diagnosis for Chinese patients. In other words, I believe that we helped save a lot of lives" (*ibid.*), said Dr. Chengquan Zhao, associate director of cytopathology at UPMC, professor of pathology at the University of Pittsburgh School of Medicine, and coordinator of UPMC's telepathology program with KingMed.

Not only does this partnership result in better care for cancer patients in China, it promotes continuing learning and educational experiences for physicians and other staff of both parties. This success story of tele-health is just one example of how health IT can add synergistic values to all stakeholders involved. As the technology gets more advanced, possibilities to realize global healthcare benefits could become endless.

▶ I. Introduction

As the world shrinks and nations become increasingly more interconnected, no one nation can afford to turn inward and focus solely on health status, health professions education, or health system development and enhancement simply for the sake of its own citizenry.

—Roger J. Bulger, David Hawkins, and John Wyn Owen[2]

Globalization is a comprehensive phenomenon exhibited throughout the long history of the growth of population and the advancement of civilization. Although it may be traced as far back as the 14th century,[3] the phenomenon of the global exchange of ideas, goods, and services has gained much popularity since the close of the 1980s.[4] The antecedents of globalization substantiate an understanding of the current circumstances, whereas the results and their implications are the agents that stimulate changes and future development. Globalization encompasses an array of interactive factors that greatly affect the world in different ways. The term generally has an application on at least six major diverse discourses: economic, technological, environmental, political, social, and cultural contexts.[5,6] It is the intertwined connection among these facets that has transformed the world into its new millennial era.

The world has recognized extensive advantages of globalization. The most common benefits revolve around economics. Economists assert that globalization can lead to free trade, greater competition, economies of scale, more efficient approaches for resource allocation, and increases in economic prosperity, which in turn result in poverty reduction.[7-9] Through the globalized system, nations and their citizens are engaged in exchanging information, embodying cross-cultural diffusion, and creating unprecedented global cultures. As a result of the economic and social globalization, nations have formed relationships in which agreements must take place. Therefore, international political organizations, such as the United Nations (UN)[10] and the World Trade Organization (WTO), provide rules and regulations that are utilized to manage the rights of, and relationships among, nations.

To date, many international initiatives have been established to address global degradations in our environment, such as air and water pollution, as well as global warming.[11,12] Such examples of integral efforts have informed us that globalization is an imperative process to which we must pay close attention. As the achievement of any process requires the right tool, globalization cannot occur without technological advancements. Technology acts as both the catalyst and the enabler of globalization. The introduction of logistics and information technologies allows the world population to connect and access resources around the globe, but the need for more effective and efficient means to achieve other purposes have prompted ongoing creation of innovative technologies. The world has continued to experience disruptive technologies, such as Blockchain,[13] Artificial Intelligence (AI),[14] and Internet of Things (IoT),[15] which may potentially create transformational values across industries.

Paradoxically, some people have argued that globalization has given rise to some detrimental effects, such as inequality and vulnerability.[16] However, empirical studies have shown that developing countries that have open policies for globalization exhibit lower poverty rates than those that are using inward-oriented policies.[17] Moreover, the World Bank[18] reported that the openness to international integration is a vital factor that contributes to less inequality among countries. Evidence also shows that even though the effect of gross domestic product (GDP) volatility on developing countries was greater than that of developed countries, the overall volatility on both GDP and export growth for developing countries significantly decreased during the 1990s, except for the East Asia region due to the 1997–1998 financial crisis.[19] Accordingly, these negative effects should not be perceived as adverse consequences of globalization, but rather a result of the unorganized involvement of nations in the global network.

Ideas from globalization in the major contexts have been adopted in the healthcare services industry.[20] Particularly, calls for the globalization of health care started to gain momentum in the mid-1990s when information and communications technologies (ICT) came to be employed as a new channel to deliver care to patients in remote locations. This industry can wholly benefit from globalization and take advantage of the advancements in ICT, particularly health information technology (health IT).

A number of empirical studies show that health IT plays a prominent part in the solution to various predicaments confronting the global healthcare environment, such as an upward spiral of medical costs, unacceptably low quality of care in many countries, increasing medical errors, and administrative inefficiencies.[21-23] The world of health IT has advanced, nearly on a daily basis, and various terms, such as tele-care, telemedicine, tele-health, mobile health (mHealth), and eHealth, have been used to define an innovative approach with use of various health IT applications to rendering healthcare services. More recently, the industry has coined the new term "smart health," which covers the most comprehensive set of concepts and stakeholder viewpoints of healthcare services delivery.[24,25] While the ultimate goal of these nomenclatures is to build an integrated, technology-enabled healthcare system that creates value (i.e., affordable and high quality care) for all populations of the world, they have certain differences in their characteristics and scope. The differences will be explained shortly. To this point, various organizations in both public and private sectors at local and federal levels across the globe have continued to make progress in collaborating their efforts toward the same goal. The synergy through the integrated healthcare system[26] would permit developed, developing, and under developed countries to contribute both tangible (i.e., human resources, money, and technology) and intangible (i.e., infrastructural shifts, knowledge, and skills) assets that would otherwise be limited.

We utilize two economic applications—the production possibilities frontier and positive externalities—to analyze the economic perspectives of health IT deployment in health care. This chapter also investigates the barriers to e-health adoption through four different theoretical models. Using the e-health strategic framework developed by the World Bank[27] and the WHO, the current status of telemedicine and e-health adoption in developed, developing, and underdeveloped countries is explored. Moreover, we propose methods by which developed and developing countries can contribute to this supreme health IT-enabled globalization initiative.

▶ II. Tele-Care, Telemedicine, Tele-Health, and E-Health

Health IT, as a global term, fundamentally identifies ICT deployment in health care. There is now a vast array of health information technologies [e.g., electronic medical records (EMR), clinical decision support (CDS), analytics platforms, and health information exchange (HIE)] in use to support relevant stakeholders in the care delivery processes.

However, this specific section focuses on the use of health IT in the context of making healthcare services efficiently and effectively accessible to patients in need, especially in the areas where healthcare services have been historically and usually scarce. Specifically, numerous definitions have been used to identify ICT deployment in such healthcare delivery practice. However, no one definition has been universally accepted. Even though many of these terms share common and overlapping characteristics, each one conveys a different semantic and covers a different scope or boundary.

Barlow, Bayer, and Curry[28](p.397) define *tele-care* as "a set of services bringing care directly to the end-user" at a remote location via ICT deployment. Among the most commonly cited definitions of *telemedicine* is that given by Dr. Salah H. Mandil, WHO Director of Health Informatics and Telematics, as "the practice of medical care using audio, visual, and data communications: this includes medical care delivery, consultation, diagnosis, treatment, education, and the transfer of medical data."[29](p. 4) As referenced by the American College of Nurse Practitioners, *tele-health* refers to "the removal of time and distance barriers for the delivery of health care services or related health care activities. Some of the technologies used in tele-health include telephones, computers, interactive video transmissions, direct links to health care instruments, transmission

of images, and teleconferencing by telephone or video."[30] Basically, one can think of tele-health as a healthcare services provision that is directly enabled by health IT while a clinician and a patient are in different physical locations. To bring these interrelated terms into harmony, Norris[31] defined the three terms in similar technological aspects, yet each focuses on different users and recipients of the services. While *tele-care* is central to medical services provided to patients, *telemedicine* involves services benefiting both patients and physicians. In addition, *tele-health* serves patients, physicians, and administrators. Readers who are interested in an in-depth treatment of how these various terminologies relate to each other may also refer to Tan.[32] For completeness of this review, we elaborate on the prevailing view of telemedicine in the next section.

▶ III. Types of Telemedicine

Norris[33] identifies four major current categories of telemedicine; the categorization is not meant to provide an exhaustive list of services provided through telemedicine. Whether or not the scope of telemedicine can be expanded depends heavily on the innovative progression of health IT.

Tele-Consultation

This type of telemedicine can occur in the context of real-time provider–provider or provider–patient interactions. Telephone and videoconferencing are the basic ICT used to deliver these services. The more advanced technologies used for *tele-consultation* are mHealth[34,35] and a combination of "a high-speed network, a medical image database, a super-high-definition imaging system, and an IP-based video conferencing system."[36] The main application is tele-radiology in which

X-ray files are transmitted 24/7 to obtain result interpretations and consultations around the world. Some other applications include tele-ophthalmology, tele-dermatology, and tele-oncology. Illustrated by their names, these applications represent the utilization of tele-medicine in a particular branch of medicine, such as ophthalmology, dermatology, and retinology. For example, *tele-opthalmology* refers to the use of ICT to facilitate the provision of care to patients with visual pathway diseases.[37] Some applications of tele-opthalmology are ophthalmic imaging and visual rehabilitation consultations.[38] Basically, tele-opthalmology is the practice of telemedicine of eye care. *Tele-dermatology* is the use of ICT to assist dermatologists and other related health professions to provide care to patients with skin diseases.[39] *Tele-oncology* is used to facilitate the delivery of cancer care covering the entire episode of care ranging from diagnosis to supportive care and follow-up services.[40] As the industry has moved forward, this type of tele-medicine has become the most common form.

Tele-Education

Knowledge is power. Being able to access and retrieve information and knowledge anywhere, anytime is another service of telemedicine. The most common use of *tele-education* is continuing medical education (CME) in which physicians are not required to participate in live conferences or workshops, but can learn and gain the most up-to-date information or practice guidelines about particular diseases through accessing materials on the Internet. In the United States, the Accreditation Council for Continuing Medical Education (ACCME) is the accrediting body of continuing medical education, ensuring the quality and reliability of information utilized by physicians to maintain their competence and incorporate new knowledge.[41] Therefore, physicians can rely on ACCME-accredited programs that are offered online. Tele-education may be realized as a by-product of tele-consultation, where local

providers learn from remote providers during the care provision processes. Tele-education benefits not only practitioners, but also consumers. Patients are able to access information regarding their symptoms and diseases from multiple legitimate websites, which are provided by highly reputed healthcare services organizations, such as world-renowned academic health centers and governmental health-related institutions. The indirect advantage for the patients is that they can have some control over their own health and participate in the shared medical decision-making and practice.[42,43] Moreover, this application can act as a new conveyor of medical education, adding value to conventional text-based classrooms. The academics can also benefit from the availability of online publishing and literature searching, as well as collaboration, which will enhance the diffusion of knowledge. The quality of publications can be ascertained among the peer-reviewed journals, popular publications, and authoritative academic databases.

Tele-Monitoring

This type of telemedicine is important; through its use, patients can be consistently monitored even after they are discharged from an acute care setting or after a visit. They can communicate with their physicians concerning their current status, and the ongoing treatment scheme can be modified accordingly. Patients are able to recover in their place of residence rather than being institutionalized in hospitals or other healthcare delivery settings. *Tele-monitoring* can play an important role in life-threatening and time-sensitive conditions, such as those arising from a heart attack. One of the tele-monitoring applications is tele-cardiology. *Tele-cardiology* can be used to facilitate disease management among patients with coronary artery disease and chronic heart failure.[44] The patients can self-monitor electrocardiogram (EKG), body weight, or blood pressure at home and share the results with physicians or nurse practitioners. Researchers have found that tele-cardiology is effective in improving patient compliance, increasing the quality of life, and potentially reducing costs.[45] Nowadays, this type of telemedicine has converged with the concept of mHealth because of the worldwide growth of mobile communication devices and availability of abundant mHealth applications.[46,47]

Tele-Surgery

While tele-surgery is a relatively new concept compared with the others just mentioned, its use has become more widespread and practical.[48,49] There are two types of *tele-surgery*: tele-mentoring, where specialists provide assistance to the surgeons from a remote location, and tele-presence surgery, where surgeons utilize robotic arms to carry out surgical procedures from a distance. International evidence has confirmed the benefits of both types of tele-surgery. Anvari[50] observed the utilization of tele-mentoring and tele-robotic surgery and reported that knowledge from these practices can be translated rapidly and effectively. He also predicted that these services would eventually transform the surgical world because more advanced health IT can be deployed. A group of Japanese surgeons and researchers also reported the safety and efficacy of tele-robotic surgery in patients with mucosal or submucosal lesions.[51]

Connecting Telemedicine to E-Health

Apart from the aforementioned nomenclatures, *e-health* is another commonly used term that combines everything related to the use of ICT and computers in medical practice and health care. Similar to telemedicine, there are many definitions of e-health. In fact, a review of the literature yields more than 50 unique definitions of e-health.[52] Eysenbach[53] provides a broad definition of this new concept:

E-health is an emerging field in the intersection of medical informatics, public health and business, referring to health services and information delivered or enhanced through the Internet and related technologies. In a broader sense, the term characterizes not only a technical development, but also a state of mind, a way of thinking, an attitude, and a commitment for networked, global thinking, to improve health care locally, regionally, and worldwide by using information and communication technology.

Since 2005, the WHO has focused on e-health as a central theme that connects ICT and health care. Thus, it simply defines e-health as "the use of information and communication technologies (ICT) for health."[54(p. 1)] The WHO categorizes the application of e-health into three broad areas. These areas are related to the types of telemedicine identified earlier. The categorization also places an emphasis on the services provided to patients and practitioners.

1. *Public services.* These services provide information to people via the Internet.
2. *Knowledge services.* These services are comparable to tele-education in that they aim at conveying medical information, knowledge, and education to the healthcare professionals who are in training and practice.
3. *Provider services.* These services focus on the utilization of e-health applications to deliver healthcare services to others.

For conciseness, we now present these four major terms in the same diagram, as illustrated in **FIGURE 14-1**. As shown, *tele-care* is a subset of *telemedicine*, and *telemedicine* is a smaller level of *tele-health*. *E-health*

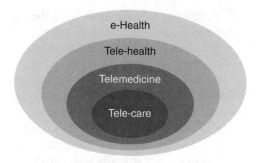

FIGURE 14-1 Tele-care, Telemedicine, Tele-Health, and E-Health in Perspective.

is an umbrella term that embraces the entire medical-related interventions being delivered and connected through ICT. For this reason, the term *e-health* will be used throughout this chapter, as it is the most encompassing term in the globalization of health care.

▶ IV. The Economic Perspectives of ICT and E-Health

Through the innovative advancement of ICT, the world is getting smaller, yet more dynamic. While individuals are connected around the globe by means of IT networks, health systems organizations have adopted health IT for both strategic and operational purposes. As a consequence, health IT has become an integral part of the healthcare services industry. With a rapid increase in IT adoption rates, the tremendous advantages of IT have been extensively recognized. Atkinson and McKay[55(p.1)] stated that "[t]he integration of IT into virtually all aspects of the economy and society is creating a digitally enabled economy." In effect, IT provides social and economic benefits to the adopters and society as a whole. Therefore, this notion reflects the beneficial implications of the integration of ICT into health care and offers increasingly robust opportunities for globalized e-health.

However, as society strives to attain maximum utilization from limited resources, at least two concerns arise among economists: efficiency and equity.[56] Economists are concerned with production efficiency because it identifies "whether the [products or] services (for a given level of quality) are produced at the lowest cost."[57(p. 405)] To reach such a goal, products and services must be produced in the most effective way. The other issue is how limited resources can be equitably distributed to the population. As previously discussed, the World Bank found that there is less inequality among nations participating in globalization. Therefore, nations adopting healthcare globalization should permit their citizens to have equal opportunities to access better medical care. Research also supports the notion that telemedicine provides social efficiency.[58] Two theoretical, economic tools—production possibilities frontier and positive externalities—are employed to demonstrate the economic benefits of health IT or ICT in health care.

Before these two tools are discussed, we make an assumption to differentiate two periods of e-health adoption. Based on Roger's S-curve and rate of adoption over time,[59] the first period starts off slow and is followed by a rapid growth. The second period begins where the adoption rate moves into the stabilization and eventually declines. We argue that both quality and quantity of care increase in the first period, while the second period experiences an increase in quality and a decrease in quantity. These arguments are further incorporated in the production possibility frontier (PPF) discussion.

Production Possibility Frontier

Under the assumption that the society only produces two goods and all factors related to production are completely utilized, the PPF model or curve represents all efficient combinations of outputs.[60] The PPF model also illustrates the concepts of "trade-off" and "opportunity costs." In this particular circumstance, we use a PPF curve to explain

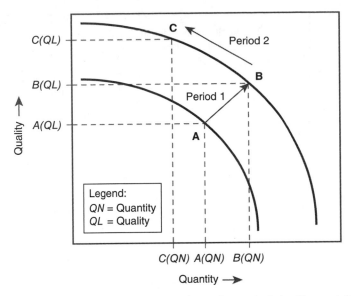

FIGURE 14-2 Production possibility frontier between quality and quantity in healthcare delivery system at the first and second periods.

the trade-off between quality and quantity of care provided to people in the society. As depicted in **FIGURE 14-2**, the *x*- and *y*-axes represent the quantity and quality of healthcare services delivered in society, respectively.

The assumption is that at point *A*, e-health globalization does not exist. The global healthcare system provides *A(QL)* amount of quality to *A(QN)* people. Once health IT is brought into the system, and the benefits of health IT are realized, the PPF curve is shifted upward and outward. At the new PPF curve, the system can increase the quality of care to *B(QL)* and increase the number of people receiving care to *B(QN)*. This phenomenon takes place in the first period because the production of quality and quantity of medical services provided without health IT is limited. But once health IT is introduced and its adoption starts to take off, the society as a whole will benefit from the efficiency that health IT brings to the healthcare system. This trend will continue until the society moves into the second period, in which the utilization of health IT in health care becomes a commodity and adoption levels off.

Thus, with health IT adoption and diffusion, we have the scenario in the second period, where the quality of care continues to increase to *C(QL)*, but the quantity provided will decrease to *C(QN)* because at this point e-health has become an ordinary practice in the global healthcare system from which the majority of citizens in nations can benefit. As the majority of people have had access to better healthcare services, they arc likely to be healthy. Healthy people in turn require less care, and thus lead to the reduction in the amount of medical services produced. This process should be perceived as a cycle. Whenever the new application of health IT is employed in health care, people would continue to gain benefits from it. The notion of positive externality can also be used to substantiate our call for globalization of health care through e-health implementation.

Positive Externality

Goods or services with positive externalities provide benefit to members of society who

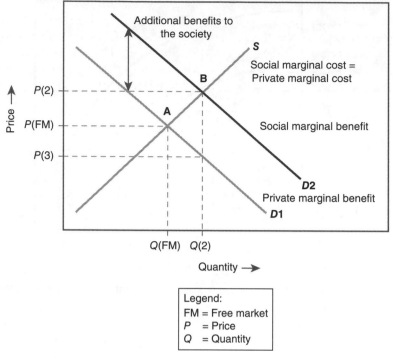

FIGURE 14-3 E-Health as a Good with Positive Externality.

Note: This figure illustrates the increase in social benefit when a good with positive externality is present in the market.

Adapted from B. Sen, "Externalities" University of Alabama at Birmingham, September 13, 2005.

are not directly involved in the production, transaction, and consumption of the goods or services.[61] Presented in **FIGURE 14-3**, the supply curve *S* is treated as a social marginal cost, which is also equivalent to private marginal cost, and the demand curve *D*1 represents an individual benefit.[62] Point *A* represents the free market (i.e., actual equilibrium), where private marginal cost equals private marginal benefit. When a good with positive externalities is present in the market, which results in the socially optimal level or point *B* (i.e., ideal equilibrium), the problem becomes that there is a discrepancy between the demand curve *D*1 at the free market and the social marginal benefit curve, which is *D*2. While we want the society to have *Q*(2) of e-health and its benefits, the demand at the free market is only *D*1. For that reason, a public and international policy regarding the price and supply of goods or services with positive externalities is among

one of the top priorities of nations and related international organizations.

E-health is considered to be a service with positive externalities that will bring value to the society. The positive externalities of e-health can be derived from two major sources: health IT and health care. Atkinson[63] provided the case that the necessary applications of ICT utilized in e-health, such as broadband telecommunications, lead to positive externalities. An obvious example of how e-health produces positive externalities in healthcare services settings is the increase in preventive care and reduction in infectious disease.[64] If individuals receive care for their infectious disease at the early stage of the contagion, they reduce the risk of infection for other members of the society. In essence, these individuals do not only produce a positive externality by getting care of their conditions, but also avoid a negative externality that could have occurred. Some other benefits to the society include, but are not limited to, the increase in productivity of healthy people and the federal budget savings from fewer needs in healthcare services that can be utilized in other social programs, such as education and transportation. While the benefits are initially accrued at the individual level, the positive consequences of these benefits will lead to the socially optimal level. At point *A*, e-health (a good with positive externality) gets under-traded, and the society would like to reach the ideal level at point *B*. However, the problem at point *B* is that an investment in e-health costs *P*(2), while the market is only willing to pay *P*(3). The amount that healthcare delivery organizations, or even the government of developing and undeveloped nations, are willing to pay for e-health infrastructures might be limited due to scarce resources. In this situation, international organizations, such as the World Bank and WHO, would play a vital role in providing the global society with the optimal benefit level.

V. Factors Influencing the Adoption of E-Health

To study adoption of innovation, researchers have extensively utilized four different theoretical paradigms from which they draw antecedent factors. These frameworks include the technology adoption model, the theory of planned behavior, the diffusion of innovation theory, and the technology-organization-environment framework. Based on these models, a number of technological and non-technological antecedents influencing the adoption of e-health are discussed.

Technology Acceptance Model

Developed by Davis,[65] the technology acceptance model (TAM) has become one of the most influential theoretical foundations used in studying the acceptance of new technology at the individual level. Two main constructs included in this model—perceived usefulness (PU) and perceived ease-of-use (PEOU)—are related to the perception of users toward the new technology.[66,67] This model is used to study the acceptance of telemedicine technology among physicians in Hong Kong and was found to have a reasonable prediction.[68] TAM has also been modified based on studies in developing countries that identified accessibility as a factor that played a major role in adoption of technology.[69] In another related study, TAM was extended to study sustainable adoption of technologies for human development in developing countries.[70] Some studies in the healthcare context included additional factors to the original TAM and still found PU and PEOU to be strong determinants of intention to use Internet-based health applications or telemedicine.[71,72] Over the past several years, numerous studies have shown that TAM is a valid and parsimonious theoretical framework for examining adoption of technological innovation.[73,74]

Theory of Planned Behavior

Extended from the psychological theory of reasoned action (TRA) by Ajzen and Fishbein,[75] the theory of planned behavior (TPB)[76-78] suggests that an individual's intentions to adopt and use technology can be explained by three factors:

1. *Attitudes toward behavior*, or an individual's perceptions toward his or her performance of particular behavior (i.e., adopting technology).
2. *Subjective norms*, or an individual's perceptions about particular behavior that are influenced by social normative pressures (i.e., significant other's beliefs on whether an individual should or should not adopt technology).

3. *Perceived behavioral control*, or an individual's perceptions about ease or difficulty of performing a particular behavior (i.e., adoption of technology can be influenced by his or her efforts).

Utilizing a theory comparison approach, Chau and Hu[79] employed both TAM and TPB in examining physicians' intentions to accept telemedicine technology. Their findings suggest that TPB may be less applicable than TAM in a study of ICT innovation acceptance.

Diffusion of Innovation Theory

Initially introduced in 1962, Rogers's diffusion of innovation theory (DOIT) has become a seminal theory employed among researchers in studying adoption of innovation.[80] Unlike TAM and TPB, DOIT focuses on the attributes of innovation as predictors of adoption and may be applied at an organizational level. To lend itself more readily to adoption, an innovation must contain five attributes: relative advantage, compatibility, complexity, trialability, and observability. Menachemi, Burke, and Ayers[81] provide an informative analysis of how these attributes can affect adoption of telemedicine among physicians, patients, hospital administrators, and payers.

Apart from these attributes, Rogers also emphasizes several other important factors that play a major role in adoption of innovation. Rogers asserts that a *communication channel* is an important means through which messages are passed along from one individual to another. He further explains that even though *mass media* are a great means to rapidly communicate with the public and potential adopters, *interpersonal communication* or word-of-mouth is more effective in persuading people to espouse an innovation. The interpersonal communication channel is even more powerful if individuals share similar socioeconomic status and educational level.[82] In addition, because potential adopters are a member of *society*, *social norms*, *behaviors*,

structures, and *systems* are inevitable factors that researchers must take into considerations when studying adoption of innovation.

Technology-Organization-Environment Model

Tornatzky and Fleischer[83] developed the technology-organization-environment (TOE) model, a comprehensive framework, to study adoption of technological innovation at an organizational level. They argue that technological, organizational, and environmental aspects of an organization influence its adoption and implementation of innovative technology.

The *technological* facet refers to the availability of technologies that an organization can access internally and externally. These include existing technologies currently available in-house and other technologies that an organization can acquire in the market. The *organizational* facet describes the characteristics of an organization, such as firm size, type of organization structure, complexity of managerial structure, and the amount of slack resources. The *environmental* aspect encompasses many factors regarding the industry structure, competition, suppliers, and politics and regulations.

One of the advantages of this model is that it more closely reflects the nature of an organization's operation. While researchers utilized this model as a theoretical framework to conduct studies of adoption of innovation in other industries,[84–86] it has not been employed for such studies in the healthcare services industry.

VI. Barriers to E-Health Adoption

Researchers have classified different types of barriers to the diffusion and adoption of e-health.[87] This discussion focuses on four major issues: financial, technological, social/cultural, and legal. The awareness and comprehension of these barriers are important because they prevent society from achieving the ultimate goal of healthcare globalization through initiatives such as e-health.

Financial Barriers

Even though health IT development costs have significantly dropped over the past decade, some nations still find it difficult to acquire the necessary infrastructure. Some developing countries argue that an investment in health IT is not prudent or possible when their citizens still lack basic necessities, such as water, food, housing, and basic education. Lam[88] stated that the limited resources, different needs, and healthcare settings in developing countries should serve as an urgent need for us to search for new treatment methods that are more effective and efficient than existing practices utilized in developed countries. Even for developed nations that have the means, the cost of fully implementing e-health and telemedicine in all locales and regions is considered a major undertaking.

Another financial barrier is rooted in the cost-effectiveness analysis. Researchers have attempted to conduct cost-effectiveness analysis of telemedicine, but they are confronting some uncertainties, such as the rapid change of and the costs of implementing such systems, joint costs among different ICT used in health care, and multiple uses of health IT.[89,90]

However, recent research studies have found that widespread utilization of telemedicine can contribute to a considerable reduction in costs. Spaulding[91] and his research team reported that the cost of tele-consultation dropped from $7328 when only one tele-consultation was performed to below $150 when 200 tele-consultations were achieved. As a result, the true financial benefits of telemedicine or health IT can be realized when there is an economy of scale. Thus, e-health makes complete sense if it is globalized.

Technological Barriers

Whenever technologies, especially health IT, become the center of discussion, we must deal with the problems of infrastructure, standardization, compatibility, reliability, capacity, availability, assistance, and maintenance. E-health and telemedicine cannot be accomplished unless a telecommunications infrastructure is sufficiently available to handle the transmission of tele-medical data and information. Even though standardization and compatibility are critical issues for health IT implementation, assistance and maintenance are inevitable for ongoing operations. The initial investment in health IT infrastructure is more problematic in underdeveloped and developing countries than developed countries. The strategies used to overcome this barrier are covered in a later section.

Social and Cultural Barriers

Obviously, there are social and cultural differences among nations around the world. As neither ICT nor health IT are artifacts, it is almost impossible to ensure that a specific e-health application would be acceptable similarly across various societies and cultures. Therefore, most such applications would normally need to be modified to fit local contexts. This requires that healthcare processes that affect interactions among global, regional, and local levels be understood.[92] Moreover, countries take different approaches in handling and managing healthcare planning and policies. Lack of political will is another important issue. Whether an e-health system will be fully implemented depends on the commitment among various groups in the society, especially the political group and the government that leads the country. These fragmented systems only obstruct the growth and successful development of global e-health.

Legal Barriers

Legal conundrums are the top concern among physicians, healthcare managers, and policy makers. An overwhelming list of key issues includes "confidentiality and security, patients' right of access, data protection, duty of care, standards of care, malpractice, suitability and failure of equipment, physician licensure and accreditation, physician reimbursement, intellectual property rights," and income taxes.[93(p.37)] These obstacles add another critical facet to the complexity of e-health at a global level.

Altogether, these various barriers imply a high need for an establishment of a central entity that will act as a strong advocate of global e-health, organize the collaborative efforts among nations of the world, and provide a practical strategic framework. The framework can then be utilized as a map and a compass that would guide all nations of the world to the same destination of healthcare globalization. Because e-health processes involve various stakeholders, we now present some of the key constituents with a major stake in e-health.

▶ VII. Stakeholder Analysis

E-health is a system-wide integrated process innovation; thus, the level of success in its widespread adoption must be accelerated by various stakeholders and is dependent upon multiple factors. The power of e-health to affect healthcare services delivery systems at the global level not only is beneficial to humanity, but also contributes to the complexity of its adoption. Therefore, the involvement of major stakeholders and their perspectives concerning this process innovation must be addressed.

This section illustrates an extensive, but not exhaustive, list of important stakeholders involved in the process of planning, adoption, and implementation of e-health. No single group of stakeholders is more important than another. Each and every stakeholder plays an important and unique role in the process of adoption.

International Organizations

Because e-health is a worldwide paradigm shift in healthcare delivery systems, the major

international entities such as WHO, the World Bank, and the United Nations take on key roles in setting the strategic directions; acting as central collaborating organizations; providing both monetary and nonmonetary resources; and enacting international policies regarding the adoption, implementation, and utilization of e-health. WHO has identified e-health as an integral tool in achieving universal health coverage (i.e., all citizens of the world have access to affordable and good quality healthcare services), which is a shared goal of health reform efforts across various countries, and also one of the WHO's priorities. The WHO built a strategic framework that nations could employ as a guideline in adopting and implementing e-health.[94] Details of the WHO strategic framework are presented in a later section.

Government

At the national level, the government of each country is an influential body that can support and expedite the development of e-health policies and their standards, as well as the adoption and implementation of e-health among other relevant stakeholders. A number of countries, such as the United States, Canada, and the United Kingdom, are placing e-health or use of health IT at the top priority of their national agendas. The political willpower shared among the members of the government leadership is inevitable to the success of this system-wide process innovation. However, even though the government is playing a highly supportive role, the federal government of various countries, including both developed and developing countries, is confronting the most fragile issue of minimal available funding. Nevertheless, some countries, such as Canada and Ireland, are heavily investing in e-health.[95,96]

Physicians/Clinical Providers

Physicians and other clinicians, such as nurses, form another group of vital stakeholders of the e-health system because they are the direct users of the system and are arguably assumed to have a share in taking the responsibility for such an investment. Physicians and nurses must be directly involved in the design process of any e-health platform simply because this system will eventually replace their routine activities. Moreover, they have to contribute the medical knowledge that will be incorporated into the system. One of the major barriers among the care providers is the lack of time,[97] which might prevent them from participating in the various steps of e-health adoption and implementation. Moreover, the alteration of routine practices might lead to the decrease in productivity and efficiency for both administrative and clinical staff—at least for a time.

Hospitals

Hospitals have a comprehensive awareness of e-health and have been a leading entity in its investment. Hospitals are a major provider of healthcare services, are most ready in terms of facility and infrastructure, and thus are assumed to acquire ICT needed for e-health. As with other stakeholders, limited funding and increasing IT costs are the major concerns for all hospitals. Moreover, most hospitals, especially those with for-profit status, are reluctant to share information that could benefit competitors. However, if fully implemented, e-health could help reduce the asymmetric pattern of information distribution among all hospitals, as well as between the hospitals/providers and consumers/patients. In effect, if the hospitals and providers have access to the same types and amounts of information and are not concerned too much about using unrevealed information to create competitive advantages, they may turn their attention, time, and effort to focus on improving quality of care and saving lives.

Patients

As the world moves farther into the information age, patients and health consumers have better awareness of information regarding diagnosis, symptoms, and available treatment alternatives. They tend to support the concept and completion of e-health. However, a large percentage of the world's population is living in underserved areas that bar them from necessary infrastructure, as well as the knowledge and information about e-health. Although patients are more likely to support this innovation, they are still addressing some imperative concerns. The most critical concern is privacy protection because with this system, patients' individual information and personal health records are transmitted electronically and can be accessed by multiple people, ranging from bill collectors to physicians associated with various types of healthcare services organizations. In some countries, such as the United States, where the majority of the population relies on the provision of private or employer-sponsored health insurance, consumers are also concerned that insurance companies will use their information to limit benefits, increase premiums, or possibly eliminate their insurance coverage policy. Under employer-sponsored health plans, employees are afraid that their employers will terminate employment once they have knowledge of their adverse health status.

Application Vendors

This group takes a completely supportive role in the e-health system because it has a direct benefit from developing an e-health platform. However, the competition among vendors is a major concern. In most geographic markets, there are many components related to the applications of e-health, so it is unlikely that any one vendor will have a dominant market share. However, the first mover will be able to take advantage of initial occupant of a market segment. As many entities are trying to set a standard for e-health, vendors are uncertain about what will happen to their existing or in-development platforms and products. Also, many pending policies on e-health standards and products in different countries might be threatening the stability of many vendors. Because of the fact that different medical services providers might have different needs for their system and might require some customization, vendors cannot take advantage of fixed cost allocation for mass production.

Third-Party Payers

Third-party payers include different entities, such as insurance companies, government agencies, and employers. These groups have important stakes in the development of e-health. First, when patients do not directly pay for their medical services, the third-party payers are the source of reimbursement of payment for medical bills charged to the patients by hospitals and physicians. Thus, they indirectly act as the provider of funding of any programs in which hospitals or physician practices want to invest. Second, third-party payers play a vital role in the successful implementation of e-health because they are involved in the daily transaction of an innumerable amount of health information. The data they collect can benefit both providers and patients in numerous ways, such as elimination of repeated diagnostic orders, prevention of prescription errors, and improvement of overall quality. However, similar to hospitals, insurers are concerned about availability of information to competitors, which could be manipulated against their competitive advantages.

Even so, while government agencies are inclined to publicly support e-health, some private insurance companies are still suspicious about the financial and time benefits.[98] The principal goal of insurance companies is to keep the "medical loss ratio" as low as possible. The medical loss ratio is "the percentage of the insurer's premiums paid out in medical claims" and is used by Wall Street for judging their performance.[99(p. 1250)] Therefore, the lower the medical loss ratio, the higher the profits insurance companies will make. Whether or not e-health can really reduce the amount paid out in medical claims is uncertain and requires

further evidence-based studies or more business cases. Regarding the time savings for medical claim processing, insurers argue that slow adjudication is caused by the presumption that every claim is subject to errors and misrepresentation and thus requires scrutiny for potential frauds and abuses. However, insurance companies should benefit a great deal from using the administrative portion of e-health to track frauds and abuses.

▶ VIII. WHO's Strategic Framework for E-Health Development

Based on the World Bank's logical framework on e-strategies, the WHO has developed the e-health development model,[100] which is illustrated in **FIGURE 14-4**. The model encompasses three tiers and constructs a solid foundation for enacting policies and actions toward the provision of e-health systems. Specifically, it is a guideline for strategic planning and implementation, as well as monitoring and control. It also offers assistance to nations in terms of preparation for the aforementioned challenges.

The bottom tier in Figure 14-4 is the basis for e-health implementation in nations. The national commitment to this innovation is vital to further development at the top two tiers. Established at a national level, a governing entity must include multiple stakeholders, delineate the vision, and bestow leadership and directions. It is also responsible for creating e-health policies and funding approaches and mechanisms for infrastructure development that supports e-health systems.

The second tier defines enabling actions that link foundation policies and strategies to the e-health applications. This level addresses the barriers and quests for strategic solutions that are appropriate and practical. The enabling actions involve citizen protection, equity promotion, multilingual capabilities,

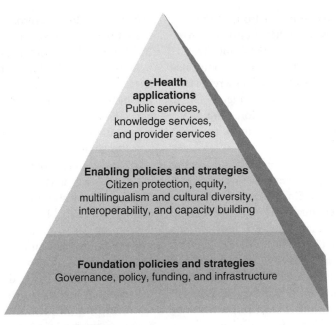

FIGURE 14-4 Framework for Strategic E-Health Development.
Adapted from WHO, 2007, p. 15.

groundwork for cultural diversity, assurance of interoperability among e-health systems, and enhancement of health IT and ICT capacity and capabilities among healthcare professionals and students.

The top tier is the linkage between the e-health systems and the citizens of the nations. It is the e-health services that are delivered to consumers and providers. The success of e-health applications relies heavily on the strong foundation and proper execution in policies and strategies determined in the first two tiers.

In 2005–2006, the WHO utilized this model as a background framework to conduct a global survey to examine the current status of e-health across various countries.[101] The WHO emphasizes the components in all three tiers. The participating countries are divided into income groups defined by the World Bank[102]: high, upper-middle, lower-middle, and low. The WHO conducted two additional global surveys in 2010 and 2015 in order to explore further developments of e-health strategies and adoption among its member states.

The results from the third and latest survey[103] indicated "impressive progress," even though some may have not reflected the trend anticipated in the first global survey report. For example, the third survey found that 58% of the responding member countries have an e-health strategy in place, which was lower than the projected 85% based on the first survey. However, such country-level policies have occurred across both large or small and developed or developing countries. Additionally, 90% of those countries also reported that they have set aside funding to implement their e-health strategies. The high-income countries reported public funding as the main source, whereas lower-income countries relied more on donor and nonpublic support.

In terms of the tele-health, 57% of the responding countries have developed or included tele-health policies as a national agenda. Teleradiology was the most common form of tele-health, and remote patient monitoring has made it a growing trend. More than 80% reported having a national mHealth program and recognized that their healthcare organizations used social media for health promotion. Approximately 47% of countries have national EMR systems, and 54% reported enacting legislation to protect patients' electronic health data and information. Only 17% indicated use of analytical capabilities to mine and analyze big data.

In order to continue the adoption trend, the WHO has urged countries to recognize the importance of health IT as an integrated component of healthcare delivery processes. Furthermore, the early adopters must work toward improving the quality of data collected in order to promote effective use of analytical capabilities to generate meaningful use information in not only diagnoses and treatments for patients, but also an improvement of healthcare organizations' efficiency and effectiveness.

▶ IX. Flow of Resources Between Developed and Developing Countries

This section briefly discusses the possible flow of tangible and intangible resources between developed and developing countries. Although the results of the WHO global survey imply higher needs among developing and undeveloped countries, they can—at the same time—contribute to the development of healthcare globalization. While the developed countries have advantages in supplying tangible resources, such as capital for investment, they can in turn gain knowledge, which is the most powerful intangible asset, from developing and undeveloped countries.

The World Bank focuses on development through knowledge. It identifies the importance of knowledge in the process of

transforming limited resources into things that meet our needs. Knowledge-sharing through ICT is the highlight of e-health that is expected by both international organizations and countries. Through continuous knowledge-sharing, the healthcare system will gain inner coherence because scientific medicine is enforced by accountability and legitimacy.[104]

Researchers in developed countries can learn and benefit from the studies conducted in developing and undeveloped countries. Many empirical studies related to telemedicine as well as health IT have been conducted in developing parts of the world, and the results from these studies can lead to more care and research and may introduce alternative treatments for some existing diseases.[105,106] Along with a rapid increase in international travel, the emergence of serious infectious diseases, such as human immunodeficiency virus (HIV) and the recent international outbreaks of severe acute respiratory syndrome (SARS), has prompted countries around the world to prepare for these global threats. We believe that e-health globalization would provide some much-needed intervention in these circumstances and countless other scenarios.

The use of directly observed therapy, short-term (DOTS) for treating tuberculosis is a good example of how developed countries can learn and adopt the practices from developing countries. This particular treatment for tuberculosis was found to be effective in Africa and Asia in the early 1950s and has since become the standard method of treatment, but the U.S. Centers for Disease Control and Prevention (CDC) first recommended it for tuberculosis patients only in 1993.[107] Even though developing countries might lack sophisticated technology and hefty research and development funds, they do have some natural resources and can conduct efficient but innovative research that can produce a lot of knowledge that could be shared with the rest of the world. Research experience can also be transferred among various contexts across the world.

▶ X. Conclusion

E-health has widely opened more channels for distributing medical information and knowledge across international boundaries. We suggest that the PPF economic tool theoretically demonstrates that e-health can improve the wellness of the world population and increase efficiency and effectiveness in the healthcare delivery system. The implication of external, positive effects of e-health calls for urgent political support and investment from private sectors. To help accelerate the adoption of e-health development, international entities, such as the WHO and World Bank, should take action in monitoring the price of health IT solutions, co-fund research and major international efforts in health IT implementations, and encourage developing and undeveloped countries to adopt and invest in e-health by providing some levels of subsidies and transferred expertise.

The international agenda should increase the emphasis on social values, while maintaining the focus on the economic value of trade. Through this combination, policies and actions can aim toward maximizing the economic values without imposing negative consequences on citizens of the world. Several theories that help with the understanding of the factors that influence e-health adoption were presented, as well as some of the barriers to e-health adoption. We also presented a discussion on key stakeholders in e-health, because understanding each stakeholder's perspective and role enhances the implementation and adoption process. The strategic framework set forth by the WHO can serve as a strong foundation for the healthcare globalization through e-health. Furthermore, the current status of e-health development in developed and developing countries shows a positive trend. The collaboration among countries and international entities is imperative in the process of design, implementation, and evaluation of e-health endeavors.

While developed countries have the ability to provide tangible supports to this global health and wellness initiative, developing countries are also able to contribute in terms of natural resources and knowledge sharing. Research has shown that developed countries can attain benefits from innovative research studies conducted in developing countries. Through mutual exchange, the world can achieve the ultimate goal of an integrated, globalized healthcare system with effective and efficient use of health IT.

Notes

1. UPMC International Services. (2015). *Establishing second-opinion pathology consultations in China*. Retrieved from upmcinternational.com/casestudy/kingmed-case-study
2. Bulger, R. J., Hawkins, D., & Owen, J. W. (1999). Forward. In D. E. Holmes (Ed.), *Reflections of globalization of health: Consequences of the 3rd Trilateral Conference* (pp. v–vi). Washington, DC: Association of Academic Health Centers.
3. Ludden, D. (2007). *A quick guide to the world history of globalization*. Retrieved from www.sas.upenn.edu/~dludden/global1.htm
4. Riggs, F. W. (2000, July 29). *Globalization: Key concepts*. Retrieved from www2.hawaii.edu/~fredr/glocon.htm
5. Raskin, P., Banuri, T., Gallopín, G., Gutman, P., Hammond, A., Kates, R., & Swart, R. (2002). *The great transition: The promise and the lure of the times ahead*. Boston, MA: Stockholm Environment Institute.
6. International Monetary Fund. (2000, April 12). *Globalization: Threat or opportunity?* Retrieved from www.imf.org/external/np/exr/ib/2000/041200.htm
7. Levitt, T. (1983). The globalization of markets. *Harvard Business Review, 61*(3), 92–102.
8. Masson, P. (2001). Globalization: Facts and figures. *International Monetary Fund*. Retrieved from www.imf.org/external/pubs/ft/pdp/2001/pdp04.pdf
9. Sachs, J. D. (2005). *The end of poverty: Economic possibilities for our time*. New York, NY: Penguin Press.
10. United Nations. (2007). *Definition of developed and developing countries*. Retrieved from http://unstats.un.org/unsd/cdb/cdb_dict_xrxx.asp?def_code=491

11. World Health Organization. (2007). Global environmental change. *World Health Organization.* Retrieved from www.who.int/globalchange/en/

12. Charles, J. A. (2004, July 14). *The environmental benefits of globalization: Rising global affluence is a good thing for environmental sustainability.* Retrieved from www.globalenvision.org/library/1/645/

13. Till, B. M., Peters, A. W., Afshar, S., & Meara, J. (2017). From blockchain technology to global health equity: Can cryptocurrencies finance universal health coverage? *BMJ Global Health, 2*(4), e000570. doi:10.1136/bmjgh-2017-000570

14. Panch, T., Szolovits, P., & Atun, R. (2018). Artificial intelligence, machine learning and health systems. *Journal of Global Health, 8*(2), 020303.

15. O'Halloran, D., & Kvochko, E. (2015). *Industrial internet of things: Unleashing the potential of connected products and services.* Davos-Klosters, Switzerland: World Economic Forum.

16. World Bank. (2000). Poverty in an age of globalization. *World Bank.* Retrieved from www1.worldbank.org/economicpolicy /globalization/documents/povertyglobalization.pdf

17. Sachs, (2005), *ibid.*

18. World Bank, (2000), *ibid.*

19. *Ibid.*

20. Mittelman, M., & Hanaway, P. (Eds.). (2012). Globalization of healthcare. *Global Advances in Health and Medicine, 1*(2), 5–7.

21. Walker, J., Pan, E., Johnston, D., Adler-Milstein, J., Bates, D. W., & Middleton, B. (2005). The value of health care information exchange and interoperability. *Health Affairs, 2005*(January–June), W5-10–W5-18 (Suppl. Web Exclusives).

22. Low, A. F., Phillips, A. B., Ancker, J. S., Patel, A. R., Kern, L. M., & Kaushal, R. (2013). Financial effects of health information technology: A systematic review. *The American Journal of Managed Care, 19*(10 Spec No), SP369–SP376.

23. Kruse, C. S., & Beane, A. (2018). Health information technology continues to show positive effect on medical outcomes: Systematic review. *Journal of Medical Internet Research, 20*(2), e41. doi:10.2196 /jmir.8793

24. Lasi, H., Fettke, P., Feld, T., & Hoffmann, M. (2014). Industry 4.0. *Business & Information Systems Engineering, 6,* 239–242.

25. Kang, M., Park, E., Cho, B. H., & Lee, K.-S. (2018). Recent patient health monitoring platforms incorporating internet of things-enabled smart devices. *International Neurourology Journal, 22*(Suppl. 2), S76–S82.

26. Tan, J. (Ed.). (2005). *E-health information systems: Introduction to students and professionals.* San Francisco, CA: Jossey-Bass.

27. World Bank. (1999). *World Development Report 1998/99: Knowledge for Development* [electronic version]. Oxford, UK: Oxford University Press.

28. Barlow, J., Bayer, S., & Curry, R. (2006). Implementing complex innovations in fluid multi-stakeholder environments: Experiences of 'Telecare.' *Technovation, 26*(3), 396–406.

29. Al-Shorbaji, N. (2000). Health informatics and telematics with reference to the work of WHO/EMRO. *World Health Organization,* 4. Retrieved from www.emro.who.int/publications/IT.pdf

30. American College of Nurse Practitioners. (2007). What is telehealth? Retrieved from www.acnpweb .org/i4a/pages/Index.cfm?pageID=3470

31. Norris, A. C. (2002). *Essentials of telemedicine and telecare.* West Sussex, UK; New York NY: John Wiley & Sons, Ltd.

32. Tan, (2005), *ibid.*

33. Norris, (2002), *ibid.*

34. Olla, P., & Tan, J. (2006, April–June). The M-health reference model: An organizing framework for conceptualizing mobile health systems. *International Journal of Health Information Systems & Informatics, 1*(2), 1–19.

35. Olla, P. Mobile health technology of the future: Creation of an M-health taxonomy based on proximity. *International Journal of Healthcare Technology and Management, 8*(3/4), 370–387.

36. Yamaguchi, T., Sakano, T., Fujii, T., Ando, Y., & Kitamura, M. (2002). Design of medical teleconsultation support system using super-high-definition imaging system. *Systems and Computers in Japan, 33*(8), 9–18.

37. Kifle, M., Mbarika, V., & Datta, P. (2006). Telemedicine in Sub-Saharan Africa: The case of teleopthalmology and eye care in Ethiopia. *Journal of the American Society for Information Science and Technology, 57*(10), 1383–1393.

38. *Ibid.*

39. Watson, A. J., Bergman, H., & Kvedar, J. C. (2007). *Teledermatology.* Retrieved from http://www .emedicine.com/derm/topic527.htm

40. Weinstein, R. S., Lopez, A. M., Barker, G. P., Krupinski, E. A., Descour, M. R., Scott, K. M. ... Bhattacharyya, A. K. (2007). The innovative bundling of teleradiology, telepathology, and teleoncology services. *IBM Systems Journal, 46*(1), 69–84.

41. Accreditation Council for Continuing Medical Education. (2007). *About Us.* Retrieved from www.accme.org/index.cfm/fa/about.home/About .cfm

42. Kaplan, R. M. (1999). Shared medical decision-making: A new paradigm for behavioral medicine—1997 presidential address. *The Society of Behavioral Medicine, 21,* 3–11.

43. Kaplan, R. M., & Frosch, D. L. (2005). Decision making in medicine and health care. *Annual Review of Clinical Psychology, 1,* 525–556.

44. Roth, A., Korb, H., Gadot, R., & Kalter, E. (2006). Telecardiology for patients with acute or chronic cardiac complaints: The 'SHL' experience in Israel and Germany. *International Journal of Medical Informatics, 75*(9), 643–645.

45. Giallauria, F., Lucci, R., Pilerci, F., De Lorenzo, A., Manakos, A., Psaroudaki, M., … Vigorito, C. (2006). Efficacy of telecardiology in improving the results of cardiac rehabilitation after acute myocardial infarction. *Monaldi Archives for Chest Disease, 66*(1), 8–12 (Abstract retrieved August 10, 2007, from PubMed database).

46. 2016 Top Markets Report Health IT A Market Assessment Tool for U.S. Exporters U.S. Department of Commerce | International Trade Administration | Industry & Analysis (I&A) July 2016.

47. U.S. Department of Commerce | International Trade Administration | Industry & Analysis (I&A).

48. Cazac, C., & Radu, G. (2014). Telesurgery—An efficient interdisciplinary approach used to improve the health care system. *Journal of Medicine and Life, 7*(Special Issue 3), 137–141.

49. Choi, P. J., Oskouian, R. J., & Tubbs, R. S. (2018, May). Telesurgery: Past, present, and future. *Cureus, 10*(5), e2716.

50. Anvari, M. (2007). Telesurgery: Remote knowledge translation in clinical surgery. *World Journal of Surgery, 31*(8), 1545–1550.

51. Hirano, Y., Ishikawa, N., Omura, K., Inaki, N., Hiranuma, C., Waseda, R., & Watanabe, G. (2007). Robotic intragastric surgery: A new surgical approach for the gastric lesion [electronic version]. *Surgical Endoscopy* (online publication ahead of print).

52. Oh, H., Rizo, C., Enkin, M., & Jadad, A. (2005). What is eHealth (3): A systematic review of published definitions [electronic version]. *Journal of Medical Internet Research, 7*(1), e1.

53. Eysenbach, G. (2001). What is e-Health? [electronic version]. *Journal of Medical Internet Research, 3*(2), e20.

54. World Health Organization. (2007). Global observatory for eHealth. *World Health Organization.* Retrieved from http://www.who.int/ehealth/resources/bf_full.pdf

55. Atkinson, R. D., & McKay, A. S. (2007). Digital prosperity: Understanding the economic benefits of the information technology revolution. *Information Technology & Innovation Foundation.* Retrieved from www.itif.org/files/digital_prosperity.pdf

56. Feldstein, P. J. (2003). *Health policy issues: An economic perspective* (3rd ed.). Chicago, IL: Health Administration Press.

57. *Ibid.*

58. Stolyar, V., Selkov, A., Atkov, O., & Chueva, E. (2004, April 21). *Social efficiency of modern telemedicine.* Paper presented at the Med-e-Tel 2004 Conference. Retrieved from www.medetel.lu/index.php?rub=educational_program&page=parallel_sessions_2004

59. Rogers, E. M. (2003). *Diffusion of innovations* (5th ed.). New York, NY: Free Press.

60. Folland, S., Goodman, A. C., & Stano, M. (2004). *The economics of health and health care* (4th ed.). Upper Saddle River, NJ: Pearson Education.

61. McPake, B., Normand, C., & Kumaranayake, L. (2002). *Health economics: An international perspective.* New York, NY: Routledge.

62. Sen, B. (2005, September 13). *Externalities.* Birmingham, UK: University of Alabama at Birmingham.

63. Atkinson, R. D. (2007). *The case for a national broadband policy.* Retrieved from www.itif.org/files/CaseForNationalBroadbandPolicy.pdf

64. Androuchko, L., & Nakajima, I. (2004). *Developing countries and e-health services.* Retrieved from http://ieeexplore.ieee.org/iel5/9246/29313/01324524.pdf

65. Davis, F. D. (1989). Perceived usefulness, perceived ease of use, and user acceptance of information technology. *MIS Quarterly, 13*(3), 319–340.

66. Davis, F. D., Bagozzi, R. P., & Warshaw, P. R. (1989). User acceptance of computer technology: A comparison of two theoretical models. *Management Science, 35,* 982–1003.

67. Bagozzi, R. P., Davis, F. D., & Warshaw, P. R. (1992). Development and test of a theory of technological learning and usage. *Human Relations, 45*(7), 660–686.

68. Hu, P. J., Chau, P. Y. K., Sheng, O. R. L., & Tam, K. Y. (1999). Examining the technology acceptance model using physician acceptance of telemedicine technology. *Journal of Management Information Systems, 16*(2), 91–112.

69. Musa, P. F. (2006). Making a case for modifying the technology acceptance model to account for limited accessibility in developing countries. *Information Technology for Development, 12*(3), 213–224.

70. Musa, P. F., Meso, P., & Mbarika, V. Toward sustainable adoption of technologies for human development in Sub-Saharan Africa: Precursors, diagnostics, and prescriptions. *Communications of the Association for Information Systems, 15*(33), 592–608.

71. Chismar, W. G., & Wiley-Patton, S. (2002, January). *Does the extended technology acceptance model apply to physicians.* Proceedings of the 36th Annual Hawaii International Conference on System Sciences (HICSS'03), 160a. Retrieved from http://csdl2.computer.org/comp/proceedings/hicss/2003/1874/06/187460160a.pdf

72. Vieru, D. (2001).A model for telemedicine adoption: A survey of physicians in the provinces of Quebec and Nova Scotia (M.Sc. dissertation, Concordia University, Canada). Retrieved from ProQuest Digital Dissertations database (Publication No. AAT MQ59291).

73. Venkatesh, V., Morris, M. G., Davis, G. B., & Davis, F. D. (2003). User acceptance of information technology: Toward a unified view. *MIS Quarterly, 27*(3), 425–478.

74. Venkatesh, V., & Davis, F. D. (2000). A theoretical extension of the technology acceptance model: Four longitudinal studies. *Management Science, 46*(2), 186–204.

75. Ajzen, I., & Fishbein, M. (1980). *Understanding attitudes and predicting social behavior.* Englewood Cliffs, NJ: Prentice-Hall.

76. Ajzen, I. (1985). From intention to actions: A theory of planned behavior. In J. Kuhl & J. Bechmann (Eds.), *Action control: From cognition to behavior* (pp. 11–39). New York, NY: Springer.

77. Fishbein, M., & Ajzen, I. (1975). *Belief, attitude, intention, and behavior: An introduction to theory and research.* Reading, MA: Addison-Wesley.

78. Ajzen, I. (1991). The theory of planned behavior. *Organizational Behavior and Human Decision Processes, 50,* 179–211.

79. Chau, P. Y. K., & Hu, P. J. (2002). Investigating healthcare professionals' decisions to accept telemedicine technology: An empirical test of competing theories. *Information and Management, 39,* 297–311.

80. Rogers, (2003), *ibid.*

81. Menachemi, N., Burke, D. E., & Ayers, D. J. (2004). Factors affecting the adoption of telemedicine—A multiple adopter perspective. *Journal of Medical Systems, 28*(6), 617–632.

82. Rogers, (2003), *ibid.*

83. Tornatzky, L. G., & Fleischer, M. (1990). *The process of technology innovation.* Lexington, MA: Lexington Books.

84. Zhu, K., Kraemer, K. L., Xu, S., & Dedrick, J. (2004). Information technology payoff in e-business environments: An international perspective on value creation of e-business in the financial services industry. *Journal of Management Information Systems, 21*(1), 17–54.

85. Zhu, K., Kraemer, K. L., & Xu, S. (2002, December). *A cross-country study of electronic business adoption using the technology-organization-environment framework.* ICIS 2002: 23rd Annual International Conference on Information Systems, 337–348. Retrieved from www.crito.uci.edu/publications/pdf /CrossCountryStudy.pdf

86. Kuan, K. K. Y., & Chau, P. Y. K. (2001). A perception-based model for EDI adoption in small businesses using a technology-organization-environment framework. *Information & Management, 38*(8), 507–512.

87. Tanriverdi, H., & Iacona, C. S. (1999). Diffusion of telemedicine: A knowledge barrier perspective. *Telemedicine Journal, 5*(3), 223–244.

88. Lam, C. L. K. (2000). Knowledge can flow from developing to developed countries. *British Medical Journal, 312,* 830.

89. Sisk, J. E., & Sanders, J. H. (1998). A proposed framework for economic evaluation of telemedicine. *Telemedicine Journal, 4*(1), 31–37.

90. Beach, M., Miller, P., & Goodall, I. (2001). Evaluating telemedicine in an accident and emergency setting. *Computer Methods and Programs in Biomedicine, 64*(3), 215–223.

91. Spaulding, R. J. (2007). *Cost analysis: Does telemedicine cost more, less, or about the same as traditional methods of consulting with patients?* Retrieved from www2.kumc.edu/telemedicine /research/costanalysis.htm

92. Shuaib, F., Musa, P. F., Muhammad, A. Musa, E., Nyanti, S., Mkanda, P., … Ali Pate, M. (2017). Containment of Ebola and polio in low-resource settings using principles and practices of emergency operations centers in public health. *Journal of Public Health Management and Practice, 23*(1), 3–10.

93. Norris, (2002), *ibid.,* 37.

94. WHO, (2007), *ibid.*

95. E-Health-Media. (2007, August 8). *Ireland to invest euros 500m in e-health.* Retrieved from http://ehealtheurope.net/News/2935/ireland _to_invest_euros_500m_in_e-health

96. Canada Ministry of Health. (2006, May). *$150M investment in e-health to improve patient care.* Retrieved from www2.news.gov.bc.ca/news_releases _2005-2009/2006HEALTH0028-000518.htm

97. Audet, A. M., Doty, M. M., Peugh, J., Shamasdin, J., Zapert, K., & Schoenbaum, S. (2004). Information technologies: When will they make it into physicians' black bags? *Medscape General Medicine, 6*(4), 2.

98. Kleinke, J. D. (2000). Vaporware.com: The failed promise of the health care internet. *Health Affairs, 19*(6), 57–71.

99. Kleinke, J. D. (2005). Dot-gov: Market failure and the creation of a national health information technology system. *Health Affairs, 24*(5), 1246–1262.

100. World Bank. (2007). What is stakeholder analysis? *The World Bank.* www1.worldbank.org/publicsector /anticorrupt/PoliticalEconomy/PDFVersion.pdf

101. Kaplan, (1999), *ibid.*

102. World Bank, (2007), *ibid.*

103. World Health Organization. (2016). *Global diffusion of eHealth: Making universal health coverage achievable. Report of the third global survey on eHealth.* Geneva, Switzerland: World Health Organization (License: CC BY-NC-SA 3.0 IGO).

104. Miscione, G. (2007). Telemedicine in the upper amazon: Interplay with local health care practices. *MIS Quarterly, 31*(2), 403–425.
105. Mitka, M. (1998). Developing countries find telemedicine forges links to more care and research. *Journal of the American Medical Association, 280*(15), 1295–1296.
106. Nakajima, I., & Chida, S. (2000). Telehealth in the Pacific: Current status and analysis report (1999–2000). *Journal of Medical Systems, 24*(6), 321–331.
107. Morse, D. I. (1996). Directly observed therapy for tuberculosis—Spend now or pay later. *British Medical Journal, 312,* 719–720.

Chapter Questions

14-1 Define *tele-care, telemedicine, tele-health*, and *e-health*. Discuss the similarities and differences among these terms.

14-2 Name four major types of telemedicine and provide some applications of each.

14-3 Discuss the production possibility frontier (PPF) and positive externality economic perspectives and their implications on e-health.

14-4 Identify factors and barriers influencing the adoption of e-health among healthcare organizations and providers.

14-5 Discuss the importance of the process of stakeholder analysis, and identify the major stakeholders in globalized e-health.

14-6 Discuss the relevance of each tier in the World Health Organization (WHO) framework for strategic e-health development presented in this chapter.

Biographies

Anantachai Panjamapirom is an Independent Consultant in healthcare management and health information technology. He earned a PhD in Health Services Administration, an MBA from the University of Alabama at Birmingham (UAB), and an MS in Information and Communication Sciences from Ball State University. He has published research articles in academic journals (e.g., *Health Care Management Review, Preventive Medicine, Journal of General Internal Medicine, Studies in Health Technology and Informatics)* and presented at a number of conferences (e.g., *Healthcare Information and Management Systems Society, Academy of Management, American Medical Informatics Association, Academy Health*).

Dr. Panjamapirom was a research Director with the Health Care Information Technology Advisory and Quality Reporting Roundtable research programs at the Advisory Board Company. He led strategic and best practice research, served as a subject matter expert, and provided policy analysis and strategic and operational guidance in support of hospital and health system executives. His principal areas of expertise included CMS quality reporting programs (e.g., Promoting Interoperability, Quality Payment Program, MACRA), value-based payment models, IT performance management, and IT implications in accountable care environment. He is a Certified Professional in Healthcare Information and Management Systems (CPHIMS).

Philip F. Musa is the Director of Management Programs and Associate Professor of Management and Information Systems in the Collat School of Business at The University of Alabama at Birmingham. His earned degrees include: PhD (in ISQS), MPH (in Epidemiology), MSEE, and MBA. He has published dozens of research in journals and academic conferences (e.g., *European Journal of Information Systems, Communications of the AIS,*

Information Systems Journal, Journal of Public Health Management and Practice, Journal of Medical Systems, Communications of the ACM, Journal of Global Information Management, Journal of Information Systems Education, Journal of Information Technology for Development, etc.)

Dr. Musa has taught courses in Project Management, Supply Chain Management, Quality Management, Strategic Information Systems in HealthCare, Systems Analysis and Database, Electrical Engineering, Operations Management, etc. He has served on special projects at other universities and on editorial boards of several academic journals, and on program committees of many professional conferences and dissertation committees. He is a licensed professional Engineer and a Senior Member of the Institute of Electrical and Electronics Engineers (IEEE). He is a Member of the Association of Information Systems (AIS), and a lifetime member of Phi Kappa Phi and Public Health's Delta Omega Honor Society.

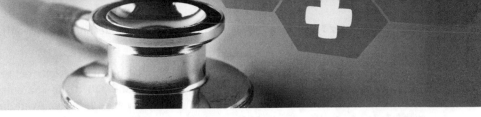

CHAPTER 15

Exploring Healthcare Futures: Emerging Technology in Health Care

Phillip Olla, Rajib Biswas, and Joseph Tan

LEARNING OBJECTIVES

- Overview Developments of Big Data Analytics (BDA)
- Speculate Emerging Technology for the Next 5–10 Years
- Rationalize the need for continually innovating health care
- Recognize how different categories of emerging technology may impact the kinetics of digital health adoption
- Explore healthcare futures

CHAPTER OUTLINE

Scenario: Orbita Driving Innovation in Conversational Artificial Intelligence (AI) and Voice Technology Solutions for Health Systems[1]

O rbita, a U.S. company dedicated to creating a platform for managing voice experiences in health care, partnered with Amazon in 2017 to create the *Alexa Diabetes Challenge* on behalf of Merck. Today, it is further leveraging the transformative power of conversational AI interfaces, such as voice assistants, chat-bots, and other conversational user interfaces, to create solutions for patient engagement, improved business and clinical processes, and future health care (e.g., remote care). Orbita, for example, has also worked with the Mayo Clinic to generate a consumer-skill guide for answering general first aid questions and is looking to work with clinical research organizations and large pharmaceutical companies to implement voice-activated data collection systems for clinical trials. More recently, in collaboration with team members from Brigham and Women's Hospital (BWH), Orbita has formed a *Digital Innovation Hub* to promote and explore the use of conversational AI interfaces to implement convenient health systems voice-enabled digital health solutions.

The BWH–Orbita collaboration was made possible via MassChallenge HealthTech, a Massachusetts-based accelerator matching digital health companies with industry partners to promote digital transformation in health care. The managing director of MassChallenge HealthTech, Nick Dougherty, commented: "Orbita and Brigham are two of the industry leaders in health innovation. Their collaboration was inevitable and it thrills us that we helped accelerate getting such an amazing relationship off the ground." (*Ibid.*)

Essentially, *Orbita Voice*™ will be developed as a cloud-based platform to allow BWH to pilot test, prototype, and explore voice and chat-bot interactions between BWH caregivers and patients in and outside of the hospital as well as at home. According to a 2018 press release: "Orbita Voice™ is the most widely used enterprise-grade platform for designing, building and maintaining HIPAA-compliant voice and chatbot healthcare applications, where data security and integrating with existing systems and processes are mission critical."[2]

Adam Landman, MD, chief information officer (CIO) at BWH noted: "Voice and chat-bot interfaces have the potential to reshape healthcare delivery. We're seeing strong interest in voice among our internal researchers and innovators who work continuously to champion new uses of technology to improve care delivery…We look forward to exploring the applications of voice in health care, while also being thoughtful and measured about the unique privacy and security challenges these new technologies represent."[1]

Orbita founder and chief executive officer (CEO), Bill Rogers, commented: "…Voice changes the game. Everyone has a voice and it is one of the last facilities you lose as you age. Voice-powered digital health solutions dramatically reduce the barriers to engagement by providing an intuitive, hands-free care experience…Whether focused on pharma, payers, providers, or device makers, these partners are most valuable to us and our clients."[1] Nathan Treloar, president and cofounder of Orbita, admitted: "The Brigham is an exceptional partner and has played a pivotal role in helping us understand where the Orbita Voice platform can solve real-world problems…This esteemed organization has had true success in advancing health care by adopting and scaling new technologies across their system. We're thrilled to collaborate with the Brigham to drive innovation in the use of voice in powerful new ways that we cannot yet even imagine."[1]

Based on your reading of this scenario, what is your vision of future health care in your locality? Do you see ways in which non-emergency care services may be conveniently transformed to closer-to-home services and connecting to your family physician via voice-activated systems? How do you rationalize third-party payers, such as major healthcare insurance companies, footing the bills for remote care services and even for lifestyle changes educational programs supported with Orbita technology?

▶ I. Introduction

Global healthcare systems are being confronted with exceptional challenges. One of the most pressing issues is longevity; people are living longer and the elderly population continues to increase. This positive health indicator is creating an increasing strain on health systems around the world due to the more complicated and resource-demanding conditions. Delivering health care is becoming more complex, and the costs are increasing at an alarming rate. There is an urgent need for disruptive technology to address these challenges.

On a positive note, health care is undergoing a tremendous change due to the accumulation of massive data and the plethora of emerging technologies that are being adapted to address healthcare challenges. There are many factors that will contribute to the beginning of a period of the rapid diffusing of technological advancements and emerging technology into healthcare systems. The key factors for the adoption include the following.

Innovation Maturity[3]

Technological advances are clearly needed in health care, many of which may be reaching maturity in other sectors. The growing need for innovative and disruptive solutions to meet healthcare delivery challenges implies opportunities to apply new thinking in traditional workflow and routine business processes. This is especially true when applying convenient technological solutions that follow the principles of lean thinking incrementally to

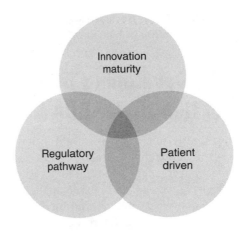

transform complex activities and poorly coordinated processes incrementally.

Regulatory Guidance[4]

Regulators are now more open than in the past to provide guidance on the adoption of new technology into the health systems, making it easier for innovators to understand the pathway for approval and clinical adoption. With increased willingness of policymakers to be opened to new paradigms in healthcare services delivery, new forms of care interventions via emerging technologies can be accommodated.

Patient Driven Innovation[5]

Better informed patients are now driving demands for new treatments, procedures, and technologies, putting a lot of pressure on healthcare systems. These factors are also driving patient engagement and empowerment, which is fundamentally changing how to prevent, diagnose, and cure diseases.

Prior to discussing the various classes of emerging technologies with the potential to disrupt the healthcare delivery systems, let us review the fundamental shift and developing trends in big data analytics (BDA) that relates to the different themes and thinking of this revised edition, so as to better project how best the solutions of various emerging technologies can facilitate the future health and wellbeing of the next generation of human beings.

▶ II. Developing Trends of Healthcare BDA

As previously noted, BDA will aid in unveiling where new technological capabilities, such as the convergence of advances in capturing devices, sensors, and mobile applications with integrative capabilities, can be optimally applied in addressing future healthcare systems challenges. Some key benefits of BDA include:

- More efficient ways of collecting massive datasets; for example, genomic information;
- Increasing patient social communications in digital forms; that is, allowing patients to view, share, and interact with others about their own health information; and
- Revelation of hidden medical knowledge, even the streaming of knowledge discoveries.

FIGURE 15-1 illustrates the modus operandi of BDA. As shown, there are components spanning from lab to pharmacy entailing data collection processes and interactions among patient, physician, and research and development (R&D). In order to build up a synergistic effort in resource optimization, the collection of these data is accompanied by the social networking data of the patient. The overarching idea is to make health care accessible to all with the optimal output, while simultaneously saving precious time and lowering costs to funders of the systems.

BDA Key Components

As the name implies, BDA in health care is dependent on several key elements. For instance, patient data from electronic health records (EHRs) is a vital element. Again when we look at the data, two key questions arise:

(a) Are these data structured or unstructured? and (b) How easy it is to establish and draw out relationships among the sourced data elements that may be coming from multiple channels (thereby making it very difficult to extract useful and meaningful information in terms of the overall message(s) hidden within the data)?

Simply put, two sorts of databases exist: (a) structured or (b) unstructured health records. Additionally, there is the necessity of a supporting system which can handle the large amounts of data generated in an efficient and intelligent manner. For instance, the clinical data must be interpreted separately for individuals and cohorts (or even populations) in the context of available social networking data linked to these individuals and cohorts (or even populations).

BDA Transforming Effects

BDA is revolutionizing the healthcare industry. Multiple impacts of BDA's transformative effects are summarized in this section vis-à-vis the different aspects of the care systems delivery (as discussed throughout this revised edition) in order to ensure the ultimate health and wellbeing of patients, the primary consumers of the health systems.

Patient Healthy Lifestyle Changes and Wellbeing

One of the beneficial effects of BDA in health care is the ability to provide valuable diagnostic, therapeutic, and predictive tools, which can impact the need for lifestyle behavioral changes of patients. As an example, we can cite mobile health (m-Health) as a means to consciously streamline a patient's lifestyle data, which are linked to his or her nutrition, physical activities, sleeping habits, and more; furthermore, the BDA tools can integrate the different sets of big healthcare data with large, factual reference data. Additionally, these BDA tools can personalize interventions for specific patient(s) being monitored.

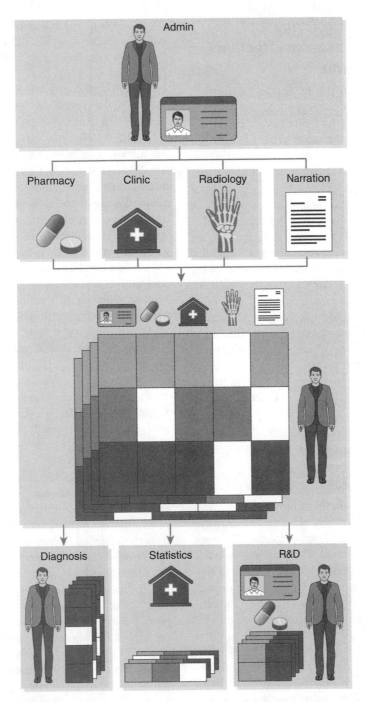

FIGURE 15-1 Schematic of BDA in Healthcare Systems.

Purportedly, these tools will furnish valuable information over time to enable the proper identification of appropriate and effective medication, thereby giving a detailed overview of progresses and setbacks encountered in therapies and more.

Understanding Triggers of Chronic Diseases for Effective Early Detection

In fact, BDA can unveil, in early diagnosis, the most probable triggers of chronic diseases. These data analytical processes can propel ongoing research toward a deeper understanding between social and other parameters, given that these data comprise a complex mix of physical behaviors, nutrition, genetic factors, environmental factors, and any signs of developing mental or physical diseases. At this time, the interfacing between different systems controlling disease propagation still baffles researchers. As such, we have to rely on BDA, which can provide us insights, to build an integrated view of changing health and well-being status of individuals and groups, encompassing various biomarkers. Eventually, these data (i.e., omics or quantified self-data) can aid in improving early detection of diseases and long-term management of adverse health factors, thereby reducing costs to the systems (and the patients).

Population Health

Public health policy is largely influenced by regional and national socioeconomic status. Together, these policies in turn define societal action whose main goal should be to improve population health and care outcomes. Through specific interventions, BDA can act as guidance toward addressing policies pertinent to a certain population. These policies are dependent on the quality of research and interventions. Again, there is a dearth of methods for validating certain interventions, such as those employed within the mental health domain or other critical illness domains (e.g., diabetes, cancer, and more). Although BDA work toward supporting health policies, there still exist several obstructions and challenges. For instance, patient privacy and the protection of data hinder analysis through a combined approach of healthcare provider and services.

Likewise, unstructured health records can be challenging for BDA. When and if methodological scalability and privacy friendliness can be achieved with outcomes more intelligently deduced via advanced statistical methods, the pathway for the development of precise and effective interventions can then be realized. With the advent of technological advances in BDA, one can synergistically amalgamate data from the healthcare environment and information from society. Social networks, forums, and blogs can then be used to retrofit our health environment by providing a wealth of data from which appropriate decisions can be made to benefit public health. When one combines information from informal sources and data emerging from diagnosis and surveillance, it is conceivably possible to achieve an early detection of disease outbreaks and transmission.

Indeed, the *AutoRegression with Google information* or ARGO project, which was essentially devising a predictive model to accurately estimate the influenza epidemics via Google search data,[6] provides a timely example. The ARGO project was accomplished through the amalgamation of tracking of disease, spread dynamics, and surveillance by adopting a popular social networking means, such as Twitter. Based on a well-planned analysis of these data with travel details incorporated, including changes in trade and climate, it is possible to attain a predictive model for population-based interventions, as well as identify improved treatment pathways for individual patients. Beyond this, with early detection of disease outbreak, experts from private, as well as government-funded, research institutions can assist in planning and coordinating key effective strategies, such as quarantine and vaccination, to promote public health and wellbeing.

Precision Medicine

Unlike a fee-for-service (FFS) model where physicians are incentivized to provide more services, value-based health care is a payment model based on patient health outcomes and may be treated as a guiding principle for sustainable health care.[7] This payment model actually comprises units, such as patient reported outcome, the amount of cost incurred during care and the eventual decision of payment varies based on the outcome achieved. Essentially, the incentives for health care being offered rely on the care services surpassing some measurable performance index as linked to patient related outcome, which is the underlying premise for personalized medicine or precision medicine (PM). For a proper implementation and tracking of progressive effects of PM interventions, there must be a streamlined flow of collection, analysis, and aggregation of data by inclusion of total care path, cost, and other measures as they relate to patient care outcome. In fact, such patient-linked health outcomes would require monitoring at three stages: (a) during; (b) before; and (c) after treatment. Key challenges in this paradigm may include the lack of an updated administrative care map, which can cater to associated specific care pathways to produce an accurate estimate of incurred expenditures. In the case where there is a succinct connection of care processes as well as care pathways with the assistance of BDA, empirical, evidence-based decisions for specific therapies may materialize. Notwithstanding, there is also the necessity for standardized and authenticated methods in order to achieve proper tracking of measurable outcomes.

Optimizing Healthcare Workflows

In industrial sectors, most of the processes are predictable; hence, workflow priorities and objectives can be well structured and defined. In the healthcare sector, however, many of the clinical procedures are complex and subjective, making the processes completely ill defined and thereby exhibiting a volatile and somewhat chaotic system. Influenced by patients

and their changing needs as communicated to their service providers, the productivity of the systems as a whole becomes a lot more challenging unless the various stakeholders are well apprised of the functionalities of the healthcare domain. This calls for the requirement of necessary and intelligent tools which will pave the way for an integrated multi-stream flow of data spanning EHRs, patient monitoring data, laboratory data, nursing operation data, and more in order to achieve a seamless connectivity for the provision of healthcare workflows and services within the framework of optimal resource utilization.

Privacy, Ethics, and Security

Privacy and security are fundamentals in safeguarding and protecting the rights of those whose data have been collected by third parties. With the advent of increasing data services, many people need access to data from multiple sources. With the potential for these various sorts of data to be integrated meaningfully and intelligently, substantial information previously unknown or unconnected about individual(s) or group(s) may be revealed. This has led to potential misuse, and even the intentional abuse of the collected data. Accordingly, ethical questions on the use of collected data arise, such as the appropriate dissemination of data; sales of data without the permission of the person providing the data; or hacking of user identification, passwords, and other key private information vis-à-vis unannounced motivation behind the collection and use of data. Consequently, there has been a growing number of nationwide, and even international, regulatory bodies coming up with new rules and acts, such as the General Data Protection Act[8] (GDPR) from the European Union, the Canadian Personal Information Protection and Electronic Documents Act of Canada (PIPEDA) and the Privacy Act, as well as the Health Insurance Portability and Accountability Act of 1996 (HIPAA) and HIPAA security ruling from the United States. Together, the ultimate intention of these Acts is to cater all public and private sectors, regardless of where a company or individual may be operating in the world, bringing all private and organizational sectors under their rules.

Blockchain Technology

Initially linked to Bitcoin,[9] the blockchain notion presents a distributed ledger technology with the beneficial characteristics of being able to connect all distributed stakeholders directly without the need of a trusted third party (TTP). Briefly, blockchain entails the use of distributed consensus protocols, such as the proof-of-work (PoW) protocol,[10] to generate fast, inexpensive, and more efficient ways of data sharing among distributed stakeholders in contrast to the cumbersome traditional operations deployed in the United States' distributed regional health information organizations (RHIOs).[11] As the distributed stakeholders in health care operate independently (i.e., patients, providers, insurers), the benefits of a blockchain-based decentralization include: (a) having these stakeholders connect directly with each other, providing access to the same patient information without a third-party intermediary; (b) having medical data sharing capabilities among the stakeholders at substantially reduced cost; (c) eliminating the challenge of duplicate testing when patients' test results have to be stored separately in different interoperable databases, further lowering costs to the systems; (d) having the ability to resolve disagreement among stakeholders due to deploying the PoW consensus protocol; and (e) having all stakeholders avoid data redundancy with a complete set of medical records that helps to protect the data from accidental losses, corruption, and malicious attacks.[12]

Evidently, blockchain's immutability property guarantees the integrity, transparency, and auditability of the stored data. The data, once saved on the generated blockchain, cannot be further altered and could therefore be checked or verified conveniently for any claimed alterations. Together, these particular characteristics of blockchain create trust among collaborating stakeholders; for example, should any records on the blockchain need to be altered, the time-stamping and corresponding changes in the hash outputs of the block containing that record would break the original chain, unless such changes were previously endorsed by every blockchain-linked stakeholders. Conceivably, the blockchain notion and properties align consistently with the strict requirements of big healthcare data analytics and data sharing applications.

Technical and Representational Challenges and Opportunities

We close this section with a look not only at the technical challenges and opportunities for BDA in health care, but also the need for better representation and preserved integrity of the big healthcare datasets being discussed.

Data Quality and Integrity

The quality and integrity of data is vital due to the expensive processes involved in medical and pharmaceutical big data processing. Moreover, the consistency, reliability, and reproducibility are key measures of data integrity and quality. Hence, vigilance must be maintained in how data is generated, executed, and transformed before readying them for storing and sharing. With constant upgrading of analytical methods and increased complexity of big data processing operations, the sourcing of data is critical, as this can significantly affect the quality of data being captured and the concluding interpretation of the information processed from the captured data.

Data Quantity and Visualization

Another vital consideration for effective and efficient BDA is data quantity and its visualization. Notably, BDA is dependent not only on voluminous data, but the resulting interpretability of the derived information from the datasets. Since BDA span across clinical, genetic, behavioral, environmental, financial, and operational data, there should be an effective mechanism to tackle the large wealth of information to retrieve valuable insights toward the improvement of health care in terms of quality, cost-effectiveness, and efficiency. This will require not only having sufficient and adequate amounts of the right sets of data, but also a way to visualize the resulting analysis so as to ensure not only optimization of the use of existing healthcare products and services, but also the continuous propositions of new rules, procedures, and visualization mechanisms to better disseminate the data for improved expert interpretation of the analysis.

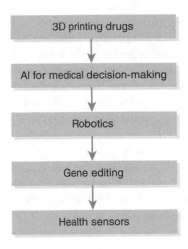

▶ III. Key Emerging Technologies in the Next 5–10 Years

Emerging technologies are technologies that may be new or old, but have the potential to be disruptive; that is, these technologies will and can transform how things are performed. Many of these technologies may be considered to be radical, evolving relatively quickly, and have a prominent impact on a domain. Examples include gene editing, AI, robotics, and nanotechnology.

The furthermost impact of emerging technologies are realized in the future; therefore, the emergence phase may be considered to be risky and ambiguous.[13] In the past, new and innovative technological advancements have resulted in technological convergence of dissimilar technologies advancing toward analogous objectives and then becoming integrated. An example of technological convergence is the integration of voice and data services to create a suite of productivity applications. In health care, we are seeing the innovative convergence

of robotics and AI, AI and radiology, and 3D printing and pharmacology to create new and novel technologies for the purpose of improving health care.

Today, emerging technology is playing a pivotal role in the transformation of health care and will continue to do so with more advances expected in the near future. Readers should have an appreciation of what emerging technologies to expect over the next 5–10 years, and to understand some of the hurdles that will accelerate or hinder the adoption of these technologies.

3D Printed Drugs

3D printing is a manufacturing process that creates three-dimensional objects through layering of the ingredient material. One of these materials that could have considerable benefits in the future is drug formulation. The adoption of 3D printing of drugs would improve patient-specific drug therapies.[14] This is sometimes referred to as personalized medicine. Drugs usually come in standardized dosages and chemical compositions; however, patients are different and may respond differently to the same drugs. In the future, customizing the drugs to each patient[15] could deliver better outcomes. The existing drug manufacturing process does not allow for customization of drugs, and this approach is very expensive. Conversely, 3D printing forms create limitless drug formulas and complex release profiles. A release profile refers to adjusting the way the drug chemicals are bound so that the active ingredients in the drug can be released at a predefined, controlled rate and in a targeted manner.[16] 3D printing drugs will also allow for on-demand manufacturing of drugs,[17] which means that drugs could be printed at the point of care. This would be beneficial in emergency scenarios or in regions with limited medical resources and storage capabilities.

Some of the challenges of 3D printing include:

- *Raw material risks*: Generally, the risks include variability in layer thickness, inaccurate chemicals positioning during printing, improper layering due to environmental conditions, compositional variation, and thermal variation, among other things.[18]
- *Product liability*: If 3D printing of drugs is widely adopted, pharmaceutical companies would become licensers of drugs blueprints rather creators and sellers of drugs. One of the key issues to address would be who assumes product liability.[19] 3D printing drugs will eventually make therapeutic pharmaceuticals cheaper, more effective, and widely available. The counter argument is the potential increased risk of the proliferation of counterfeit medicines, since printers are easier to hack than traditional manufacturing processes.[20]

In 2015, the Food and Drug Administration (FDA) approved the first 3D printed drug, Spritam tablets for oral suspension.[21] Spritam is used for treating seizures in children and adults who have particular types of epilepsy.[22] The drug is manufactured by Aprecia Pharmaceuticals who used ZipDose Technology to create the drug. An important benefit of the 3D printing process is the rapid disintegration while in the mouth, while also having great taste-masking ability, as well as a high drug load. This fast-melt dosage form can reach up to 1000 mg of drug load compared to other fast-melt dosage forms that usually range between 50 and 200 mg.[23]

The future will see more 3D printed drugs being created and seeking approval, and they will be more widely adopted.[24] A more robust regulatory framework from the FDA is required to cover future plans for regulation and the oversight required. Apart from the printer, a collection of active pharmaceutical ingredients (APIs) is required to be kept in storage for the printing to be done on demand. While common APIs like acetaminophen can be kept in storage easily, many others that are more obscure and may be difficult to keep, as they may require specialized storage that could be costly and not easily available. The next area of research concerns applicability of 3D printing for specialized drug development. 3D printing drugs is expected to have the most impact on generic drugs but specialized drugs are more complicated, expensive, and dangerous.

AI for Medical Decision-Making

AI has long been promised to provide the next disruptive solutions for healthcare woes, but has typically fallen short of the hype—until now.[25] There is now strong evidence that AI can provide significant improvements over manual processes. Although the evidence is typically generated from research, there are now commercially available AI-enabled platforms that are being positioned to slowly transform various critical domains of the medical practice. With technological advances of digitized data acquisition (via electronic medical record or EMR systems and sensors), machine learning techniques, and advanced computing infrastructure, AI clinical applications are now expanding to encompass problems that were previously thought to be exclusively within the domain of a human expert's capabilities. In the next section, we highlight some of the clinical applications of AI in health care.

Clinical Applications of AI

Image Analysis. To date, much progress has been made in improving efficiencies of image analysis by rapidly and precisely identifying anomalies for a radiologist to review via the use of an AI pattern and image. An example of this technique has reportedly been applied to *Computed Tomography* or CT images to identify specific lung nodules; in some instances, the AI image recognition algorithm was 97% faster than a panel of radiologists. On a similar note, specialized AI-empowered algorithmic solutions have been implemented via *Machine Learning* (ML) and *Deep Learning* (DL) platforms for analyzing radiological images for cancer patients with results found to be faster and more accurate than radiologists.[26] Such accurate readings and analysis will facilitate the early detection of true positives, thereby avoiding the negative experience of patients who may be given a false positive result, which is reportedly typical for one in four patients.[27] In the future, this technique will be embedded into the imaging to automatically provide real-time opinions, thereby achieving greater efficiencies and improved accuracy in image readings, analysis, and interpretation.

More recently, online solutions via dermatology apps to detect skin conditions where users can contact their physicians quickly (and remotely) have emerged.[28] For example, an AI-enabled app can be trained to recognize smartphone photo format. In this instance, anyone using a smartphone can freely deploy the app to match certain skin conditions to over 300,000 images of skin ailments.

Robotic Assisted Surgery. AI-assisted robotic surgery is an area of potential growth in the near future. AI is being adopted in orthopedic surgery to analyze data from pre-operation medical records and guide a real-time surgical instrument to improve the accuracies of a medical surgical procedure. AI can also learn from various past surgical procedures and provide recommendation of best treatment procedures based on prior outcomes for similar surgeries.

Past research[29] has demonstrated that AI-assisted robotic technique can be leveraged via using minimally invasive techniques, which can often also result in a reduction of blood loss, needed blood transfusion, potential complications, potential postoperative pain, length of hospital stays, and length of recovery times. Improved ergonomics also help physicians and surgeons in managing the surgical processes such as having visualization in 3-D and the freedom and/or intuitiveness of movement-enabled hand-eye coordination that may be difficult to achieve with traditional surgeries.

AI Dosing. AI techniques have also demonstrated improvements in the reduction of medication dosage errors. Past research[30,31] has suggested that AI could generate $16 billion in savings from adverse events related to errors in medicine dosing, which account for over 30% of all preventable medical errors. AI has been used to prevent overdose, providing the correct dose of immunosuppressant drugs administered to organ patients, thereby removing the educated guesswork. Note that dosing errors can make up to 37% of all preventable medical errors.

AI Diagnosing. Increasingly, emerging AI techniques have been applied to provide decision-aiding capabilities to augment clinical judgment and diagnosis. Examples of such case studies include using AI to diagnose skin cancers, heart defects, and other critical illnesses. Recent research published in *Nature*[32] revealed that AI neural networks for skin-cancer diagnosis can easily match the performance of medical experts. Indeed, it has been further predicted that AI, by doing a preliminary diagnosis before a patient enters the emergency department (ER), could yield $5 billion in annual savings.[33]

Virtual Nurse Assistant. A variety of AI-powered virtual assistants[34] have now been developed to support and service those people who may be in need; for example, the elderly and handicapped. A practical example is the AI-powered nurse avatars—these systems can be, and have been, used to assess symptoms and direct patients to the most effective care setting.

AI for Security and Administration. AI has proven to be effective in improving administrative inefficiencies. These activities are largely related to the back office support activities in healthcare institutions that can consume 51% of a nurse's workload and 16% of physician activities. AI-based technologies, such electronic document, digital workflow processes, and voice-to-text transcription, can improve administrative burdens and reduce time required for non-patient-care activities, such as writing reports, charting health status and tracking key performance measures, prescriptions processing, and ordering tests.

Another activity that can be reduced by AI technology is fraud and error monitoring. Healthcare breaches[35] have been purported to cost organizations $380 per patient record. Using AI to monitor and detect abnormal interactions with proprietary data could create $2 billion in annual savings by reducing health record breaches.[36] Traditional means of fraud detection is dependent on computerized rules-based detection with humans manually reviewing the flagged medical claims. Such human-assisted monitoring activity is time-consuming and prone to error as it relies on accurately detecting anomalies after the event has occurred. Health insurers are now experimenting with AI-supported data mining, along with AI-based neural networks (NNs) and non-traditional hybrid mining methods to review medical claims, reimbursements, and suspicious activities.[37,38] With NNs (which are AI-based models that rapidly mimic the processes of the human brain), it has been estimated that AI could create $17 billion in annual savings by improving the speed and accuracy of fraud detection in Medicare claims.[39]

Robots in Health Care

Robots have been successfully deployed across a growing number of high technology industries such as automotive, manufacturing, and aerospace. Today, health care is also experiencing an influx of advanced robots. Some of the most prominent examples are explored here.

Surgical Precision

The da Vinci robotic surgical platform is the most prominent surgical robot. It has been adapted to a variety of surgeries with greater reach, flexibility, smaller incisions, and shorter recovery times. The da Vinci is frequently used for prostatectomies, cardiac valve repair, and gynecologic surgical procedures.[40]

There is a misconception about robotic surgery that the robot conducts the medical procedure. What the da Vinci surgical system does is not autonomous, nor does it have any decision-making capabilities. The system is dependent initially on a surgeon for the starting input; then, all the interaction with the vision and motor functions are performed via the remote human–computer interaction.

The da Vinci is designed to replicate the movement of the surgeon with microinstruments; however, it is not designed to make decisions or move without the surgeon's direct input. This system does enable the possibility of telesurgery, or remote surgical operations.[41]

Remote Consultation

Robots can now autonomously navigate into hospital rooms to conduct a remote consultation. The FDA approved RP-VITA autonomous medical telepresence robot that allows doctors to remotely interact with patients on the hospital wards. These new generation of robots have AI that supports autonomous movement. The doctors can remotely direct the robot to anywhere in a hospital. The robot has advanced mapping; obstacle detection; avoidance technology; and uses lasers, sonar, and sensors for navigation.[42]

Robotic Exoskeletons

Exoskeletons used in the medical field are controlled by AI and integrated with smart robotics.[43] They are created to enhance body movements for patients who have lost mobility, such as in spinal cord injuries. The exoskeletons use transducers to harness the strength and motion of the patient. The robots can be classified by the purpose the serve; for example, the Hybrid Assisted Limb uses the hands movement to enhance strength in the hands.[44] The Ekso Bionics exoskeleton is used during a patient's rehabilitation to assist patient with mobility enhancement.[45]

Companion Robots

Loneliness and social isolation are now considered to be an epidemic and a predictor of ill health.[46] Social companion robots have been on the increase due to the advancements in robotics and AI.[47] These robots can either be fashioned as a humanoid or an animal. They can also vary in size and interaction capabilities. PARO,[48] for example, is an interactive baby seal therapeutic robot that provides benefits of animal therapy to patients in medical facilities.

The Luvozo PBC has created a robotic concierge called Sam to improve the quality of care in senior living communities. Sam is a human-sized robot that delivers frequent check-ins on patients related to nonmedical care for residents in long-term care settings. By doing so, it reduces the costs of care and improves patient satisfaction.

Gene Editing (or Genome Engineering)

This is a form of genetic engineering in which deoxyribonucleic acid (DNA) can be manipulated. DNA is contained in the cells. It is a long, double chain of molecules called nucleotides. Genes are made of DNA that transfer our traits through generations. They act as the "instruction books" while the ribonucleic acid (RNA) and proteins do most of the work.[49] In certain instances, genes may contain a typographical error in the DNA. It can be a change, gap, or duplication; also referred to as a mutation. These mutations can cause the gene to work incorrectly or not work at all. Scientists have discovered ways to delete, modify, or replace DNA in the genome of a living organism. Previous attempts at genetic engineering techniques randomly inserted genetic material into a host genome. New techniques allow the genetic material to accurately be inserted at a targeted location.[50]

Clustered regularly interspaced short palindromic repeats (CRSIPR)[51] is a new genetic engineering technique for gene editing that allows for alteration of gene functions. CRISPR may also called CRISPR/Cas9. According to Lundberg & Novak,[52(p. 38)] "These easy and accessible methods are making DNA programmable in a way that is already having a profound impact on human, animal, and crop plant biology." CRISPR has the power to change the genetic makeup of a cell. It also has the power to change an entire ecosystem. However, the current focus of this technology has been on health care. CRISPR has the power to cure diseases caused by genetic disorders,[53] including diseases such as cancer, cystic fibrosis, anemia, and high cholesterol.

Seen as a major advancement, gene editing can now potentially alter multiple genes in one sitting, whereas only one gene at a time could be edited in the past. Scientists around the world are locked into "CRISPR race" to find gene edits to cure diseases. Still, due to the ethical aspect of gene editing (as it is unethical and prohibited to alter human DNA), all testing is currently being conducted on animals. Scientists experiment with regular mice, mate them with genetically altered mice, and then study the offspring. This allows the scientists to study gene alteration. Beyond the ethical issues, CRISPR does have other issues; for example, CRISPR is not 100% accurate. In different studies, it can vary from 50% to 80%

accuracy.[54] The Cas9 enzyme could possibly cut the wrong piece or part of a DNA strand. This would result in unintended mutations. Scientists have used CRISPR to "eliminate disease in animal model systems" and plan to pursue human germline editing.[55] There is a risk that altering one gene could affect others and causes unintended harm.

CRISPR presents unprecedented ethical concerns, that impact how humanity evolves. If a scientist edits an embryo or an adult gene, both affect future generations. If there is a mistake in the gene editing, it is also passed on to the future generations. There are concerns that eventually the appeal to stray away from therapeutics usage would be too great. Scientists and biotechnology companies would promote the use for human enhancement that could provide advantages in human intelligence and physical characteristics or improve resistance to biological pathogens. The idea of creating a designer baby that is disease resistant, attractive, and strong is a hot topic of discussion for ethicists. Unfortunately, the simplicity and affordability of CRISPR could also put it into the hands of people who wouldn't prioritize ethics, the environment, or public safety.[56] We have already been confronted with claims by a scientist that CRISPR has been used to edit the DNA of a baby in China to make the baby resistant to HIV.

Health Sensors[57]

A health sensor is any device that can monitor-record any health or wellness related information in real-time by capturing physiological, behavioral, or physical activities. The popularity and adoption of health sensors have risen over the years due to the availability of consumer products, such as FitBits and Apple watches. Indeed, these sensors come in many forms and shapes, including wearable devices (e.g., clothing, watches, bracelets), implanted devices (e.g., pacemakers), and ingestible sensors (e.g., the Proteous smart pill). In addition to physiological parameters, a health sensor

can also be fabricated to detect micro-electro-mechanical system (MEMS) motion sensors activity such as accelerometers and gyroscopes. Magnetic field sensors are widely used for measuring related activities.

Signals

This refers to the ability to combine different sensing capabilities with the analytical power of AI, thereby providing the capabilities to support continuous disease monitoring. The AI can provide advanced monitoring capabilities to provide real-time interpretation of physiological signals to support early diagnosis of diseases, such as cardiovascular, neurological, and pulmonary diseases, at their early onset.

Owing to the discovery of new materials, health sensors are becoming more advanced. These sensors comprise different types of flexible material capable of being integrated into various objects, such as textile fiber, clothes, and elastic bands or embedded into organs and tissue within the human body. Sensors can also be programmed to a variety of different physiological parameters, such as electrocardiogram (ECG), electromyogram (EMG), heart rate (HR), respiration rate (RR), body temperature, blood pressure (BP), electrodermal activity (EDA), and arterial oxygen saturation (SpO_2). More specifically, the continued advancement in battery, non-toxic material, and enhanced biosensing capabilities will be a key enabler for the next generation of advanced wearable and implantable sensors adopted as prognostic tools. These next generation sensors will have cutting-edge diagnostic capabilities that lead to more proactive diagnosis, such as being able to detect poisonous compounds in the air or dangerous pathogens in meals, or predicting allergic reactions from drugs or food before they occur, reducing incidences of serious illness before they happen. The ability to detect toxic pathogens and contagions is an expensive and time-consuming process that typically occurs after multiple people have fallen ill. Hence, early detection will prevent food-borne and environmental disease outbreaks.

One of the prominent technological advancements that will enable sensors to transform health care is that of nanosensors. Nanosensors are constructed from nanoparticles or nanostructured materials, such as carbon nanotubes. These miniaturized enzymatic sensors are ideal for health, environmental, and chemical analysis. Currently, use of nanosensors such as implantable devices is costly; also, their utility is limited due to the potential cytotoxic effects embedded in them. With new material advances, manufacturing approaches, and 3D printing capabilities, innovative approaches to investigate biocompatibility will soon become available. Overcoming the biocompatibility challenge will foster a new generation of health sensors that perform intelligent tasks, such as monitoring organs, wounds, or implants and the effects of drug.

All in all, the significance of health sensors for clinical applications is on the rise, and this trend is predicted to continue. Both the clinical staff and healthcare researchers now acknowledge the importance and potential benefits of these sensors. In the coming years, sensors will be responsible for innovations and scientific discoveries in the areas of point-of-care diagnostics, therapeutics, drug discovery, genomics, and PM. In fact, the increase in the adoption of sensors is already leading to the rapid improvements in advanced diagnostics, precision treatment, and continuous patient monitoring. The demand for consumer-based health sensors is increasing due to trends in personal wellness applications and digital health monitoring. Today's consumers are more health conscious with an educated interest in using medical grade health and fitness tools. The adoption of sophisticated multi-sensing health sensors will improve disease management and enhance the quality of health care delivered by hospitals. As such, the future health sensor market will provide real-time personalized advanced physiological monitoring that will reduce the need for hospitalization, resulting in lower healthcare costs and better quality of life for the patient.

▶ IV. Reinventing Healthcare Futures[58]

Many developed as well as developing countries across the globe are finding that healthcare expenditure is becoming or has become unsustainable due to globalization (i.e., sedentary lifestyles as a result of urbanization and economic development) and demographic reality (i.e., growth in aging populations). As such, policymakers and researchers alike believe two key factors will largely redefine our healthcare futures: continuous digital disruption in health care and health solutions that are economically sustainable.

The ultimate goal of an ideal healthcare system is to increase its accessibility, lower its delivery costs, and improve its quality, all within the framework of economic sustainability. Fortunately, digital health, as discussed throughout this revised text (e.g., PM, AI and social media, sensors and wearables, mobile health apps, telemedicine and tele homecare, 3D printing, and big healthcare data analytics), is paving a way to enable new modalities of healthcare delivery in the near future that is both transformative and more cost-effective.

Healthcare Innovations in Different Countries

The motivation to sustain healthcare costs across different countries is creating innovative approaches vis-à-vis the historical evolution and recent transformation of individual countries healthcare delivery systems. Access to health coverage in the United States, for example, has significantly improved with the ACA (Affordable Care Act), leading to the abandonment of traditional fee-for-service

(FFS) care delivery model toward a value-based (pay-for-performance) model.

Other developed countries, such as Canada and the United Kingdom, have attempted to improve the interoperability of health data systems, employing big healthcare data analytics to drive policies and decision-making to achieve more connected healthcare systems where duplicate testing and unnecessary medical services are eliminated through better gatekeeping by family physicians with faster, more well-coordinated and meaningful access to relevant and timely diagnostic and therapeutic data on their patients. Meanwhile, mobile health solutions are being implemented to improve accessibility across sparsely populated rural areas and remote regions in rapidly developing economies, such as India, China, and even Africa.

Health 2.0

Today, we are beginning to hear of news of major technological companies, such as Apple, Google, and Amazon, investing heavily into developing sustainable and transformative approaches for healthcare futures, apart from the traditional players and third-party funders, such as governments, major pharmaceuticals, regional hospitals and health systems delivery chains, health monitoring and medical devices companies, as well as large health insurance companies. The new landscape for healthcare futures is changing rapidly and will therefore involve multi-sectorial partnering, which can bring together varied skills and expertise from app development to big data analytics as well as customer engagement. It is believed that these megatrends will evolve over time to Health 2.0, a radically different model for the future healthcare delivery systems available anytime, anywhere.

On the one hand, patients will act as empowered consumers—they will be more informed and have more control over their health decisions rather than behaving as passive recipients of care, actively sharing their thoughts into their ongoing treatment processes. On the other hand, care providers will have access to more intelligent information via powerful analytics to focus on optimal preventive procedures, appropriate medication, and disease management. Other than the traditional ability to deliver health care in specific locations, patients will eventually have the option to access an increasing range of healthcare services delivered anywhere, anytime.

▶ V. Conclusion

To summarize, the emerging technology we have presented in this chapter promises even greater change. Here, we review some of the disruptive potential of these emerging technologies and their impact on healthcare futures.

- *BDA in health care*: Sensors employed in healthcare monitoring of patients will further add to the abundance of real-time, real-world data, requiring intelligent analysis and meaningful interpretations. As we have noted, BDA in health care have been applied to analyze social media and health records from EHRs, but the "gold mine" of sensor data remains largely untapped. Soon, the ability to integrate the information in the EHRs with round-the-clock sensor data on diet, fitness activity levels, and medication adherence of patients will be a sea change in comprehensively decoding the causes of various health problems in these patients.

- *3D Printing*: Bioprinting of human tissue, skin, and internal organs may sound futuristic; yet in some research facilities, it already is happening. In fact, such printed organs are often being considered as viable treatment alternatives as they can be generated from "the very cells of the body they will reenter."[59] In other words, these printed organs can be matched specifically to the size and exact requirements of the individual patient needing them. People are literally dying on a daily basis while waiting for the right donors with matching organs due to the longstanding shortage of organ donors across the globe. It is hoped that human bodies will not reject these printed organs when transplanted, with the entire process only taking a few hours.

- *AI, Robots, Sensors*: AI and robots can have a significant impact on future health if virtual doctors deployed via devices, such as our smart phones and smartwatches or as mechanical robots, can alert us to potential emergencies (e.g., an oncoming stroke or heart attack) before such events occur. Such decision aiding applications are fertile ground for AI complex machine-learning and pattern-recognition algorithms that will be able to diagnose and prescribe more intelligently than humans given the decreasing doctor-to-patient ratio worldwide. Moreover, physicians, empowered with augmented visualization through the use of 3D holographic scenarios, will be able to better diagnose patients while touching and interacting with objects in front of them. Professor Dian Tjondronegoro of Southern Cross University claimed:

Imagine in the future if healthcare professionals were able to look at a graphical summary of patients' physiological data and medical images being mapped and overlaid on top of the actual body parts using sensor and monitoring technology... They would be able to make better

decisions and more accurate diagnoses....The real future potential of AI will be to keep us healthy and well—not just monitor us when we are sick, particularly when coupled to genetic specific biology and pharmaceutical or robotic interventions.[60]

Put together, the key barriers facing the current healthcare systems so as to evolve seamlessly into Health 2.0 are fragmentation and slow adoption of disruptive innovations. Moreover, with a growing body of wide-ranging stakeholders (patients, care providers, funders, investors, and other players such as researchers and policymakers), realizing the vision of Health 2.0 becomes even more difficult. Not only do the barriers of fragmentation and slow adoption have to be overcome, but diverse perspectives, data, and innovative approaches also have to be integrated, ultimately creating a learning system of connected health care. This will never be easy, particularly in health care, with its limited interoperability of legacy systems and restricted data sharing capabilities as a result of longstanding regulations and expressed concerns over patients' rights to data confidentiality, privacy, and security. Digital health, with its rapid dissemination of large amounts of data, will make these noted challenges even more difficult and complex. It is now the job of our next generation health information systems analysts, informaticians, scientists, researchers, and all other stakeholders who have a stake in the success of healthcare futures, to work together in unison to achieve Health 2.0.

Notes

1. Retrieved from www.luminary-labs.com/using-voice-technology-power-engaging-digital-health-experiences/
2. Retrieved from www.prweb.com/releases/orbita_takes_steps_to_drive_innovation_in_conversational_ai_and_voice_technology_solutions_for_health_care/prweb15854439.htm
3. Consoli, D., & Mina, A. (2009). An evolutionary perspective on health innovation systems. *Journal of Evolutionary Economics, 19*, 297. doi:10.1007/s00191-008-0127-3
4. Hwang, J., & Christensen, C. M. (2008, September/October). Disruptive innovation in health care delivery: A framework for business-model innovation. *Health Affairs, 27*(5), 1329–1335. Retrieved from www.healthaffairs.org/doi/10.1377/hlthaff.27.5.1329
5. Akenroye, T. O. (2012). Factors influencing innovation in healthcare: A conceptual synthesis. *The Innovation*

Journal: *The Public Sector Innovation Journal*,
17(2), article 3. Retrieved from www.innovation.cc
/scholarly-style/2012_17_2_3_akenroye_innovate
_healthcare.pdf

6. Shihao, Y., Santillana, M., & Kou, S. C. (2015, May).
ARGO: A model for accurate estimation of influenza
epidemics using Google search data. *Proceedings of the
National Academy of Sciences, 112*(47), 14473–14478.
doi:10.1073/pnas.1515373112

7. Canadian Foundation for Health Improvement:
What Is Value-Based Healthcare (VBHC). Retrieved
from www.cfhi-fcass.ca/WhatWeDo/health-system
-transformation/value-based-healthcare

8. Bradbury, D. (2017, April 24). Getting ready for
GDPR. *Canadian Lawyer*. Retrieved from www
.canadianlawyermag.com/article/getting-ready
-for-gdpr-3607/

9. Nakamoto, S. (2008). Bitcoin: A peer-to-peer
electronic cash system. White Paper from Satoshi
Nakamoto Institute. Retrieved from https://bitcoin
.org/bitcoin.pdf

10. *Ibid.*

11. Adler-Milstein, J., Bates, D. W., & Jha, A. K. (2009). U.S.
regional health information organizations: Progress &
challenges. *Health Affairs (Millwood), 28*(2), 483–492.
doi:10.1377/hlthaff.28.2.483. Retrieved from www
.ncbi.nlm.nih.gov/pubmed/19276008

12. Fedak, V. (2018). *Blockchain and Big Data: The
match made in heavens*. Retrieved from https://
towardsdatascience.com/blockchain-and-big-data
-the-match-made-in-heavens-337887a0ce73

13. Gross, B. C., Erkal, J. L., Lockwood, S. Y., Chen, C.,
& Spence, D. M. (2014, March 20). Evaluation of 3D
printing and its potential impact on biotechnology
and the chemical sciences. *Analytical Chemistry,
86*(7), 3240–3253.

14. Palo, M., Holländer, J., Suominen, J., Yliruusi, J.,
& Sandler, N. (2017, September 2). 3D printed
drug delivery devices: Perspectives and technical
challenges. *Expert Review of Medical Devices, 14*(9),
685–696.

15. Ventola, C. L. (2014, January 1). Medical applications
for 3D printing: Current and projected uses. *P & T:
A Peer-Reviewed Journal for Formulary Management,
39*(10), 704–711.

16. Gross et al., (2014), *ibid.*

17. Norman, J., Madurawe, R. D., Moore, C. M. V., Khan,
M. A., & Khairuzzaman, A. (2017, January 1). A new
chapter in pharmaceutical manufacturing: 3D-printed
drug products. *Advanced Drug Delivery Reviews, 108*,
39–50.

18. *Ibid.*

19. Alhnan, M. A., Okwuosa, T. C., Sadia, M., Wan,
K.-W., Ahmed, W., & Arafat, B. (2016, August 18).
Emergence of 3D printed dosage forms: Opportunities

and challenges. *Pharmaceutical Research, 33*(8),
1817–1832.

20. Zeltmann, S. E., Gupta, N., Tsoutsos, N. G.,
Maniatakos, M., Rajendran, J., & Karri, R. (2016,
January 1). Manufacturing and security challenges in
3D printing. *Jom Warrendale, 68*(7), 1872–1881.

21. FDA. (2016, May 10). *Draft guidance for industry
and food and drug administration staff: Technical
considerations for additive manufactured devices*.
Gross, B. C. Retrieved from www.fda.gov/media
/97633/download

22. Markarian, J. (2016, January 1). Using 3D printing for
solid-dosage drugs. *Pharmaceutical Technology, 40*(8),
34–36.

23. *Ibid.*

24. Oyewumi, O. M. (2015, January 1). 3D printing
technology in pharmaceutical drug delivery:
Prospects and challenges. *Journal of Biomolecular
Research & Therapeutics, 4*, 4.

25. The Medical Futurist. (2016). *AI will redesign
healthcare*. Retrieved from https://medicalfuturist.
com/artificial-intelligence-will-redesign-healthcare

26. Al-Shamasneh, A., & Obaidellah, U. (2017, February).
Artificial intelligence techniques for cancer detection
and classification: Review study. *European Scientific
Journal, 13*(3), 1857–7881. doi:10.19044/esj.2016
.v13n3p342

27. Median Blogs. (2018, March 14). *Industry trends:
AI revolutionizes imaging analysis*. Retrieved from
http://mediantechnologies.com/industry-trends
-ai-revolutionizes-imaging-analysis/

28. Akgül, C. B., Rubin, D. L., Napel, S., Beaulieu, C. F.,
Greenspan, H., & Acar, B. (2011). Content-based
image retrieval in radiology: Current status and
future directions. *Journal of Digital Imaging, 24*(2),
208–222.

29. Ho, C., Tsakonas, E., Tran, K., Cimon, K., Severn,
M., Mierzwinski-Urban, M., … Pautler, S. (2012).
Robot-assisted surgery compared with open surgery
and laparoscopic surgery. *CADTH Technology
Overview, 2*(2), e2203. Retrieved from www.ncbi.nlm
.nih.gov/pmc/articles/PMC3442615/

30. Solomon, M. (2018, October 24). *Beyond the
hype: Real applications of artificial intelligence
in medication management*. Retrieved from
www.pocp.com/real-applications-artificial
-intelligence-in-medication-management/

31. Chatterjee, A. (2017, July 17). *Use of artificial
intelligence to reduce medical errors*. Retrived from
http://blog.myhealthvectors.com/index.php/tag
/reduced-errors/

32. Esteva, A., Kuprel, B., Novoa, R. A., Ko, J., Swetter, S.
M., Blau, H. M., & Thrun, S. (2017). Dermatologist-
level classification of skin cancer with deep neural
networks. *Nature, 542*, 115–118.

33. Kalis, B., Collier, M., & Fu, R. (2018). 10 promising AI applications in health care. *HBR*. Retrieved from https://hbr.org/2018/05/10-promising-ai-applications-in-health-care

34. D'Mello, Y. (2018, May). *How virtual nurses are elevating patient care*. Retrieved from https://aithority.com/robots/automation/how-virtual-nurses-are-elevating-patient-care/

35. Cost of a Data Breach Study: Essential report on today's security landscape. *IBM Security Report*. Retrieved from https://www.ibm.com/security/data-breach

36. *Ibid.*

37. Joudaki, H., Rashidian, A., Minaei-Bidgoli, B., Mahmoodi, M., Geraili, B., Nasiri, M., & Arab, M. (2015). Using data mining to detect health care fraud and abuse: A review of literature. *Global Journal of Health Science, 7*(1), 194–202. doi:10.5539/gjhs.v7n1p19

38. Tan, J., & Wang, J. (2017). Non-traditional data mining applications in Taiwan National Health Insurance (NHI) databases: A Hybrid Mining (HM) case for the framing of NHI decisions. *IJHISI, 12*(4), 31–51.

39. Joudaki et al., (2015), *ibid.*

40. MarketWatch. (2005, February 3). *Robots as surgical enablers*. Retrieved from www.marketwatch.com/story/a-fascinating-visit-to-a-high-tech-operating-room?dist=msr_2

41. Peters, B. S., Armijo, P. R., Krause, C., Choudhury, S. A., & Oleynikov, D. (2018). Review of emerging surgical robotic technology. *Surgical Endoscopy, 32*(4), 1636–1655. doi:10.1007/s00464-018-6079-2

42. Owano, N. (2013, January 25). FDA gives green light to RP-VITA hospital robot. *Phys.org*. Retrieved from https://phys.org/news/2013-01-fda-green-rp-vita-hospital-robot.html#jCp

43. Dr. Hempal Digital Health Network. (2018, July 9). *Helping people walk with exoskeletons: The growth of wearable robots in healthcare*. Retrieved from https://www.dr-hempel-network.com/digital-health-technolgy/wearable-robots-in-healthcare/

44. Miura, K., Kadone, H., Koda, M., Abe, T., Endo, H., Murakami, H., … Yamazaki M. (2018). The hybrid assisted limb (HAL) for care support, a motion assisting robot providing exoskeletal lumbar support, can potentially reduce lumbar load in repetitive snow-shoveling movements. *Journal of Clinical Neuroscience, 49*, 83–86. doi:10.1016/j.jocn.2017.11.020. Retrieved from www.ncbi.nlm.nih.gov/pubmed/29254733

45. Innovation Meets Neuro-rehabilitation. (video, n.d.). Retrieved from https://eksobionics.com/eksohealth/

46. Researchers Confront an Epidemic of Loneliness. (2016, September 7). *The New York Times in Education*. Retrieved from https://nytimesineducation.com/researchers-confront-an-epidemic-of-loneliness/

47. The Medical Futurist. (2018, July 31). *The top 12 social companion robots*. Retrieved from https://medicalfuturist.com/the-top-12-social-companion-robots

48. Paro: Therapeutic Robot. (n.d.). Retrieved from www.parorobots.com/

49. Smith, A. (n.d.). *DNA: Form, function, and ethics*. Retrieved from www.stgabrielcarlisle.org/dna-form-function-ethics/

50. Loewe, L. (2008). Genetic mutation. *Nature Education, 1*(1), 113. Retrieved from www.nature.com/scitable/topicpage/genetic-mutation-1127

51. CRISPR/Cas9, *Gene Editing Tool by ORIGENE*. (n.d.). Retrieved from www.origene.com/products/gene-expression/crispr-cas9?gclid=Cj0KCQiA-c_iBRChARIsAGCOpB0qaUbcCHywabEB31KLeYPoLo_bPKL2jbsXiYa0laoAJhXAoJOMKxwaAomnEALw_wcB

52. Lundberg, A. S., & Novak, R. (2015). CRISPR-Cas gene editing to cure serious diseases: Treat the patient, not the germ line. *American Journal of Bioethics, 15*(12), 38–40. doi:10.1080/15265161.2015.1103817

53. Vidyasagar, A. (2018, April 20). What is CRISPR? *Live Science*. Retrieved from www.livescience.com/58790-crispr-explained.html

54. Evitt, N. H., Mascharak, S., & Altman, R. B. (2015). Human germline CRISPR-Cas modification: Toward a regulatory framework. *American Journal of Bioethics, 15*(12), 25–29.

55. *Ibid.*

56. Lefferts, J. A. (2016, February). CRISPR: Changing the way we modify DNA. *Clinical Chemistry*. doi:10.1373/clinchem.2015.246983. Retrieved from http://clinchem.aaccjnls.org/content/62/3/536

57. The Medical Futurist. (2018, September 6). *The body map of digital health sensors*. Retrieved from https://medicalfuturist.com/the-body-map-of-digital-health-sensors

58. *EY-Building a better working world. (n.d.). With growing health needs, is digital the best medicine?* Retrieved from www.ey.com/gl/en/issues/business-environment/ey-megatrends-health-reimagined

59. Wnuk, P. (2018, July 9). Bio-printing organs and the future of healthcare. *Pharmaphorum*. Retrieved from https://pharmaphorum.com/views-and-analysis/bioprinting-organs-and-the-future-of-healthcare/

60. Bedo, S. (2018, October 24). What the future of healthcare will look like with artificial intelligence. *News.com.au*. Retrieved from www.news.com.au/lifestyle/health/health-problems/what-the-future-of-healthcare-will-look-like-with-artificial-intelligence/news-story/6927dd8a81c77dcb03a94f352ebe91cc

Chapter Questions

15-1 What are examples of "emerging technology in health care" today?

15-2 How do you see big healthcare data analytics developments impacting the future of health care?

15-3 Why is 3D printing unique for future patient survival?

15-4 Provide some case examples of AI, robots, and sensors in health care.

15-5 How do you think the futures of health care would be sustainable economically with the rapid adoption of disruptive technologies when the process of innovation is never easy nor cheap?

Biography

Dr. Rajib Biswas received his MSc degree in Physics from Dibrugarh University, India, and received his PhD from North East Institute of Science & Technology, India. Since 2010, he has been serving as a faculty member in Department of Physics, Tezpur University, India. He has been editorial board member of several peer reviewed journals. His current research interests are Optoelectronics, Fiber-Optics and Instrumentation, Nano materials, Heavy metal ion detection, Contamination, Big data analytics, etc.

MINI-CASE (PART IV)

The Leadership of Future Health

Joseph Tan with Joshia Tan

▶ The Leadership of Future Health[1]

Introduction

In recent conversations telescoping on future health, the notion of health and wellbeing becoming a central societal concern appears to come from a major and profound cultural shift; that is, there is a paradigm of adopting innovative programming for bringing up children while changing their lifestyle and behaviors, impacting the health and wellbeing of next generation of the human race. A profound example to demonstrate the concept of health and wellbeing encompassing nutrition, housing, and education is the Harlem Children's Zone.

Here, the smart community-dwelling concept is to stimulate access to locally grown, affordable, healthy food via a breakthrough community strategy; that is, the implementation of an open-source platforms, such as CreativeCommons.org, to allow the visualization of social problems and community-based solutions amalgamated by converging resources in community neighborhoods to achieve the "healthy people, healthy places" vision. In this sense, the communities, including even the poorer neighborhoods, will soon have access to healthier food sources while shifting consciously towards adopting healthier lifestyle changes.

Vision of 2032

Illustratively, by 2032, it is argued that advances in emerging technologies will empower social connectivity among willing members of these communities to draw on resources needed to transform investments at the local level. Essentially, it provides a starting point for healthier lifestyle behavioral changes as well as reorienting entertainment and other services towards healthy lifestyle enhancement. Such ideas will in turn encourage major support from well-endowed nonprofit charitable organizations, such as the Bill & Melinda Gates foundation, and all participating citizens with the commitment and mandate to improve health from the cradle to the grave. Likewise, the new education system will be redesigned to produce a workforce primed to work smarter while living a healthier work-life balance.

Soon, a health-social equity correlation will highlight the success of such health-oriented trending communities; additional success will be realized via the application of powerful analytics software resolving complex problems by feeding massive data on where best to deploy limited community resources and assets. The discoveries of hidden knowledge and new insights will also propagate and diffuse through the sharing of innovative thinking so that idle community resources may be more effectively, efficiently, and productively deployed towards galvanizing a broad-based commitment in achieving a more equitable and healthy society.

Healthy People 2020, 2030 Initiatives

Initiatives such as Healthy People 2020 and 2030 will increasingly shape the common dialogues among the millennials, academics, and trained healthcare professionals to highlight the central role of societal health and well-being. By drawing on big data analytics, and with input from individual health records, environmental, and national statistical data, it is purported that such examination will offer complex solutions for transforming ways to better deliver care for all people, especially the elderly as well as the disabled. Indeed, such an orientation with properly channeled leadership will undoubtedly provide a means towards achieving more responsible fiscal management, economic vitality, greater

national security, and privacy for human rights so people can live healthier, safer lives and stay healthy.

At the individual level, big data will drive personal health agendas, facilitate self-care management, especially for those who may have to deal with chronic diseases, and offer the potential of personalized medicine and therapies in order to restore these individuals back to a healthy state. Similarly, the individual big data clouds could eventually be aggregated so as to feed into the generation of community health status reports for evaluating the differing health statuses across participating communities.

▶ Conclusion

Imagine that you have been chosen to head and champion a community program with participants from various Detroit neighborhoods who want to be part of the Healthy 2030 initiative, with the vision of moving towards a healthier society, as previously envisioned. How would you go about attracting buy-ins from community members, leaders, academics, and businesses in the greater Detroit area to work together towards the aforementioned scenario? What types of digital or physical assets, big data applications, and other resources such as IoT (Internet of Things)-assistive devices like community Robots you believe may be shared in smart communities to empower all participating individuals, including community leaders, with insights towards achieving the vision of "healthy people, healthy places" throughout the greater Detroit area?

Note

1. Tsouros, A. (2013, October) City leadership for health and well-being: Back to the future. *Journal of Urban Health, 90*(Suppl 1), 4–13. Published online August 30, 2013. doi:10.1007/s11524-013-9825-8. Retrieved from www.ncbi.nlm.nih.gov/pmc/articles /PMC3764264/

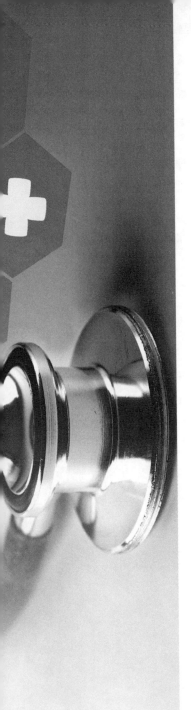

PART V

HMIS Practices and Cases

CASE 1

Digital Health Technology Commercialization Strategies

Greg Moon and Phillip Olla

▶ Digital Health

Digital health (d-health) relates to the convergence of digital technologies with wellness, health care, or lifestyle modifications to improve the efficiency of the healthcare system. D-health utilizes information and digital communication technologies to alleviate the health challenges faced by institutions and consumers. D-health encompasses hardware, software, and services to bring about the transformation.[1] Hardware components include items such as wearables, tablets, robots, gaming consoles, sensors, and glasses. Software solutions include applications, artificial intelligence (AI) bots, and programs that run on the healthcare infrastructure. D-health services include components such as telemedicine, integrated communication, image archiving services, and remote monitoring services.[2,3] The unique feature of D-health is the use of these three components to create an interconnected health system.

D-health involves stakeholders from different disciplines, including biomedical engineers, clinicians, public health experts, epidemiologists, entrepreneurs, and technology innovators, with a wide range of expertise.

▶ Categories of Global D-Health Solutions

The World Health Organization (WHO) has recently classified d-health solutions, based on how the digital and mobile approaches are being used to support health system needs and which stakeholders receive the benefits. Specifically, the categories are:

- Interventions for healthcare "clients"
- Interventions for healthcare providers
- Interventions for health system or resource managers
- Interventions for data services

- *Interventions for clients*: Clients are the patients or members of the public who use the d-health technology to manage a health condition. Solutions could be used for education, diagnosis, treatment, or communication. Solutions, which are incorporated into digital data servicing

1	2	3	4
Interventions for clients	Interventions for healthcare providers	Interventions for health system or resource managers	Interventions for data services

for users, may be targeted as apps and/or platforms provided by caregivers to patients.

- *Interventions for healthcare providers*: This grouping contains d-health solutions created for healthcare workers, including doctors, nurses, and the general healthcare workforce.
- *Health system and resource managers*: These applications are created to support administrative functions and to manage the operations of health systems. Some of the solutions in this category include supply chain management (SCM), financing, and human resource management.
- *Interventions for data services*: This category consists of applications that enable a wide range of activities related to data collection, data analytics, clinical systems, and data use and exchanges.

▶ Categories for Commercial D-Health Systems

In addition to the aforementioned WHO categories, it is helpful to delineate d-health solutions based on how they are being commercialized. From this perspective, d-health includes mobile health (m-health),[4] health information technology (IT), genomics, wearable devices, AI, telehealth and telemedicine, as well as personalized medicine. There are now research findings that suggest that d-health can provide the following benefits:

- Reduce inefficiencies
- Improve access
- Reduce costs
- Increase quality
- Make medicine more personalized for patients

Both patients and consumers are now using d-health to manage health conditions and track health and wellness related behaviors. D-health incorporates the use of technologies, such as smartphones, social networks, and Internet applications, essentially creating innovative approaches to monitor health and gain access to health information at the right time and have it be presented in the right context. Together, these advancements are leading to a convergence of people, information, technology, and connectivity to improve health care and health outcomes.

The United States Food and Drug Administration (FDA) is now proactively focusing on d-health. Under the FDA's Center for Devices and Radiological Health, their role has expanded as the medical devices now have connectivity, AI algorithms, and additional digital features. The FDA provides guidance and clarity in the following areas in the d-health field to ensure the benefits are balanced with the potential risks[5]:

- Wireless medical devices
- Mobile medical apps
- Health IT

- Telemedicine
- Medical device data systems
- Medical device interoperability
- Software as a Medical Device (SaMD)
- General wellness
- Cybersecurity

▶ Commercialization Strategies

Despite the challenging d-health marketplace, several strategies for commercialization have proven to be effective. Three primary commercialization strategies have emerged:

- Strategy 1. Continued focus on health systems—with more intelligent sales approaches
- Strategy 2. Go around the health systems—target alternative customers
- Strategy 3. Co-opt the health systems—become a vertically integrated care provider

Strategy 1. Continued Focus on Health Systems—With More Intelligent Sales Approaches

Far from mysterious, this strategy relies on standard good business practice: (a) create offerings that customers want to buy; (b) be well prepared for the commercialization stage; and (c) make it hard for these risk-averse customers to say no. While this may sound overly simplistic, a surprising number of d-health companies neglect these fundamentals.

Create Offerings that Customers Want to Buy

The most critical early objective is to understand the target customers' specific business and clinical needs in order to inform product development and downstream marketing efforts. One best way to achieve such an understanding is to gather insights from primary sources and to engage these sources in a collaborative process of product definition. The effort may range from simple interviews, at minimum, to more sophisticated ethnographic techniques and user-centered design (UCD), budget, and resources permitting. The stakeholders providing insights should be those who directly influence future purchasing decisions as their opinions are the most critical for defining a salable product. Such stakeholders generally come from two camps: (i) those accountable for care delivery and clinical outcomes and (ii) those accountable for the organization's business success.

For the care delivery stakeholders, if a potential solution envisioned for use in the outpatient setting exists, the primary stakeholder is generally the doctor; if the inpatient setting is targeted, the nurse or case manager is likely the primary stakeholder. The discussions should focus on significantly unmet clinical needs and operational pain points. If a product or service is already envisioned, it should be put forth for consideration, with the goal of open feedback; this feedback is then used to drive the development of a revised product description (for reconsideration by the stakeholders). Simply put, the process should be iterative, using the hypothesis-testing paradigm that is at the heart of both UCD and the lean startup techniques espoused by Eric Ries[6]—techniques already familiar to most software-oriented companies. In contrast, for the business stakeholders, the exploration should ideally be informed by real, quantitative data, if and where possible. Obtaining such data from potential customers at this early stage is not often possible, but as IBM's Turner explains, "Getting your hands on utilization and outcomes data is like gold. Not only does it help you to model the business case, it involves the customer as a co-creator from the outset. How are they going to say no to an offering that they helped create?"[7] The main takeaway is that ascertainment of specific customer needs is essential *before* significant expenditure of developmental resources.

One helpful "hack" can allow a company to leapfrog far ahead in the product definition process, but it applies to a relatively narrow set of offerings. Namely, it involves digitally enabling clinical protocols that are widely known to provide better outcomes or decrease costs. Omada Health impressively executed such an approach during the early stages of its business. Omada's first offering was a mobile-centric, digital version of the lifestyle intervention used in the Diabetes Prevention Protocol (DPP).[8] Strong evidence supported the effectiveness of the DPP to reduce weight and prevent or delay the onset of Type 2 diabetes in at-risk individuals—so much so that the U.S. Preventive Services Task Force[9] called it out as an exemplar of a strong behavioral health intervention. However, it is known to be very resource intensive, with multiple in-person coaching, education, and exercise sessions. Omada Health's Founder and CEO, Sean Duffy, explains: "[Directly leveraging the DPP] made those first sales so much easier since providers and health systems had already embraced the intervention but were also concerned about the resources required. We didn't need our own data at first, since the customers already assumed a digitized version of the DPP would work."[10]

Be Well Prepared for Stage Commercialization

Appropriate preparation requires sufficient time, money, and, more than anything, great diligence. The main areas of preparation are the development of technical and process solutions (to facilitate integration) and stage-appropriate evidence (to facilitate the sale). Regarding the former, Omada's Duffy advises, "When you want to commercialize, you need to be 'enterprise ready.' In addition to having reliable technology and support systems, you need to have built in all the things the customer's IT team requires, like SOC 2 and HL7

compliance, etc. That takes upfront work, but it pays off."[11]

As for clinical evidence, there is wide agreement among leaders of successful d-health companies that the more high-value proof points that a company has, the better. Ginger.io's Singh recommends taking a stage-appropriate approach: "When you are starting out, you might go for more accessible endpoints, like engagement and satisfaction. While low hanging fruit, these data help conversations with customers. As your company matures, target the more substantial endpoints, like clinical outcomes and cost savings." He also adds a very practical tip: "Remember, you're generating tons of data with your customer populations. If you, very appropriately, conduct data analysis under the umbrella of quality improvement, you have an evidence generating machine."[12] Pear Therapeutics, pioneers of "digital therapeutics," has taken evidence generation to a logical, effective extreme. Digital therapeutics involves the use of innovative, clinically-validated disease management and direct treatment applications to enhance, and in some cases, replace, current medical practices and treatments[13]; it is important to note that a companion medication may or may not be part of the offering. As Pear's Vice President of Corporate Development, Antoun Nabhan explains, "We want digital therapeutics to look as much like pharmaceuticals as possible to the purchaser. What gives pharmaceuticals their value?—the volumes of clinical evidence. We get our apps approved with pharmaceutical-level effectiveness data, and then sell them based upon the power of that evidence."

Make It Hard for These Risk-Averse Customers to Say No

The path of least resistance for a health system decision maker is to say no to innovation, for all the reasons described previously. Savvy digital health companies therefore reduce perceived risk in the sales process. "The simplest thing we did was to avoid calling ourselves a 'start up.' We were always a 'digital health company focused on reducing the impact of chronic conditions,'" says Omada's Duffy.[14] Another key tactic is to leverage an internal or external champion, trusted by the customer organization, to help make the sale. A frequently employed method is to focus first and foremost on developing an enthusiastic clinical champion. Leaders at Omada, Ginger.io, and Pear all spoke of the power of a physician evangelist to shape purchasing decisions. Pear's Nabhan describes as follows: "We use our clinical data to convince the physician of a product's value. He or she then does the internal advocacy to get it on formulary."[15] Regarding trusted external parties, professional societies and key opinion leaders can be valuable allies. As IBM's Turner explains, "Health systems don't trust '.coms,' but they do trust '.orgs.'"[16]

A d-health company can also use innovative financial arrangements to reduce both perceived and real risk. Outcomes-based contracting (OBC) originally emerged in the pharmaceutical industry to manage concerns around rising drug costs, in particular specialty pharmaceuticals. OBCs are risk-sharing arrangements between medical product manufacturers and payers in which the performance of the product is tracked in a defined patient population over a specified period of time and the level of reimbursement is tied by formula to the outcome.[17] These arrangements can be temporary, as part of an initial evaluation period, or ongoing. They also do not need to be all-or-nothing and can instead be part of a hybrid scheme, in which there is a baseline payment combined with upside payments when outcomes are met. Additionally, outcomes targets can be population- or individual patient-based. Regardless of the particular structure, OBCs can significantly reduce barriers to implementing a relatively untested (or very expensive) innovation as payment is directly tied to value; they also create explicit alignment around the goals of the implementation. One caution is that they should only

be entered into if the innovator company has a fairly clear estimation of projected outcomes, usually achieved through preceding clinical studies.

D-health companies have started to embrace these arrangements, too. Proteus Digital Health is once such company. "The particular clinical scenario determines the appropriate outcome target, which in our case can be behavioral or clinical," says George Savage, Proteus' Co-founder and Chief Medical Officer (CMO). "For instance, some of our contracts focus on a threshold level of adherence, which is measured by our digital medicine's platform, and total payment is contingent upon hitting that threshold."[18] Omada Health also uses such contracts. "We get paid for engagement, based upon uptake of the Omada solution by users," explains Omada's Duffy. "We also get paid a higher amount if sustained weight loss is achieved." Given the overall healthcare industry's shift to value-based payment (VBP) models, it is anticipated that OBCs—which are very aligned with VBP—will continue to proliferate in d-health.

It should be noted that all of the Strategy 1 approaches discussed simply represent good business practices. As such, they are recommended for *all* d-health ventures, including companies that follow the two alternative strategies, described next.

Strategy 2. Go Around the Health Systems—Target Alternative Customers

- Given the challenge of selling to health systems, many d-health companies have elected to address other healthcare stakeholders as their primary customers. To that end, d-health offerings have proliferated for a range of alternative customers, including health and wellness consumers, employers, pharmaceutical companies, and traditional payers.

Business to Consumer (B2C)

Consumer-targeted d-health products focus on applications with a non-medical intended use, such as fitness and physical and mental well-being. Some of these offerings have a device component, like Fitbit (wearable devices) and Peloton (exercise bikes plus subscription), and hardware sales constitute a major portion of revenue. There are also myriad software-based d-health solutions for a variety of non-medical purposes, including diet and weight loss, work-outs, medication management, fertility, and stress management.

The consumer segment can seem quite attractive due to minimal regulatory burden; for example, prescriptions are not necessary and the potential for rapid scalability exists. Unfortunately, the space has become crowded, resulting in few standouts while customer acquisition costs can be prohibitive. These conditions may explain why, according to a recent Rock Health report, only a small minority (14%) of d-health companies employs the consumer-pay model. Furthermore, 61% of those companies who start with a B2C model moved to another model [B2B (business-to-business) or B2B2C (business-to-business-to-consumer)].[19]

Self-Insured Employers (SIEs)

Eighty percent of U.S. companies with greater than 500 employees and thirty percent of those with 100–500 employees are self-insured.[20] Self-insurance means that a company assumes 100% liability for the cost of health care for their employees. The C-suite tends to be acutely aware of the total cost of care, since this substantial line item directly affects a company's profitability. It is therefore no surprise that SIEs are quite motivated to reduce their healthcare costs. This motivation represents significant opportunity for d-health companies.

SIEs have the reputation for a readiness to experiment with innovative healthcare solutions, even if validation is limited. Jeff, a healthcare and benefits strategist at a Fortune 50 company, captures the situation well. "Large employers do not have the luxury to wait for perfect validation. If we see a solution related to our focus areas that could plausibly provide benefit, we often go with our gut to get the ball rolling."[21] Bill Ihrie, former Senior Vice President of benefits and health care at Lowe's, similarly describes an iterative built-test-learn process for engaging with innovator companies. "You could wait around forever for definitive evidence before implementation. At Lowe's, we did the opposite. If something seemed promising, we would roll it out among 20,000–30,000 people, gather data, and look at outcomes like engagement, biometric endpoints, and ROI. If trends looked positive, we would scale it to our entire workforce and continue our analysis with subsequent data." On a cautionary note for innovator companies, though, he adds, "Of course, in return for our willingness to experiment, the companies must be open to doing things 'the Lowe's way' and be flexible with their business models."[22] For instance, Lowe's avoids payment on a per-member, per-period basis for d-health solutions, instead paying based on engagement or outcomes, as is the case for the company's engagement with Omada.

In an effort to reduce costs, SIEs have adopted d-health offerings that address both the demand and supply sides of their benefit programs. On the demand side, the goal is to eliminate unnecessary resource utilization. Healthcare navigator applications have been a mainstay in this arena, enabling more informed decision-making by employee-healthcare consumers. For instance, Castlight combines virtual and human assistants—fueled by large datasets of benefit plan details, service costs, and provider quality ratings—to help employees choose higher-quality, lower-cost options when they are seeking care. Such a service benefits both the employer and the employee, who is increasingly enrolled in a high-deductible health plan. Collective Health also helps employees navigate the healthcare experience. More so than Castlight, though, the company's platform facilitates employer operations related to self-insurance, with tools to integrate various benefit programs, streamline financial operations, and analyze population health and utilization.

On the supply side, employers are seeking d-health solutions that prevent, delay, or better manage conditions known to be major company cost drivers. Although the mix varies by industry and company, diabetes, cardiovascular disease, depression, and musculoskeletal disorders typically generate the highest expenses for employers; these expenses result from a combination of direct medical expenditures, absenteeism, and presenteeism.[23] It is therefore not a surprise that many employer-oriented d-health solutions address these conditions, as part of wellness and population health programs (for prevention and identification) or as tools for the management of existing conditions. Some standouts include Omada and Livongo (diabetes), Ginger.io, Lyra, Headspace (mental health and wellness), and Hinge Health (musculoskeletal). Currently, no d-health products exist that have been widely adopted by employers to help manage *established* cardiovascular disease, but many offerings exist to address modifiable cardiovascular risk factors, especially obesity and inactivity (e.g., Fitbit and Omada).

Unifying these offerings is that they all directly address SIE's economic pain points, which echoes the earlier premise that d-health companies must, first and foremost, understand their target customers' business needs.

Traditional Payers

While health insurance companies may, at first blush, appear to be promising target customers for d-health companies, they can be inaccessible in reality. As traditional payers control massive amounts of healthcare information and have the capital to invest in large technology and data science teams, they have an incomparable capacity for analytics-based data arbitrage. As a result, they generally create in-house d-health solutions and supporting services, rather than source them from third parties. The archetypal 800-lb gorilla in this regard is UnitedHealthcare, or more specifically, its Optum division. Optum has enormous reach, using technology to power a wide range of services, including health economics-related data analytics, pharmacy management, population health management, healthcare delivery, and healthcare operational management. With this multi-faceted portfolio, the company caters to essentially every healthcare stakeholder, including consumers, providers, employers, health plans, government, and life sciences companies.

Even so, traditional payer-related opportunities still exist for d-health innovator companies. First, traditional payers appear loath to internalize the development of hardware devices, such as wearables and other sensors, and continue to purchase or partner to access devices and the resulting biometric data. For instance, UnitedHealth's Motion program leverages wearables from Garmin, Samsung, Fitbit, and Striiv, which the company purchases from these vendors.[24] Additionally, payers are beginning to deploy capital for d-health investments. UnitedHealthcare established Optum Ventures in late 2017, a $250 million fund dedicated to d-health.[25] Extrapolating, it is reasonable to assume that UnitedHealthcare and other traditional payers will pursue a mergers and acquisitions (M&A) strategy related to promising d-health technology, so these entities may increasingly present exit opportunities for smaller d-health companies.

Pharmaceutical Companies

The traditional pharma business model—sell as many pills, at the highest price, for as long as possible—is widely expected to disappear. As drug prices soar, healthcare reimbursement is moving toward value-based payment

(VBP), for which quality, patient satisfaction, outcomes, and costs are coming sharply into focus. Hence, pharma and biotech companies are actively pursuing alternative business models that leverage data, patient engagement, and services—a dynamic for which d-health solutions are extremely well-suited.

Some compelling examples of pharmaceutical-digital health partnerships can be cited. When Otsuka's flagship antipsychotic medication Abilify—at one point the top selling drug in the United States[26]—was hitting its "patent cliff" (i.e., when patent protection, and hence premium pricing, end), they partnered with Proteus Digital Health to create the world's first digital drug. The resulting product system comprised medications with an embedded ingestion sensor, a wearable patch, a smartphone app for patients, and web-based portals for providers and caregivers. Approved in late 2017, the product was commercially released in 2018, priced significantly above generic levels.[27] Another example is the Boehringer Ingelheim-Propeller Health partnership around asthma and chronic obstructive pulmonary disease. Boehringer Ingelheim produces respiratory medications for use with an inhaler whereas Propeller's d-health platform uses a combination of inhaler sensors, apps, analytics, personal feedback, and education. Results from a recent $n = 497$ patient study demonstrated a 78% reduction in use of a rescue inhaler and a 48% increase in symptom-free days.[28] A lighter-touch integration is Takeda's partnership with Cognition Kit around depression. This collaboration combines the use of antidepressant medications and an Apple Watch-based app that captures daily self-reported patient mood and measurements of cognitive function. "This initiative is an excellent example of the pilot work being done at Takeda to build a body of evidence for new ways of measuring outcomes in mental health," says Nicole Mowad-Nasser, Vice President of External Partnerships at Takeda.[29] Despite these success stories, however, a digital revolution in the pharmaceutical industry will

likely not happen overnight, due to a cultural mismatch between d-health companies and pharmaceutical companies. Says Pete Masloski, a principal at ZS Associates, a global technology marketing firm, "One of the challenges is that [d-health] is a different world than pharma. The world of Silicon Valley, high-tech apps, and consumers is a very different world. It moves at 1000 miles an hour compared to healthcare. It's a different culture."[30]

In summary, other than health systems, d-health companies may also effectively target a variety of other customers.

Strategy 3. Co-Opt the Health Systems—Become a Vertically Integrated Care Provider

Recall that in the early days of commercialization, Gingio.io senior management discovered a flaw in their initial model that was outside of their control. Specifically, the lack of access to follow-up mental health care negated the value of their depression identification technology. They also noted that case managers within their customers' organizations—responsible for facilitating follow-up care within the respective health systems—were highly variable from the standpoints of protocols used and quality of service. Singh relates wryly, "It was a pretty memorable board meeting when we presented our conclusion: that Ginger needed to add the delivery of care to our plate. We knew that we couldn't change the health systems, so we needed to innovate around them." The company thereafter internalized case managers and coaches and created a network of clinicians. Interestingly, the company found the added operations both economically fruitful and freeing. "Once we became a vertically integrated system, we controlled everything, and we could completely reenvision the delivery of mental health care."[31] The company was also much better positioned to address self-insured employers as customers, and could monetize their offering in two ways: by charging on a per-member-per-month basis and also billing for clinical services delivered.

Vertically Integrated Care Provider Strategy

Following a different path toward vertical integration, *telehealth companies* are vertically integrated by design. These companies utilize Internet-based telecommunications technology to enable remote, device-agnostic consultations with a network of clinicians. The value proposition is clear for the patient user: obtain care, typically on-demand, 24/7, from the convenience of home. The earliest telehealth companies, such as Teledoc, were designed for lower-acuity, non-chronic conditions. Their customers were primarily self-insured employers, who benefited from lower-cost alternatives to urgent care or emergency room visits, as well as potentially minimizing time away from work. More recently, however, there has been a surge in interest from providers and health systems in implementing telehealth services as an extension of their brick-and-mortar offerings. As a result, patients could have the same convenience but could see familiar doctors and experience a greater continuity of care. Some newer entrants, like SnapMD, have focused on this provider-based demand, while Teledoc addresses both sets of customers (SIEs and providers).[32] By increasing payer willingness to reimburse remote patient visits, the provider-oriented business model has been buoyed. Furthermore, telehealth companies have begun using technology to augment care beyond mere telecommunication capabilities. For instance, HealthTap launched "Dr. AI," a chatbot trained with data from millions of encounters on the platform, which provides relevant answers to health questions and helps to triage care. Similarly, Lyra Health uses intelligence to connect people with personalized mental health resources, including self-help tools and referral to its network of providers for telemetric or in-person care. It remains to be seen if the delivery of telemetric, coordinated

chronic care is feasible at scale, but this is the logical next step for health systems and telehealth companies.

Finally, some unexpected entities have or may become digitally-enabled, vertically-integrated care providers at scale. UnitedHealthcare's Optum has aggressively entered into the care delivery business, with hundreds of urgent and primary care locations, as well as 30,000 employed and affiliated physicians.[33] There is also increasing speculation that technology giant Amazon will become a direct healthcare provider, potentially leveraging its well-honed distribution systems to provide pharmacy benefits services and its Alexa platform to bring voice technologies into the home, clinic, and hospital.[34] Apple has also made intriguing moves related to health care. In addition to its Health app, which captures biometrics from a variety of sources, the company entered into a recent agreement with 13 major health systems to download electronic health record (EHR) data onto patients' personal Apple devices.[35] With this in mind, it is reasonable to imagine personalized, mobile, AI-based patient education and care solutions, powered by one's medical history and physiologic data.

▶ A Note on Financing Digital Health Companies

Given the major hurdles to development, validation, and commercialization of products in this space, d-health companies often lack the capital to go the distance, irrespective of their go-to-market strategy. As noted, investment in this space is at an all-time high, but the bulk of this financing is large, follow-on investing going to a handful of standout companies.[36] Omada's Duffy puts it very succinctly: "If you are going to try to do anything disruptive in healthcare, you better raise a boatload of cash."[37] Karan Singh from Ginger.io expanded on this theme: "You need to pick investors who aren't in it for a quick win. They need to understand that d-health requires the long game."[38]

Case Questions

In today's d-health marketplace, you are asked to champion a new innovative product for detecting oncoming stroke with a digital monitoring device that would be wearable, so that potential patients can be alerted prior to the stroke's onset. How would you go about setting up such a venture? Discuss the different strategies that would be wise to consider. Provide a recommendation for how you would proceed if you had just received joint two millions dollar funding from both the National Institute of Health (NIH) and the National Science Foundation (NSF).

Notes

1. Bhavnani, S. P., Narula, J., & Sengupta, P. P. (2016, May 7). Mobile technology and the digitization of healthcare. *European Heart Journal, 37*(18), 1428–1438. doi:10.1093/eurheartj/ehv770
2. Widmer, R. J., Collins, N. M., Collins, C. S., West, C. P., Lerman, L. O., & Lerman, A. (2015, April). Digital health interventions for the prevention of cardiovascular disease: A systematic review and meta-analysis. *Mayo Clinic Proceedings, 90*(4), 469–480. doi:10.1016/j.mayocp.2014.12.026. PMC 4551455. PMID 25841251.
3. "Digital health." Food and Drug Administration. US Department of Health and Human Services. 30 August 2016. Archived from the original on 12 November 2016.
4. Retrieved from www.who.int/reproductivehealth/publications/mhealth/classification-digital-health-interventions/en/
5. Retrieved from www.fda.gov/medicaldevices/digitalhealth/
6. Ries, E. Personal Communications.
7. Don Turner, personal communication.
8. The Diabetes Prevention Program (DPP) Research Group. (2002). The Diabetes Prevention Program (DPP): Description of lifestyle intervention. *Diabetes Care, 25*(12), 2165–2171.
9. US Preventive Services Task Force. (2014). Final recommendation statement regarding healthful diet and physical activity for cardiovascular disease prevention in adults with cardiovascular risk factors: Behavioral counseling. Retrieved from www.uspreventiveservicestaskforce.org/Page/Document/RecommendationStatementFinal/healthy-diet-and-physical-activity-counseling-adults-with-high-risk-of-cvd
10. Sean Duffy, personal communication.
11. *Ibid.*
12. Karan Singh, personal communication.
13. Digital Therapeutics Alliance. (2018). Retrieved from www.dtxalliance.org/
14. Sean Duffy, *ibid.*
15. Antoun Nabhan, personal communication.
16. Don Turner, *ibid.*
17. Carlson, J. J., Garrison, L. P., & Sullivan, S. (2009). Paying for outcomes: Innovative coverage and reimbursement schemes for pharmaceuticals. *Journal of Managed Care and Specialty Pharmacy, 15*(8), 683–687.
18. George Savage, personal communication.
19. Rock Health. (2017). *The rumors about digital health business models are true.* Retrieved from https://rockhealth.com/rock-weekly/the-rumors-about-digital-health-business-models-are-true/
20. Fronstin, P. (2016). Self-insured health plans: Recent trends by firm size, 1996-2015. *Employee Benefits Research Institute Notes, 37*(7), 2–6.
21. Jeff W., personal communication.
22. Bob Ihrie, personal communication.
23. Goetzl, R. Z., Long, S. R., Ozminkowski, R. J., Hawkins, K., Wang, S., & Lynch, W. (2004). Health, absence, disability, and presenteeism cost estimates of certain physical and mental health conditions affecting U.S. employers. *Journal of Occupational and Environmental Medicine, 46*(6), 398–412.
24. UnitedHealthcare. (2017). UnitedHealthcare and Qualcomm integrate wearable devices from Samsung and Garmin into wellness program. Retrieved from https://newsroom.uhc.com/news-releases/motion-update.html
25. Optum. (2017). Optum announces $250 million fund to invest in next generation of health care innovation. Retrieved from www.optum.com/about/news/optum-announces-250-million-fund-invest-next-generation-health-care-innovation.html
26. IMS Health. (2014). *Top 100 most prescribed, top-selling drugs.* Retrieved from www.medscape.com/viewarticle/829246

27. Otsuka America Pharmaceutical, Inc. (2017). Retrieved from www.otsuka-us.com/discover/articles -1075

28. Barrett, M., Combs, V., Su, J. G., Henderson, K., & Tuffli, M. (2018). AIR Louisville: Addressing asthma with technology, crowdsourcing, cross-sector collaboration, and policy. *Health Affairs, 37*(4), 525–534.

29. Takeda Pharmaceuticals USA. (2017). Takeda and Cognition Kit present results from digital wearable technology study in patients with major depressive disorder (MDD). Retrieved from www .prnewswire.com/news-releases/takeda-and -cognition-kit-present-results-from-digital-wearable -technology-study-in-patients-with-major-depressive -disorder-mdd-300558846.html

30. Pete Masloski, personal communication.

31. Karan Singh, *ibid.*

32. Mobihealth News. (2018). In-depth: Who owns telemedicine delivery—Payers or providers? Retrieved from www.mobihealthnews.com/content /depth-who-owns-telemedicine-delivery-payers-or -providers

33. Bloomberg. (2018). *30,000 strong and counting, UnitedHealth gathers a doctor army.* Retrieved from https://www.bloomberg.com/news/articles/2018 -04-09/30-000-strong-and-counting-unitedhealth -gathers-a-doctor-army

34. CNBC. (2017). As Amazon moves into health care, here's what we know—And what we suspect—About its plans. Retrieved from www.cnbc.com/2018/03/27 /amazons-moves-into-health-what-we-know.html

35. Blumenthal, D., & Chopra, A. (2018). Apple's pact with 13 health care systems might actually disrupt the industry. *Harvard Business Review.* Retrieved from https://hbr.org/2018/03/apples-pact-with-13-health -care-systems-might-actually-disrupt-the-industry

36. Rock Health. (2018). Digital health funding: 2017 year in review. *loc. cit.*

37. Sean Duffy, *ibid.*

38. Karan Singh, *ibid.*

CASE 2

The Impact of Electronic Medical Records (EMRs) on Clinical Workflow and Practices: Perspectives of MS, a Physician Resident in Ottawa, Canada

Brandon Lam and Joseph Tan

▶ Introduction

Over the years, medicine has been delivered via different modalities to the public. The emergence of electronic medical records (EMRs) has significantly improved the patient interfacing in terms of reliability, convenience, and productivity of medical services delivery. Even so, challenges exist; specifically, this case attempts to shed light on the different beneficial and challenging aspects that a physician resident (MS) has noticed for a currently implemented EMR system, such as *Epic* and *vOacis*.

For years, many healthcare professionals have shifted from using paper-based records to handling patient information via EMRs. Eventually, they are so use to paperless EMRs that if they have to physically rewrite orders or transmit the same patient information to be charted on paper and are expected to look through dozens of paper documentation for specific information on particular patients, they would find it truly inconvenient. With EMRs, all that needs to happen is simply to log into the system via a pre-registered username–password combination to securely gain access to a vast amount of information about a patient and what the hospital itself has to offer.

As the patient information sought can range from past medical histories, current blood work, recent diagnostic imaging, and a lot more, almost any details about a patient appear to be possible to obtain. In fact, barring any further security checkpoints and institutional authorization verification, the life story of the patient is literally just clicks away. Notwithstanding, many physicians and physician residents (for instance, MS) have differing opinions in regards to the deployed EMRs. Specific to this case, MS therefore expresses herewith his personal perspectives on a range of topics regarding the benefits and challenges of EMRs, specifically that of *Epic* and *vOacis*.

▶ Patient Charting/ Documenting

Epic has made documenting (or charting) the hospital journey of a patient much easier than navigating through the traditional paper-based charting and documenting procedures. For example, when a patient has to be admitted from the emergency department (ED), the attending caregiver has to fill out a lot of paperwork before the patient can be assigned a hospital bed. Such paperwork includes tedious work, such as filling out admission notes and orders.

Now, instead of having to fill out multiple different papers (as in traditional orders and procedures which require hours just to write the admission notes), *Epic* simplifies the routines for patients to get admitted in that the required admission notes can be completed in minutes electronically via well-designed templates on a relatively intuitive and easy-to-handle online platform. Importantly, *Epic* includes premade templates that can be used to further reduce the amount of time needed to begin a chart on a patient. For instance, most admission order templates will have boxes that

can be checked off on things that are typically ordered and *Epic* allows the user to edit that based on preferences. If the premade templates do not suit the end user, it is possible to make a custom template and save it for later use.

MS, the physician resident using the EMRs implemented in a facility located in Ottawa, Canada, found that every way he would want to chart for a patient's hospital stay exists in *Epic*. Hence, in contrast to having binders full of paper that are difficult to sift though, it is possible to have hundreds of notes about a patient that are organized and easy-to-find with the implementation and ongoing use of these EMRs.

So, when a patient is admitted, MS needs to track the progress of that patient, which may include writing progress notes that contain the patient's overall well-being, symptoms, vitals, physical exam, assessment, and plan. *Epic* has a premade template that allows MS to quickly fill in the lines or boxes related to the respective symptoms (chest pain, shortness of breath, nausea, and more) of the patient. Also, instead of typing out the findings on the physical exam, *Epic* also has a large selection of choices that can be chosen during each individual exam. For the cardiac exam, for example, choices such as S3/S4 extra heart sounds (which are abnormal heart sounds) and crackles (fluid in the lungs) can be selected in the respiratory exam. If the patient has concerns over abdominal pain, *Epic* has a silhouette of the human body that allows physicians to distinctly mark the area of tenderness. These features of the progress note taking are especially helpful during the morning hours prior to rounding on the patients. Indeed, every morning, when the entire team of allied healthcare professionals round on their patients in their ward by going through the respective patient assessment and management plan, without an efficient and functional EMR, the rounding activities alone can take up to half a day. Thankfully with the help of *Epic*, rounding usually takes 1–2 hours.

Toward the end of a patient's hospital journey, physicians and physician residents, such as MS, need to create a discharge summary that outlines the events preceding admission to the hospital, the patient's diagnosis, their management, any relevant investigations (blood work, medical imaging), and medications to continue or discontinue following discharge. Once again, *Epic* comes in handy as this system has another premade template that can easily organize the discharge summary to be coherent and concise. Once the discharge summary is completed, it is dispatched to the respective patient's family doctor who will follow up on further necessary and future patient care services.

▶ Centralized Application to Access Patient's Medical Records

One of the challenges of having an EMR is the difficulty of communicating with other hospitals having differing and sometimes non-interoperable EMR systems. MS finds that he cannot typically access a patient's medical record in a hospital where the EMR is different or non-interoperable. Imagine a 27-year-old male (a new patient—Titus Liu) presenting to the ED with shortness of breath. When MS, working in the ED, tries to look up Titus Liu, the patient, in the hospital EMR, he finds no medical history. When MS takes a history, Titus reports that he has been short of breath for a week without fever, chills, or night sweats. Titus denies having a productive cough. He denies any chest pain, palpitations, or leg pain. Furthermore, Titus denies any past medical or surgical history. He is allergic to penicillin and is not currently on any medications. Titus has a significant family history of premature coronary artery disease (CAD) in both his parents. He has a 10 pack-year smoking history; binge drinking habits; and has a diet significant in fatty foods.

Upon a careful physical exam, Titus is found to be tachycardic and tachypneic. His blood pressure is 120/80, temperature is 37.5°C, with O_2 saturation of 100%. His chest X-ray, ECG, and blood work come back normal. MS has excluded all the common causes of shortness of breath including a heart attack, pneumonia, pneumothorax, pulmonary embolism (PE), and congestive heart failure. After ruling out all the red flags, MS decides that Titus can be discharged home safely.

Now imagine the same scenario, but this time MS has access to Titus' medical records from different hospitals with interoperable EMRs. MS sees that Titus has an extensive psychiatric history due to many ED visits for panic attacks and hallucinations. With this significant information, the most likely diagnosis could be psychogenic shortness of breath, which was not on the differential diagnosis initially. Thus, the treatment management plan for Titus would now change because MS would have referred the patient to a psychiatrist for further assessment and treatment. As demonstrated, having a lack of access to Titus' medical records can result in unnecessary diagnostic investigations, poor use of resources, and even incorrect diagnosis.

To combat issues, such as those previously noted, some regions have a centralized application within EMR systems that contain pertinent patient medical records from EMRs across the different hospitals and that can be accessed via *Epic* or *vOacis*. These important records include consultation notes, clinic notes, ED visits, and diagnostic imaging (X-rays, echocardiograms, ultrasounds). With such a centralized application, MS and other caregivers are then able to learn all about a patient's medical history to arrive at a correct diagnosis and appropriate management plan. This diminishes the cost of unnecessary investigations in the work up of a patient, such as Titus, and improves overall resource management within the hospital.

▶ Orders

Orders have been made simple as well due to implemented EMRs. For basic blood work on a patient, such as a complete blood count (CBC) or IV fluids, MS can easily type out these orders, which will then get sent to nurses as urgent tasks to complete. There is no more need for filling out requisition forms that take time out of his busy schedule, and it is possible now to fill out orders in a matter of seconds. For diagnostic imaging, MS typically had to fill out requisitions that patients needed to hand to the clerks who would then register them. Now, he can order imaging, and that patient's information gets sent right to the imaging department. The clerks will know that the patient is coming, and they will have everything set up for them as they arrive.

▶ Access to Resources

The treatment guidelines that inform MS on how best to treat patients with specific diseases are based on hundreds of clinical research data. Medicine is built on the foundation of research, which gives caregivers such as MS the best evidence possible to treat patients effectively. This research includes randomized controlled trials (RCTs) and validation of clinical decision-making tools, as well as many others. With so much data in medical society, it is difficult for MS to memorize every treatment guideline for every disease. EMRs like *vOacis* make it easier for MS by having guidelines installed into the software. Hence, when MS is unsure on how to approach a disease, he can quickly access the information on *vOacis*. For example, for the outpatient treatment of community-acquired pneumonia (CAP) in patients who were previously healthy, the recommendation is for doctors to prescribe a macrolide (azithromycin, clarithromycin, or erythromycin[1]). Conversely, for patients with the presence of comorbidities, such as chronic heart or lung diseases, the guidelines advice is

for physicians to prescribe a respiratory fluoroquinolone (moxifloxacin or levofloxacin) or a combination of a B-lactam (amoxicillin) with a macrolide.[1] And, for hospital acquired pneumonia (HAP), the antibiotics recommended to be prescribed are piperacillin-tazobactam or a respiratory fluoroquinalone.[2]

Each region in Canada differs in the prevalence of diseases and microorganisms. These microorganisms also differ in susceptibility to various types of antibiotics for various regions; accordingly, EMRs can be equipped with the ability to show physicians what antibiotics local microorganisms are susceptible to in that specific region; an example is shown in **TABLE CS2-1**.

Antibiograms like these allow MS and other caregivers to prescribe the most effective antibiotic so as to have the most successful chance at curing a patient's infection, depending on where the patient is located. Without helpful tools like antibiograms in EMRs, physicians would be prescribing endless amount of antibiotics in order to arrive at the most effective one. This increases the risk of antibiotic resistance, which is becoming a global health issue.

▶ Mobile Access (Tablets, Phones)

To further increase productivity and time management, EMRs, such as *Epic* and *vOacis*, are nowadays accessible on tablets and phones, such as iPad and iPhones.

Mobile versions of EMRs, as shown in **FIGURE CS2-1**, allow caregivers, such as MS, to access medical records rapidly.[3]

Such interfaces allow the caregivers to look at progress notes to get up-to-date on a patient's overall condition in the hospital anytime, anywhere. Orders can also be placed quickly on tablets. Where MS finds this most helpful is in looking up blood work, diagnostic imaging, and vital signs. Whenever MS

TABLE CS2-1 Antibiogram Recommendations for Toronto General Hospital Emergency Department (ED)

Gram Positive Isolates	Penicillin (%)	Ampicillin (%)	Cefazolin (%)	Cloxacillin (%)	Clindamycin (%)	Vancomycin (%)
Staphylococcus aureus (MSSA)	–	–	100	100	70	100
Enterococcus	–	70	–	–	–	100
Streptococcus pneumoniae	100	–	–	–	90	80
Group A Strep	100	–	–	–	70	100

Gram Negative Isolates	Ampicillin (%)	Amox/Clav (%)	Ceftriaxone (%)	Ciprofloxacin (%)	Gentamicin (%)	Meropenem (%)
Escherichia coli	50	80	80	70	90	99.9
Enterobacter	–	–	–	97	99	99.9
Proteus mirabilis	85	90	95	100	90	99
Pseudomonas aeruginosa	–	–	–	70	70	84.5

Example of an Antibiogram.

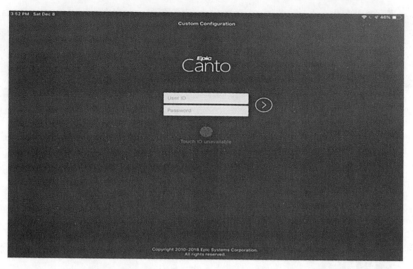

FIGURE CS2-1 Mobile interface of an EMR (electronic medical record) system.

is charting or reassessing his patients, he is always looking for these three investigations. Having the ability to access this information in such a timely manner definitely improves his clinical workflow and resulting productivity. Hence, tablets give MS and other caregivers the convenience of not having to be stuck on a computer to utilize the EMRs. The mobility improves the day-to-day hospital and clinical workflow.

▶ Clinics

EMRs have also improved the organization and workflow in the clinics. For *Epic*, the schedule of the day shows the name of the patient, time of appointment, reason for referral or chief complaint, and where the patient currently is (e.g., waiting room, examination room number). Having all this pertinent information at your fingertips is convenient and allows the clinic to run smoothly. When the nurse assigns a patient a room, it is updated on the EMR. If the patient is sent for additional testing, such as an echocardiogram, instead of having to chase down a nurse and inquire about the patient,

the physician can view the clinic schedule on *Epic* and there will be an indicator, such as a grey dot beside the patient's name, that specifically informs the physician where or what is being done on the patient.

▶ Reference Value

In most clinical settings, blood work is almost ordered for every patient. Depending on what specific blood marker you are looking for, the abnormal lab values can be elevated or low. On *Epic* and *vOacis*, physicians or physician residents compare the measured value of blood markers to reference ranges that are already embedded into the system, as illustrated in **TABLE CS2-2**. The EMR labels the specific marker as "High" or "Low" automatically based on the reference ranges it uses. Even if the value is higher or lower than the reference range by 1, the EMR automatically labels the marker as abnormal.

The problem here is what abnormal values may be considered to be significant? If the white blood cell count is elevated at 11, do we go looking for a source of infection in

					Reference	
Date	Test	Value	Units	Abnormality?	Range	Status
December 05, 2019 (15:35)	WBC	11.4	×10^9/L	High!	3.5–10.5	Completed
December 05, 2019 (15:35)	RBC	2.50	×10^12/L	Low!	3.50–5.00	Completed
December 05, 2019 (15:35)	HGB	128	g/L		115–155	Completed
December. 05, 2019 (15:35)	HCT	0.390	L/L		0.380–0.500	Completed
December 05, 2019 (15:35)	MCV	90.0	fL		80.0–100.0	Completed
December 05, 2019 (15:35)	MCH	29.8	Pg		25.0–34.0	Completed
December 05, 2019 (15:35)	MCHC	328	g/L		315–355	Completed
December 05, 2019 (15:35)	RDW	12.8	%		11.5–15.5	Completed
December 05, 2019 (15:35)	PLAT	195	×10^9/L		130–380	Completed
December 05, 2019 (15:35)	MPV	11.7	fL		9.0–14.0	Completed

TABLE CS2-2 Blood Reference Valuation on an EMR (Electronic Medical Record) System

Clinical Information System. Telus Health.

the patient? If a patient's troponin level is high at a value of 46, do we worry about a heart attack? This is where the issue of treating the patient versus treating the lab value arises. If the patient does not report fever and chills but the white count is slightly elevated, should we be worried about an infection? If a female does not report any retrosternal chest pain but her troponin is elevated, should we call cardiology for an urgent catherization? The EMR does not inform us when and how to treat the patient, it only tells us that there may or may not be something wrong with the patient. Hence, to improve this ambiguity of EMR reference ranges, the upper and lower limits of normal need to be set at a certain value where an abnormal reading is significant enough for the physician to consider further work up or treatment for the patient. By having this function, it improves the overall reliability of the EMR and allows the caregivers to be more confident when assessing their patients.

▶ Privacy of Patients

Currently, one of the biggest issues with EMRs is privacy. How can healthcare providers protect the privacy of patients when information about them is so readily accessible and available? Physicians, dieticians, and nurses as well as a wide variety of other allied healthcare professionals are involved in patient care; hence, patients can become vulnerable to a data breach of their privacy. Imagine if a high-profile patient was admitted to a hospital for a very serious condition. Any information mentioned about the patient to a person who is not taking care of them is a violation of the patient's rights to privacy and confidentiality. VIP or high-profile patient's medical records are not blocked from anyone who has access to *Epic* or *vOacis*. Hence, nothing is stopping people from inputting the patient's name or health number to gain access to information, such as their diagnosis or past medical history.

A solution to solve this problem would be to only allow healthcare providers who are taking care of the patient to have authorized access to the patient's medical record. This solution will prevent unauthorized users from accessing medical records they are not supposed to access. However, what if there was a breach of privacy? Who is to blame and what should the punishment be? Many hospitals have had violations of patient privacy but no concrete solutions have been established.[4] Should the perpetrator's punishment be equivalent to the wrongful action? Who is to decide how healthcare workers are to be punished? This is an ongoing issue and no clear answers have yet been reached.

Another issue with privacy is paper copies of patient lists. In the morning, patient lists are printed out for the entire team to update

everybody on issues, such as new patients, patients who have passed away, and floor issues that need to be managed. At the end of the day, when it is time to get rid of the list, there are designated shredder bins where these listings should be placed so that they can be properly disposed of; however, it is very common for people to misplace the patient list accidently. One solution to this problem would be to permanently ban the use of patient lists. No more patient lists mean that it would be impossible for people to misplace them. Yet, this may be impractical as printing patient lists have been done for decades.

A final issue regarding privacy is the dissemination of patient information wirelessly. In a healthcare team, members constantly communicate with each other about patients, usually on a cell phone. According to MS, a lot of healthcare workers use unsecure messaging systems, such as applications like WhatsApp, where patient data can be easily accessed if hacked. There are very few mobile applications that provide healthcare workers the security to talk about patient data. In *Epic* or *vOacis*, healthcare workers are unable to communicate with each other while actively engaged in the interface. Some applications exist that allow physicians to communicate privately, but it is inconvenient as it is a separate application from the EMR. One suggestion to fix this would be to develop an "In-EMR" messaging function that seamlessly allows caregivers to communicate with each other while they are accessing the EMR. This would be convenient and would protect the privacy of patients at the same time.

▶ EMR Implementation

The transition from paper records to an EMR in a tertiary care hospital is a complex process. This change does not happen overnight but it is typically a year or longer process. EMR implementation has to be performed strategically in order to minimize the amount of confusion and disruption to both the health-care workers and physicians. Over the course of the implementation, workshops and lessons are often held to educate healthcare workers and to train them on the proper use of the new EMR. On the day of implementation, EMR specialists are stationed in almost every department to make sure things run smoothly. If EMRs are not implemented effectively, the implementation can significantly drain hospital finances while crippling its associated clinical workflow and disrupt its routines. Conversely, if implementation is done professionally, the hospital stands to gain access to timely and relevant patient data, which can be used to support and champion excellence in patient care.

Case Questions

MS has been actively reading on the future of EMRs in Canada and came across an interesting *CMAJ* article penned by a medical student, Eric Zhao, who compared the lack of mandate to unify communications among EMR users (physicians) as the early days of Amazon, with Bezos finally resolving the challenge by changing the Amazon culture and focus.[5] If you are the Bezos in charge of future EMR developments in Canada, what would you do that may make a significant difference and further leverage the huge benefits to be had from EMRs?

Notes

1. IDSA/ATS Consensus Guidelines on the Management of Community-Acquired Pneumonia in Adults. (2007). *Clinical Infectious Diseases, 44*, 27–72.
2. Guidelines for the management of adults with hospital acquired, ventilator-associated, and healthcare-associated pneumonia. (2005). *American Journal of Respirology and Critical Care Medicine, 171*, 388–416.
3. Epic Canto EMR IPad Application. Epic Systems Corporation.
4. Beltran-Aroca, C. M, Girela-Lopez, E., Collazo-Chao, E., Montero-Perez-Barquero, M., & Munoz-Villanueva, M. C. (2016). Confidentiality breaches in clinical practice: What happens in hospitals? *BMC Medical Ethics, 17*(1), 52.
5. Zhao, E. (2019). The Future of EMRs in Canada. *CMAJ*.

Biography

Brandon Lam is a medical student at the University of Ottawa. He hopes to pursue his residency education in the FRCPC (Fellow of the Royal College of Physicians of Canada) Emergency Medicine program and subsequently a fellowship in Critical Care Medicine. His academic and research interests include emergency medicine and cardiology. He has published in anatomy textbooks that are currently used at Queen's University, Canada. He has also published in high-impact factor journals, such as *The American Journal of Cardiology and Development*. He aspires to be both an intensive care unit and emergency physician.

CASE 3

St. Joseph Mercy Oakland (SJMO): Digital Leadership in Health Care

Mohan Tanniru, Jack Weiner, and Monica Garfield

Jack Weiner, the Chief Executive Officer (CEO) and President of SJMO, wanted to develop a new vision for St. Joseph's Hospital (SJH). He knew he had to think of something that would enable him to stay competitive in the new landscape that was emerging in the healthcare industry in Southeast Michigan. He was facing a number of challenges, including cost containment inside SJH and regulatory pressures coming from outside SJMO. He was also trying to improve on the overall level of patient satisfaction provided by SJMO. In order to stay competitive in the ever-changing regulatory market, he knew he had to transform SJMO. As he thought about transformation, he considered how other companies in similar situations evolved. There were companies like Western Union that once was known for sending telegraphs who had to transform their business into one that sent money, and Nokia went from selling rubber boots to selling cell phones. While these were great examples of revolutionary changes, Jack was not interested in changing the healthcare industry, but instead wanted to become better and smarter about how he competed in the healthcare market. As he considered this, it struck him that General Motors (GM) had learned to modify its products, operations, marketing, and other parts of the company to stay competitive in the automotive market. How did GM do this? He decided to visit GM to see how they drove their transformations. While on this visit he saw how technologies were transforming the automotive industry and dashboards were being used to monitor its performance on several dimensions. He wanted to see how SJMO could use advanced digitization to help reinvent itself in addressing its many challenges.

> We are not following the traditional pathway of health IT implementation. We want to understand what is happening in each patient-healthcare staff encounter and make sure our digitization efforts are in alignment with our service goals as well as our

organizational goals as we improve quality of care, reduce costs, and improve patient satisfaction. We want to always ask the following question: How can the use of IT best serve our patients? We want the technology used to have a positive impact on our healthcare mission (quality, cost, and patient satisfaction), and we want to assess this impact both locally and at the organizational level at every step.

Jack Weiner

Jack wanted to ensure that the transformation actions impacted multiple facilities within SJMO (e.g. emergency room, operating rooms, and patient rooms), but he felt he should begin by focusing on patient rooms. A patient spends a significant amount of time in the patient room, and several events that occur in these rooms have cost and patient satisfaction implications. For example, patient falls, hospital acquired infections, food-related complications for diabetic patients, inadequate monitoring of patient conditions which can lead to complications, and more such incidents are all controllable to some degree, and they also impact both patient satisfaction and length of stay in the hospital. Therefore, he laid out the following objectives for the digital transformation of SJMO:

1. Become proactive in anticipating potential complications occurring in patient rooms to contain costs and improve patient satisfaction.
2. Support the alignment of clinical unit and hospital administration goals along a few key performance metrics (e.g., quality of patient care, unanticipated costs inside the hospital, patient satisfaction, readmission costs, etc.), so that both groups work toward the same goals.

Besides using innovative ideas to support the digital transformation of SJMO and

address the stated objectives, Jack wanted SJMO to document its innovations for both learning within the hospital and to gain recognition by external peers. In order to gain the external recognition from his peer group, he focused on gaining recognition by *Wired Magazine's Innovator of the Year* award. This is an annual award that looks at innovative applications of technology in health care across the United States. The *American Hospital Association (AHA)* and *Hospitals & Health Networks* jointly coordinate the award deliberation, with over 350 submissions each year. The submissions are evaluated by a group of hospital CEOs and Chief Information Officers (CIOs) in order to select twenty finalists and one *Innovator of the Year*. SJMO's digital transformation efforts discussed in this case won five finalist recognitions in three consecutive years (2014–2016), with one of them in winning the *Innovator of the Year* award in 2015.[1] No other community hospital has won recognition with such consistency. This journey was not the result of a single project, but was the implementation of a vision to become a digital leader in health care.

▶ Background of SJMO

SJMO is a 443-bed community teaching hospital located in Pontiac, Michigan. SJMO is a member of the Saint Joseph Health System, which is a subsidiary of Trinity Health, the fourth largest Catholic healthcare system in the United States. SJMO is ranked nationally in the top 5% for clinical experience and is among the top 50 cardiovascular programs in the nation, in addition to being a Level II trauma center. SJMO is recognized as a center of excellence and a leader for women and child services, joint care, and surgical procedures. SJMO completed a $252 million renovation and expansion of the hospital's west wing in 2014 that included the addition of a new eight-story patient tower, along with a two-story surgery center.

SJMO faces stiff competition from many well-known hospitals, such as William Beaumont, Henry Ford Health System (HFHS), St. John Health Systems (a part of a large hospital network called Ascension), Detroit Mercy, and Crittenton-Ascension in Rochester, MI (right next to Pontiac). Many of these hospitals have significant resources from private donors; moreover, these competing facilities are known to have higher bed capacity and well-recognized surgical units with patients covered by private insurers. Even though SJMO is also a part of a large healthcare chain (Trinity Health System), it is dwarfed by a much larger and well-recognized hospital in the same system: St Joseph Mercy Ann Arbor, which has higher-level visibility, a wealthier and more educated patient mix, and a higher number of patients insured by private companies.

SJMO, as well as other hospitals in the healthcare industry, has been under tremendous pressure from regulators who assess care quality and from insurers who continue to change reimbursement systems to influence care delivery behaviors. The need for transformative changes in health care is not a luxury but a necessity, and this need has become more intense as patients, just as customers in other industry sectors, have started to demand more services supported by advanced digitization tools.

▶ Healthcare Industry Landscape

Baylor University Hospital's introduction of a prepayment hospital insurance plan for a group of school teachers[2] in 1929 is considered the first instance of what evolved into our modern-day healthcare insurance. This started a major change in health care. It transformed the organizational structure and operations of hospitals, bringing an amalgamation of physicians under contract with hospitals in order to provide focused care in various specialties. This was the way health care was primarily managed until July 30, 1965, when President Lyndon B. Johnson signed into law a bill that led to Medicare and Medicaid. Medicare and Medicaid were formed to pay for health insurance for the elderly and poor. This made the federal government a major player in healthcare reimbursement and led to the further formalization of healthcare leadership and strategies, including the consolidation of many care delivery specialties to exploit impending economies of scale.

In the ensuing decades, the federal government started to look for better ways to manage payments for healthcare services. To make payment systems uniform across different hospital operations, the government started to use a program called Diagnosis Related Groups (DRGs) for financial reimbursement to hospitals. The DRGs were initially designed to measure the quality of clinical care based on a diagnosis of a patient's medical condition. Over time, hospitals have adapted to DRGs, and fee-for-service (FFS) reimbursement based on the DRG became a way to recover costs incurred in the care of patients.

Then came the Affordable Care Act (ACA)[3] in 2009. One of the goals of ACA was to bring healthcare coverage to many uninsured individuals using federal subsidies and a mandate to spread overall healthcare costs across the US citizens. It also created incentives for improving patient satisfaction, reducing 30-day readmissions, and bundling payments that spread reimbursements over a longer period (both inside and outside the hospital) to cover the costs of care. All these measures were intended to control healthcare cost increases and improve the continuity of patient care. However, they also highlighted the need for an alignment of goals among two different groups that influence hospital costs and reimbursements: the clinical group and hospital administration. These two groups have an unusual reporting structure in hospitals.

▸ Organizational Structure of Hospitals

Hospitals, unlike most other businesses, have a dual organizational structure. All clinical specialties have an organizational structure where there is a head for each clinical department leading the physician staff of that department. These heads report to the chief of staff, who reports directly to the board. The chief of staff is responsible for the quality of care provided in the hospital. The CEO is the head of the administrative structure of the hospital and reports directly to the board as well (see **FIGURE CS3-1**).

The CEO works with the Chief Financial Officer (CFO), the Chief Operations Officer (COO), the CIO, the chief of nursing, the quality manager, and the human resource (HR) manager to run the hospital's operations. The staff they manage includes clinical staff (nurses, anesthesiologists, pharmacists, lab technicians, and more) and operations staff (those who manage emergency, operating and patient rooms, lab/test facilities, and more). Conflicts that arise between clinical and administrative units are brought to the board for resolution.

This dual structure poses significant challenges when attempting to align goals between clinical units and administration. The diagnosis made by the physician staff determines the DRGs and dictates the revenues generated by the hospital, while the costs incurred by the hospital include both hospital operations and physicians' costs. Typically, many physicians have their own practices and are credentialed to operate within one or more hospitals. Even when physicians work directly for a hospital, the clinical group and the specialists have a significant say in the overall costs a hospital incurs in the treatment of a patient. With the clinical group deciding on the revenue stream and the administration responsible for managing overall costs, the alignment of goals between these two groups is often challenged with a significant difference in views. The ACA, with the introduction of incentives and penalties, suddenly made the need to address this challenge paramount.

The pressure on hospitals resulting from the evolving regulations under the ACA was further exacerbated by a severe recession in Michigan that spanned a decade, from the mid-2000s to the mid-2010s. This was the situation in 2009; accordingly, Jack had to decide on the hospital's future and embarked on a road to bring digital transformation to SJMO.

▸ Information Technology (IT), Systems, and SJMO Capabilities

For SJMO to undertake a digital transformation, it is useful to understand the IT capabilities of SJMO when its journey began in 2009. At that time, SJMO, just as other hospitals, had been using IT to drive down costs and improve quality.[4] Some of the ongoing applications included a decision support (DS) tool for

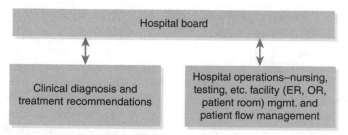

FIGURE CS3-1 Typical hospital structure.

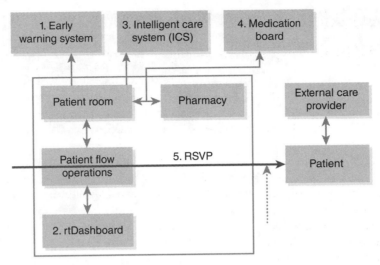

FIGURE CS3-2 Five digital transformations and their timelines.

a clinical unit (i.e., radiology), tools to speed the flow of patients in emergency departments and support a computerized physician order entry system (CPOE), and the Cerner electronic health record (EHR) system to track diagnoses, treatment processes, and patient record keeping. Most of these IT applications were leveraging software from a single vendor, Cerner, and the IT infrastructure and Cerner systems were managed by the corporate IT of Trinity Health in Novi, Michigan. SJMO maintained a handful of IT staff members who were dedicated to supporting targeted IT applications as needed. This environment was not sufficient to undertake the vision espoused by the CEO for digital transformation. Both the IT director and executive leadership recognized that digital transformation through innovations must come from resources brought from the outside, prior to making any significant investments to increase internal IT resources.

▶ SJMO's Digital Transformation

SJMOs digital transformation journey is exemplified by five information system (IS)

implementations that won national recognition and transformed patient care. **FIGURE CS3-2** highlights each of the innovations and the initial timing of these explorations.

The early warning system helps anticipate patient conditions before they became too severe (*Case Scenario 1*). The performance dashboard supports alignment of services and goals across a number of areas (*Case Scenario 2*). An intelligent care system reduces several patient room costs and addresses patient satisfaction (*Case Scenario 3*). The medication board improves productivity on the nursing floor (*Case Scenario 4*). The RSVP system addresses patient readmission costs (*Case Scenario 5*).

▶ Case Scenario 1— Early Warning System (2009–2014)

In 2009, an opportunity arose to test an early warning system for patients with deteriorating medical conditions using a technology product developed by Visensia. As shown in **FIGURE CS3-3**, clinical staff who have had previously used five independent patient readings

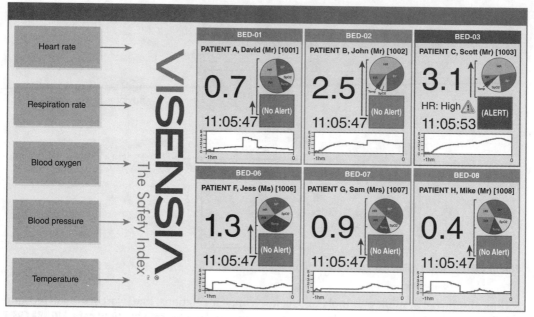

FIGURE CS3-3 SJMO color-coded vital sign monitoring.

(blood pressure, pulse rate, respiratory rate, pulse oximetry, and temperature) to assess patient conditions now could use a single index score. The color-coding scheme associated with the index (red, yellow, green, and gray) was used to alert care delivery staff to take quick action if the trends show a deteriorating patient condition.

This IS implementation transformed the way care delivery staff proactively used patient conditions to improve the rapid response team (RRT) activation rate, which measures the frequency with which staff calls the rapid response team to evaluate a patient. Both the chief medical information officer (CMIO) and CIO saw the value of the vendor technology in addressing patient care, but they also recognized the importance of nursing staff training and their engagement to effectively monitor the index and interpret the colors correctly before initiating any RRT action. The results of the early warning system pilot led to an increase in intensive care unit (ICU) up-transfers within the hospital, reduced length of stay, and reduced mortality.

The technology was adopted incrementally—with a pilot introduced in medical-surgical floors first, neurology next, and the rest in subsequent stages. Frequent reporting of results and training of staff in monitoring and interpreting the results eventually made this an integral part of patient monitoring. After four years of demonstrating accuracy and adherence to clinical guidelines, the innovation was recognized as a finalist for being one of the most innovative uses of technology in health care by *Wired* magazine in 2014.

> With these awards, our hospital has proven itself to be a regional and national leader in healthcare innovation. Our patients have benefited from these efforts and are seeing positive results first hand.
>
> Jack Weiner

The speed with which organizations need to react today to address external change means that explorations must occur constantly, sometimes while other explorations are still under review for evaluation and potential adaptation. Reflecting on the early warning system experience regarding the viability of using external vendor technology to bring digital transformations with minimal disruption to the current technology infrastructure, in 2010 the CEO decided to initiate the next digital transformation case scenario designed to bring about alignment between clinical and administrative goals.

▶ Case Scenario 2— Performance Dashboard (2010–2012)

Jack wanted clinical unit leaders to see the collective impact of their decisions and actions on overall SJMO performance and on specific metrics, such as mortality rates, length-of-stay, and patient satisfaction. As he is a strong believer in the Hoshin Kanri philosophy,[5] which advocates the alignment of unit actions and core performance metrics with a drill-down capability, an external vendor

was brought in to design a technology artifact called *rtDashboard* (rt representing "real time").

FIGURE CS3-4 provides an illustration of the visual representation of a dashboard for evaluating SJMO operations.

The CIO found a regional vendor, and the CMIO helped identify some initial projects to pilot test the dashboard (e.g. capacity management, patient throughput, and turnaround time in the emergency room or ER) that were already on the unit manager's radar. The IT staff used a number of data conversion mechanisms to bring the *rtDashboard* to functionality quickly. This was eventually achieved without disrupting the existing Cerner EHR system and several unit-level internal systems.[6]

Jack led the major SJMO cultural transformation using daily huddles where hospital unit managers were able to see their unit performance against hospital metrics and assess the need to direct actions within their own units to address variance. To support a data-driven decision-making culture and bring visibility to SJMO performance on many key metrics, the dashboards were displayed at various locations in the hospital so that all stakeholders, including patients and visitors, could see how well

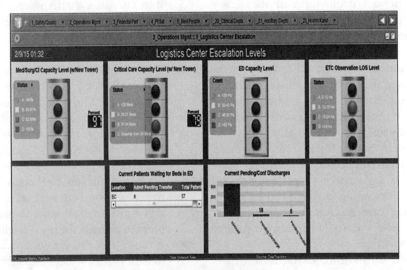

FIGURE CS3-4 An example of a dashboard visuals to evaluate operations.

the hospital was performing on these metrics. During the first phase of this transformation to the hospital unit culture, IT played a supporting role by focusing on helping unit managers understand, interpret, and act on goal and action alignment.[7]

Once the observed huddles and goal or target-based discussions became a part of the daily routine of administration and unit managers (i.e., part of regular hospital business), the second phase of the *rtDashboard* was initiated by routinizing application solicitation, prioritization, and development using a steering committee, led by the CMIO. At this time, IT staff began exploring the building of a standardized platform for importing data from the clinical units into *rtDashboard*. The *rtDashboard* was recognized as a finalist for being one of the most innovative uses of technology in health care by *Wired* magazine in 2015.

As SJMO leadership reflected on the Early Warning System and the *rtDashboard*, it became apparent that vendor and external resources could continue to supplement internal IT staff resources for exploring future digital transformations. One of the external resources SJMO found very helpful was the use of local college students to support the development and deployment of these new innovations.

Jack and the CMIO turned their attention to opportunities to digitize patient rooms in order to control costs. In 2012, an opportunity presented itself when the hospital administration requested that the board consider expanding its bed capacity to address patient needs. Jack proposed an innovative new hospital wing (the South Tower) that showcased a human-centered approach to building a hospital that creates a space for patient healing, while also leveraging advanced digitization to transform care services in all the patient rooms to reduce costs and improve patient satisfaction.

This led to the third digital transformational scenario at SJMO: The Intelligent Care System (ICS).

We didn't just construct a new building, we created a living, breathing hospital that plays an integral part in our patients' healing process.

Jack Weiner

▶ Case Scenario 3— Intelligent Care Systems (2012–2015)

The ICS was different from the first two projects in that it uses 11 different technologies to automate multiple services to support care delivery and patient–nurse communication within patient rooms.

FIGURE CS3-5 depicts how the ICS serves as a coordinating tool to connect the various educational, wellness support, monitoring, and communication systems within SJMO's patient rooms.

The ICS then is essentially a conglomeration of key technologies, comprising a suite of software components; the major software components included:

- A wrist-worn device, which pulls vital sign data from a patient's wrist and sends it to Visensia for early warning (to reduce care-related complications; recall that Visensia is the early warning system that was discussed earlier);
- A smart bed that alerts nurses when patients with high fall risk are trying to get out of bed (to reduce patient falls);
- A gel dispensing system that staff use to wash their hands as they walk in and out of a patient room (to reduce hospital acquired infections);
- An educational channel connected to patient diagnosis to help tailor education and nutritional guidance to patients (to prepare patients for post-discharge);
- A multi-level call system that allows a patient to seek select care, such as toilet, pain medication, or general information (to improve communication);

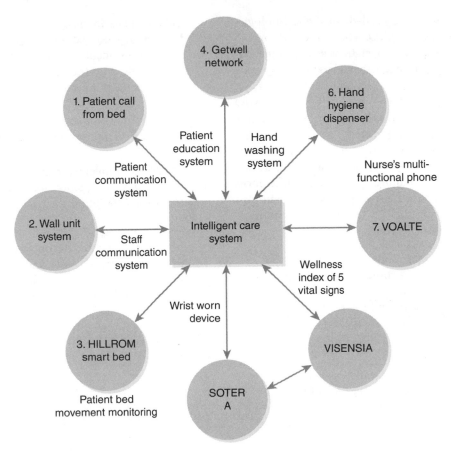

FIGURE CS3-5 Interfaces of SJMO's Intelligent Care Systems (ICS).

- A wall unit that connects care staff with catering, transport, physicians, and more (to speed up communication and set up alerts, such as administering pills for diabetic patients before serving food or administering pain management drugs at regular intervals); and
- A smartphone system that is connected to all these systems that helps the nursing staff send texts, receive alerts, and make phone calls.

This was a radical change for both the nursing and small IT staff. While funding became available to bring about these technologies, the timing of their implementation was too short to develop an incremental roll out strategy. The CIO, in partnership with the CMIO, formed a team of nursing and IT staff to explore available new technologies and to evaluate their effectiveness and maturity to support patient room services. A pilot implementation was completed in 2013 on one floor to establish its potential in reducing hospital acquired infections, reducing patient falls, and improving patient–staff communication before a decision was made to implement ICS in all the 443 patient rooms beginning in 2014 when the building was opened.

During the first phase of the ICS implementation, there was recognition on the part of the administration that this would lead to many growing pains because of its impact on the care provided. The hospital administration was concerned that even after the implementation of all these technologies, their full adoption would need to address a number of issues that arose as they rolled out the technologies further across SJMO. They were prepared to address gaps in expectations as these surfaced and even the need to address these quickly using changes in technology, processes, or training of people. While the CIO and CMIO led the digital transformation effort in the early phases, Jack entered the picture when post-implementation evaluation required process and policy-level changes, as well as during discussions required to bridge differences among vendor technologies as they attempted to work together to streamline communication and data sharing.

> From the start, the initiative was viewed as a clinical project, not an IT project. The IT people became clinical experts, and the pilot site's clinicians became IT experts.
>
> —Robert Jones, IT Director, SJMO[8]

> One challenge early on was getting the vendors of the different technologies to work together.
>
> —Fabian Fregoli, Vice President of clinical quality and patient safety and CMIO[9]

As anticipated, while the ICS was being implemented across the various floors, several issues surfaced that needed to be addressed; for example, early use of the smart bed led to too many alerts and contributed to stress among nursing staff. Adjustments had to be made to address both alerts and process changes in the workflows to support better workflow integration. Similarly, hand hygiene technology saw limited adoption at first with the staff viewing it as "big brother" watching, so processes were altered and a competition between the floors helped spur adherence to the new system.

> Nurses were given time to get accustomed to the RTLS [real time locator sensor] badges before hand-hygiene performance data were shared—first at the unit level, lastly at the shift level,

and now down to the individual level. The system resulted in a 300 percent improvement in hand-hygiene compliance, and the HAI [hospital acquired infection] rate fell to zero in the pilot's first quarter.
>
> —Fabian Fregoli, Vice President of clinical quality and patient safety and CMIO[10]

For its ICS implementation, SJMO won the *2015 Most Wired Innovator* award. Additionally, the new building was recognized for its design.

> From the integrated technology, to lights, to art, to the size and shape of patient windows, the design of the new South Patient Tower utilizes proven methods and techniques to further promote positive outcomes for our patients.
>
> —CARITAS Project's Generative Space Award[11]

The next digital transformation did not come from the C-level suites, but from the nursing staff. To improve their productivity, nurses saw the need for a way to alert them when drugs were being sent to the nursing floor. Indicative of the cultural change within SJMO, the staff began to look for opportunities for digitization to address this issue. This next digital transformation resulted in the design of a digital medication board.

▶ Case Scenario 4— Medication Board (2014–2015)

SJMO nursing staff realized that they were spending a considerable amount of time tracking drugs prescribed to a patient and sent to the pharmacy, as these medications were either on their way or deposited at a location (e.g., IV Room for the sterile preparation of intravenous medications), without the awareness of nurses. The new innovation allowed a pharmacist to use a television screen or log on to a portal to access a medication board. The medication board provided order category, priority, patient name, room, destination, drug name, location, status, and more. It showed the prescription delivery time, distributed either physically or via a tube system, and an automated text message alert was sent to the nurse via Voalte iPhone for pickup.

After its implementation, it was viewed as an easily generalizable innovation to improve productivity for many hospitals across the Trinity system. At the same time, the CMIO began exploring the use of a technology used in the patient rooms to address issues related to high risk patients post-discharge in an aim to reduce readmission costs, another key hospital metric. This led to the next digital transformation, called *Remote Specialist Visiting Physicians (RSVP)*, which was the first extension of hospital technology to patients outside the hospital.

▶ Case Scenario 5— RSVP (2014–2015)

The *RSVP* program was designed to support the continuity of care for high-risk patients using a mix of technology and care coordinators inside and outside the hospital. External care coordinators recruited from the local fire department—emergency medical technicians (EMTs)—visited patients to follow-up and engaged them in a two-way consultation with physicians using video conferencing technology (e.g., SwyMed Telemedicine). Additionally, SJMO partnered with Vivify Health to distribute 20 kits to patients so they could monitor their vital signs and consult with a hospitalist at SJMO.

The pilot project showed improvements in reducing patient readmissions and improving patient satisfaction. It was then expanded to another region. Both the Medication Board and RSVP won finalist recognition by *Wired* magazine in 2016.

> Our hospital has been active in identifying opportunities where technology may benefit our patients. We explore IT solutions that have the potential to improve quality and patient care; however, we never substitute technology for the personal connection with our patients and their families. We look for solutions that support and strengthen that personal connection.
>
> —Fabian Fregoli, VP of Clinical Quality and Safety and CMIO at SJMO[12]

▶ Looking Forward

The five digital innovations helped to transform SJMO hospital over the six years from 2009 to 2015. Today SJMO is an active user of technology that focuses on improving care within the hospital, including ER operations and specialty units like Radiology. The CIO, reflecting on these technologies said:

> Today, we expect hospitals to continue to evolve and look for new digitization opportunities, and we feel like are ready to tackle these with flexibility and speed.
>
> —Chief Information Officer

The CEO and CIO felt that they were well positioned to continue to evolve and stay competitive in the healthcare industry. They were eager to begin to roll out these technologies to other hospitals in the Saint Joseph Health System.

> Our ability to change the culture of managers and care providers in the last five years will position us to be a champion of change to other hospitals within the Trinity system as well

as others who want to see how it can be done. We received not only external recognition, but many visitors came to see what we have done.

—Jack Weiner

St. Joseph Mercy Oakland has served as the pilot program for many of our health system's technology innovations. Our health system is actively working to deploy many of these award-winning technologies across each of our five hospitals in the Metro Detroit region.

—Rob Casalou, President & CEO of
Saint Joseph Health System[13]

Case Questions

Jack was happy with the success Saint Joseph's Mercy had made in their transformation to date. Even so, he wondered if they had met the goals they set out to meet at the beginning of the transformation and how they could continue to evolve. Imagine you have been asked to consult with Jack. What new issues may arise that are most pressing as they roll out these systems and other forward-looking innovations to the other hospitals in the Metro Detroit region? How do you think Jack could anticipate the issues and help resolve them? How could Jack know how well these systems were being deployed and implemented? What should they do to continue to be competitive in the ever-changing healthcare landscape?

Notes

1. SJMO Press Release. (2015). St. Joseph Mercy Oakland wins national "2015 Most Wired Innovator" award from American Hospital Association. Retrieved from www.stjoeshealth.org/body.cfm?id=7598&action=detail&ref=5521
2. Ballard, D. J., Spreadbury, B., & Hopkins, R. S. (2004). Health care quality improvement across the Baylor Health Care System: The first century. *Proceedings (Baylor University Medical Center), 17*(3), 277–288.
3. *Civic Impulse.* (2009). H.R. 1–111th Congress: American Recovery and Reinvestment Act of 2009. Retrieved from www.govtrack.us/congress/bills/111/hr1
4. Santavicca, W. (2009). St. Joseph Mercy Oakland. Cath Lab Digest. Retrieved from www.cathlabdigest.com/articles/St-Joseph-Mercy-Oakland (17:7)
5. Kesterson, R. K. (2014). *The basics of Hoshin Kanri.* Boca Raton, FL: CRC Press.
6. Weiner, J., Tanniru, M., Khuntia, J., Bobryk, D., Naik, M., & Page, K. L. (2016, May). Digital leadership in action in a hospital through a real time dashboard system implementation and experience. *Journal of Hospital Administration, 5*(4), 34.
7. Weiner, J., Balijepally, V., & Tanniru, M. (2015, September/October). Integrating strategic to operational decision-making using data-driven dashboard implementation: The case of St. Joseph Mercy Oakland Hospital. *Journal of Healthcare Management, 60*(5), 319–331.
8. Robert Jones, personal communications.
9. Fabian Fregoli, personal communications.
10. Fabian, *ibid.*
11. SJMO Press Release, *ibid.*
12. Fabian, *ibid.*
13. Rob Casalou, personal communications.

Biographies

Monica J. Garfield is a Professor in Computer Information Systems at Bentley University, Waltham, Massachusetts. Her research focuses on the use of IT to enhance team formation and knowledge building as well as socio-technical issues that impact the use and implementation of IT systems. She has worked in the field of telemedicine and team formation for over 20 years, resulting in numerous publications, invited talks, and presentations. Her work has appeared in such journals as *Information System Research, MIS Quarterly,*

Communications of the ACM and *Journal of Management Information Systems*. She is also the international director of the IT PhD program at Addis Ababa University in Ethiopia.

Dr. Mohan Tanniru is a senior investigator at Henry Ford Health System in Detroit, Michigan and a Professor of Practice in the College of Public Health at the University of Arizona. He is also an Emeritus Professor of MIS in the Decision and Information Science Department of the School of Business Administration at Oakland University and was the former Dean of the School of Business and the founding director of Applied Technology of Business Program at Oakland University. Prior to becoming a Dean, he was the Department Head of MIS at the University of Arizona and taught at Syracuse University and the University of Wisconsin-Madison.

He has published over 90 papers in journals, such as ISR, MIS Quarterly, Decision Sciences, DSS, JMIS, IEEE Transactions in Eng. Management, and Communications of ACM. His recent work in health care has been published in Healthcare Policy and Technology, J of Patient Satisfaction, J of Hospital Administration, and J of Healthcare Management. He has coordinated numerous graduate and under-graduate projects with over 60 large companies including GM, Chrysler, EDS/HP, Lear, Comerica, Carrier-UTC, MONY, Bristol Myers-Squibb, Honeywell, Intel, and Raytheon, and several healthcare organizations, such as Kaiser Permanente, Beaumont Health Systems, St. Joseph Mercy-Oakland, and Henry Ford Health System.

Jack Weiner recently retired as President and Chief Executive Officer of St. Joseph Mercy Oakland (SJMO). He led the organization in a major cultural and technological transformation. As a 443-bed tertiary community teaching hospital in Oakland County and under his leadership, SJMO became the regional leader in clinical quality and safety. The technological transformation includes the construction of a new Patient Tower that includes state of the art technology found in only one other hospital in the country. The clinical enhancements include an extensive telemedicine program and tlle deployment of one of the first virtual medicine networks. Under his leadership St. Joseph became a major research center conducting both Phase Two and Phase Three drug studies and medical equipment and procedure evaluations.

Mr. Weiner led the implementation of the Patient Electronic Medical Record (EMR) system which expands throughout SE Michigan Trinity Hospitals and physician offices. The telemedicine-based Michigan Stroke Network, through the deployment of remote presence robots, has led an initiative that improves the care of stroke patients to hospitals throughout the state of Michigan. The program has been expanded nationwide. In response to a changing healthcare environment, he initiated the development and operation of an extensive clinically integrated delivery network of more than 700 providers and the establishment of innovative payment programs to respond to changing reimbursement requirements. Since his retirement he has continued his academic activities at Oakland University by teaching a series of courses in the Master's degree program in healthcare management. He is an active consultant in healthcare facility design and continues his work in promoting digitization of data and structural decision making.

Prior to joining SJMO in 2003, Mr. Weiner served as President and CEO of SJM of Macomb. Under his leadership, an open-heart surgery program and major expansion program were launched. He also served as Vice President for Facility and Ambulatory Operations at St. Mary's Health Services in Grand Rapids, and President and CEO of Northeastern Hospital in Philadelphia. He held several other positions at Michigan hospitals during his more than 45 years in the healthcare industry.

Mr. Weiner began his administrative career with the Upjohn pharmaceutical company where he coordinated Phase One and Phase Two clinical trials and was involved in more than 200 clinical trials. His healthcare career began as a pharmacist when he received his PharmD in clinical pharmacy in 1974 from Wayne State University. He also holds a Master in health services administration from the University of Michigan, and a Bachelor of Science degree in pharmacy from the University of Buffalo.

CASE 4

Theranos: Innovating an Industry Primed for Innovation

Chloe Nyitray, Brandon Nixon, Grace Simpson, and Joseph Tan

▶ Introduction

Like many revolutionary startup lead entrepreneurs before her, Elizabeth Holmes dropped out of a highly regarded college to pursue a bold idea that she felt was destined to change the face of health care. During her 2 years at Stanford's School of Engineering, she studied Chemical Engineering and worked in a lab with PhD students under the supervision of Channing Robertson, the Dean of Stanford's School of Engineering.[1] Additionally, she had spent a summer in Singapore performing various lab tests at the Genome Institute Lab for severe acute respiratory syndrome (SARS).[2] These experiences highlighted the opportunities for efficiency in blood diagnostics testing, and along with her personal fear of needles, Elizabeth was eventually motivated to file a patent for a portable blood analyzer in 2003.[3]

In 2004, she launched the biotech startup, Theranos, (a combination of the words therapy and diagnosis) with the intent to develop "technological innovations that will enable access to the information patients need to take control of their health, with the goal of detecting diseases in time to affect outcomes."[4] Channing had the utmost confidence in Elizabeth, and while he discouraged her from abandoning her academic studies, he recognized that "just one or two of these people come forward every generation, and she's one of them."[5] Channing joined Theranos as the first technical advisor and brought with him a few part-time lab students to begin development of the patent.[6]

▶ Elizabeth's Upbringing and History

Coming from a family with a history of medical and entrepreneurial accomplishments,[7] Elizabeth was determined to succeed at a young age. She is a descendant of Charles Fleischmann, an innovator of yeast. In the late 1800s, Fleischmann brought a superior strand of yeast to America, and became one of the wealthiest men in the nation.[8] Her great grandfather, Dr. Christian Holmes, leveraged the family's position in society to launch the *Cincinnati General Hospital* and the *University of Cincinnati Medical School*.[9] Elizabeth's parents both spent time working in government services before moving from Washington, D.C. to Houston.[10]

Looking back, Elizabeth's competitive spirit and ambition was clear from a young age. At 7, she architected detailed drawings of a time machine, and at 9 she confidently told family members she wanted to be a billionaire when she grew up.[11] By the time she was in high school, Elizabeth was fluent in Mandarin and completed a college-level 9-week Mandarin summer program at Stanford including an immersion trip to Beijing.[12] At 19, with her first patent filed, Elizabeth dropped out of Stanford to dedicate herself full-time to accomplishing her long-term vision.[13]

▶ Developing the Disruptive Technology

Theranos set out on a mission to disrupt the delivery of health care. The technology being developed at the company was designed to automate and miniaturize laboratory testing.[14] Drawing of blood, or phlebotomy, has existed for hundreds of years as a means of aiding doctors in the provision of health care.[15] Typically a patient's physician will decide to order a lab test to diagnose diseases or monitor treatments. The patient travels to a hospital or health office to have a vial of their blood extracted by a technician. This blood specimen is then packaged, shipped to a laboratory, and tested, and results are provided to the physician in 2 days to a few weeks.[16] The process, while vital, is often criticized for the long wait for times for results, inaccessibility to the patient, and high cost when tests are duplicated for multiple purposes.[17]

Elizabeth envisioned a patient-centric redesign of blood tests. She imagined that a Theranos solution could exist "within five miles of virtually every American home,"[18] offering a better way of laboratory testing for both patients and providers. In 2005, Ian Gibbons, a biochemist, joined Theranos. Ian's research focused on the development of systems that would process small amounts of fluids. Together with Ian, Elizabeth and a group of researchers created 23 patents. Elizabeth and the Theranos employees secretly worked towards reengineering the process of blood testing. In 2013, Theranos began to offer their diagnostic services in wellness centers in Phoenix, Arizona. The technology produced by Theranos was accessible, patient-friendly, and only required a finger-prick of blood from the patient.

Finger-pricking was a less invasive way of extracting blood; it is commonly used to monitor blood glucose levels in diabetic patients.[19] The process was simple. A patient would arrive at a Theranos center where a technician would increase blood flow to the finger and extract the blood using a finger prick. Only a raindrop sized droplet was required to fill the Theranos nanotainers. Nanotainers were sent for processing to a Theranos laboratory which used their own cutting-edge platform, called the "Edison," to process the droplets of blood. The Theranos technology was revolutionary in an industry that had seen limited improvement to patients or providers in recent years. Patients only had to provide a drop of blood for testing. Theranos claimed that with only a single droplet of blood, the company could run over 200 tests, reducing the need for multiple laboratory visits.[20] Elizabeth's tenacity for disrupting health care also made its way into legislation after she successfully lobbied the state of Arizona to allow patients to order a lab test without a physician order.[21] This empowered patients to achieve earlier diagnosis. Providers loved the Theranos technology because it provided faster results, sometimes in as little as 15 minutes.[22] The cost was also an attractive factor. For example, the traditional lab test for cholesterol costed $50 or more, while the Theranos test cost just $2.99.[23] A few years after its inception, Theranos was on track to become a leader in terms of cost and product differentiation in the marketplace for blood diagnostics.

▶ Seeking Partnerships

In order to fund the research, development, and commercialization of the Theranos technology, Elizabeth sought out multiple partnerships. Draper Fisher Jurvetson (DFJ), a venture capitalist (VC) firm that "invests in visionaries who make history by forging the future in consumer, enterprise and disruptive technologies" was the first to invest in the company.[24] Founded by Timothy Draper, once a neighbor whose children played with Elizabeth growing up, DFJ provided $500K and led the initial seed round of financing for the company on June 15, 2004.[25] Over the next 13 years, Theranos completed nine more rounds of funding, successfully securing a total of $1.37B via a mix of private placements and VCs at a peak valuation of $9B[26,27] (see *Appendix A*).

There were a total of 18 investors involved in all 10 rounds of financing for Theranos, of which only two were VCs.[28] The remaining 16 investors were brought on board through private placements, "fundraising that is restricted to wealthy investors and disclosed to the Securities Exchange Commission (SEC) via an exemption from registration under securities laws called Form D."[29] By restricting financing to accredited investors and individuals with a net worth of $1M or more, Elizabeth was able to reduce the visibility of Theranos within the industry and avoid SEC scrutiny that often comes from funding raised via public investment sources.

Following the initial seed investment by DFJ, Elizabeth leveraged other familial relationships to secure financing from a number of

high-profile investors including Larry Ellison, founder of Oracle, Rupert Murdoch, founder of News Corporation and Fox News, and Betsy DeVos, American businesswoman and current US Secretary of Education.[30] *Appendix B* offers a breakdown of the full investor listing. Moreover, Elizabeth had carefully chosen to establish a high-profiled board of key advisors and directors, including Henry Kissinger and George Schultz, former Secretary of States, James Mattis and William Perry, the current and former Secretary of Defense, and Senators Bill Frist and Sam Nunn.[31] The Theranos Board of Directors had astonishing credentials with strong depth of experience, but it noticeably lacked female presence and CEOs from similar industries.

In 2011, Elizabeth was demonstrating the technology at John Hopkins University where she was approached by Walgreens executives, who were considering integrating Theranos testing centers in-store. Elizabeth agreed to provide her devices to Baltimore researchers to validate the accuracy of the test results. However, numerous delays in its development meant the validation studies were overlooked and not completed before the deadline for Walgreens to launch in-store testing centers. Over the next 2 years, before officially announcing the deal publicly in 2013, executives and outside advisors to Walgreens began to grow weary with the repeated delays in rolling out in-store testing centers. However, Walgreens feared that reneging on the agreed-upon deal would lead Theranos to partner with another pharmacy chain, and the company was unwilling to miss out of the breakthrough opportunity.[32] Yet, despite Walgreens continuing demand for answers "it received few that were useful from Theranos, which closely guarded its technology and operations."[33] Even after executives visited the company to review its quality control procedures, access was severely restricted for the visitors to only within and inside the laboratory. One executive recalled "the results were actually really good, but I was never allowed to go into the lab. I have no idea that the results I saw were run on the Edison devices or not."[34]

▶ Elizabeth's Rise to Fame

In the early days of Theranos, Elizabeth kept a low profile and focused her efforts on securing private investment and working long hours at the company.[35] But, in June 2014, this changed when *Fortune* featured Elizabeth on its cover issue.[36] Elizabeth was not your typical unicorn start-up founder. The media held a particular fascination with Elizabeth Holmes. After this 2014 *Fortune* release, she graced the cover of *Forbes 400* issue on the richest people in America. *Times* followed suit, naming her as one of the Most 100 Influential People and she was also featured by *USA Today, Inc., NPR, Fox Business, CNN,* and *CBS News.*[37] Then the awards flooded in; soon, Elizabeth accepted a role from President Obama as a U.S. Ambassador for Global Entrepreneurship in addition to the *Horatio Alger* award for outstanding Americans who demonstrate exceptional personal and professional achievements.[38]

When parallels were drawn between Apple founder Steve Jobs and Elizabeth Holmes, she appeared to take the flattery to heart. Publicly, Elizabeth began emulating Jobs in his signature black turtleneck style, leaned on his management techniques described in Walter Isaacson's biography, used the same advertising firm to design the website for Theranos, and referred to the proprietary blood-testing system as the "iPod of health care."[39]

▶ Warning Signs: Myths Versus Reality

As a start-up with a bold vision, Theranos was able to attract a star cast of investors with plenty of VC funding coming its way. Along the way, Theranos was also able to attract top talent from across Silicon Valley. This was a good thing

because by 2006, the high level of employee turnover was starting to become noticeable.[40] Taking a page from Steve Jobs' playbook, Elizabeth felt it was best to silo internal groups from collaboration and instead create an isolated environment of secrecy to speed the pace of innovation.[41] Employees were asked to avoid using the company name on their LinkedIn profiles to throw off competitors, and new hires were not told their actual job responsibilities until signing the non-disclosure and starting their first day; disturbingly, legal threats were made when employees spoke publicly about the company.[42] Meanwhile, Elizabeth dedicated a lot of her time to understanding the work across the broader organization.[43] In 2017, the associated interview and job reviews posted for Theranos on Glassdoor.com, an online platform and database for employees to rate their company, yielded an overall rating of 3.1/5, with top pros attributed to smart colleagues, free catered meals, and great pay and benefits (*Appendix C*). Long working hours, poor decision-making by Senior Leaders, and lack of transparency across teams were noted as cons.[44]

While Theranos managed to acquire partnerships with key companies within the medical industry, the scientific community was beginning to question the validity of the Theranos technology.[45] Released outcomes of their blood testing services appeared too good to be true. Theranos touted that their Edison devices were able to analyze over 200 markers from a single drop of blood, contradicting sound scientific research concerning contamination and dilution challenges.[46] Moreover, questions arose about how a college dropout with no medical experience could have solved such a complex problem so quickly. Owing to a loophole that permitted labs to develop their own machines, Theranos was not required to receive FDA approval to conduct patient testing as long as they did not sell these devices in the market.[47] Since Theranos completed lab testing on patients internally and did not sell their devices, there was no need for FDA approval.[48]

▶ The Beginning of the End

On October 16, 2015, a week prior to an important conference where Elizabeth was scheduled to speak, the Wall Street Journal published a scathing expose.[49] This report speculated that Theranos' breakthrough blood diagnostic testing abilities were a far cry from reality and only about 15 of the claimed 240 tests were actually performed on proprietary Edison machines, with the rest of the tests being run through traditional machines from other big-name companies, such as Siemens.[50] Further, the report claimed there was a discrepancy with the results of the proficiency-testing samples of the proprietary Theranos Edison machine with two other control equipment types for testing involving vitamin D, two thyroid hormones, and prostate cancer.[51] When concerns around the results were raised with senior leaders and copied to Elizabeth, the employees were told to report results using the two other control equipment results and disregard the Edison results.[52]

> The former employees say they did what they were told but were concerned that the instructions violated federal rules, which state that a lab must handle "proficiency testing samples … in the same manner as it tests patient specimens" and by "using the laboratory's routine methods." In its everyday business at the time, Theranos routinely used Edison machines to test patients' blood samples for vitamin D, the two thyroid hormones and prostate cancer, the former employees say.
>
> *WSJ*[53]

Other concerns included: (a) the reliability of using diluted blood samples for multiple tests; (b) doctor and patient concerns over extremely elevated results from Theranos; and (c) that several results from Theranos were later disconfirmed by other laboratory tests.[54]

The day after the article was released, Elizabeth appeared on the television show Mad Money with Jim Cramer to address the concerns by saying "This is what happens when you work to change things. First they think you're crazy, then they fight you, and then, all of a sudden, you change the world."[55] Elizabeth was careful to take a forward-looking approach when answering the direct questions on the program. She was proactive in announcing the recent decision of the company to withdraw use of the nanocontainer used within the Edison device as a voluntary decision.[56] Elizabeth also addressed the claim that the majority of tests Theranos completed were processed on non-proprietary equipment. Here, she responded:

> This is taken completely out of context. Starting when we launched our services in 2013, we put on our website that we do venous testing, so blood draws from the arm, the traditional way, and starting in 2015 we announced and it was published in San Francisco paper, in Fortune, I talked about it in an interview I did with Forbes, that we made a decision to expand our test menu to include all of the specialty and esoteric tests that are traditionally run only very infrequently but cost a huge amount of money and we believe as part of what we do, that part of our greatest innovations is making these tests available at extremely low costs.[57]

▶ The Downfall of Theranos

The 2015 *WSJ* article was a catalyst to the demise of Elizabeth Holmes' tenure as CEO of Theranos. As a result of mounting evidence against the efficiency of Theranos lab results, the U.S. Centers for Medicare and Medicaid Services (CMS) launched a formal investigation. CMS both revoked Theranos' certificate as a laboratory and mandated that Elizabeth be banned from running a laboratory for 2 years.[58,59] Their decision was justified by the fact that Theranos posed, "immediate jeopardy to patient health and safety."[60] Shortly afterwards, Walgreens ended their partnership with Theranos.[61]

In June 2017, Theranos settled a suit brought by Walgreens for under $30 million, a far cry from the $140 million that Walgreens invested into the failed partnership.[62] The collapse of Theranos' laboratory operations was just the beginning. In March 2018, Elizabeth was charged with fraud by the SEC.[63]

▶ Theranos and Elizabeth's Future

In early June 2018, rumors were spreading that Elizabeth was wooing the venture capitalist community to form a new health-focused technology company.[64] But by June 15, 2018, the Federal Bureau of Investigation (FBI), Food and Drug Administration (FDA), and the U.S. Postal Inspection Agency (USPIS) announced that a federal grand jury had indicted Elizabeth on two counts of conspiracy to commit wire fraud and nine counts of wire fraud for deceiving hundreds of doctors and patients and defrauding investors out of hundreds of millions of dollars.[65] The basis of the claims stem from the methods in which Theranos used advertisements and solicitations to drive the usage of propriety laboratory testing even though Elizabeth was well aware that the test results were likely to be unreliable. If convicted, Elizabeth could face up to 20 years behind bars and a fine of $250,000.[66] As of the writing of this case, Elizabeth has not yet made a public statement regarding the case, but will have the option to plead guilty and settle or fight the charges publicly in court.[67]

Case Questions

From a company with a $9 billion dollar valuation, a mission to change the world of health care under the leadership of a brilliant young founder, what was the turning point where Theranos tipped the balance too far from *making* promises to *delivering* on promises? What specific risks do healthcare unicorn start-ups face that differ from pure technology focused companies? Can Elizabeth save the company given current personal circumstances? How involved should a Board of Directors be in verifying company claims?

Notes

1. Aluetta, K. (2014). Blood, simpler. *The New Yorker*.
2. Retrieved from www.straitstimes.com/business/companies-markets/former-young-us-biotech-star-charged-with-fraud-over-blood-testing-claims
3. Weisul, K. (2015). How playing the long game made Elizabeth Holmes a billionaire. Article by Inc. Magazine. Retrieved from www.pinterest.ca/pin/570690584012672385/
4. The United States Attorney's Office. (2018). Theranos founder and former chief operating officer charged in alleged wire fraud schemes. Retrieved from www.justice.gov/usao-ndca/pr/theranos-founder-and-former-chief-operating-officer-charged-alleged-wire-fraud-schemes
5. Weisul, (2015), *ibid*.
6. *Ibid*.
7. Retrieved from https://famouskin.com/famous-kin-chart.php?name=58650+elizabeth+holmes&kin=58671+charles+fleischmann
8. Carreyrou, J. (2018). *Bad blood: Secrets and lies in a Silicon Valley startup*. New York, NY: Penguin Random House.
9. *Ibid*.
10. Hartmans, A. (2019). The rise and fall of Elizabeth Holmes, Who started Theranos when she was 19 and became the world's youngest female billionaire before it all came crashing down. Retrieved from www.businessinsider.com/theranos-founder-ceo-elizabeth-holmes-life-story-bio-2018-4
11. *Ibid*.
12. Carreyrou, (2018), *ibid*.

13. Parloff, R. (2014). This CEO is out for blood. *Fortune* (with protracted correction published on 2015). Retrieved from http://fortune.com/2014/06/12/theranos-blood-holmes/

14. Rago, J. (2013). The weekend interview with Elizabeth Holmes: A drop of blood; an instant diagnosis. *The Wall Street Journal.*

15. *Ibid.*

16. *Ibid.*

17. *Ibid.*

18. *Ibid.*

19. Waltz, E. (2017). After Theranos. *Nature Biotechnology, 35,* 11. doi:10.1038/nbt.3761

20. Carreyrou, J. (2016a). A prized startup's struggles—Silicon valley lab Theranos is valued at $9 billion but isn't using its technology for all the tests it offers. *The Wall Street Journal.*

21. Carreyrou, J. (2015). Hot startup Theranos hast struggled with its blood-test technology. *Wall Street Journal* (Online).

22. Aluetta, (2014), *ibid.*

23. *Ibid.*

24. Draper Fisher Jurvetson. (2018). Portfolio | DFJ Venture Capital.

25. Abelson, R., & Creswell, J. (2015). Theranos founder faces a test of technology, and reputation. *The New York Times.*

26. Crunchbase. (2018). Theranos | Crunchbase.

27. Mirhaydari, A. (2018). Hot to not: The valuation implosion at Theranos | PitchBook.

28. Lemkin, J. (2018). How did the venture capitalists that invested in Theranos fall for Elizabeth Holmes' scam? | SaaStr.

29. Mckenna, F. (2018). The investors duped by the Theranos fraud never asked for one important thing. *MarketWatch.*

30. O'Brien, S. A. (2018). Elizabeth Holmes surrounded Theranos with powerful people. Retrieved from https://money.cnn.com/2018/03/15/technology/elizabeth-holmes-theranos/index.html

31. *Ibid.*

32. Weaver, C., & Carreyrou, J. (2016, May). Craving growth, Walgreens dismissed its doubts about Theranos—WSJ. *Wall Street Journal* (Online), 1–8.

33. *Ibid.*

34. *Ibid.*

35. Parloff, (2014), *ibid.*

36. *Ibid.*

37. Carreyrou, (2018), *ibid.*

38. *Ibid.*

39. *Ibid.*

40. *Ibid.*

41. Bilton, N. (2016). Exclusive: How Elizabeth Holmes's house of cards came tumbling down. Retrieved from www.vanityfair.com/news/2016/09/elizabeth-holmes-theranos-exclusive

42. Stevenson, A. (2015). Theranos CEO fires back at WSJ: I was shocked. Retrieved from www.cnbc.com/2015/10/15/theranos-ceo-fires-back-at-wsj-i-was-shocked.html

43. Bilton, (2016), *ibid.*

44. Glassdoor. (2018). Theranos reviews. Retrieved from www.glassdoor.ca/Reviews/Theranos-Reviews-E248889_P3.htm?countryRedirect=true

45. Waltz, (2017), *ibid.*

46. *Ibid.*

47. Carreyrou, (2016a), *ibid.*

48. Carreyrou, (2018), *ibid.*

49. Carreyrou, (2015), *ibid.*

50. *Ibid.*

51. *Ibid.*

52. *Ibid.*

53. *Ibid.*

54. *Ibid.*

55. Stevenson, (2015), *ibid.*

56. Carreyrou, (2018), *ibid.*

57. Carreyrou, (2015), *ibid.*

58. Carreyrou, J. (2016b). Under fire, Theranos CEO stifled bad news. *The Wall Street Journal.*

59. Waltz, (2017), *ibid.*

60. *Ibid.*

61. Carreyrou, (2016b), *ibid.*

62. Carreyrou, (2018), *ibid.*

63. Carreyrou, (2016b), *ibid.*

64. Hartmans. (2018). Theranos founder Elizabeth Holmes is reportedly seeking Silicon Valley investors for a new company. Retrieved from www.businessinsider.com/theranos-founder-elizabeth-holmes-new-startup-report-2018-6

65. Abelson & Creswell, (2015), *ibid.*

66. The United States Attorney's Office, (2018), *ibid.*

67. Henning, P. J. (2018). What's next for Elizabeth Holmes in the Theranos fraud case? Retrieved from www.nytimes.com/2018/06/18/business/dealbook/holmes-theranos-fraud-case.html

▶ Appendix A—Theranos Investment Rounds

Date	Round	Capital Raised
June 15, 2004	Seed	$500K
February 11, 2005	Series A	$5.8M
February 21, 2006	Series B	$9.1M
November 17, 2006	Series C	$28.5M
July 8, 2010	Venture	$45M
September 9, 2013	Funding	$50M
February 1, 2014	Private Equity	$198.9M
March 1, 2015	Private Equity	$348.5M
May 25, 2017	Secondary Market	$582.2M
December 23, 2017	Debt Financing	$100M

Reproduced from https://www.crunchbase.com/organization/theranos#section-funding-rounds.

▶ Appendix B—List of Theranos Investors

Investors

Investor Name	Lead Investor	Funding Round	Partners
Fortress Investment Group	Yes	Debt Financing - Theranos	—
Puget Sound Venture Club	—	Secondary Market - Theranos	—
Partner Fund Management	No	Private Equity Round - Thera...	—
Raymond Bingham	No	Private Equity Round - Thera...	—
Palmieri Family Trust	No	Private Equity Round - Thera...	—
Esoom Enterprise	No	Private Equity Round - Thera...	—
Jupiter Partners	No	Private Equity Round - Thera...	—
B.J. Cassin	No	Private Equity Round - Thera...	—
Continental Properties	No	Private Equity Round - Thera...	—
BlueCross BlueShield Ventur...	No	Private Equity Round - Thera...	—
Walgreens	Yes	Funding Round - Theranos	—
The Lawrence J. Ellison Revo...	—	Series C - Theranos	—
ATA Ventures	—	Series C - Theranos	—
Tako Ventures	—	Series C - Theranos	Larry Ellison
Continental Ventures	—	Series C - Theranos	—
ATA Ventures	—	Series B - Theranos	—
Rupert Murdoch	—	Series A - Theranos	—
Draper Fisher Jurvetson (DFJ)	Yes	Seed Round - Theranos	—

▶ Appendix C— Glassdoor Reviews as of July 2018

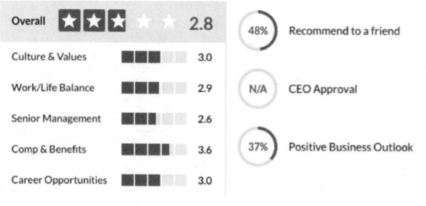

Theranos Ratings and Trends   ✕

| Overall | ★★★ ☆ ☆ | 2.8 |

Culture & Values	3.0
Work/Life Balance	2.9
Senior Management	2.6
Comp & Benefits	3.6
Career Opportunities	3.0

48% Recommend to a friend

N/A CEO Approval

37% Positive Business Outlook

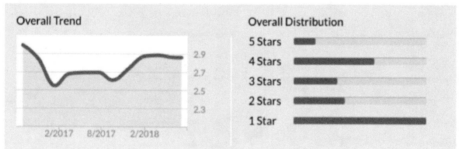

Overall Trend

2.9
2.7
2.5
2.3

2/2017   8/2017   2/2018

Overall Distribution

5 Stars
4 Stars
3 Stars
2 Stars
1 Star

Source: https://www.glassdoor.ca/Reviews/Theranos-Reviews-E248889.htm ¶
¶

Biographies

Chloe Nyitray is a graduate of the University of Waterloo's Statistics for Health Program and is on track to complete her Masters of eHealth in Summer 2019. Chloe is passionate about applying her knowledge of statistics and analytics to help drive better decision-making. She is currently working on a project to implement activity based budgeting and corporate management in one of Canada's largest hospital networks. She has always had a keen interest in data science and visual analytics and is excited to continue encouraging organizations to make data-driven decisions. Statistics and data are not her only passions—you can often find Chloe running on the trails with her adorable golden doodle, Hunter.

Brandon Nixon is a two-time graduate from the DeGroote School of Business at McMaster University. After completing his Honours B.Comm (Information Systems, Economics Minor) in 2012, he went on to complete his MBA (Management Information Systems) part-time and graduated in the summer of 2018. Brandon's passion for technology led him down the path of IT Consulting within the financial services industry, where he has worked on largescale digital transformation projects for a number of Tier 1 U.S. and Canadian banks. Prior to this, Brandon held various roles in the private and public sector working on the analysis, development, and implementation of IT systems at Manulife and the Ontario Securities Commission respectively. In his spare time Brandon likes to travel, play sports, and explore new hobbies.

Grace Simpson currently leads Amazon's North American Learning and Development team deploying authentic assessments and experiences for operations leaders across 130 locations. She deploys a customer-centric mindset to prepare university and industry graduates for the demands of Amazon's operations environment. Grace will graduate with her MBA from McMaster University in June 2019 after receiving her Honours B.Comm in 2012. Grace has also spent time exploring Human Resources at ArcelorMittal Dofasco and GeoDigital Technologies before moving into operations management where she launched (and subsequently closed) Target Canada stores.

CASE 5

Patients Like Me (PLM): Social Media in Public Health

Phillip Olla, Brianna Mozariwskyj, Vickee Le, and Ly Le

▶ Introduction

The growing prevalence of social media (SM) has fundamentally changed the way people share information and connect with the world. Widespread use of online platforms is also transforming the way public health efforts engage with the greater population.

Public health is the science and art of preventing disease, prolonging life, and promoting health through the organized efforts and choices of society, organizations, and individuals.[1] SM has made it easier for public health organizers to spread and collect valuable health data and for people to form communities to promote health and to connect with others who may have similar medical conditions.

▶ SM Adoption in Health Care

In the last decade, healthcare professionals have used SM to spread vital health information to a wider audience. Online platforms now facilitate dialogue between patients and healthcare professionals and collect data on patient experiences. Facebook, Twitter, Wikipedia, YouTube, blogs, discussion boards, forums, and online chatrooms are among the most commonly used platforms for public health-related activities.[3] These platforms allow users to promote health education, reduce stigma around illness, and stay updated on health crises and other issues taking place around the world.[2]

Below are a few examples of the ways SM can be used in health care are[4]:

- *Assessing reliability and false information*: False information about medical conditions is tremendously common. Through the use of various SM sites, users can cross-reference with other sources to eliminate unreliable and potentially harmful information.
- *Real-Time Urgent Updates*: SM allows vital information to spread widely and rapidly during emergencies. For example, Crisis Tracker is a platform that uses data from SM to track events as they occur. Crisis Tracker then compiles the data

to provide detailed summaries of the events.[3] Companies that track and analyze such data can help spread accurate information about emergency events quickly to create awareness.[5]

- *The Connection between SM and Public Health*: SM platforms can also be used as tools for health promotion. Facebook, Twitter, Instagram, and other apps allow physicians and healthcare workers to post daily messages that promote a healthy lifestyle. Expert medical practitioners can post the latest scientific facts and discoveries, organize social events, and spread public health messages to patients and to community members at large.

- *Disease Prophylaxis and Management*: Public Health organizations have begun using SM to keep people informed on the outbreak of diseases and epidemics. Innovative Support to Emergencies Disease and Disasters (InSTEDD) is an organization that is a great example of this. InSTEDD uses a tool called Riff to sift through information from multiple sources, filtering out irrelevant data to identify critical patterns. Riff uses algorithms to detect anomalies and potential health events. The patterns it detects using information from SM help aid in the prophylaxis of disease outbreaks.

- *Networking*: Common behaviors such as smoking, drinking, and poor diet cause widespread health problems. These behaviors increase the risk of developing chronic diseases such as diabetes, heart disease, and stroke. Social networks provide a common space to discuss these issues, and allow people to connect with others who struggle with the same problems. For example, organizations such as Weight Watchers (WW) and Alcoholics Anonymous (AA) form groups to lend each other support and participate in healthier behaviors together.[6]

▶ Patients Like Me (PLM)

"Patients Like Me" is a SM platform that allows patients to find a community of people like themselves, get answers about their medical conditions, and take charge of their health.[7] PLM connects patients living with similar medical conditions and diagnoses. The site gives newly diagnosed patients a place to get answers from people who have already lived through the same struggles. **FIGURE CS5-1** illustrates the options available to create a support system with a community of people who understand the unique challenges of their diagnosis.

Most healthcare data are inaccessible to the public as a result of privacy regulations. PLM has a powerful impact on patients by giving them access to health data that is often kept under lock and key. Many patients find it difficult to be actively engaged in their own care plan because they don't have all the information required. PLM gives patients the power to make their own educated decisions about their plan of care.

PLM allows patients to get advice from others who also live with their condition. Patients can track their progress and compare their experiences. By sharing the hard-earned knowledge in a public SM forum, patients have given each other a valuable gift of learning what they can do to improve their quality of life and outcomes.

One user of PLM, a patient called Mary, posts about the struggles and triumphs of living with a diagnosis of Multiple Sclerosis (MS). When she was younger, she loved playing softball, track, golf, and basketball, and she even went on to be a marathon runner and double back diamond skater. Her MS confined her to a wheelchair; but she emphasizes how she has never let her diagnosis stop her from enjoying and cherishing life. Despite her limitations, she continues to participate in everyday activities she enjoys such as volunteer work, book club, and making videos for her family and friends. Her story is just one out of many that can inspire people and give hope to

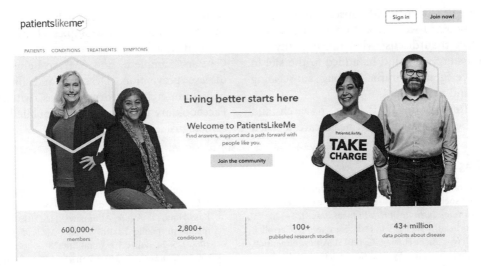

FIGURE CS5-1 Patients Like Me (PLM) Data Points.

other patients with MS. PLM showcases many stories that allow people to find answers about their diagnosis and show them what life looks like for other people with their symptoms.

Another resource that PLM offers is allowing patients to learn about their genes and how they are affecting them. Patients can track the changes in their body with signs and symptoms resulting from their disease. This further lets patients learn and understand about their condition so that they can specifically prepare before their condition worsen, connect with others just like them so that they can receive help to better manage and endure their diagnosis without being shocked.

PLM shares all information and data to the public. The availability of this public data will help advance our understanding of a disease to enable better treatment options. Its purpose is to change and advance the healthcare system so that patients' lives can be better through the collective knowledge this platform offers.

▶ Conclusion

Integrating SM into public health creates a powerful platform that allows information to

be disseminated rapidly around the world in real time. SM and public health have the capability to support vital communication channels between healthcare workers and patients to allow knowledge to be shared more easily, and to be accessible anytime, anywhere. In addition, amalgamating SM techniques with public health methods provides the capability to gather and analyze data that can be used to predict epidemics to prevent pandemics, and reduce the impact of these outbreaks and support disaster planning. Combining SM and public health also has the potential to reduce disease prophylaxis, management, and treatment. Accordingly, these two domains work cohesively to positively impact the healthcare system so that people can connect and promote a healthier life.

Case Questions

Imagine that you are the Chief Patient Officer at PLM. New investors want to sell PLM data to a pharmaceutical company and restrict patient access to the data. What are some of the potential problems that could arise from using "Patients Like Me" and how can you mitigate these problems? How would you protect the interest of current PLM subscribing patients? Visit the PLM website and review the various diseases, then discuss what functionality you would suggest should be added to the site to improve greater traffic among subscribing users and newcomers.

After reading this case, research and describe how dedicated healthcare-focused platforms are being used in public health, giving specific illustrative examples. How can SM be used in a disaster management situation? Give an example of how SM can be used for disease prevention. Describe and illustrate how commercial platforms such as Twitter and Facebook are being used as for public health campaigns.

Notes

1. Coiera, E., Lau, A., Laranjo, L., & Dunn, A. (2017). How social networks are changing health behaviour. *Australian Institute of Health Innovation, 1*, 1–12.
2. Moorhead, S. A., Hazlett, D. E., Harrison, L., Carroll, J. K., Irwin, A., & Hoving, C. (2013). A new dimension of health care: Systematic review of the uses, benefits, and limitations of social media for health communication. *Journal of Medical Internet Research, 15*(4), e85. doi:10.2196/jmir.1933
3. Giustini, D., Ali, S. M., Fraser, M., & Kamel Boulos, M. N. (2018). Effective uses of social media in public health and medicine: A systematic review of systematic reviews. *Online Journal of Public Health Informatics, 10*(2), e215. doi:10.5210/ojphi.v10i2.8270
4. Kass-Hout, T. A., & Alhinnawi, H. (2013). Social media in public health. *British Medical Bulletin, 108*(1), 5–24. doi:10.1093/bmb/ldt028
5. *Crisis Tracker*. (2019). Retrieved from https://crisistracker.org/
6. Our philosophy Openness is a good thing. (2015–2019). *Patients Like Me*. Retrieved from https://news.patientslikeme.com/
7. Westchester. (2008). *Patients Like Me*. Retrieved from www.patientslikeme.com/members/westchester

Biographies

Vickee Le is a research assistant at the Center for Research at Madonna University. She is on track to obtain her BSN with hopes of pursuing a DNP in the future. Her research interest is in Digital Health. She has interned with St. John's Providence Hospital in Livonia and Novi, Michigan, in the Occupational Health Department and at St. Joe's in Ann Arbor, Michigan, on the Mother and Baby floor.

Brianna Mozariwskyj is a BSN nursing candidate at Madonna University. She is a research assistant at the Center for Research at Madonna University. She is a student-athlete and is captain of the Women's Soccer Team at Madonna University. She also participates in research and clinical trial planning.

Ly Le, a native Californian, received her Bachelor of Science in Marketing at Woodbury University. After graduation, she embarked on an entrepreneurial journey, started three business in Michigan and continuing her education as a pre-med student at Wayne State University.

Index